Fungal Immunology:

From an Organ Perspective

Fungal Immunology:

From an Organ Perspective

Edited by

Paul L. Fidel, Jr.
Department of Microbiology, Immunology, and Parasitology
Louisiana State University Health Sciences Center
New Orleans, Louisiana

and

Gary B. Huffnagle
Department of Internal Medicine
University of Michigan
Ann Arbor, Michigan

Springer

Library of Congress Cataloging-in-Publication Data

Fungal immunology from an organ perspective / edited by Paul L. Fidel, Jr, Gary B. Huffnagle.
p. ; cm.
Includes bibliographical references and index.
ISBN 0-387-24092-6
1. Mycoses–Immunological aspects. 2. Pathogenic fungi. I. Fidel, Paul L. II. Huffnagle, Gary B.
[DNLM: 1. Mycoses–immunology. 2. Fungi–immunology. WC 450 F97889 2005]
QR245.F8533 2005
616.9′6901–dc22

2004063196

ISBN-10: 0-387-24092-6 e-ISBN: 0-387-25445-5 Printed on acid-free paper.

ISBN-13: 978-0387-24092-3

Printed in the United States of America. (SPI/EB)

9 8 7 6 5 4 3 2 1

springeronline.com

To my father, Paul Fidel, Sr., who has followed my career progress
with tremendous interest and enthusiasm

P.L.F

Special thanks to Beatric Finkel-Jimenez, Ph.D. for her efforts in
helping prepare the chapters for submission

Preface

Knowledge of how the human immune system defends against infections caused by the medically important fungi continues to evolve as an increasing amount of data accumulate from both clinical studies and animal models. It has been 10 years since a volume of chapters dedicated to fungal immunology has been published. Thus, when the opportunity presented to edit a new volume in fungal immunology, we were both honored and excited about the prospects. However, in considering a layout and format, we strived for a unique angle by which to showcase the immense data accumulated over the past 10 years. Accordingly, rather than simply separate the book by organism with chapters on each type of response or separate the book by type of response with inclusion of chapters for each organism, we decided on a layout based on organ systems, recognizing that each medically important fungal organism often causes disease in distinct organ systems, together with the contemporary concept that innate and adaptive immune reactivity is not mutually exclusive, but highly linked and networked for optimal function. Thus, we feel we have succeeded in providing a unique format that did not sacrifice content. Furthermore, the organ-specific approach has the potential to better serve infectious disease physicians and researchers working in specific organ systems without loss of any information of interest to immunologists and medical mycologists. The organs inclusive are: oral cavity, brain/CNS, lung, skin, vagina, and blood. Included in each organ section are chapters detailing the most contemporary host response mechanisms against the fungal pathogens most often affecting those organs, including local and regional host response mechanisms now recognized to be as critical as systemic immune mechanisms. Also included are chapters on fungal hypersensitivity, fungal sinusitis, and fungal–endothelial cell interactions. As immunity to fungi are often not mentioned in discussions of immunology and infectious diseases, this compilation will provide easy access to information that may stimulate the inclusion of fungi in future discussions.

It has become quite apparent in compiling the chapters for this book that despite each fungal organism having distinct properties, it is uncanny how similar the host responses are against each organism. Moreover, the host response patterns can be quite distinct to other types of organisms (i.e., bacteria, viruses, parasites). Thus, the book provides the medium to fully realize the unique yet highly uniform means by which the host responds to these diverse eukaryotic human pathogens—the fungi.

Paul L. Fidel, Jr., Ph.D.
Gary Huffnagle, Ph.D.

Contributors

Robert B. Ashman, Department of Oral Biology and Pathology, University of Queensland School of Dentistry, Brisbane, Queensland, Australia

James M. Beck, Division of Pulmonary and Critical Care Medicine, University of Michigan Medical School and Veterans Affairs Medical Center, Ann Arbor, MI, USA

Maria H. S. L. Blotta, Department of Clinical Pathology, State University of Campinas (UNICAMP) Faculty of Medical Sciences, São Paulo, Brazil

Maria Boccanera, Department of Infectious, Parasitic and Immune-Mediated Diseases, Istituto Superiore di Sanità, Rome, Italy

Kent L. Buchanan, Department of Microbiology and Immunology, Tulane University School of Medicine, New Orleans, LA, USA

Vera L. G. Calich, Department of Immunology, University of São Paulo (USP) Institute of Biomedical Sciences, São Paulo, Brazil

Arturo Casadevall, Division of Infectious Diseases, Department of Internal Medicine, Albert Einstein College of Medicine, Bronx, NY, USA

Antonio Cassone, Department of Infectious, Parasitic and Immune-mediated Diseases, Istituto Superiore di Sanità, Rome, Italy

Stephen J. Challacombe, Division of Oral Medicine, Pathology & Immunology, GKT Dental Institute, King's College London, United Kingdom

Flavia De Bernardis, Department of Infectious, Parasitic and Immune-mediated Diseases, Istituto Superiore di Sanità, Rome, Italy

George S. Deepe, Jr., Division of Infectious Diseases, Department of Internal Medicine, University of Cincinnati College of Medicine, Cincinnati, OH, USA

Anna Dongari-Bagtzoglou, Department of Oral Health and Diagnostic Sciences, University of Connecticut School of Dental Medicine, Farmington, CT, USA

Paul L. Fidel, Jr., Department of Microbiology, Immunology, and Parasitology, Louisiana State University Health Sciences Center, New Orleans, LA, USA

Camile S. Farah, Department of Oral Biology and Pathology, University of Queensland School of Dentistry, Brisbane, Queensland, Australia

Marta Feldmesser, Division of Infectious Diseases, Department of Internal Medicine, Albert Einstein College of Medicine, Bronx, NY, USA

Scott G. Filler, Harbor-UCLA Research and Education Institute, Torrance, CA, USA

Masutaka Furue, Department of Dermatology, Kyushu University Graduate School of Medical Sciences, Fukuoka, Japan

Beth A. Garvy, Departments of Microbiology, Immunology, and Molecular Genetics and Internal Medicine, University of Kentucky Chandler Medical Center, Lexington, KY, USA

Francis Gigliotti, Departments of Pediatrics and Microbiology and Immunology, University of Rochester Medical Center, Rochester, NY, USA

Jack R. Harkema, Department of Pathobiology and Diagnostic Investigation, Michigan State University, East Lansing, MI, USA

Cory M. Hogaboam, Department of Pathology, University of Michigan Medical School, Ann Arbor, MI, USA

Gary B. Huffnagle, Division of Pulmonary and Critical Care Medicine, Department of Internal Medicine, University of Michigan Medical School, Ann Arbor, MI, USA

Kazuyoshi Kawakami, Department of Microbiology and Immunology, School of Health Sciences, Faculty of Medicine, Tohoku University, Sendai, Japan

Bruce S. Klein, Department of Pediatrics, University of Wisconsin Medical School, Madison, WI, USA

Alan P. Knutsen, Pediatrics Research Institute, St. Louis University Health Sciences, St. Louis, MO, USA

Tetsuya Koga, Department of Dermatology, Fukuoka Red Cross Hospital, Fukuoka, Japan

Thomas R. Kozel, Department of Microbiology and Immunology, University of Nevada School of Medicine, Reno, NV, USA

Viswanath P. Kurup, Allergy-Immunology Division, Department of Pediatrics, Medical College of Wisconsin and Veterans Affairs Medical Center, Milwaukee, WI, USA

Dennis M. Lindell, Division of Pulmonary and Critical Care Medicine, Department of Internal Medicine, University of Michigan Medical School, Ann Arbor, MI, USA

Tetsuo Matsuda, Department of Dermatology, Kyushu University Graduate School of Medical Sciences, Fukuoka, Japan

Mukesh Mistry, Division of Oral Medicine, Pathology & Immunology, GKT Dental Institute, King's College London, United Kingdom

Julian R. Naglik, Division of Oral Medicine, Pathology & Immunology, GKT Dental Institute, King's College London, United Kingdom

Durdana Rahman, Division of Oral Medicine, Pathology & Immunology, GKT Dental Institute, King's College London, United Kingdom

Tobias E. Rodriguez, Division of Pulmonary and Critical Care Medicine, Department of Internal Medicine, University of Michigan Medical School, Ann Arbor, MI, USA

Luigina Romani, Department of Experimental Medicine and Biochemical Sciences, University of Perugia, Perugia, Italy

Jane M. Schuh, Department of Veterinary and Microbiology Sciences, North Dakota State University, Fargo, ND, USA

Judd E. Shellito, Division of Pulmonary and Critical Care Medicine, Louisiana State University Health Sciences Center, New Orleans, LA, USA

Donald C. Sheppard, McGill University, Montreal, Quebec, Canada

Peter G. Sohnle, Division of Infectious Diseases, Department of Medicine, Medical College of Wisconsin and Veterans Affairs Medical Center, Milwaukee, WI, USA

Srividya Srinivasan, Division of Infectious Diseases, Department of Medicine, Medical College of Wisconsin and Veterans Affairs Medical Center, Milwaukee, WI, USA

Takeshi Uenotsuchi, Department of Dermatology, Kyushu University Graduate School of Medical Sciences, Fukuoka, Japan

David K. Wagner, Division of Infectious Diseases, Department of Medicine, Medical College of Wisconsin and Veterans Affairs Medical Center, Milwaukee, WI, USA

Robert D. Wagner, Microbiology Division, National Center for Toxicological Research, Jefferson, AR, USA

Marcel Wüthrich, Department of Pediatrics, University of Wisconsin Medical School, Madison, WI, USA

Contents

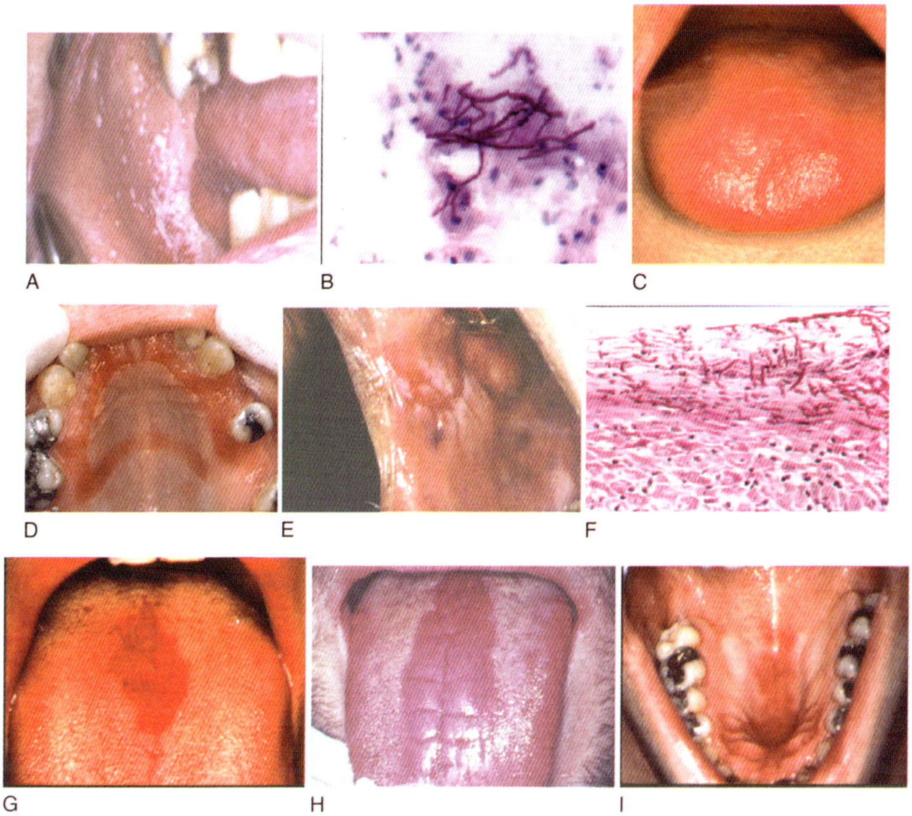

Figure 3.1. (A) *Acute pseudomembranous candidiasis*. Note the white plaques, which consist of hyphae, desquamated epithelial cells, and polymorphonuclear leukocytes. (B) Cytological smear from pseudomembranous candidiasis showing hyphae, desquamated epithelial cells, and polymorphonuclear leukocytes (Periodic acid Shiff stain). (C) *Acute atrophic candidiasis* (antibiotic sore tongue) showing generalised depapillation of the dorsum of the tongue secondary to *Candida* overgrowth. (D) *Chronic atrophic candidiasis*. Chronic atrophic candidiasis in a patient who wears a cobalt chrome partial upper denture. The mid-portion of the palate is of normal color, but the mucosa under the denture is very erythematous. (E) *Chronic hyperplastic candidiasis*. Mixed red and white plaques inside the buccal mucosa in the commissure areas. These are often slightly raised and histologically show hyphal invasion. (F) Section from chronic hyperplastic candidiasis showing invading hypha forms of *Candida* (PAS stain). (G) Median rhomboid glossitis, a form of chronic hyperplastic candidiasis of the tongue, usually found at the junction of the anterior two thirds and posterior third of the tongue. (H) *Erythematous candidiasis*. The central portion of this tongue is very erythematous as well as depapillated. This patient has AIDS. (I) *Erythematous candidiasis*. The central portion of the palate is very erythematous. No white plaques are seen. This patient has AIDS.

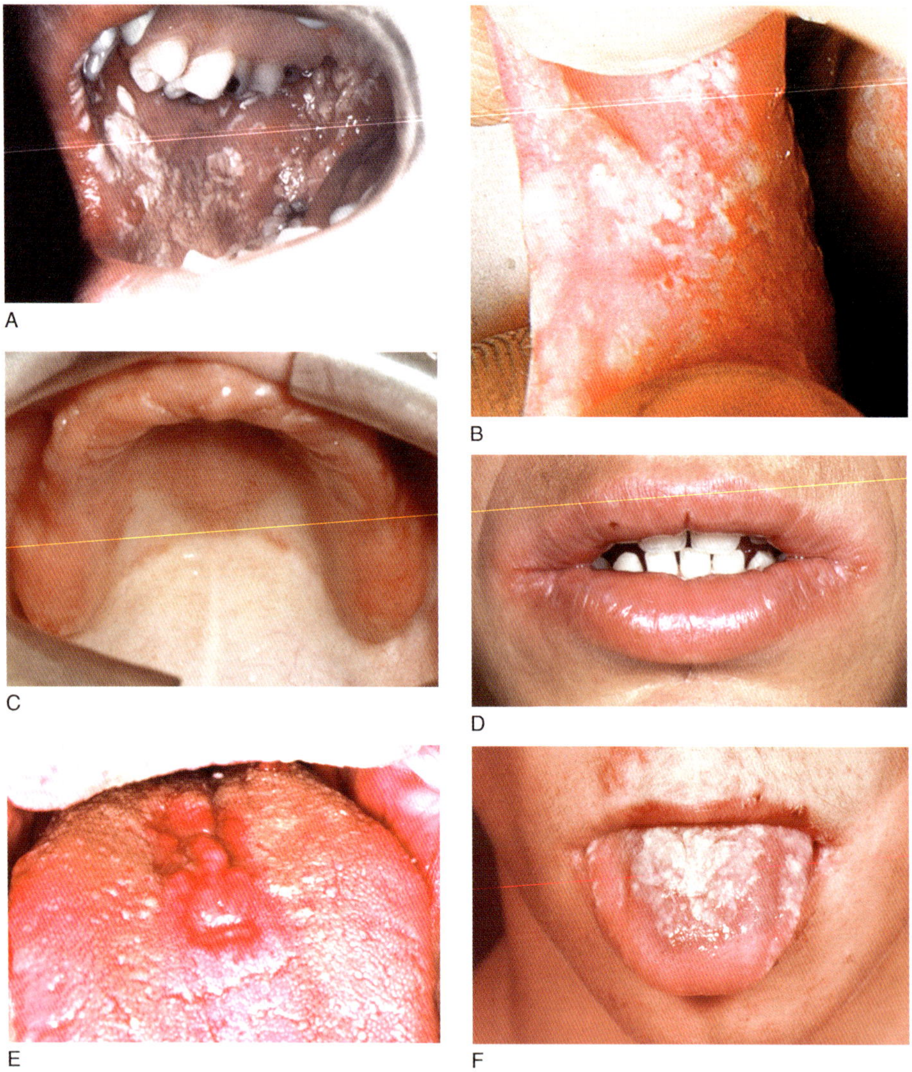

Figure 4.1. Clinical presentation of acute pseudomembranous candidiasis (A), chronic mucocutaneous candidiasis (B), Candida-associated denture stomatitis (C), angular cheilitis (D), median rhomboid glossitis (E), and hyperplastic candidiasis (F). (Reprinted from publication *Clinics in Dermatology*, 18: 553–562, Farah, et al. "Oral Candidosis" © 2000 with permission from Elsevier Inc.)

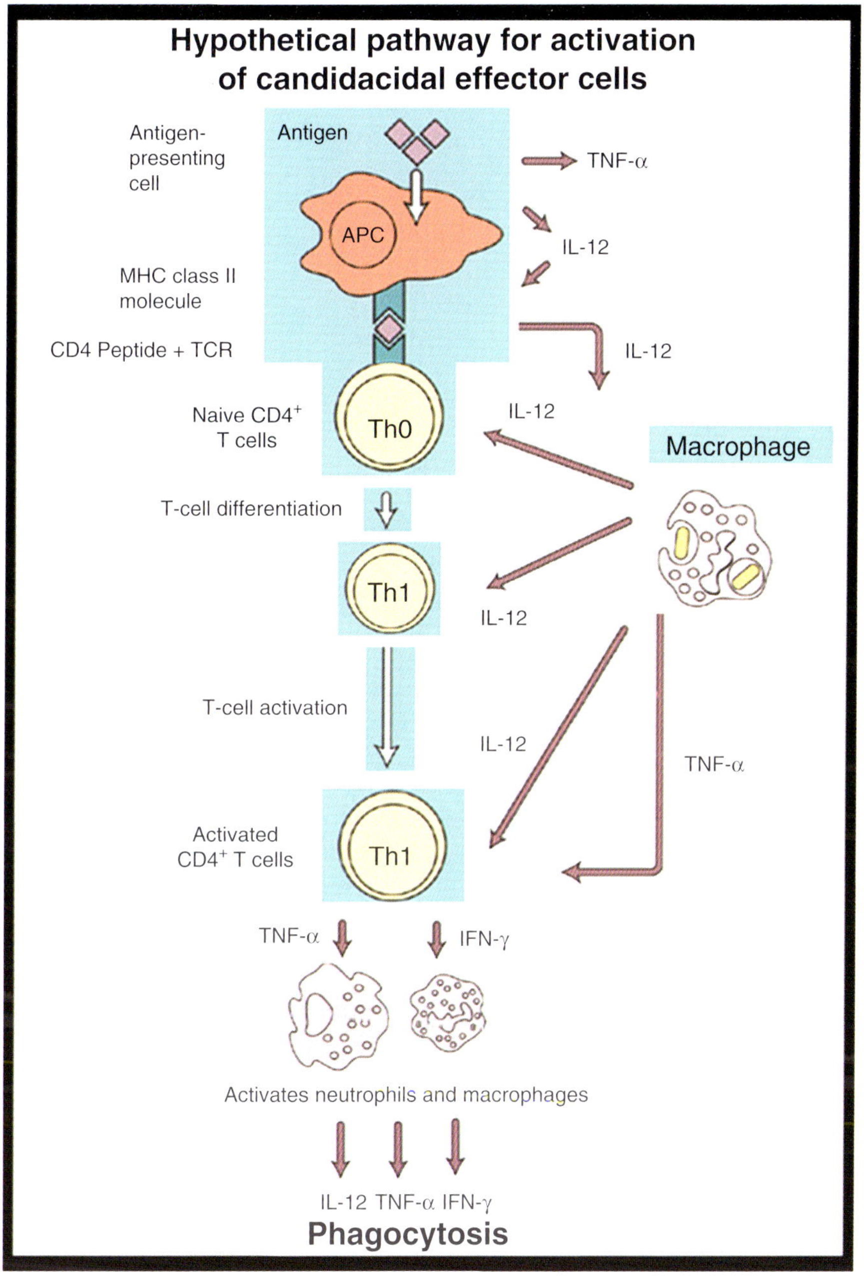

Figure 4.2. Hypothetical pathway for activation of effector cells in oral candidiasis. Stimulation of antigen-presenting cells (APC) by antigen(s) of *Candida* results in the production of TNF-α, which increases recruitment of inflammatory cells, and augments the candidacidal activity of phagocytic cells early in the course of infection. The APCs secrete IL-12, which drives the differentiation of naïve $CD4^+$ T cells, and induces a Th1-type cellular immune response. The Th1 cytokines (IFN-γ and TNF-α) act both separately and synergistically to promote *Candida* killing by both neutrophils and macrophages; while both IL-12 and IFN-γ act on the APC in a feedback loop to enhance their activation.

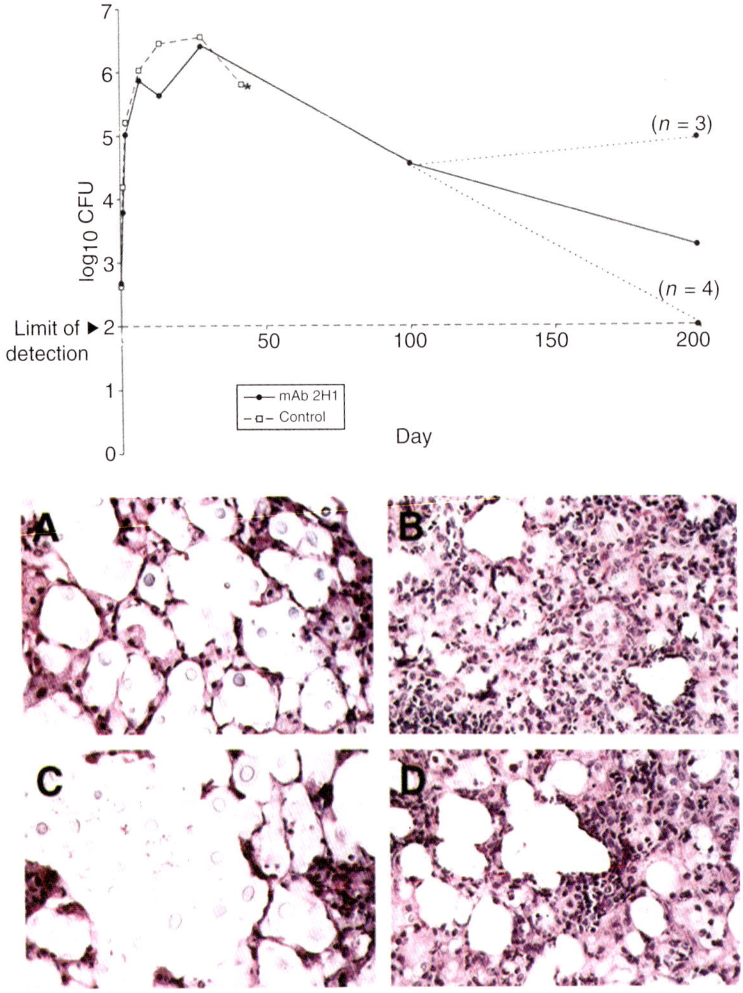

Figure 9.1. Top: The relationship between lung CFU and time in control and mAb 2H1-treated mice following i.t. infection with 10^4 *C. neoformans* yeast. MAb 2H1 (1 mg/mouse) was given intraperitoneally 24 h prior to infection. Values represent means. Broken lines from day 100 to day 199 represent the curves when day 199 mice were separated into those with detectable lung CFU (upper line) and those for whom CFU were not detectable (lower line). Asterisk (*) indicates point after which CFU data could not be obtained from control animals because they began to die rapidly. For control mice, n = 10, 9, 8, 10, 12, 13, and 4 at 2, 24, 48 h, 7, 14, 28, and 42 days, respectively. For mAb 2H1-treated mice, n = 10, 10, 10, 11, 10, 27, 4, and 7 at 2, 24, 48 h, 7, 14, 28, 100, and 199 days, respectively. Because the curves are derived from multiple experiments, statistical analysis was not included. Bottom: A and C, day 28 lungs of two control mice show a predominance of extracellular *C. neoformans*. Organisms were able to grow freely in the alveolar space outside of inflammatory foci. B and D, day 28 lungs of two mAb 2H1-treated mice show granulomatous inflammation and predominantly intracellular *C. neoformans* (arrows). In mAb 2H1-treated mice, organisms were usually contained within foci of inflammation; H&E stain, X250. Reproduced with permission from *J. Immunol.* 1997; 158: 790–799. Copyright 1997. The American Association of Immunologists, Inc.

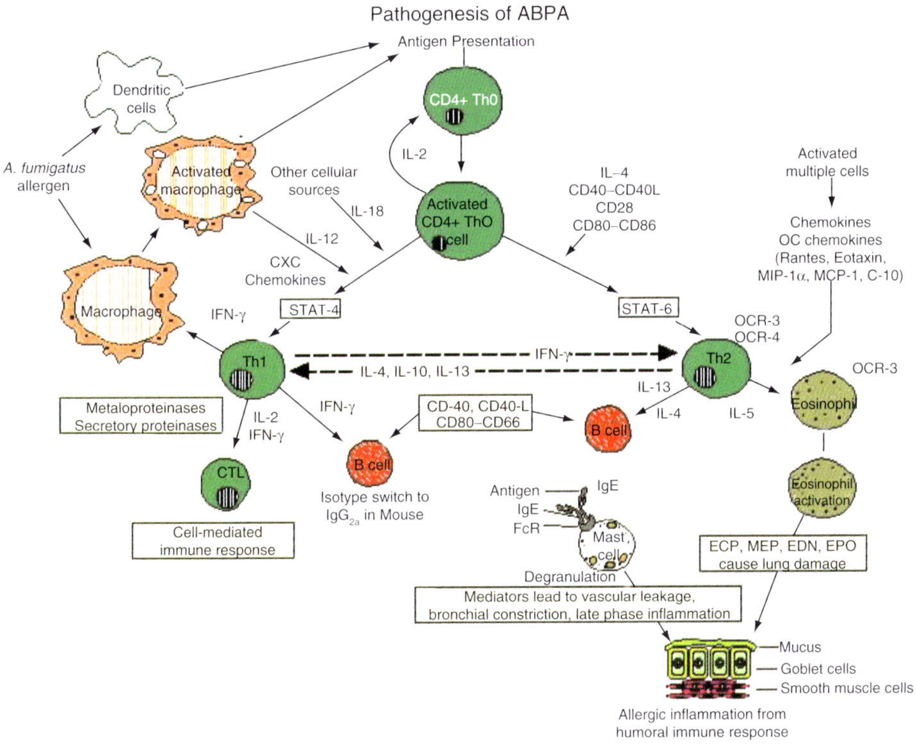

Figure 12.1. Schematic illustration of the current understanding of the pathogenesis of ABPA.

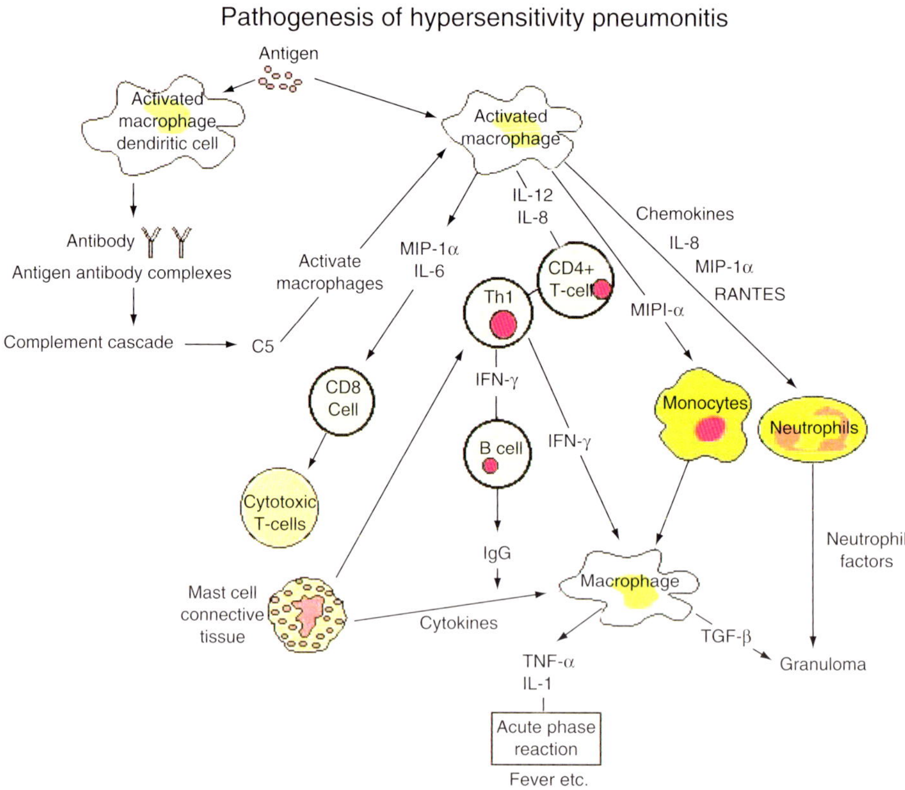

Figure 12.2. Schematic presentation of the current understanding of the pathogenesis of hypersensitivity pneumonitis.

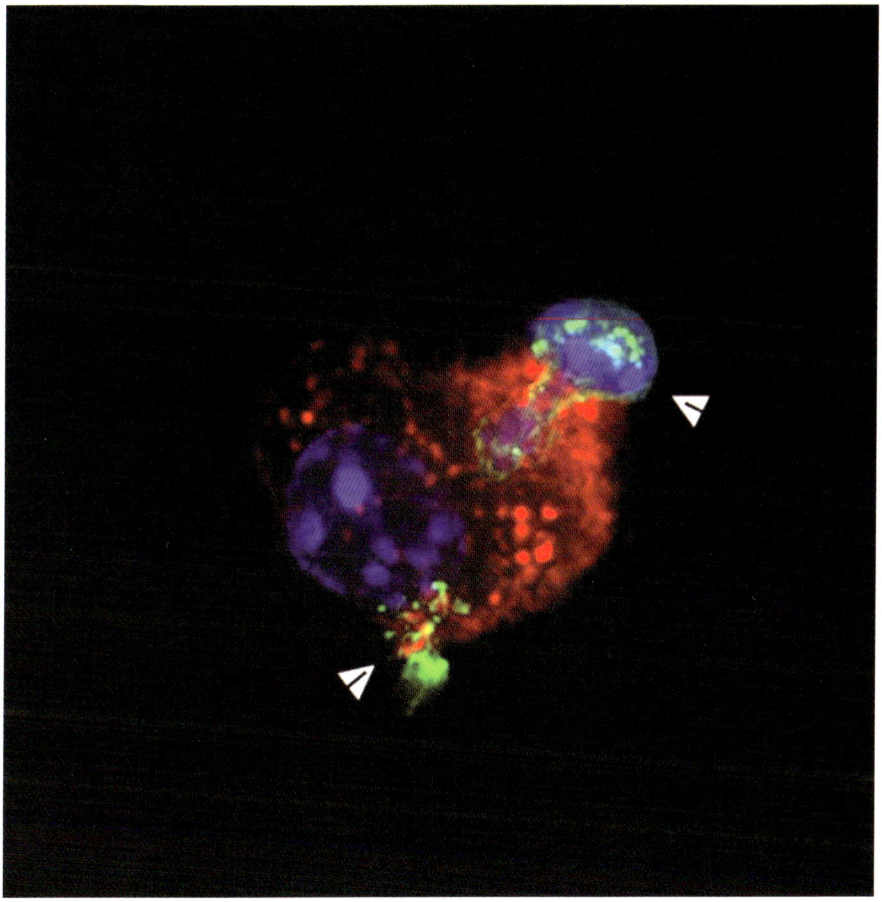

Figure 13.1. Phagocytosis of *Pneumocystis* by a murine alveolar macrophage (deconvolution microscopy, 630×). The DNA-specific dye 4′,6-diamidino-2-phenylindole dihydrochloride (DAPI) was used to stain both alveolar nuclei and fungal DNA. The green indicates surface labeling of both cyst and trophozoite (arrowheads) forms of *Pneumocystis* with fluorescein isothiocyanate (FITC). F-actin filaments within the alveolar cytoskeleton were counterstained with Phalloidin Alexa 568. Copied with permission from Steele, C., Marrero, L., Swain, S., Harmsen, A. G., Zheng, M., Brown, G. D., Gordon, S., Shellito, J. E., and Kolls, J. K. (2003). Alveolar macrophage-mediated killing of *Pneumocystis carinii f. sp. muris* involves molecular recognition by the Dectin-1 beta-glucan receptor. *J. Exp. Med.* 198: 1677–1688.

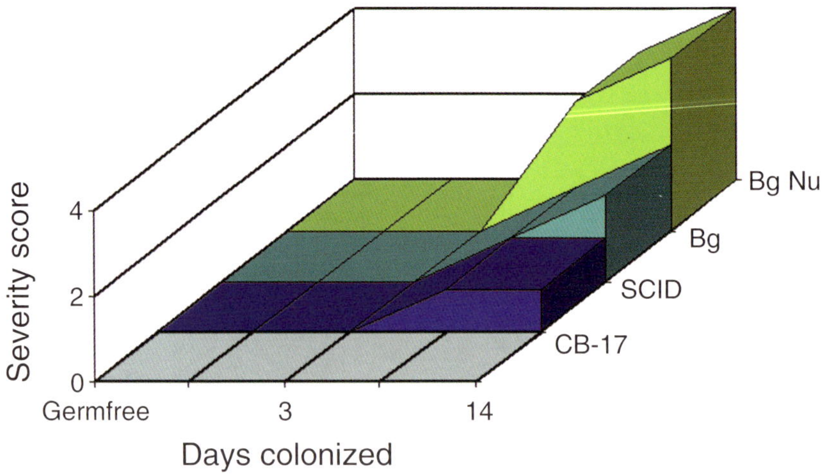

Figure 15.2. Severity of gastric candidiasis in immunodeficient mouse strains monoassociated with *Candida albicans*. Mice were monoassociated with *C. albicans* and groups of four mice of each strain were euthanized and scored for severity of gastric lesions at each time point ($n = 80$). The average severity scores are represented, with 0, no signs of disease to 4, most severe lesions with inflammation and fungal tissue invasion. The CB-17 mice were immunocompetent controls, SCID mice have T cell-mediated immune defects, Bg, beige defect mice have deficient phagocytic cell functions and Bg Nu, beige-nude mice are athymic beige defect mice lacking T cell and phagocytic cell functions.

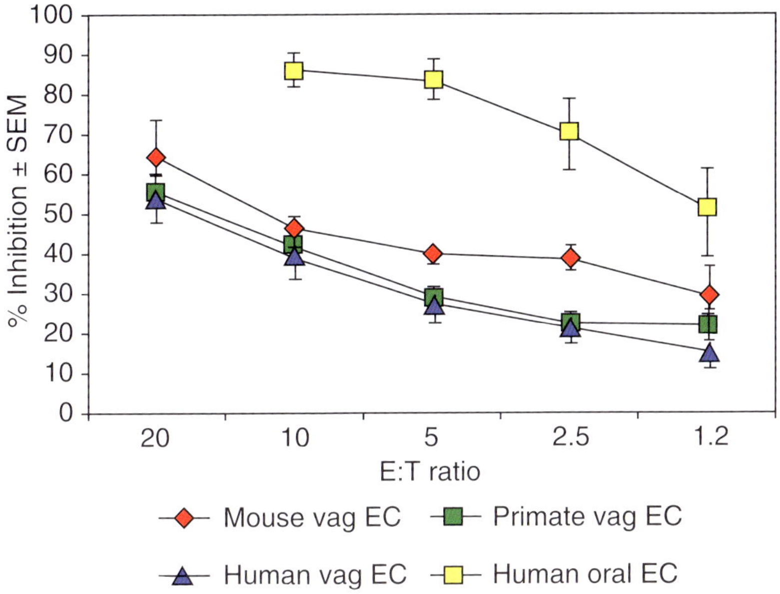

Figure 16.2. Vaginal and oral epithelial cell anti-*Candida* activity. Vaginal epithelial cells from humans (vaginal lavage), nonhuman primates (vaginal lavage), and mouse (vaginal tissue extraction) and oral epithelial cells (collected from saliva) were cocultured with *C. albicans* at various effector to target (E:T) ratios for 9 h. Controls included epithelial cells and *Candida* cultured alone. Growth of *Candida* was determined by ^{3}H-glucose uptake and percent inhibition in the coculture was determined.

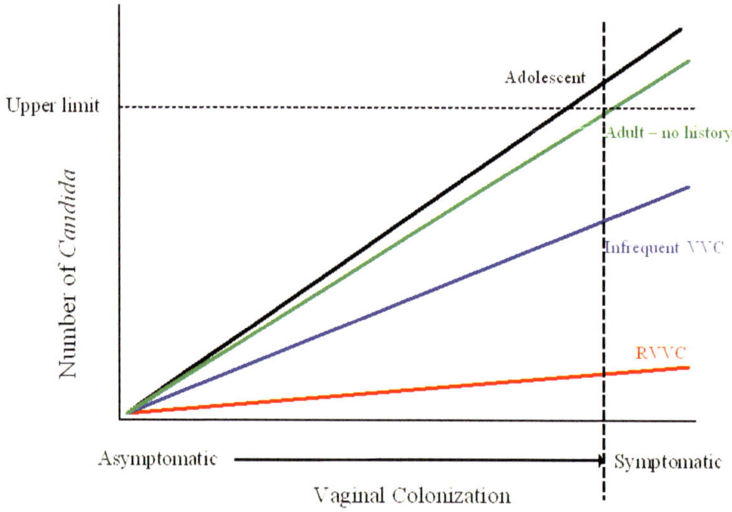

Figure 16.3. Hypothesis for acquisition of symptomatic vulvovaginal candidiasis. The hypothesis centers on the acquisition of vulvovaginal candidiasis by achieving a threshold of *Candida* organisms in the vagina. Under the threshold the vaginal presence of *Candida* is considered commensal and asymptomatic. Once the threshold is crossed (vertical dotted line), the signals are initiated that allow for migration of PMNs into the vagina that cause the symptoms associated with vaginitis. Accordingly, there is a different threshold for different groups of women. For women with RVVC the threshold is very low and increases incrementally in those with infrequent episodes of VVC, no history of VVC, and adolescents. The upper limit is an arbitrary level of organism number that would be considered unattainable.

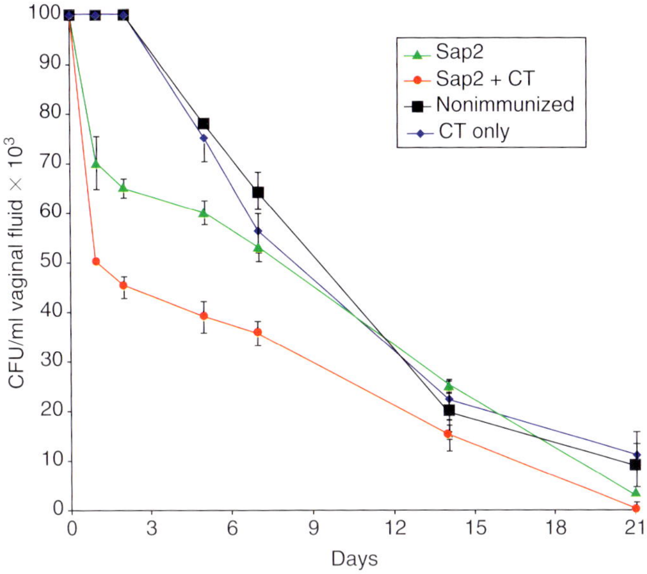

Figure 17.1. Outcome of vaginal infection by *C. albicans* in rats intravaginally immunized with proteinase (Saps) 2 plus or minus mucosal adjuvant cholera toxin (CT). Each curve represents the mean (± standard error of the mean) of the number of fungal CFU for five rats. Statistical significance was assessed by Student's *t* test (two tailed).

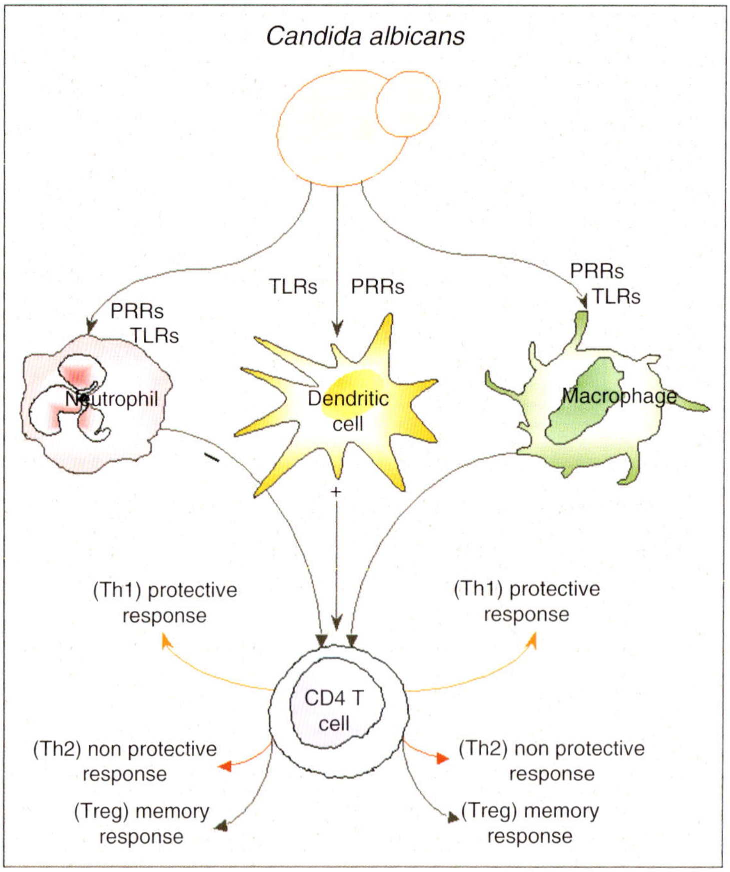

Figure 19.1. The immune response to *Candida albicans*, involving the "cross-talk" among many immune cells, including dendritic cells, macrophages, neutrophils, and $CD4^+$ T cells. Cells of the innate immune system discriminate between different forms of the fungus and produce sets of chemokines, cytokines, and costimulatory molecules through which signals to the adaptive T helper (Th) immune system. Protective and nonprotective Th cells release a distinct panel of cytokines, capable of delivering activating and inhibitory feedback signals to effector phagocytes. Together, the innate and adaptive immune systems contribute to the inflammatory response. Counter-regulatory T cells (Treg) may serve to dampen the excessive inflammatory reactions and to contribute to the development of memory antifungal immunity. (+) and (–) refer to positive and negative signals, respectively.

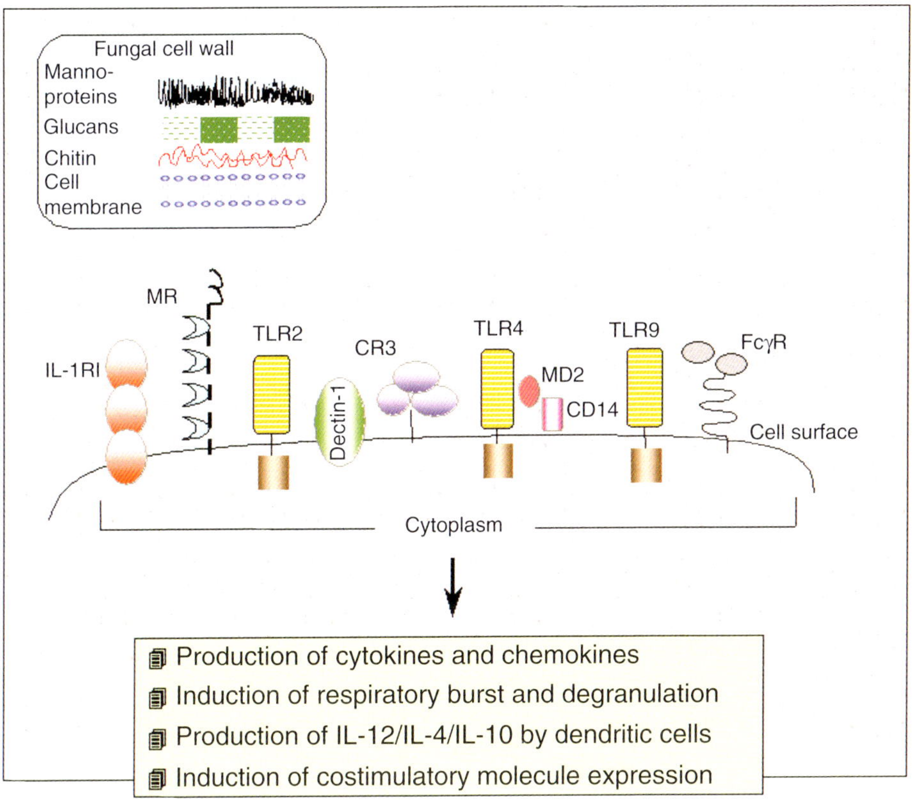

Figure 19.2. Pattern recognition receptors as activators of innate and adaptive immunity to fungi. Recognition of *Candida albicans* and fungal PAMPs, mainly associated with fungal cell wall (top left schematic icon) by Toll-like receptors (TLRs), mannose receptor (MR), complement receptor (CR3), and receptors for Fc (FcγR) leads to activation of specialized antifungal effector functions in neutrophils, such as respiratory burst and degranulation, and production of IL-12 p70 by dendritic cells (see text). As dendritic cells are equipped with pattern recognition receptors and TLRs, they are uniquely able at decoding the fungus-associated information and translating it in qualitatively different adaptive Th-immune responses. The engagement of distinct receptors by yeasts and hyphae translates into downstream signaling events, ultimately regulating costimulation, cytokine production, and development of Th and regulatory T cells. The functional plasticity of DCs at the pathogen–immune system interface may offer new interpretative clues to fungal virulence.

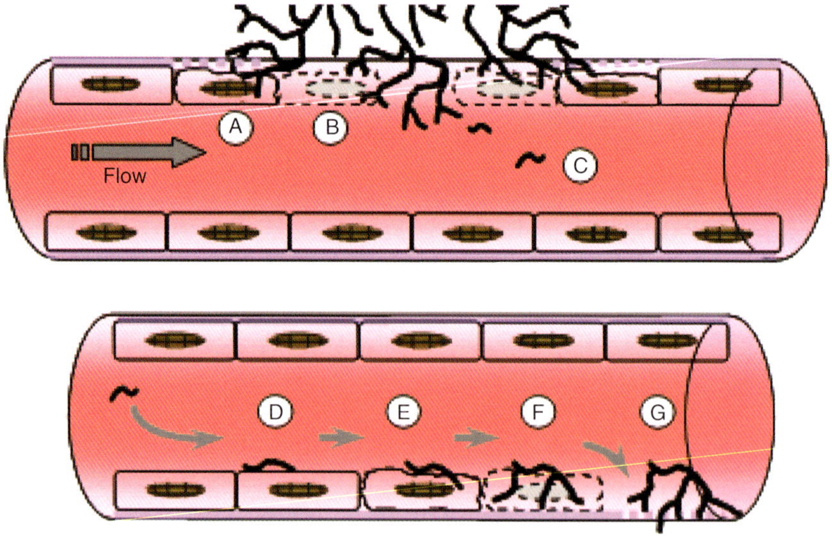

Figure 20.1. Model of angioinvasion and dissemination by *A. fumigatus*. These processes occur via the following steps: (A) abluminal endothelial cell invasion, (B) endothelial cell injury from the abluminal surface, (C) hematogenous dissemination of hyphal fragments, (D) hyphal adherence to the luminal endothelial cell surface, (E) luminal endothelial cell invasion, (F) endothelial cell injury from the luminal surface, and (G) extravascular invasion of deep organs. Steps (A)–(C) occur in the pulmonary blood vessels while steps (D)–(G) occur in the systemic blood vessels.

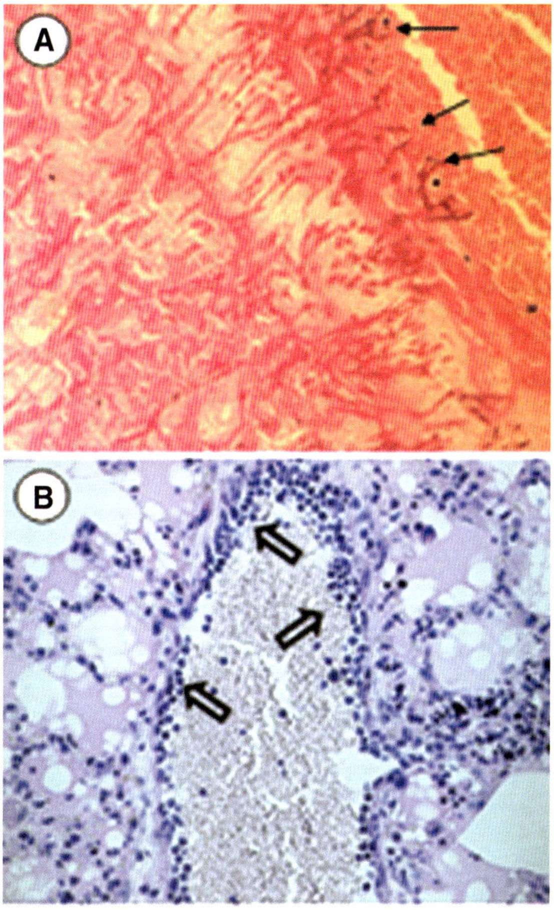

Figure 20.2. Histopathology of invasive pulmonary aspergillosis. Periodic-acid Schiff (PAS) stained thin sections from lungs of mice infected with *A. fumigatus* for 7 and 10 days respectively. (A) Abluminal angioinvasion by hyphae. Note that endothelial cells are absent at the site of the invading hyphae (arrows). (B) Neutrophil margination (open arrows) occurs in the vicinity of *A. fumigatus* lesions. Note that neutrophils have attached to the vessel wall in large numbers, suggesting that these endothelial cells are activated to express leukocyte adhesion molecules.

1

Fungal Sinusitis

Tobias E. Rodriguez[1,2], Jack R. Harkema[3], and Gary B. Huffnagle[1,2]

1. Introduction

Sinusitis afflicts 37 million people yearly, resulting in billions spent on physician visits and treatments (NIAID, 2002; CDC, 2003). Occurring in both immunocompetent and immunocompromised individuals, sinusitis is often found in the context of other chronic diseases such as allergies, asthma, inflammatory bowel disease, Crohn's disease, and cystic fibrosis (CF) (Book et al., 2003).

A number of different etiological agents and pathologies are associated with sinusitis. The incidence of fungal sinusitis is increasing and diagnosis is often delayed, recognized only after failure of antibiotic treatments. Cases of fungal sinusitis are associated with significant morbidity, or in untreated invasive cases, mortality (Benninger, 1992; deShazo and Swain, 1995; Ferguson, 2000a; NIAID, 2002; Pleis, 2003). Much remains to be learned about the pathogenesis and

[1] Division of Pulmonary and Critical Care Medicine, Department of Internal Medicine, University of Michigan Medical School, Ann Arbor, MI.
[2] Department of Microbiology and Immunology, University of Michigan Medical School, Ann Arbor, MI.
[3] Department of Pathobiology and Diagnostic Investigation, Michigan State University, East Lansing, MI.

immunology of fungal sinusitis. Most of what is currently known is limited to clinical observation. The focus of this chapter is to give a background on fungal sinusitis, the anatomy affected, the fungi involved, and the host immune response to the fungus.

2. Anatomy, Architecture, and Function

2.1. The Nasal Cavity

The nasal cavity connects the nares to the nasopharynx by way of the posterior nasal aperture (Cooper, 1994). In humans the nasal cavity is estimated to be 16 cm^3 in volume (Harkema, 1992). The cavity is divided laterally by the nasal septum, which is comprised of cartilage more distally and bone more proximally. The cavity itself is enclosed by the lateral walls, a complicated structure containing portions of several bones; three of which form the foundation for the nasal turbinates (see Fig. 1.1). These turbinates (conchae) are rounded protrusions of these three bones and extend and furl throughout the nasal cavity. They function to direct air through the hollow space, promoting filtration, humidification, and temperature regulation (Dykewicz, 2003). The bottom most of these three protrusions is the inferior turbinate, which is the largest of the three and contains numerous venous spaces in its tissues. The other two turbinates, middle and superior (with the superior being smaller and located above the middle), are formed from portions of the ethmoid bone and actually form two of the four paranasal sinus cavities. Located between each of the turbinates lies an open air space called a meatus. Each is named for the analogous turbinate (inferior, middle, or superior), and contains openings from different sources of the nasal cavity. Though each meatus serves a specific role, their general function is receiving drainage from the sinus cavities and

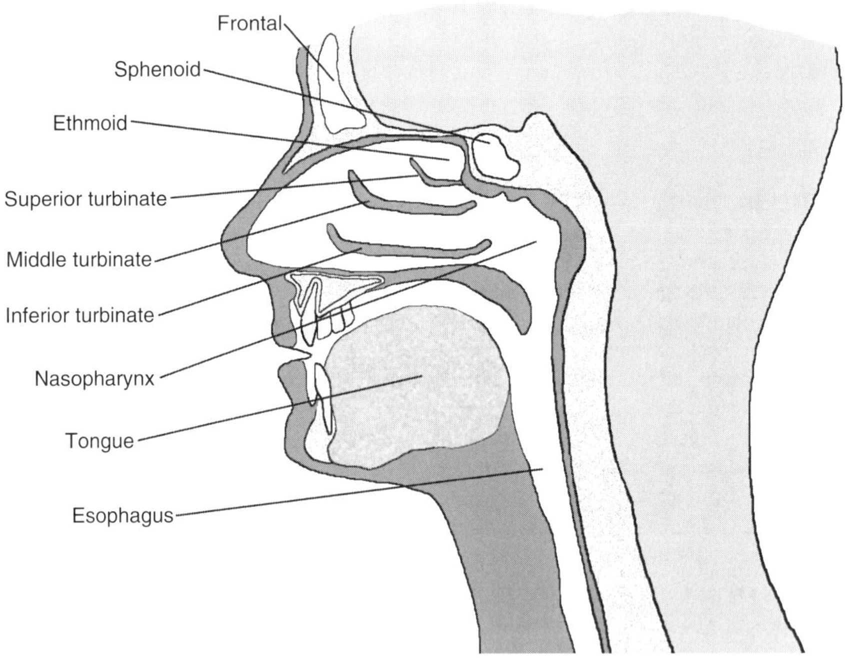

Figure 1.1. Diagram of human nasal architecture.

providing passageway for blood vessels and nervous tissue. An example of this process is the nasolacrimal duct that opens to the inferior meatus. This duct functions to drain tears away from the orbits, resulting in congestion when an individual cries (Cooper, 1994; Citardi, 2003; Dykewicz, 2003).

2.2. The Paranasal Sinuses

Located within this framework of cartilage, bones, and turbinates are the four sinus cavities of the paranasal region. They function to humidify incoming air, filter out particulate matter present in respiration, aid in resonance, lighten the weight of the skull, and protect the brain and tissues from direct trauma. All the paranasal sinuses are connected to the nasal cavity via an opening in their tissue called the ostium. This small aperture allows for release of pressure and for drainage of superfluous liquid and mucus from each of the cavities. Since the ostium is the only means by which mucus and fluid can drain from the sinus, if this opening narrows or becomes blocked due to inflammation or disease state, opportunistic organisms can flourish in the cavities, resulting in an infection (Van Alyea, 1939; Baraniuk, 1994; Citardi, 2003).

Each sinus is named by the bone it rests in or on, resulting in the frontal, sphenoid, ethmoid, and maxillary cavities (Fig. 1.1). The frontal cavities, small to medium in size, rest above the eye orbits on both sides of the face and drain into the middle meatus via the frontomasal duct and ethmoidal infindibulum. The two cavities usually lie asymmetrical to one another, though cases have been seen in which the cavities lie behind one another or are connected (Cooper, 1994).

The next set of sinuses are the ethmoid cavities which have a honeycomb appearance and contain anywhere from 6 to 12 air cells within their structure (Van Alyea, 1939; Citardi, 2003). They flank the upper area of the nose and lie in close proximity to the frontal sinuses. They drain into the ethmoidal infindibulum via several openings.

Posterior to the ethmoid sinuses, near the middle of the skull, rest the two asymmetrical sphenoid cavities. Drainage occurs via the sphenoidal ostium into the sphenoethmoid recess, which is the space between the superior turbinate, septum, and sphenoid sinus wall (Citardi, 2003).

Lastly, the largest sinus, the maxillary, lies beneath the cheeks on each side of the face. The sinus drains into the ethmoid infindibulum just as the other cavities, however, the ostium on the maxillary tends to be reasonably smaller due to the surrounding mucosa on the bone (Cooper, 1994).

2.3. Cellular Anatomy and Physiology

The nasal cavity, turbinates, and paranasal sinuses are lined with mucosa comprised of four distinct nasal epithelium populations: olfactory epithelium (OE), stratified squamous epithelium (SE), respiratory epithelium (RE), and nonciliated cuboidal/columnar epithelium (NCE), also known as transitional epithelium. Each type has its own unique cell populations and distribution throughout the nasal cavity. SE lines the external nares and vestibule of the nose, RE covers most of the nasoturbinates, maxiloturbinates, septum, and maxillary sinus cavities, OE lines the ethmoid turbinates, and NCE is found in narrow zones of transition between each type (Harkema, 1992; Herbert, 1999). In studies involving rats, Gross et al. (1982) showed the percentage of these epithelium types to be 7% for SE, 46% for RE, and 47% for OE. When compared to humans these values would shift, as OE in humans is restricted to a very small area covering the mid-dorsal aspect of the nasal cavity. Additionally, rodents only possess maxillary and ethmoid sinus cavities, as opposed to the four found in humans.

The external nares and vestibule are completely lined by SE. In rats and mice there are

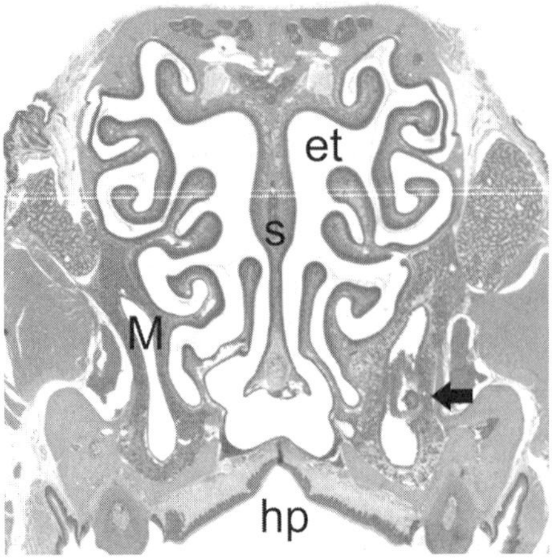

Figure 1.2. Histological analysis of murine sinuses in a model of acute invasive fungal sinusitis. The arrow indicates hyphal A. fumigatus becoming invasive in the right maxillary cavity. Tissue invasion has occurred in addition to the necrotic tissue surrounding the mass. et = ethmoid turbinates; hp = hard palate; M = maxillary sinus cavity; s = septum.

predominantly basal cells along the basal lamina and several layers of squamous cells, which become progressively flatter toward the luminal surface. This group contains the largest quantity of cells in S phase of the cell cycle, meaning it possesses larger cellular turnover. There are no mucociliary mechanisms in this population as the region most likely functions to protect the subsequent tissues and physiology.

Respiratory epithelium, the predominant cell type in humans, covers most of the turbinates (except for the ethmoid region) as well as the septum and maxillary sinus cavities. In rodents the principle cell types found within the RE are cuboidal cells, goblet cells, brush cells, basal cells, and ciliated and non-ciliated columnar cells. The lamina propria of the RE contains collagen fibers, nerves, mucus, and serous glands, as well as venous sinuses, which dilate to alter the airflow through the passageway (Harkema, 1992).

The OE in humans is limited to a small portion of the nasal cavity and lines the ethmoid nasal turbinates. In rodents the epithelium is pseudo-stratified and consists of three primary cell types including supporting cells, olfactory neurons, and basal cells. The lamina propria of OE has blood vessels, unmyelinated nerve bundles, and Bowman's glands responsible for the secretion of mucus to moisten the surrounding tissue. Microvilli are present on the epithelium and help move mucus around the region (Herbert, 1999).

Lastly the NCE lies in the transitional zones between different regions, primarily between the SE and RE. It consists of microvilli-covered epithelium, nonciliated cubodial/columnar cells, and basal cells (Harkema, 1992).

2.4. The Role of Nasal Physiology in Immunity

This mechanism accounts for how a majority of foreign debris is cleared from the nasal region, though the process is hindered when the ostium becomes blocked or the mucus becomes too viscous to move. Particulates are inhaled and become trapped in the viscous mucus overlaying the respiratory epithelium. Using coordinated mucociliary beat, the mucus is swept through the cavities and is pushed into the nasopharynx where it is then swallowed and digested (Baraniuk, 1994; Herbert, 1999). This accounts for how a majority of foreign debris is cleared from the nasal region, though the process becomes complicated when the ostium becomes blocked, or the mucus becomes too viscous to move. This thickening is seen in several disease states within the sinuses, though the mechanism behind this physiology is not yet discerned. Overall, the epithelium of the nasal cavity acts as an anatomical barrier by not only preventing antigens from directly reaching superficial tissue but also by secreting lysozyme and defensins to counter nominal pathogenic microbial colonization (Baraniuk, 1994).

In addition to the anatomical barriers, leukocytes play an indispensable role in the paranasal region innate immunity. Since each variant of fungal sinusitis carries its own specific host response, further information regarding the role of nasal physiology in innate and adaptive immunity will be discussed with each of the different classifications of fungal sinusitis.

3. Classifications of Fungal Sinusitis

As mentioned before, sinusitis is defined as a disease state localized to any of the four paranasal sinus cavities. Within the context of these diseases, the subject of fungal sinusitis can be divided into four categories: noninvasive fungal masses (commonly called fungal balls), invasive sinusitis (with acute and chronic subtypes), chronic sinusitis, and allergic fungal rhinosinusitis (AFRS). The basis for these manifestations is dependent on the immune status of the host. Depending on whether the host is immunocompetent, immunocompromised, or is atopic, the type of disease and severity encountered can shift based on fluctuations in the host status.

3.1. Noninvasive Fungal Masses (Fungal Balls)

Fungal balls of the paranasal sinuses are commonly referred to as mycetomas in the literature (though this is a misnomer as mycetomas technically represent superficial fungal infections on the feet) (Ferguson, 2000c). Fungal balls are noninvasive, non-immunogenic types of fungal sinusitis. Patients are immunocompetent and generally are neither atopic nor do they suffer from other disorders specific to the respiratory tract.

The masses themselves are mycelial mats which can rest in the sinus cavities for months or years without any sort of tissue invasion. They are described as cheeselike, gritty, rubbery, or greasy masses that are easily discernible from the surrounding mucosa. They may be black or brownish in color, and often have a fetid odor associated with them. A small, localized inflammatory response may be seen, but the integrity of the nasal architecture is unchanged (Washburn, 1994). The benign mass is usually limited to the maxillary sinus cavity, with infections occurring infrequently in the sphenoid cavity as well. Symptoms include chronic nasal congestion, pain localized to the maxillary sinus, and a postnasal drip. Often a superimposed acute bacterial infection will occur, though the infection is opportunistic and not directly integrated with the fungal sinusitis.

Several species of fungi have been reported in clinical settings as etiological agents involved with noninvasive fungal sinusitis (Table 1.1). The most predominant organisms seen within this disease state are

Table 1.1. Fungal Etiological Agents Associated with Types of Fungal Sinusitis

Type of fungal sinusitis	Fungal etiological agents
Noninvasive fungal masses (fungal balls)	*A. fumigatus, A. flavus, Alternaria* species, *Penicillium* (Ferguson, 2000b)
Invasive (acute and chronic subtypes)	*A. fumigatus, A. flavus, Alternaria* species, *C. neoformans* and *C. albicans* (Ferguson 2000a, Schell 2000)
Chronic rhinosinusitis	*A. fumigatus, A. flavus, Alternaria* species, *C. albicans, Penicillium, Fusarium* (Ponikau Sherris et al., 1999)
Allergic fungal rhinosinusitis (AFRS)	*A. fumigatus, Alternaria, Bipolaris, Curvularia* (Ferguson, 2000a; Houser and Corey, 2000)

Aspergillus fumigatus, *A. flavus*, and species of *Alternaria*, with *Penicillium* being seen in extremely rare cases (Schell, 2000). The prevalence of *Aspergillus* in noninvasive fungal sinusitis parallels the prevalence of this organism as one of the most common airborne fungal pathogens (Latgé, 1999).

The exact pathogenesis of noninvasive fungal masses is currently unknown, though the most likely cause is the persistence of the fungal spores within the nasal cavity (Ferguson, 2000c). Normally factors such as mucociliary beat are responsible for clearing fungal spores from the sinus region; however when an antigen is not removed, for reasons that are unclear, it may undergo germination (Baraniuk, 1994). Once hyphal extension transpires, the organism can become too large to be cleared by normal physiological means and is then able to establish an infection, though a nonimmunomodulatory one (Ferguson, 2000c).

Currently the only treatment available for noninvasive fungal sinusitis is surgery to remove the obstruction (Ferguson, 2000c). Irrigation can be useful in washing out small mycelial masses, but in the case of larger masses endoscopic surgery is preferred in targeting both the maxillary and sphenoid sinuses.

3.2. Invasive Fungal Sinusitis

Within invasive fungal sinusitis there are two distinct subtypes, acute and chronic. Acute sinusitis occurs in immunocompromised hosts (bone marrow transplant patients, HIV, etc.) and generally lasts for less than 4 weeks. In the literature it is commonly referred to as fulminant sinusitis, conveying the rapid disease progression and destruction affiliated with the infection (Ferguson, 2000a). Characteristically the disease progresses in a matter of days, with hyphal growth and extension pushing out of the sinus cavities and invading the surrounding mucosa, vascular system, and in severe cases, the cranium. Histological analysis reveals prominent hyphal extension, an influx of cellular exudates, and necrotic tissue surrounding the area. If patients presenting symptoms of acute invasive sinusitis fail to receive proper medical treatment, severe damage can occur to the nasal cavity, bone structure, and death can ensue (Fig. 1.2).

In studies performed by Rudack on mucosa samples from acute invasive sinusitis patients, concentrations of proinflammatory cytokines interleukin (IL)-1β and IL-6 were shown to be increased compared to control mucosa, but not seen at levels high enough to merit statistical significance (Rudack et al., 1998). However in analyzing levels of IL-3 and IL-8, values were significantly higher than controls, indicating an innate immune response against the invading fungus.

Most cases of acute sinusitis begin with the onset of the common cold (NIAID, 2002). These viral colds do not cause acute sinusitis per se, but rather act to inflame the sinuses and surrounding mucosa. Even if immunocompromised, most hosts would still be able to clear fungal spores from the nasal cavity via ciliated cells (Baraniuk, 1994). However with the overproduction of mucus and increased inflammation caused by the cold, the size of the ostium becomes limited, and any fungi present in the sinuses can no longer be mediated effectively. This is also the case for other opportunistic organisms such as *Haemophilus influenzae* and *Streptococcus pneumoniae* (NIAID, 2002).

Again, the most predominant organisms seen within this disease state are *A. fumigatus*, *A. flavus*, and species of *Alternaria* (Table 1.1). Additionally rare cases of *Cryptococcus neoformans* and *Candida albicans* have been seen in cases of acute invasive fungal sinusitis (Schell, 2000).

Chronic fungal sinusitis differs from the acute variation in that the host is for the most part immunocompetent and the symptoms affiliated with the disease last longer than 4 weeks (Washburn, 1994).

These patients typically suffer from a longstanding history of upper respiratory allergies, asthma, and nasal polyposis. The disease can take months or years to progress and symptoms include the erosion of barriers separating the paranasal cavities, as well as adjacent structures such as the orbits, brain, and pituitary gland (Stringer, 2000). Additionally patients suffer from mycotic aneurysms, carotid artery ruptures, erosion of the maxillary floor which results in palatal degradation, and erosion of the cribriform plate which results in chronic headaches, seizures, and decreased mental status. Etiological agents found in clinical cases are the same as those in the noninvasive and the acute invasive forms (Schell, 2000).

In studies performed by Rudack and others on samples taken from chronic fungal sinusitis patients, the only cytokine shown at elevated levels was IL-3 (Rudack et al., 1998). This is contrasted against more recent work which indicates the increased expression of IL-1β, IL-5, IL-6, IL-8, and TNF-α in the sinonasal mucosa of patients with chronic sinusitis (Lennard et al., 2000).

The exact etiology of what causes chronic invasive fungal sinusitis is unknown. Most patients are immunologically intact and contain no cellular level defects that contribute to the overall morbidity of the disease (Washburn, 1994). The chronic inflammation results in rearrangement of the normal sinus architecture, which impedes drainage and can lead to superimposed bacterial sinusitis (Ferguson, 2000a). However, the notion of this pathophysiology being sufficient to cause chronicity is unfounded. One report suggests that the fungus is simply acting as an opportunist and taking advantage of a weakened and diseased sinus and yet others point to the not yet fully elucidated fungal virulence factors as rationale (Jahrsdoerfer et al., 1979).

Chronic invasive fungal sinusitis is usually misdiagnosed and is only recognized after patients take antibiotics for a long period without cessation of symptoms (Stringer, 2000). Current therapy uses the prescription of steroids to initially decrease inflammation, and if no change is seen in the patient's progress, a combination of endoscopic surgery and antifungal chemotherapy is applied. Even with these procedures the disease state recurs quite frequently postsurgery and posttreatment (Washburn, 1994; Stringer, 2000; NIAID, 2002).

3.3. Chronic Rhinosinusitis

Chronic rhinosinusitis (CRS) is an inflammatory condition of the paranasal mucosa and nasal cavity that persists longer than 3 months. Typically medical or surgical treatments offer very little assistance to these patients, a reflection of the general morbidity caused by this disorder. There has been much controversy regarding the specific pathogenesis of CRS in the literature, as there are currently several competing theories as to what the mechanism of disease might be. Additionally, all studies have been analyzed with different parameters and with different methods, adding a great deal of discrepancy to the field, and not allowing all work to be directly comparable.

Histopathology reveals inflammation of the mucosal lining, goblet cell hyperplasia, subepithelial edema, and mononuclear cell infiltration as hallmarks of CRS (Bachert et al., 2004). The major leukocyte affiliated with inflammation in CRS is the eosinophil, differing from the invasive forms of sinusitis where neutrophils (PMNs) are predominantly seen (Harlin et al., 1988; Wei et al., 2003). However an increase in IL-8 (a PMN chemokine) has been seen in CRS patients, suggesting neutrophils may aid in the local immunity of the nasal cavity, but are not the primary effector cells in this condition (Suzuki et al., 1996). In addition to IL-8, other proinflammatory mediators such as IL-1β, IL-6, MCP-1, TNF-α, and the eicosanoid PGE2 have all been seen in CRS and appear to play a role in the persistence of inflammation (Kuehnemund et al., 2004). In CRS patients, histopathology reveals inflammation of the mucosal lining, goblet cell hyperplasia, subepithelial edema, and mononuclear cell infiltration (Bachert et al., 2004).

Another direct symptom of CRS is the development of polyposis that is almost always correlated with the disease (Ferguson, 2000a). Polyps form from edematous tissue stemming from the middle meatus and can cause disruption of respiration, or, in severe cases, facial deformity (Moloney, 1977; Drake-Lee, 1997; Settipaine, 1994). The polyps are usually pale in color due to poor blood supply, but in the presence of inflammation can appear more reddish. One theory on the early formation of polyps is the "epithelial rupture theory" put forward by Tos (1997). He posits that formation starts with a rupture along the nasal epithelium caused by pressure from edematous and infiltrated lamina propria. The lamina propria projects beyond the fault and is slowly covered by expanding epithelial cells. As the polyp grows in length, it starts to become vascularized and eventually is completely enveloped by nasal epithelium. Another hypothesis based on work from Bernstein and others, builds upon the ulceration and re-epitheliazation proposed by Tos, and explains polyp formation and persistence begins with the upregulation of GM-CSF and G-CSF by macrophages within the nasosinal cavity (Bernstein, 1997). These cytokines are responsible for the recruitment of eosinophils, mast cells, and PMNs to the site of inflammation, resulting in the release of various inflammatory intermediates such as prostaglandins, leukotrienes, and major basic protein (MBP) (Bernstein, 1997). This eventually leads to a further amplification of the response, altering ion transport (Na^+ and Ca^{2+}), and resulting in water retention within the epithelium and lamina propria. This water retention results in edema and aids in the growth of the polyps themselves.

Though the mechanism of chronicity behind CRS is unknown, recent work by Ponikau et al. (1999) suggests that a hypersensitive reaction to a fungal etiological agent may be responsible. In a sample of 210 CRS patients, they found 96% (202/210) tested positive for the presence of fungi in their nasal samples. The predominant fungi isolated were species of *Aspergillus, Alternaria, Candida*, and *Penicillium* (Table 1.1). Additionally the study also found 100% (14/14) of healthy volunteers tested positive for fungal colonies. This suggests that while the fungi themselves are probably not the sole mediator of CRS, the hypersensitive response demonstrated by CRS patients may be caused by the fungi. This etiology is parallel to the known disease allergic fungal rhinosinusitis (AFRS, discussed later in the chapter), though Ponikau et al. failed to find significant levels of IgE in the study, traditionally a characteristic of AFRS. Thus the authors suggest the term "eosinophilic fungal rhinosinusitis" be used in lieu of AFRS so as to describe the onset of eosinophilia, without the foundation of IgE being a mechanistic process in the disease (Ponikau et al., 1999). This work was supported by Braun and others who used similar techniques and found comparable results (Braun et al., 2003).

Contrasted against this theory is the work done by Ferguson who suggests that CRS be divided into two distinct subcategories; those patients with AFRS and those with a similar, but distinct clinicopathological entity, eosinophilic mucin rhinosinusitis (EMRS) (Ferguson, 2000b). EMRS is described as histopathologically similar to AFRS with the distinct absence of fungi in the samples. In a review of the literature and from patient studies, Ferguson compared 431 patients with AFRS to 69 with EMRS and found that patients with AFRS tended to have a lower incidence of asthma (41% vs. 93%), decreased aspirin sensitivity (13% vs. 54%), and increased total IgE levels. Additionally AFRS patients were more likely to have allergic rhinitis (84% vs. 63%) and were also younger in age (30.7 vs. 48.0). All values were found to have statistical significance. Ferguson concluded these disorders were different enough from one another and that their characteristics should denote these distinctions; AFRS should be characterized by fungal isolation and is mediated by IgE hypersensitivity (Type 1), and EMRS be characterized by the presence of allergic mucus, lack of fungal isolation, and mediated by general immune dysregulation.

While the exact pathogenesis of CRS is unclear, it is understood that the altered nasal environment lends itself to frequent acute bacterial and viral co-infections (Davis and Kita, 2004). In this scenario microbes are able to act as opportunists and take advantage of the host's weakened immune state. The inflammatory response responsible for altering the nasal environment (interruption of mucociliary beat, remodeling of nasal architecture, obstruction of sinonasal ostia, etc.) is believed to be a key factor in contributing to the persistence of CRS.

3.4. Allergic Fungal Rhinosinusitis

Allergic fungal rhinosinusitis (AFRS or AFS in the literature) is a hypersensitivity disease of the paranasal sinuses afflicting patients who are immunocompetent albeit with a history of atopy and allergic rhinitis to fungi. The disease process begins as the fungi become entrapped within the nasal cavity, presumably because of ostium obstruction or mucociliary disorder, and initiate a hypersensitive immune response. Just as with the other forms of fungal sinusitis, *A. fumigatus* is the most common etiological agent associated with AFRS (Table 1.1).

Traditionally it has been believed the mechanistic process underlying this disorder was IgE and IgG (Type I and Type III) mediated (Bent and Kuhn, 1997; Stewart and Hunsaker, 2002). However, as mentioned earlier, recent observations concerning patients who exhibit AFRS without increased IgE levels have questioned this mechanism, and has led to the suggestion of renaming AFRS to "eosinophilic fungal rhinosinusitis" to account for this disparity (Ponikau et al., 1999; Braun et al., 2003; Corradini et al., 2003). It is important to note that AFRS is most likely a multifactoral process, though the decisive factor is almost certainly the patients' hyperimmune response to the fungus (Stewart and Hunsaker, 2002). The production of an allergic mucin develops, which contains high levels of eosinophils, Charcot-Leyden crystals (by-products of eosinophilia) and noninvasive hyphal bodies (Washburn, 1994; Houser and Corey, 2000). The mucin is a thick, greenish-brown, viscous material that traps the fungi, not allowing it to be cleared from the sinuses. This leads to a cyclical immune response as more eosinophilia occurs in response to the fungus, thereby overwhelming the nasal cavity and adding to the chronicity of this disease. Additionally, as AFRS is a form of CRS, nasal polyposis is almost always associated with patients suffering from this disease.

Strong parallels have been made between AFRS and allergic bronchopulmonary aspergillosis (ABPA), a hypersensitivity disorder limited to the lungs and specific to *A. fumigatus*. ABPA is a late-phase allergic inflammatory response occurring in patients diagnosed with asthma or Cystic Fibrosis (Knutsen, 2003). In patients with ABPA, hyphal *Aspergillus* can be found in the airspaces and parenchyma of the lungs. Increased IgE levels, as well as systemic and pulmonary eosinophilia, characterize the disease. The disease can have a number of clinical presentations including hemoptysis (in which patients cough up large amounts of blood) as well as bronchietasis (a condition where large amounts of fibrous tissue are formed within the lungs). In humans the $CD4^+$ T-cell population in ABPA produces increased levels of IL-4, -5, -10, and -13 (Grünig, 1997; Houser and Corey, 2000; Knutsen, 2003). This response increases class switching of B cells to stimulate IgE production as well as maturation and activation of eosinophils, resulting in skewing the immune response towards a Th2 reaction. Additionally there is increased adhesion molecule (VCAM) production, an increase in mast cell degranulation, and eventually anergy to *A. fumigatus* is reached via delayed type hypersensitivity (DTH).

Recent findings by Shah and others examined the incidence of AFRS in ABPA patients. Ninety-five patients with diagnosed ABPA were assessed radiologically for AFRS. Of those 95, 22 patients scored positive for having fungal rhinosinusitis (23%). All patients demonstrated positive skin tests and had increased total and specific IgE levels. In addition, allergic mucin was seen in all patients, with five patients having hyphal development within the paranasal region (Shah et al., 2001).

Therapy for AFRS includes reduction of fungal burden and restoration of normal sinus drainage. To achieve the latter goal, abnormal soft tissue masses are extirpated with endoscopic surgery, however, reports suggest surgery alone results in recurrence of the diseased state (Washburn, 1994; Kupferberg et al., 1997; Marple et al., 2002). In a study put forward by Kupferberg, 19 of 24 patients who had undergone surgery for AFRS suffered a recurrence of symptoms postsurgery (Kupferberg et al., 1997). Similar studies noted patients who were given fungal immunotherapy postoperatively were more likely to experience remittance than those patients who received no immunotherapy (Marple et al., 2002). In addition to surgery and antifungal treatments, long-term topical nasal corticosteroids are also utilized, though steroid therapy is thought to increase the likelihood of a secondary fungal invasion (Washburn, 1994).

4. Summary

Fungal sinusitis is an emerging family of fungal diseases, which has been thus far understudied. Though widely recognized in clinical setting and thoroughly reported in the literature, studies to corroborate these observations are yet to be done. In addition, few or no animal models have been developed to study the pathogenic process of fungal sinusitis. Future studies will need to explore the underlying host defense anomalies that predispose individuals to fungal infection of the sinuses and also examine the microbial factors that facilitate colonization, infection, and invasion.

References

Bachert, C., Vignola, A.M., Gevaert, P., Leynaert, B., Van Cauwenberge, P., and Bousquet, J. (2004). Allergic rhinitis, rhinosinusitis, and asthma: One airway disease. *Immunol. Allergy Clin. North Am.* 24(1): 19–43.

Baraniuk, J. (1994). In H.M. Druce (ed.), *Physiology of Sinusitis. Sinusitis: Pathophysiology and Treatment*, Vol. 1. Marcel Dekker, New York, pp. 19–39.

Benninger, M.S. (1992). Rhintis, sinusitis, and their relationships to allergies. *Am. J. Rhinol.* 6(March–April): 37–43.

Bent, J.P. and Kuhn, F.A. (1997). Allergic fungal sinusitis/polyposis. In G.A. Settipaine (ed.), *Nasal Polyps: Epidemiology, Pathogenesis and Treatment*. OceanSide Publications, Providence, pp. 127–136.

Bernstein, J.M. (1997). The immuno histopathology and pathophysiology of nasal polyps (the differential diagnosis of nasal polyposis). In G.A. Settipaine (ed.), *Nasal Polyps: Epidemiology, Pathogenesis and Treatment*. OceanSide Publications, Providence, pp. 85–95.

Book, D.T., Smith, T.L., McNamar, J.P., Saeian, K., Binion, D.G., and Toohill, R.J. (2003). Chronic sinonasal disease in patients with inflammatory bowel disease. *Am. J. Rhinol.* 17(2): 87–90.

Braun, H., Buzina, W., Freudenschuss, K., Beham, A., and Stammberger, H. (2003).

Eosinophilic fungal rhinosinusitis': A common disorder in Europe? *Laryngoscope* 113(2): 264–269.

CDC (2003). *Fast Stats A–Z—Sinus Conditions*, Centers for Disease Control and Prevention, 2003.

Citardi, M. (2003). *Brief Overview of Sinus and Nasal Anatomy*; American Rhinologic Society, 2003.

Cooper, M. (1994). Anatomy of the nasal cavity and the paranasal sinuses. In H.M. Druce (ed.), *Sinusitis: Pathophysiology and Treatment*, Vol. 1. Marcel Dekker, New York, pp. 5–18.

Corradini, C., Del Ninno, M., Schiavino, D., Patriarca, G., and Paludetti, G. (2003). Allergic fungal sinusitis. A naso-sinusal specific hyperreactivity for an infectious disease? *Acta Otorhinolaryngol. Ital.* 23(3): 168–174.

Davis, L.J. and Kita, H. (2004). Pathogenesis of chronic rhinosinusitis: role of airborne fungi and bacteria. *Immunol. Allergy Clin. North Am.* 24(1): 59–73.

deShazo, R.D. and Swain, R.E. (1995). Diagnostic criteria for allergic fungal sinusitis. *J. Allergy Clin. Immunol.* 96(1): 24–35.

Drake-Lee, A. (1997). The pathogenesis of nasal polyps. In G.A. Settipaine (ed.), *Nasal Polyps: Epidemiology, Pathogenesis and Treatment*. OceanSide Publications, Providence, pp. 57–64.

Dykewicz, M.S. (2003). Rhinitis and sinusitis. *J. Allergy Clin. Immunol.* 111(2 Suppl.): S520–S529.

Ferguson, B.J. (2000a). Definitions of fungal rhinosinusitis. *Otolaryngol. Clin. North. Am.* 33(2): 227–235.

Ferguson, B.J. (2000b). Eosinophilic mucin rhinosinusitis: A distinct clinicopathological entity. *Laryngoscope* 110(5 Pt 1): 799–813.

Ferguson, B.J. (2000c). Fungus balls of the paranasal sinuses. *Otolaryngol. Clin. North Am.* 33(2): 389–398.

Gross, E.A., Swenberg, J.A., Fields, S., and Popp, J.A. (1982). Comparative morphometry of the nasal cavity in rats and mice. *J. Anat.* 135(Pt 1): 83–88.

Grünig, G., Corry, D.B., Leach, M.W., Seymour, B.W.P., Kurup, V.P., and Rennick, D.M. (1997). Interleukin-10 is a natural suppressor of cytokine production and inflammation in a murine model of allergic bronchopulmonary aspergillosis. *J. Exp. Med.* 185(6): 1089–1099.

Harkema, J.R. (1992). Epithelial cells of the nasal passages. In R.A. Parent (ed.), *Comprehensive Treatise on Pulmonary Toxicology*, Vol. 1. CRC Press, Boca Raton, pp. 27–36.

Harlin, S.L., Ansel, D.G., Lane, S.R., Myers, J., Kephart, G.M., and Gleich, G.J. (1988). A clinical and pathologic study of chronic sinusitis: The role of the eosinophil. *J. Allergy Clin. Immunol.* 81(5 Pt 1): 867–875.

Herbert, R.A. and Leininger, J.R. (1999). Nose, larynx and trachea. In R. Maronpot (ed.), *Pathology of the Mouse*. Cache River Press, Vienna, IL, pp. 259–292.

Houser, S.M. and Corey, J.P. (2000). Allergic fungal rhinosinusitis: Pathophysiology, epidemiology, and diagnosis. *Otolaryngol. Clin. North Am.* 33(2): 399–409.

Jahrsdoerfer, R.A., Ejercito, V.S., Johns, M.M., Cantrell, R.W., and Sydnor, J.B. (1979). Aspergillosis of the nose and paranasal sinuses. *Am. J. Otolaryngol.* 1(1): 6–14.

Knutsen, A.P. (2003). Lymphocytes in allergic bronchopulmonary aspergillosis. *Front Biosci.* 8: d589–d602.

Kuehnemund, M., Ismail, C., Brieger, J., Schaefer, D., and Mann, W.J. (2004). Untreated chronic rhinosinusitis: A comparison of symptoms and mediator profiles. *Laryngoscope* 114(3): 561–565.

Kupferberg, S.B., Bent III, J.P., and Kuhn, F.A. (1997). Prognosis for allergic fungal sinusitis. *Otolaryngol. Head Neck Surg.* 117(1): 35–41.

Latgé, J.P. (1999). *Aspergillus fumigatus* and aspergillosis. *Clin Microbiol Rev* 12(2): 310–350.

Lennard, C.M., Mann, E.A., Sun, L.L., Chang, A.S., and Bolger, W.E. (2000). Interleukin-1 beta, interleukin-5, interleukin-6, interleukin-8, and tumor necrosis factor-alpha in chronic sinusitis: response to systemic corticosteroids. *Am. J. Rhinol.* 14(6): 367–373.

Marple, B., Newcomer, M., Schwade, N., and Mabry, R. (2002). Natural history of allergic fungal rhinosinusitis: a 4- to 10-year follow-up. *Otolaryngol. Head Neck Surg.* 127(5): 361–366.

Moloney, J.R. (1977). Nasal polyps, nasal polypectomy, asthma, and aspirin sensitivity. Their association in 445 cases of nasal polyps. *J. Laryngol. Otol.* 91(10): 837–846.

NIAID (2002). Sinusitis, Office of Communications and Public Liaison, 2003.

Pleis, J. and Coles, R. (2003). Summary Health Statistics for U.S. Adults: National Health Interview Survey, 1999; National Center for Health Statistics. Vital Health Stat 10 (212).

Ponikau, J.U., Sherris, D.A., Kern, E.B., Homburger, H.A., Frigas, E., Gaffey, T.A., and Roberts, G.D. (1999). The diagnosis and incidence of allergic fungal sinusitis. *Mayo Clin. Proc.* 74(9): 877–884.

Rudack, C., Stoll, W., and Bachert, C. (1998). Cytokines in nasal polyposis, acute and chronic sinusitis. *Am. J. Rhinol.* 12(6): 383–388.

Schell, W.A. (2000). Unusual fungal pathogens in fungal rhinosinusitis. *Otolaryngol. Clin. North Am.* 33(2): 367–373.

Settipaine, G.A. and Settipane, R.A. (1994). Tetrad of nasal polyps, asprin sensitivity, asthma, and rhinosinusitis. In H.M. Druce (ed.), *Sinusititis: Pathophysiology and Treatment,* Vol. 1. Marcel Dekker, New York, pp. 227–246.

Shah, A., Panchal, N., and Agarwal, A.K. (2001). Concomitant allergic bronchopulmonary aspergillosis and allergic Aspergillus sinusitis: A review of an uncommon association. *Clin. Exp. Allergy* 31(12): 1896–1905.

Stewart, A.E. and Hunsaker, D.H. (2002). Fungus-specific IgG and IgE in allergic fungal rhinosinusitis. *Otolaryngol. Head Neck Surg.* 127(4): 324–332.

Stringer, S.P. and Ryan, M.W. (2000). Chronic invasive fungal rhinosinusitis. *Otolaryngol. Clin. North Am.* 33(2): 375–387.

Suzuki, H., Takahashi, Y., Wataya, H., Ikeda, K., Nakabayashi, S., Shimomura, A., and Takasaka, T. (1996). Mechanism of neutrophil recruitment induced by IL-8 in chronic sinusitis. *J. Allergy Clin. Immunol.* 98(3): 659–670.

Tos, M. (1997). Early stages of polyp formation. In G.A. Settipaine (ed.), *Nasal Polyps: Epidemiology, Pathogenesis and Treatment.* OceanSide Publications, Providence, pp. 65–72.

Van Alyea, O. (1939). Ethmoid labyrinth. *Arch. Otolaryngol.* 29: 881–902.

Washburn, R.G. (1994). Chronic fungal sinusitis in the nonimmunocompromised host. In H.M. Druce (ed.), *Sinusitis: Pathophysiology and Treatment,* Vol. 1. Marcel Dekker, New York, pp. 205–226.

Wei, J.L., Kita, H., Sherris, D.A., Kern, E.B., Weaver, A., and Ponikau, J.U. (2003). The chemotactic behavior of eosinophils in patients with chronic rhinosinusitis. *Laryngoscope* 113(2): 303–306.

2

Innate Defense Mechanisms in Oral Candidiasis

Anna Dongari-Bagtzoglou

Department of Oral Health and Diagnostic Sciences, School of Dental Medicine, University of Connecticut, Farmington, CT 06030-1710.

1. Introduction

Candida species can be isolated from the oral cavity of up to 80% of healthy individuals as a commensal organism (Odds, 1988; Wilkieson et al., 1991). Despite these extremely high reported carriage rates, very few healthy carriers will develop clinical signs of the oral infection. This commensal relationship however can change in response to a change in the local oral microenvironment. Breakdown of mucosal integrity, qualitative or quantitative shifts in oral microbial flora, or an inadequate innate host response can lead to increased fungal burden, which can cause a chronic oral mucosal inflammatory response to the organism, also known as *Candida* stomatitis (reviewed in Scully et al., 1994). Perhaps the most important host defense strategy against *Candida albicans* is the activation of the innate arm of the immune system, principally represented by the polymorphonuclear leukocyte (PMN) or neutrophil. This is evidenced by the fact that neutropenic patients are highly susceptible to the fungus, and that the disappearance of yeast cells from tissues parallels the appearance of neutrophils (reviewed in Ashman and Papadimitriou, 1995). Although PMN are considered important in the resistance to and eradication of fungi, it appears that these functions in vivo require stimulation with an activating agent. $CD4^+$ T cells maintain a central role in the defense against *Candida* since they provide such activating signals to PMN through the release of specific cytokines (Ashman and Papadimitriou, 1995). The importance of the $CD4^+$ T helper cell in the eradication or control of *Candida* growth in vivo is evidenced by the increased incidence of oral mucosal candidiasis in patients affected by HIV disease or immunosuppressive treatment, which primarily targets the $CD4^+$ T cell subset (Coleman et al., 1997; O'Daniels et al., 2000). Thus it appears that oral candidiasis emerges at later stages of HIV infection or during chronic pharmacological immunosuppression, when *Candida*-specific $CD4^+$ T cell clones are materially or functionally depleted, as innate immunoeffectors are faced with a remarkably increased burden of commensal microorganisms, and with essentially minimal activating help from circulating T helper cells. Interestingly, even though PMN activation may be compromised in these individuals, cases of oral invasive candidiasis or disseminating candidiasis through the oral mucosa are rare among these patients and seem to be associated only with additional risk factors such as severe neutropenia or high doses of corticosteroid treatment (Imam et al., 1990). Thus it is possible that either (a) unique innate defense mechanisms operate in the oral mucosa, which control invasive infection and are independent of T cell or neutrophil function; or (b) a certain degree of PMN activation still takes place at the infection site, which may be due to cytokines released from structural oral mucosal cells. This chapter will focus on the innate immune and nonimmune defense mechanisms, which may play a role in limiting oral *Candida* infections. Finally a critical evaluation of the inherent defense mechanisms unique to the oral mucosa that may prevent invasive infection in the immunocompromised host will be presented.

2. Unique Structural and Ecological Features of the Oral Mucosa

2.1. Structure of the Oral Mucosa

The oral mucosa is a highly permeable tissue, with regional variations, as the type and keratinization status of the epithelial cell layer varies in different locations of the oral cavity. The oral cavity is lined by at least four different types of mucosa (Squier and Finkelstein, 2003). While nonkeratinized epithelium lines the majority of the oral cavity, covering the hard palate and gingiva is the masticatory mucosa, which receives the most severe mechanical forces and has stratified keratinized epithelium. The dorsal surface of the tongue is covered by specialized mucosa and is also lined by keratinized epithelium, which specializes in taste and other neurophysiologic functions. Junctional epithelium is a relatively undifferentiated and nonkeratinized epithelium, which forms the junction between the oral mucosa and the teeth. Another unique structural feature of the oral cavity is the localized presence of submucosa containing adipose tissue and minor salivary glands (Squier and Finkelstein, 2003).

The most common form of *Candida* stomatitis affects the palatal and dorsal tongue mucosa (Samaranayake and MacFarlane, 1990), and therefore this infection mostly relates to oral stratified keratinized squamous epithelium. In general, stratified squamous epithelia are thought to protect the underlying tissues by the process of keratinization, which decreases the mucosal permeability, and also by the process of desquamation of keratinized cells, which is thought to play an important role in the clearance of adherent bacteria and fungi (Samaranayake and Samaranayake, 2001).

2.2. Oral Microbial Ecology

The oral mucosa is colonized by over 200 microbial species. Thus, the potential for bacterial and fungal infections is high, with a need for innate defense mechanisms. The oral cavity is comprised of at least four microbial ecological niches with a certain degree of variability in the composition of their indigenous flora: the saliva, the tongue, and the tooth-associated supragingival and subgingival plaques (Slots, 1992). The most predominant indigenous bacterial flora in saliva, tongue and supragingival plaque are members of the *Streptococcus* species. These commensal bacteria may modulate yeast colonization by competing for nutrients and adhesion sites. Evidence for a protective role of the oral bacterial flora against fungal infection is derived from the fact that use of broad-spectrum antibiotics in humans and animals promotes oral *Candida* infection (Samaranayake et al., 1994; Deslauriers et al., 1995). In fact, many animal and in vitro studies have shown that oral *Candida* colonization can be inhibited by oral *Streptococci* (Liljemark and Gibbons, 1973; Samaranayake et al., 1994). Coaggregation of *C. albicans* or *C. dubliniensis* with the oral bacterium *Fusobacterium nucleatum* has been described in subgingival plaque, and may play a role in the pathogenesis of periodontal infections. The extent of coaggregation varied between the two *Candida* species, was inhibitable by mannose or α-methyl mannoside in both cases, and appeared to be due to the presence of a heat-stable *Candida* receptor (Jabra-Rizk et al., 1999).

Candida species are also part of the commensal flora in the oral cavity, with oral asymptomatic *Candida* carriage rates varying among different age groups. The highest asymptomatic *Candida* carriage rates (65–80%) were reported for healthy children

(Odds, 1988), the elderly (Wilkieson et al., 1991), and HIV+ patients (Campisi et al., 2002; Myers et al., 2003). *C. albicans* colonizes the oral mucosa at higher rates than many other mucosal sites in humans, but very few healthy carriers develop clinical signs of the oral infection (Odds, 1988). This is in contrast to other mucosal sites such as the vagina, where the carriage rate by healthy individuals is approximately 25% and clinical infection can be observed in otherwise healthy women (Sobel, 1988). *C. albicans* is frequently isolated from the saliva, tongue, and subgingival plaque (Redding et al., 1988, 2002; Phelan et al., 1997), and it is a change in the oral host environment that determines whether colonization will progress to infection.

3. Epidemiology, Clinical, and Histopathologic Characteristics of Oral Candidiasis

3.1. Epidemiology

General risk factors for oropharyngeal candidiasis (OPC) are the two extremes of age (Odds, 1988), trauma (O'Grady and Reade, 1993), salivary gland hypofunction (Scully et al., 1994), dental prostheses (Odds, 1988), broad-spectrum antibiotic therapy, and topical use of corticosteroids (Deslauriers et al., 1995), as well as nutritional factors (Rennie et al., 1983; Samaranayake, 1986). Among the systemic conditions that predispose patients to OPC are diabetes mellitus, HIV infection, immunosuppressive therapy, Sjogren's syndrome, and radiation therapy for head and neck cancer (reviewed in Scully et al., 1994). In most types of high-risk patients, *C. albicans* is still the main etiologic agent of oral candidiasis (Scully et al., 1994). However, over the last 15 years new *Candida* species have emerged as the infectious agent responsible for some of these infections in special patient categories, such as HIV+ patients and patients receiving radiation treatment of head and neck tumors (Redding et al., 1999; O'Daniels et al., 2000). The most commonly reported non-*albicans Candida* species involved are *C. dubliniensis*, *C. glabrata*, *C. krusei*, and *C. tropicalis* (O'Daniels et al., 2000; Redding, 2001).

Interestingly, up to 90% of HIV+ patients have had at least one episode of OPC, and their susceptibility to oral candidiasis is not paralleled by susceptibility to vaginal or disseminated infection (Scully et al., 1994). Although HIV-associated OPC is predominantly caused by *C. albicans* (Vargas and Joly, 2002; Myers et al., 2003), non-*albicans Candida* species have emerged as etiologic agents of oral candidiasis in certain HIV+ patients (O'Daniels et al., 2000; Redding, 2001). *C. dubliniensis* was isolated from as many as 32% of HIV+ patients with clinical signs of this infection (Coleman et al., 1997) and it can apparently be the sole causative agent detectable in some of these patients (O'Daniels et al., 2000; Vargas and Joly, 2002). More recent epidemiologic evidence suggests that the prevalence of *C. dubliniensis* infection in this patient population is much lower than originally proposed and ranges between 5% and 10% (Giammanco et al., 2002; Vargas and Joly, 2002). Because typically *C. dubliniensis* shows the same pattern of antifungal susceptibility as *C. albicans*, in the vast majority of cases distinction between the two species is not required for successful treatment (Redding, 2001).

OPC is also a common infection in patients receiving radiation treatment of head and neck tumors (Redding et al., 1999). This infection is thought to be due to destruction of salivary gland tissue and hyposalivation (Fotos and Hellstein, 1992). Recently, an increase in oral candidiasis has been reported in head and neck cancer patients receiving radiation therapy, which is due to infection with one or more non-*albicans Candida* species (Redding, 2001).

In fact, fungi other than *C. albicans* were detected in 59% of the head and neck cancer patients with positive cultures, whereas 27% of the culture-positive patients harbored *C. albicans* in combination with other species (Redding et al., 1999, 2001). One of the most frequently isolated *Candida* species from these patients is *C. glabrata* (Redding et al., 1999). In recent years *C. glabrata* has emerged as an important pathogen in humans, being the second or third leading agent of candidiasis at all sites (reviewed in Fidel et al., 1999). Because *C. glabrata* is most often co-isolated with *C. albicans*, its role as a causative agent in OPC has been controversial. Also, its pathogenicity has been difficult to demonstrate experimentally due to its much lower virulence in animal models of infection (reviewed in Fidel et al., 1999). However, oral infection with mixed *C. albicans* and *C. glabrata* may be clinically more severe (Redding et al., 2002) and reports of *C. glabrata* as the only detectable species from oral lesions have been rising steadily (Redding et al., 1999, 2001, 2002). This is particularly important since unlike *C. dubliniensis*, *C. glabrata* isolated from oral lesions is much more resistant to standard antifungal treatment than *C. albicans* (Redding et al., 1999, 2001). As a result, *C. glabrata* oral infection is suspected in most cases when the patient does not respond to routine doses of fluconazole (Redding et al., 2002). Interestingly, *C. glabrata* is also associated with increased oral carriage rates among the elderly, especially the ones wearing oral prostheses (Lockhart et al., 1999). In the elderly, denture stomatitis and angular cheilitis are the most common denture-related infections (Espinoza et al., 2003), and the most frequently isolated species from these lesions is *C. albicans* (Leigh et al., 2002; Dar-Odeh and Shehabi, 2003).

3.2. Clinical Features of Oral Candidiasis

All *Candida* species form the same type of oral lesions clinically (Redding, 2001). However, recent evidence suggests that mixed infections with more than one species may be associated with more severe symptoms and are more difficult to treat (Redding et al., 2002). There are three main clinical variants of oral candidiasis: the pseudomembranous (also known as thrush), the hyperplastic, and the erythematous (Axell et al., 1997). The hyperplastic form is accompanied by extensive epithelial hyperplasia and hyperkeratosis, also termed candidal leukoplakia. The erythematous form has been the predominant clinical form in HIV^+ patients with $CD4^+$ lymphocytes >400, whereas as the lymphocyte counts drop, the lesions appear to become more of the pseudomembranous type (Weinert et al., 1996). Frequently all three forms coexist and the term "multifocal candidiasis" is used to describe the lesions. *Candida* is also frequently responsible for inflammatory lesions found between the lips (angular cheilitis), under dentures (denture stomatitis), and on the dorsal surface of the tongue (median rhomboid glossitis). Symptoms associated with this infection are pain, burning mouth, and dysphagia, which can lead to poor nutrition and significant patient morbidity (Fotos and Hellstein, 1992).

3.3. Histopathologic Characteristics

Chronic hyperplastic or pseudomembranous candidiasis is a form of infection with distinct clinical and histopathological characteristics. The histologic features of this infection include a hyperplastic and parakeratotic response of the surface epithelium, which is invaded by hyphal organisms. The inflammatory infiltrate consists primarily of PMN, which form microabscesses within the epithelium, whereas very few PMN are found within the lamina propria in association with blood vessels (Eversole et al., 1997). A chronic inflammatory infiltrate is also present in the superficial lamina propria close to the epithelial border, with a characteristic high presence of IgA-expressing lymphocytes (Williams et al., 1997).

In HIV^+ patients, neutrophils appear to be a rare finding in oral candidiasis lesions and are only encountered in a limited number of erythematous forms. The inflammatory cell infiltrate is primarily mononuclear in both pseudomembranous and erythematous cases of HIV-associated infection (Romagnoli et al., 1997). Few *Candida* hyphae are associated with the atrophic epithelium in erythematous candidiasis, whereas numerous organisms are found invading into the prickle cell layer of oral epithelium in pseudomembranous candidiasis. In HIV^+ patients the inflammatory infiltrate is heavier in erythematous candidiasis and consists of $CD8^+$ lymphocytes and $CD1a^+$ Langerhans cells (Romagnoli et al., 1997). In fact, in this study $CD1a^+$ dendritic cells were the only cell type to be significantly increased in HIV^+ oral candidiasis as compared to HIV^+ or HIV^- controls. These cells were almost exclusively restricted to the basal layer of the oral epithelium. Overall a change in localization of inflammatory cells such as macrophages and dendritic cells from the lamina propria into the basal epithelial cell layer was observed, as opposed to an increase in cell number (Romagnoli et al., 1997). A more recent immunohistochemical analysis of the T cell populations in HIV-associated oral candidiasis showed an intriguing accumulation of high numbers of $CD8^+$ T cells at the lamina propria–epithelium interface of the infected sites as compared to uninfected controls, and a positive correlation between the numbers of $CD8^+$ T cells and oral fungal burden in HIV^+OPC^- individuals (Myers et al., 2003). Interestingly, $CD4^+$ cells were also found in these lesions. These cells did not colocalize with $CD3^+$ cells and were highly irregular in shape, suggesting that the majority were not T cells but macrophages or dendritic cells (Myers et al., 2003).

4. Role of Oral Fluids in the Control of *Candida* Infection

4.1. Saliva

Whole saliva is comprised of a mixture of molecules and cells derived from the major and minor salivary glands, with mucosal epithelium and the serus exudate originating in the gingival crevices (gingival crevicular fluid (GCF)). Collectively, these components form a strong innate defense barrier to infection. Abnormal salivary function, caused by reduced salivary flow or altered composition, leads to increased levels of *C. albicans* in the oral cavity, often culminating in overt OPC (Fotos and Hellstein, 1992). This is largely due to the fact that *C. albicans* species colonizing the oral cavity are constantly bathed in saliva and interact with salivary constituents, which can significantly modulate their growth, metabolic activity, and adhesion to oral mucosa.

In general, both unstimulated and stimulated salivary flow rates are decreased in patients with oral candidiasis (Ueta et al., 2000) and reduced salivary flow rates, associated with senescence, have been reported to be a risk factor for oral candidiasis (Tanida et al., 2001), believed mainly to be due to compromised mechanical clearance. Xerostomia due to pathologic changes in salivary glands from disease (e.g. Sjogren's syndrome) or treatment (e.g., head and neck radiation therapy) promotes chronic *Candida* colonization and predisposes patients to oral infection (MacFarlane, 1975), an effect that has been confirmed in sialoadenectomized animals (Jorge et al., 1993). However, history of recurrent oral candidiasis was not found to be associated with reduced salivary flow rates, but rather with a significantly more acidic saliva in a small group of patients as compared to healthy controls (Bercier et al., 1999). In general, saliva inhibits adhesion of *C. albicans* to oral epithelial cells (Ueta et al., 2000), at least partly due to the inhibitory activity of salivary mucins (de Repentigny et al., 2000) and in oral candidiasis patients this inhibitory activity appears to be somewhat suppressed (Ueta et al., 2000). Several other innate effector molecules with direct antifungal activity are contained in human saliva such as histatins, calprotectin, defensins, secretory leukocyte protease inhibitor (SLPI) and others, which are listed in Table 2.1, and will be discussed in more detail later in this chapter.

4.2. Gingival Crevicular Fluid

GCF is an inflammatory exudate originating from the leaky venules next to the oral sulcular and junctional epithelia. An increase in the flow rate of GCF has been associated with inflammatory changes in the gingival tissues, secondary to bacterial infection (reviewed in Tonetti et al., 1998). In addition to salivary PMN and macrophages that exude through the oral junctional and sulcular epithelia into the GCF, the GCF also contains relatively high levels of

Table 2.1. Oral Innate Effector Molecules with Anti-*Candida* Function

Effector	Source	Mechanism of action	Reference
Salivary mucins and proteolytic derivatives	Mucous salivary gland cells	Modulate adhesion, candidacidal activity via electrostatic interactions with yeast membrane	de Repentigny et al. (2000), Gururaja et al. (1999)
Histatins	Salivary gland epithelium	Efflux of *Candida* ATP, deprivation of energy stores	Koshlukova et al. (1999)
β-Defensins	Oral mucosal and salivary gland epithelia	Pore-forming cationic peptides	Lehrer and Ganz (1996)
Calprotectin	Neutrophils, monocytes, and oral mucosal epithelium	Zinc deprivation	Sohnle et al. (2000)
Peroxidase/MPO	Salivary gland acinar cells, neutrophils, and monocytes	Oxidative damage	Lehrer and Cline (1969)
Lysozyme	Salivary gland epithelium, neutrophils, and monocytes	Insertion of cationic regions into yeast membrane	During et al. (1999)
Lactoferrin	Acinar cells in major salivary glands, neutrophils, and monocytes	Possibly by iron deprivation	Wakabayashi et al. (1996)
Secretory leukoprotease inhibitor	Oral mucosal epithelium	Candidacidal mechanism unknown	Tomee et al. (1997)

serum-derived complement components and the antimicrobial enzymes lactoferrin and peroxidase, presumably derived from these leukocytes (Miyauchi et al., 1998; Tonetti et al., 1998).

In conjunction with PMN, the complement system may play an important role in the innate immune protection of the oral mucosa. Complement activation takes place in the gingival crevice via the classical and alternative pathways (Cutler et al., 1991). Although formation of membrane attack complex (MAC) on the surface of *C. albicans* has been demonstrated (Lukasser-Vogl et al., 2000), direct killing of pathogenic fungi through this mechanism has not been conclusively proven (Kozel, 1996). In addition, although C5-deficient mice were extremely susceptible to systemic challenge with *C. albicans*, they cleared the oral infection at the same rate as controls (Ashman et al., 2003). Therefore it appears that complement is less crucial in the clearance of oral infection than it is for disseminated disease, thus affirming the localized nature of protective host responses in *Candida* infections.

5. Cellular Components of Innate Defense Mechanisms against Oral Candidiasis

5.1. Oral Epithelial Cells

5.1.1. Immune Regulatory Function

In oral mucosal infections, *C. albicans* organisms colonize the uppermost layers of epithelium, rarely invading past the spinous cell layer (Reichart et al., 1995; Eversole et al., 1997). As a result, the oral mucosa is chronically inflamed with intense intraepithelial and subepithelial infiltration by leukocytes (Reichart et al., 1995; Eversole et al., 1997; Myers et al., 2003). Although the role of epithelial cells as an infection barrier against *Candida* is well recognized (Hahn and Sohnle, 1988), new information is emerging about the role of these cells in orchestrating the oral mucosal inflammatory response to this pathogen by synthesizing immunoregulatory cytokines.

Oral epithelial cells respond to infection with the release of a number of proinflammatory cytokines (Bickel et al., 1996), which can initiate and perpetuate mucosal inflammation. The response of oral epithelial cells to *C. albicans* infection in vitro includes an array of proinflammatory cytokines, namely interleukin (IL)-1α, IL-1β, IL-8, IL-18, tumor necrosis factor alpha (TNF-α), and granulocyte-macrophage colony-stimulating factor (GM-CSF), which have been detected at the protein and/or mRNA level (Rouabhia et al., 2002; Schaller et al., 2002; Steele and Fidel, 2002; Dongari-Bagtzoglou and Kashleva 2003a,b; Dongari-Bagtzoglou et al., 2004). These cytokine responses of oral epithelial cells to *C. albicans* infection are strain-specific, require direct epithelial cell–fungal cell contact, and are optimal when viable yeast, germinating into hyphae, are used in cell interactions (Schaller et al., 2002; Dongari-Bagtzoglou and Kashleva, 2003a,b). Strong evidence also supports the fact that IL-1α, resulting from the interactions of oral epithelial cells with *C. albicans*, autoregulates other cytokines secreted in response to this pathogen (Dongari-Bagtzoglou and Kashleva, 2003a).

IL-1α is a major constitutive and inducible proinflammatory product of epithelial cells, which can act as a key cytokine to amplify the inflammatory response by neighboring mucosal cells, or activate local leukocyte antifungal activities (reviewed in Dinarello, 1997). Studies screening cell supernatants or lysates of *C. albicans*-infected epithelia for various proinflammatory cytokines have identified IL-1α as one of the major cytokines upregulated at both the mRNA and protein levels (Schaller et al., 2002; Dongari-Bagtzoglou et al., 2004). Epithelial cell IL-1α has also been found to be present in human oral mucosal candidiasis lesions (Eversole et al., 1997). As our laboratory has shown, *Candida*-infected oral epithelial cells release this proinflammatory cytokine in its mature protein form in their microenvironment upon cell lysis. We have hypothesized that most of the IL-1α processing in the epithelial cell–*C. albicans* coculture system takes place at the plasma membrane where the cytolytic actions of *C. albicans* phospholipases and proteases trigger a release of membrane phospholipids. Membrane phospholipids may in turn activate the IL-1 convertase, which cleaves membrane-associated pro-IL-1α and triggers the release of the mature protein in culture supernatants (Kobayashi et al., 1990). Similarly, the ability of *C. albicans* to induce cleavage of the inactive IL-18 pro-peptide and trigger release of the active mature IL-18 protein has been demonstrated, an event temporally associated with the presence of the active form of the IL-1 convertase in these cells (Rouabhia et al., 2002).

IL-1α released by injured epithelial cells increases the proinflammatory cytokine production (IL-8, GM-CSF) by neighboring uninfected mucosal and stromal cells (Dongari-Bagtzoglou et al., 2004). Such a mechanism could serve to amplify and extend the local inflammatory response, even in the absence of direct fungal invasion of the deeper mucosal and submucosal tissues. The local release of cytokines such as IL-1α, IL-8, and GM-CSF by oral epithelial cells and fibroblasts could explain the histopathologic finding of neutrophilic microabscesses in these lesions (Eversole et al., 1997), since these cytokines are potent chemoattractants and/or activators of PMNs (Baggiolini et al., 1989; Blanchard et al., 1991). Recently, we established that the activation of PMN antifungal activity can take place in response to cytokines from *C. albicans*-infected oral epithelial cells in vitro. Hyphal growth inhibition experiments with human PMN from multiple donors revealed that the antifungal activity of PMN can be enhanced by two- to threefold over basal levels by *C. albicans*-infected oral epithelial cell supernatants, an effect largely dependent on the presence of bioactive IL-1α in these supernatants (Dongari-Bagtzoglou and Kashleva, in press).

We and other researchers have shown that only live, germinating organisms are capable of stimulating proinflammatory cytokine responses by oral epithelial cells, consistent with reports in endothelial cells (Orozco et al., 2000; Schaller et al., 2002; Dongari-Bagtzoglou and Kashleva, 2003a,b). *C. albicans* is a polymorphic organism which undergoes morphological transition between yeast, pseudohyphal, and hyphal forms. All three morphogenetic forms of *C. albicans* are frequently encountered in the oral mucosa (Cox et al., 1996) and in most oral infections both yeast and filamentous organisms can be found in the infected tissues (Olsen and Birkeland, 1977). Although in animal models of disseminated infection it has been established that the ability to change from yeast form to hyphae is crucial for virulence (Saville et al., 2003), the exact role of hyphal transition during the development of oral candidiasis is still unclear. However, clinicopathologic findings have correlated the presence of filamentous forms with localized tissue invasion in oral candidiasis (Reinhart et al., 1995; Cox et al., 1996). Recently we studied the interactions of oral epithelial cells with the three different morphotypes of this pathogenic organism. More specifically, we compared the ability of yeast, pseudohyphal, and hyphal organisms to adhere to and lyse oral epithelial cells, as well as their ability to trigger a proinflammatory cytokine (IL-8, IL-1α) response. By using mutant strains with defects in hyphal transformation or by applying environmental pressure, which affected filamentation in wild-type organisms, we found that morphogenesis is an important determinant of the outcome from the interactions between oral epithelial cells and *C. albicans*. When germination-deficient *C. albicans* mutants that form exclusively yeast (*efg1/efg1 cph1/cph1* mutant, Lo et al., 1997) or pseudohyphae (*tup1/tup1* mutant, Braun and Johnson, 1997) were cocultured with oral epithelial cells, they exhibited a significantly reduced capacity to adhere to oral epithelial cells and disrupt their cell membrane (Fig. 2.1). Also, in sharp contrast to strains, which formed true hyphae under these coculture conditions, germination mutants and oral strains naturally deficient in germination, triggered essentially no proinflammatory cytokine responses by these cells (Villar et al., 2004). In addition to morphogenesis, invasion of oral epithelial cells and tissues is a critical determinant of the oral mucosal inflammatory response to infection. Highly invasive *C. albicans* strains trigger a wider array and overall greater levels of proinflammatory cytokines in oral epithelial cells compared to invasion-deficient organisms (Villar et al., in press).

5.1.2. Innate Immune Effector Function

Oral epithelial cells are constantly exposed to microbial challenge and therefore play an important role as the first line of defense against infection. In addition to secretion of natural antibiotic peptides (i.e., calprotectin and defensins) with antifungal

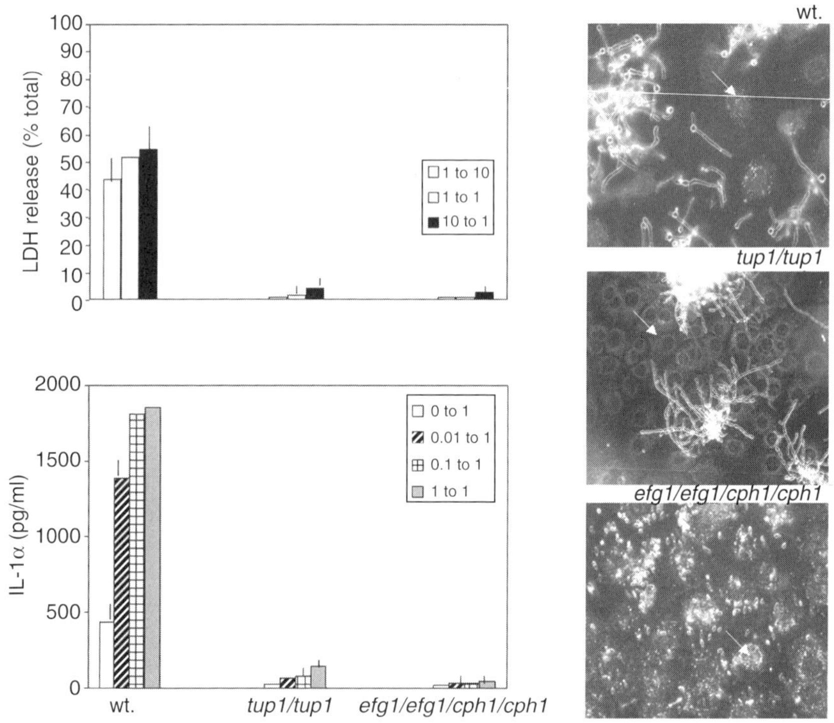

Figure 2.1. Yeast and pseudohyphal forms of *C. albicans* do not injure oral epithelial cells or trigger a proinflammatory cytokine response. SCC15 oral epithelial cells were cocultured with *C. albicans* SC5314 (wt.), or its congenic yeast (*efg1/efg1/cph1/cph*) and pseudohyphal mutants (*tup1/tup1*), at increasing fungal cell to epithelial cell ratios, for up to 20 h. IL-1α and lactate dehydrogenase (LDH) release were quantified in culture supernatants using colorimetric assays (left panel). The cellular morphology of these strains, cocultured with oral epithelial cells for 5 h, is shown on the right panel. Cultures were stained with Calcofluor White and epithelial cells are indicated by the white arrows.

activity, recently, a contact-dependent oral epithelial cell anti-*Candida* activity was described, which was significantly greater than that of vaginal epithelial cells (Steele et al., 2000). More specifically, primary human oral epithelial cells inhibited the growth of 40–85% of *C. albicans* at ratios ranging between 0.6 and 1, and 5:1 effector to target. This antimicrobial activity extended to other *Candida* species, including *C. glabrata*, *C. dubliniensis*, and *C. krusei*. Saliva appeared to have no effect on growth inhibition and cells isolated from HIV^+ patients with OPC had reduced antifungal activity as compared to HIV^+OPC^- controls (Steele et al., 2000). Mechanistic studies also confirmed a growth inhibitory rather than a fungicidal effect (Nomanbhoy et al., 2002), and further demonstrated that an acid labile molecule was involved in the growth-inhibiting interactions (Steele et al., 2001; Yano et al., in press), although the specific molecule was not identified.

5.2. Neutrophils

Neutropenia has long been recognized as the primary risk factor for invasive candidiasis, the mortality rate of which rises up to 90%, even with maximal antifungal treatment (Rodriguez-Adrian et al., 1998). Recently it has become evident that apart from neutropenia, a decrease in function of circulating neutrophils may also be responsible for reduced resistance to infection, thus cytokine treatment combined with white blood cell transfusions have been successfully tested in neutropenic patients with refractory-invasive fungal infections (Rodriguez-Adrian et al., 1998). Like G-CSF, GM-CSF is a cytokine, which also augments neutrophil antifungal activities in vitro and may have a protective function in oral candidiasis in vivo. It has been reported that administration of rhGM-CSF, as adjunctive treatment of fluconazole-refractory OPC in AIDS patients, exerts a significant beneficial effect on the oral mycoflora and may help to clear the infection in these patients (Vazquez et al., 2000).

PMN and macrophages are constantly entering the oral cavity by transepithelial migration through the oral mucosal epithelium, as well as through the oral sulcular and junctional epithelia in the gingival crevice (Tonetti et al., 1998). Salivary PMN (sPMN) is the most abundant salivary immune cell type and can be easily isolated from human saliva (Ueta et al., 1993). Although there is no information on the functional status of the macrophages in saliva, a number of investigations have examined the functional role of sPMN. It has been shown that the activation potential of sPMN is inferior to that of peripheral blood PMN, and more specifically sPMN produce reactive oxygen metabolites and possess candidacidal activity equivalent to 65% of the peripheral blood PMN (Ueta et al., 1993). Even greater sPMN hypofunction (reduced superoxide generation and candidacidal activity) has been described in patients with oral candidiasis (Ueta et al., 2000) and in high-risk individuals such as cancer patients receiving chemoradiotherapy (Ueta et al., 1993), or the elderly (Tanida et al., 2001), and thus sPMN hypofunction can be considered a possible risk factor for oral candidiasis.

5.3. Other Cell Types

Quantification of immunolabeled cells in lesions from HIV^+ persons with OPC showed that the inflammatory infiltrate consisted mainly of $CD1a^+$ Langerhans cells and macrophages, both of which moved from the lamina propria into the basal epithelial cell layer (Romagnoli et al., 1997). In this study, $CD1a^+$ cells were the only cell type, which increased considerably in numbers, as compared to healthy controls (Romagnoli et al., 1997). A significant increase in the number of $CD8^+$ cells was observed at the lamina propria–epithelial cell interface in *C. albicans*-infected oral tissues of HIV^+ individuals in a more recent study (Myers et al., 2003). The functional role of these cells in oral candidiasis is currently unknown, however, it is tempting to speculate that they may be directly involved in the clearance of the microorganism acting as innate effectors in an major histocompatibility complex (MHC)-unrestricted manner, similar to the IL-2-activated $CD8^+$ cells in mice (Beno et al., 1995).

$CD4^+$ T cells and NK cells maintain a central role in the defense against *Candida* in vivo since they provide activating signals to PMN through the release of specific cytokines (Ashman and Papadimitriou, 1995). Although NK cells are unable to kill *C. albicans* directly (Djeu and Blanchard, 1987; Zunino and Hudig, 1988; Arancia et al., 1995), in a mouse model of OPC, these cells could substitute for T cells in phagocytic cell activation and protect the animals from lethal oral infection (Balish et al., 2001). Invasive oral infection in otherwise immunocompetent mice was demonstrated using a combined neutrophil and macrophage depletion approach, implying a synergistic role of these phagocytic cell types in clearing the oral infection (Farah et al., 2001).

6. Effector Molecules with Anti-*Candida* Function in the Oral Mucosa

6.1. Salivary Mucins

These are high molecular weight glycoproteins, synthesized by mucous cells in submandibular, sublingual, and minor salivary glands. Mucins are natural lubricants of the oral mucosa, which form a protective barrier and may act as potent agglutinators of potentially pathogenic microbes. Among the salivary constituents that have been shown to serve as binding ligands for *C. albicans* in vitro, salivary mucins appear to have a particularly high binding affinity to *C. albicans* (Hoffman and Haidaris, 1993). After binding, *C. albicans* enzymatically digests mucins by the action of secreted aspartyl proteinases (de Repentigny et al., 2000). Enzymatic degradation of mucins may facilitate adhesion to buccal epithelium since intact mucins normally block the adherence of the microorganism to these cells (de Repentigny et al., 2000). Microbial proteolysis of the low molecular weight salivary mucin MUC7 in the oral cavity may also result in the release of smaller, bioactive candidacidal peptides, which share sequence and functional similarities with histatins (Gururaja et al., 1999). Based on extensive biochemical analyses of these molecules, it has been hypothesized that the candidacidal activity of cationic MUC7 histatin-like peptides probably involves electrostatic adsorption to the negatively charged phospholipid polar groups in the yeast cell membrane, followed by membrane instability, and abnormal distribution of the cytoplasm (Gururaja et al., 1999).

6.2. Histatins

These are histidine-rich proteins, which originate in the salivary glands of humans and higher primates (Oppenheim et al., 1988). Histatins 1 and 3 are synthesized in the parotid and submandibular glands, and together with histatin 5, which is a proteolytic product of histatin 3, represent about 80% of the total histatin content in human saliva (Edgerton and Koshlukova, 2000). Histatin 5 is the most effective candidacidal peptide within the histatin family, killing both yeast and hyphal organisms in vitro when used within a physiologic range of concentrations (Raj et al., 1990; Xu et al., 1991). Unlike other cationic antimicrobial peptides, histatin 5 does not kill target cells by insertion into fungal cell membranes and pore formation (Raj et al., 1998). Edgerton and coworkers (2000) have demonstrated that *C. albicans* expresses a 67-kDa histatin-binding protein receptor, detectable in the cytoplasm and cell membrane, but not the cell wall (Edgerton et al., 2000), which may provide the basis of selectivity in the killing of fungal but not mammalian cells. Biochemical and pharmacological studies of this group further demonstrated that binding of histatin 5 to its receptor triggers massive efflux of intracellular ATP without loss of membrane integrity (Koshlukova et al., 1999). Based on these findings it was further hypothesized that binding of the newly released ATP to yeast membrane ATP receptors would initiate a cascade of cytotoxic events, analogous to ATP-triggered apoptosis in mammalian cells.

The relationship between salivary levels of histatins and protection from oral *Candida* infection in vivo is unclear. Quite unexpectedly, the concentration of total histatins was elevated in a small group of clinically healthy patients with recurrent oral candidiasis as compared to controls with no history of infection (Bercier et al., 1999), a finding which suggests that repeated infection may trigger a rise in histatin synthesis by salivary gland cells. Investigators in this study explained the absence of protection despite high salivary histatin concentrations to a significantly more acidic pH of the saliva of these patients, as histatin antifungal activities are pH-dependent (Santarpia et al., 1990).

6.3. Defensins

Defensins are pore-forming cationic peptides with broad antimicrobial activity against bacteria and fungi (reviewed in Lehrer and Ganz, 1996; Diamond and Bevins, 1998). There are 28 types of human beta defensins, but only four have so far been fully characterized. Defensins are divided into α and β classes. The α defensins are expressed in neutrophils and intestinal Paneth cells, whereas the β defensins are expressed by epithelial cells of multiple organs, including but not limited to the lung, pancreas, kidney, salivary glands, skin, and oral mucosa (Diamond and Bevins, 1998).

Oral mucosal and salivary gland epithelia synthesize beta defensin 1 (hBD-1), which is constitutively expressed and is effective in killing Gram($^+$) and Gram($^-$) bacteria (Bals et al., 1998; Krisanaprakornkit et al., 1998). This defensin is believed to be involved in homeostatic interactions between the oral mucosa and the commensal flora. Another type of hBD, hBD-2, which is transcriptionally upregulated in oral epithelia in response to infectious and inflammatory stimuli (Krisanaprakornkit et al., 2003), is very effective against Gram($^-$) bacteria and fungi. hBD-2 Protein expression is absent in poorly differentiated oral epithelia, such as the junctional epithelium, or nonkeratinized oral epithelia, such as the buccal epithelium and the epithelium lining the floor of the mouth (Abiko et al., 2001, 2002; Dale et al., 2001). Human alpha defensins colocalized with elastase in the oral mucosa, indicating that they are expressed by neutrophils (Dale et al., 2001).

An immunohistochemical study of human oral candidiasis biopsies showed that hBD-2 is expressed in infected as well as adjacent uninfected epithelium, although the staining intensity was much more pronounced in the presence of *Candida* (Sawaki et al., 2002). Neutrophils and oral epithelial cells present in infected tissues only expressed alpha defensins (human neutrophil peptide (HNP)-1, HNP-2, and HNP-3). However, interpretation of the findings of this study are limited by the fact that it did not include control biopsies from healthy subjects (Sawaki et al., 2002).

Expression levels of hBD-1 vary from person to person. A single-nucleotide polymorphism (SNP) at site 668 of the hBD-1 gene exhibited a significant association with oral *Candida* carriage levels. Individuals carrying one or two copies of this SNP are predisposed to a lower *Candida* carriage in the oral mucosa (Jurevic et al., 2003). However, the biological relevance of this finding is uncertain since this

SNP does not confer a change in the amino acid composition of the peptide as it lies within the 5′ untranslated region of the gene and not within the coding region.

6.4. Calprotectin

Calprotectin is a protein complex consisting of two noncovalently linked peptide chains that are abundantly synthesized by neutrophils, monocytes, certain subpopulations of macrophages, and squamous epithelia, such as oral epithelium and activated epidermal keratinocytes (reviewed in Brandtzaeg et al., 1995). In situ hybridization studies revealed that calprotectin is synthesized in the upper and middle spinous cell layers in the oral mucosa in oral candidiasis as well as normal tissues, with no clear quantitative differences between infected and uninfected tissues (Eversole et al., 1997). This protein complex is also found in many human body fluids, including saliva (Kleinegger et al., 2001).

Calprotectin has candidastatic activity and inhibits yeast to hyphal transformation (Murthy et al., 1993). The mechanism of the antifungal function of calprotectin is unknown, however it has been suggested that it is based on zinc binding via histidine-containing sequences, which deprives the organism from this essential metal (Sohnle et al., 1991, 2000). In fact, zinc deficiency has a negative effect on *C. albicans* growth and germination in vitro (Yamaguchi, 1975). The individual peptide calprotectin chains do not exhibit antifungal activity even though they both have zinc-binding capabilities (Sohnle et al., 2000). To explain this finding it was suggested that formation of a stable heterodimer is necessary for maximum zinc affinity (Sohnle et al., 2000). Absence of a requirement for direct contact between calprotectin and the microorganism and reversibility of the antimicrobial activity in the presence of zinc also support zinc scavenging from a distance as a likely mechanism of action (Sohnle et al., 1991).

Although variability in study design and methods make it difficult to compare clinical studies, results comparing salivary calprotectin levels in health and oral candidiasis appear to be in conflict with one another. It has been reported that patients with HIV who develop oral candidiasis have significantly lower levels of calprotectin in saliva than those who do not (Muller et al., 1993). On the contrary, two other studies reported higher salivary calprotectin levels associated with higher *Candida* counts, or presence of oral infection (Kleinegger et al., 2001; Sweet et al., 2001). Inadequate control for confounding factors such as concurrent presence of active periodontal infection, and oral hygiene practices, as well as limited number of subjects examined, may have been the source of these discrepant results. Recently clinical evidence has emerged supporting the notion that salivary calprotectin levels are nonspecifically increased secondary to mucosal inflammation and that HIV infection may negatively affect calprotectin synthesis (Sweet et al., 2001).

6.5. Peroxidase and Myeloperoxidase

Peroxidase originates from two main sources in the oral cavity. Salivary peroxidase is synthesized by acinar cells in major salivary glands and myeloperoxidase (MPO) is derived from the neutrophil primary granules. Monocytes also contain MPO in their primary granules, whereas macrophages are known to lack this enzyme (Marodi et al., 1991). These enzymes combine with H_2O_2 and thiocyanate or iodide ions to produce hypothiocyanate, or hypoiodite, which are powerful oxidizing agents. In the presence of chloride ion, MPO also converts H_2O_2 into hypochlorous acid and monochloramine, the two potent microbiocidal agents. MPO plays a critical role in the fungicidal activity of PMN in vitro, and phagocytes genetically deficient in MPO fail to kill *C. albicans* (Lehrer and Cline, 1969). Exogenously supplied MPO also elevates the ability of human macrophages to kill *C. albicans* (Weber et al., 1987) and activates cytokine secretion and the respiratory burst of these cells (Lefkowitz et al., 1996; Marodi et al., 1998).

Salivary peroxidase has potent fungicidal activity in vitro (Majerus and Courtois, 1992; Bosch et al., 2000). However the role of salivary peroxidase in oral *Candida* clearance in vivo is unclear since the presence of phosphate at concentrations equivalent to those found in saliva suppresses its fungicidal activity (Lenander-Lumikari, 1992). Human MPO deficiency is the most frequently encountered neutrophilic lysosomal enzyme deficiency. The importance of MPO in clearing *Candida* infections in vivo has been suggested by case reports, which have demonstrated that patients with this deficiency may develop rapidly disseminated cutaneous *C. albicans* infection (Nguyen and Katner, 1997). Similarly, patients with hereditary MPO deficiency have an increased susceptibility to oral thrush and invasive oral candidiasis (Okuda et al., 1991), therefore it appears that MPO activity may also play a role in limiting oral infection in vivo.

6.6. Lysozyme and Lactoferrin

Salivary lysozyme is a product of the ductal epithelium of major and minor salivary glands, in addition to being potentially synthesized by sPMN. The muramidase activity of lysozyme causing degradation of the murein in bacterial cell walls is mainly responsible for its potent bactericidal activity, which has mostly been characterized for oral streptococci (Laible and Germaine, 1985). Recently, small cationic amphipathic regions were identified in the peptide sequence of lysozyme that exhibited fungicidal activity by inserting into and damaging the fungal cell membrane (During et al., 1999). Exposure of *C. albicans* oral isolates from HIV-infected patients to physiological concentrations of lysozyme triggered a rapid loss of viability to a variable extent among isolates (Samaranayake et al., 2001). On a limited number of genotypically defined strains, there was a significant negative correlation between lysozyme resistance and the duration of HIV disease, potentially implying that certain strains of *C. albicans* may develop progressive resistance over time to innate antifungal defenses such as lysozyme (Samaranayake et al., 2001).

The major sources of lactoferrin in the oral mucosa are the serous cells in salivary glands and the secondary granules of PMN. Although several antimicrobial mechanisms have been identified for lactoferrin, the classical mechanism involves high affinity for iron, which causes inhibition of microbial iron-dependent metabolism (Bellamy et al., 1992). While the iron-binding domain of this molecule is located at the carboxyterminus, the aminoterminus contains a microbicidal peptide sequence, known as lactoferricin (Bellamy et al., 1992). This peptide may be released by enzymatic degradation, which takes place in the gastrointestinal (GI) tract, and is active against fungi like *C. albicans* (Wakabayashi et al., 1996), although the exact mechanism of its fungicidal activity is still unknown. The fungicidal role of lactoferrin in saliva has been questioned by certain investigators since phosphate and bicarbonate ions at physiological salivary concentrations completely blocked its antifungal activity in vitro (Soukka et al., 1992). However, other studies dispute these findings by showing that addition of whole saliva in this in vitro system does not reduce its antifungal activities (Kuipers et al., 2002). As with salivary lysozyme, clinical or animal data supporting a role of lactoferrin in oral candidiasis are lacking.

6.7. Secretory Leukoprotease Inhibitor

SLPI is a natural anti-inflammatory and antimicrobial peptide found in mucous secretions of the oral, respiratory, and genital mucosa, and is secreted by epithelial cells lining these mucosal surfaces (reviewed in Tomee et al., 1998). SLPI is a relatively small cationic peptide (12 kDa), which acts primarily as an endogenous inhibitor of neutrophil elastase, thus limiting tissue injury and inflammation (Bingle and Tetley, 1996). In addition, SLPI has antiretroviral activity and can kill bacterial and fungal targets, through mechanisms that have not yet been defined (reviewed in Tomee et al., 1998). A pronounced fungicidal and fungistatic activity against metabolically active *C. albicans* yeast organisms has been demonstrated at physiologic concentrations of this peptide, which was localized primarily in the NH_2-terminal domain. On a molar basis this activity was similar with that of defensins and lysozyme (Tomee et al., 1997).

Although the first report on the in vitro antimicrobial activity of SLPI was in saliva (McNeely et al., 1995), to date only one study has addressed the functional role of salivary SLPI during oral infection in vivo (Chattopadhyay et al., 2004). This report on HIV-associated oral candidiasis found significantly higher levels of SLPI among participants with a history of OPC as compared to those with no history of this oral infection, but failed to show significantly higher levels in individuals with current oral infection as compared to uninfected controls. In an attempt to explain these findings the authors suggested that elevated levels of SLPI in response to recurrent infection is an attempt of the host to limit oral infection, a response that may persist long after the infection is resolved (Chattopadhyay et al., 2004).

7. Summary and Future Directions

Oral candidiasis is characterized by a recurrent, persistent, acute inflammatory reaction to *Candida* infection, which is limited to the uppermost epithelial layers of the oral mucosa. The inflammatory response to this pathogen elicits chronic pain and discomfort upon mastication, but it may also be responsible for activation of immunoeffector cells and the prevention of invasive infection. Although this chapter has concentrated on the innate immune and nonimmune mechanisms of the oral mucosal defense against *Candida*, it is well recognized that an intact arm of the adaptive immunity, represented mainly by Th1 cells, plays an instrumental role in regulating the clearance of this infection by innate immunoeffectors. The mechanisms that trigger the acute inflammatory response in the oral mucosa are currently unknown. However, dissection of this process is critical to the understanding of the pathogenesis of this fungal infection and may be important for the development of strategies to prevent invasive infection in immunocompromised hosts. Evidence is accumulating that demonstrates that the acute host response to oral infection with *Candida* is initiated and perpetuated by oral epithelial cells, the first and principal targets of infection. A number of studies support the hypothesis that oral epithelial cells, just like epithelial cells from other mucosal sites that normally harbor a great number of commensal organisms (e.g., colon, vagina), require contact with the microorganism and active invasion of the host cell cytoplasm, possibly via destruction of the plasma membrane, for a proinflammatory response. Further studies are needed to demonstrate that induction of specific cytokines in oral epithelial cells in vivo may promote the ability of PMN, monocyte, and/or keratinocyte antifungal activities. Increased production of proinflammatory cytokines by oral epithelial cells combined with the cytolytic activity of the inflammation-inducing hyphal forms of *C. albicans*, are also likely responsible for the clinical findings of redness and surface ulceration of the oral mucosa during this superficial oral infection. Further studies are also necessary to explore the contribution of other *Candida* species such as *C. glabrata* or *C. krusei* to the oral mucosal inflammatory response and epithelial cell damage in a monoinfection as well coinfection model system with *C. albi-*

cans. Future animal studies are also needed to determine whether mitigation of these proinflammatory cytokine responses and the ensuing acute inflammation would ameliorate the clinical symptoms of oral candidiasis, and/or promote invasion into the submucosal tissues. Limited knowledge is available about the contribution of salivary and oral epithelial cell antifungal peptides in the innate defense mechanisms in oral candidiasis in vivo. Knockout animal model systems will be instrumental in fully elucidating the role of such antifungal peptides (histatins, defensins, calprotectin) in the innate immune protection of the oral mucosa from this microorganism in vivo.

Acknowledgments

This work was supported in part by USPHS Research Grants RO1 DE13986 and RO3 DE12668 from the National Institute of Dental and Craniofacial Research, National Institutes of Health. The author would like to thank Dr. A. Mitchell and Dr. A. Johnson for providing the microorganisms used in some of these studies.

References

Abiko, Y., Suraweera, A.K., Nishimura, M., Arakawa, T., Takuma, T., Mizoguchi, I., and Kaku, T. (2001). Differential expression of human beta-defensin 2 in keratinized and non-keratinized oral epithelial lesions; immunohistochemistry and in situ hybridization. *Virchows Arch*. 438: 248–253.

Abiko, Y., Jinbu, Y., Noguchi, T., Nishimura, M., Kusano, K., Amaratunga, P., Shibata, T., and Kaku, T. (2002). Upregulation of human beta-defensin 2 peptide expression in oral lichen planus, leukoplakia and candidiasis: An immunohistochemical study. *Pathol. Res. Pract*. 198: 537–542.

Arancia, G., Molinari, A., Crateri, P., Stringaro, A., Ramoni, C., Dupuis, M.L., Gomez, M.J., Torosantucci, A., and Cassone, A. (1995). Noninhibitory binding of human interleukin-2-activated natural killer cells to the germ tube forms of *Candida albicans*. *Infect. Immun*. 63: 280–288.

Ashman, R.B. and Papadimitriou, J.M. (1995). Production and function of cytokines in natural and acquired immunity to *Candida albicans* infection. *Microbiol. Rev*. 59: 646–672.

Ashman, R.B., Papadimitriou, J.M., Fulurija, A., Drysdale, K.E., Farah, C.S., Naidoo, O., and Gotjamanos, T. (2003). Role of complement C5 and T lymphocytes in pathogenesis of disseminated and mucosal candidiasis in susceptible DBA/2 mice. *Microb. Pathog*. 34: 103–113.

Axell, T., Samaranayake, L.P., Reichart, P.A., and Olsen, I. (1997). A proposal for reclassification of oral candidosis. *Oral Surg. Oral Med. Oral Pathol. Oral Radiol. Endod*. 84: 111–112.

Baggiolini, M., Walz, A., and Kunkel, S.L. (1989). Neutrophil-activating peptide-1/interleukin 8, a novel cytokine that activates neutrophils. *J. Clin. Invest*. 84: 1045–1049.

Balish, E., Warner, T., Pierson, C.J., Bock, D.M., and Wagner, R.D. (2001). Oroesophageal candidiasis is lethal for transgenic mice with combined natural killer and T-cell defects. *Med. Mycol*. 39: 261–268.

Bals, R., Goldman, M.J., and Wilson, J.M. (1998). Mouse beta-defensin 1 is a salt-sensitive antimicrobial peptide present in epithelia of the lung and urogenital tract. *Infect. Immun*. 66: 1225–1232.

Bellamy, W., Takase, M., Wakabayashi, H., Kawase, K., and Tomita, M. (1992). Antibacterial spectrum of lactoferricin B, a potent bactericidal peptide derived from the N-terminal region of bovine lactoferrin. *J. Appl. Bacteriol*. 73: 472–479.

Beno, D.W., Stover, A.G., and Mathews, H.L. (1995). Growth inhibition of *Candida albicans* hyphae by $CD8^+$ lymphocytes. *J. Immunol*. 154: 5273–5281.

Bercier, J.G., Al-Hashimi, I., Haghighat, N., Rees, T.D., and Oppenheim, F.G. (1999). Salivary histatins in patients with recurrent oral candidiasis. *J. Oral Pathol. Med*. 28: 26–29.

Bickel, M., Nothen, S.M., Freiburghaus, K., and Shire, D. (1996). Chemokine expression in human oral keratinocyte cell lines and keratinized mucosa. *J. Dent. Res*. 75: 1827–1834.

Bingle, L. and Tetley, T.D. (1996). Secretory leukoprotease inhibitor: Partnering α_1-proteinase inhibitor to combat pulmonary inflammation. *Thorax* 51: 1273–1274.

Blanchard, D.K., Michelini-Norris, M.B., and Djeu, J.Y. (1991). Production of granulocyte-macrophage colony-stimulating factor by large granular lymphocytes stimulated with *Candida albicans*: Role in activation of human neutrophil function. *Blood* 77: 2259–2265.

Bosch, E.H., van Doorne, H., and de Vries, S. (2000). The lactoperoxidase system: the influence of iodide and the chemical and antimicrobial stability over the period of about 18 months. *J. Appl. Microbiol.* 89: 215–224.

Brandtzaeg, P., Gabrielsen, T.O., Dale, I., Muller, F., Steinbakk, M., and Fagerhol, M.K. (1995). The leucocyte protein L1 (calprotectin): A putative nonspecific defence factor at epithelial surfaces. *Adv. Exp. Med. Biol.* 371A: 201–206.

Braun, B.R. and Johnson, A.D. (1997). Control of filament formation in *Candida albicans* by the transcriptional repressor TUP1. *Science* 277: 105–109.

Campisi, G., Pizzo, G., Milici, M.E., and Mancuso S. (2002). Candidal carriage in the oral cavity of human immunodeficiency virus-infected participants. *Oral Surg. Oral Med. Oral Pathol. Oral Radiol. Endod.* 93: 281–286.

Chattopadhyay, A., Gray, L.R., Patton, L.L., Caplan, D.J., Slade, G.D., Tien, H.C., and Shugars, D.C. (2004). Salivary secretory leukocyte protease inhibitor and oral candidiasis in human immunodeficiency virus type 1-infected persons. *Infect. Immun.* 72: 1956–1963.

Coleman, D., Sullivan, D., Harrington, B., Haynes, K., Henman, M., Shanley, D., Bennett, D., Moran, G., McCreary, C., and O'Neill, L. (1997). Molecular and phenotypic analysis of *Candida dubliniensis*: A recently identified species linked with oral candidosis in HIV-infected and AIDS patients. *Oral Dis.* 3 (Suppl. 1): S96–S101.

Cox, D.T., Allen, C.M., and Plouffe, J.F. (1996). Locally invasive oral candidiasis mimicking zygomycosis in a patient with diabetic ketoacidosis. *Oral Surg. Oral Med. Oral Pathol. Oral Radiol. Endod.* 81: 70–73.

Cutler, C.W., Kalmar, J.R., and Arnold, R.R. (1991). Antibody-dependent alternate pathway of complement activation in opsonophagocytosis of *Porphyromonas gingivalis*. *Infect. Immun.* 59: 2105–2109.

Dale, B.A., Kimball, J.R., Krisanaprakornkit, S., Roberts, F., Robinovitch, M., O'Neal, R., Valore, E.V., Ganz, T., Anderson, G.M., and Weinberg, A. (2001). Localized antimicrobial peptide expression in human gingiva. *J. Periodontal. Res.* 36: 285–294.

Dar-Odeh, N.S. and Shehabi, A.A. (2003). Oral candidosis in patients with removable dentures. *Mycoses* 46: 187–191.

de Repentigny, L., Aumont, F., Bernard, K., and Belhumeur, P. (2000). Characterization of binding of *Candida albicans* to small intestinal mucin and its role in adherence to mucosal epithelial cells. *Infect. Immun.* 68: 3172–3179.

Deslauriers, N., Coulombe, C., Carre, B., and Goulet, J.P. (1995). Topical application of a corticosteroid destabilizes the host-parasite relationship in an experimental model of the oral carrier state of *Candida albicans*. *FEMS Immunol. Med. Microbiol.* 11: 45–55.

Diamond, G. and Bevins, C.L. (1998). β-Defensins: endogenous antibiotics of the innate host defense response. *Clin. Immunol. Immunopathol.* 88: 221–225.

Dinarello, C.A. (1997). Interleukin-1. *Cytokine Growth Factor Rev.* 8: 253–265.

Djeu, J.Y. and Blanchard, D.K. (1987). Regulation of human polymorphonuclear neutrophil (PMN) activity against *Candida albicans* by large granular lymphocytes via release of a PMN-activating factor. *J. Immunol.* 139: 2761–2767.

Dongari-Bagtzoglou, A. and Kashleva, H. (2003a). *Candida albicans* triggers interleukin-8 secretion by oral epithelial cells. *Microb. Pathog.* 34: 169–177.

Dongari-Bagtzoglou, A. and Kashleva, H. (2003b). Granulocyte-macrophage colony-stimulating factor responses of oral epithelial cells to *Candida albicans*. *Oral Microbiol. Immunol.* 18: 165–170.

Dongari-Bagtzoglou, A. and Kashleva, H. (in press) Oral epithelial cells activate neutrophil antifungal activities *in vitro*.

Dongari-Bagtzoglou, A., Kashleva, H., and Villar, C.C. (2004) Bioactive interleukin-1α is cytolytically released from *Candida albicans*-infected oral epithelial cells. *Med. Mycol.* 42: 531–541.

During, K., Porsch, P., Mahn, A., Brinkmann, O., and Gieffers, W. (1999). The non-enzymatic microbicidal activity of lysozymes. *FEBS Lett.* 449: 93–100.

Edgerton, M. and Koshlukova, S.E. (2000). Salivary histatin 5 and its similarities to the other antimicrobial proteins in human saliva. *Adv. Dent. Res.* 14: 16–21.

Edgerton, M., Koshlukova, S.E., Araujo, M.W., Patel, R.C., Dong, J., and Bruenn, J.A. (2000). Salivary histatin 5 and human neutrophil defensin 1 kill *Candida albicans* via shared pathways. *Antimicrob. Agents Chemother.* 44: 3310–3316.

Espinoza, I., Rojas, R., Aranda, W., and Gamonal, J. (2003). Prevalence of oral mucosal lesions in elderly people in Santiago, Chile. *J. Oral Pathol. Med.* 32: 571–575.

Eversole, L.R., Reichart, P.A., Ficarra, G., Schmidt-Westhausen, A., Romagnoli, P., and Pimpinelli, N. (1997). Oral keratinocyte immune responses in HIV-associated candidiasis. *Oral Surg. Oral Med. Oral Pathol. Oral Radiol. Endod.* 84: 372–380.

Farah, C.S., Elahi, S., Pang, G., Gotjamanos, T., Seymour, G.J., Clancy, R.L., and Ashman, R.B. (2001). T cells augment monocyte and neutrophil function in host resistance against oropharyngeal candidiasis. *Infect. Immun.* 69: 6110–6118.

Fidel, P.L. Jr., Vazquez, J.A., and Sobel, J.D. (1999). *Candida glabrata*: review of epidemiology, pathogenesis, and clinical disease with comparison to *C. albicans*. *Clin. Microbiol. Rev.* 12: 80–96.

Fotos, P.G. and Hellstein, J.W. (1992). *Candida* and candidosis. Epidemiology, diagnosis and therapeutic management. *Dent. Clin. North. Am.* 36: 857–878.

Giammanco, G.M, Pizzo, G., Pecorella, S., Distefano, S., Pecoraro, V., and Milici, M.E. (2002). Identification of *Candida dubliniensis* among oral yeast isolates from an Italian population of human immunodeficiency virus-infected subjects. *Oral Microbiol. Immunol.* 17: 89–94.

Gururaja, T.L., Levine, J.H., Tran, D.T., Naganagowda, G.A., Ramalingam, K., Ramasubbu, N., and Levine, M.J. (1999). Candidacidal activity prompted by N-terminus histatin-like domain of human salivary mucin (MUC7). *Biochim. Biophys. Acta* 1431: 107–119.

Hahn, B.L. and Sohnle, P.G. (1988). Characteristics of dermal invasion in experimental cutaneous candidiasis of leucopenic mice. *J. Invest. Dermatol.* 91: 233–237.

Hoffman, M.P. and Haidaris, C.G. (1993). Analysis of *Candida albicans* adhesion to salivary mucin. *Infect. Immun.* 61: 1940–1949.

Imam, I., Carpenter, C.C.J., Mayer, K.H., Fisher, A., Stein, M., and Danforth, S. (1990). Hierarchical pattern of mucosal *Candida* infections in HIV-seropositive women. *Am. J. Med.* 89: 142–147.

Jabra-Rizk, M.A., Falkler, W.A. Jr., Merz, W.G., Kelley, J.I., Baqui, A.A., and Meiller, T.F. (1999). Coaggregation of *Candida dubliniensis* with *Fusobacterium nucleatum*. *J. Clin. Microbiol.* 37: 1464–1468.

Jorge, A.O., Totti, M.A., de Almeida, O.P., and Scully, C. (1993). Oral candidiasis established in the sialoadenectomised rat. *J. Oral Pathol. Med.* 22: 54–56.

Jurevic, R.J., Bai, M., Chadwick, R.B., White, T.C., and Dale, B.A. (2003). Single-nucleotide polymorphisms (SNPs) in human beta-defensin 1: High-throughput SNP assays and association with *Candida* carriage in type I diabetics and nondiabetic controls. *J. Clin. Microbiol.* 41: 90–96.

Kleinegger, C.L., Stoeckel, D.C., and Kurago, Z.B. (2001). A comparison of salivary calprotectin levels in subjects with and without oral candidiasis. *Oral Surg. Oral Med. Oral Pathol. Oral Radiol. Endod.* 92: 62–67.

Kobayashi, Y., Yamamoto, K., Saido, T., Kawasaki, H., Oppenheim, J.J., and Matsushima, K. (1990). Identification of calcium-activated neutral protease as a processing enzyme of human interleukin 1 alpha. *Proc. Natl. Acad. Sci. USA* 87: 5548–5552.

Koshlukova, S.E., Lloyd, T.L., Araujo, M.W., and Edgerton, M. (1999). Salivary histatin 5 induces non-lytic release of ATP from *Candida albicans* leading to cell death. *J. Biol. Chem.* 274: 18872–18879.

Kozel, T.R. (1996). Activation of the complement system by pathogenic fungi. *Clin. Microbiol. Rev.* 9: 34–46.

Krisanaprakornkit, S., Weinberg, A., Perez, C.N., and Dale, B.A. (1998). Expression of the peptide antibiotic human beta-defensin 1 in cultured gingival epithelial cells and gingival tissue. *Infect. Immun.* 66: 4222–4228.

Krisanaprakornkit, S., Jotikasthira, D., and Dale, B.A. (2003). Intracellular calcium in signaling human beta-defensin-2 expression in oral epithelial cells. *J. Dent. Res.* 82: 877–882.

Kuipers, M.E., Beljaars, L., Van Beek, N., De Vries, H.G., Heegsma, J., Van Den Berg, J.J., Meijer, D.K., and Swart, P.J. (2002). Conditions influencing the in vitro antifungal activity of lactoferrin combined with antimycotics against clinical isolates of *Candida*. Impact on the development of buccal preparations of lactoferrin. *APMIS* 110: 290–298.

Laible, N.J. and Germaine, G.R. (1985). Bactericidal activity of human lysozyme, muramidase-inactive lysozyme, and cationic polypeptides against *Streptococcus sanguis* and *Streptococcus faecalis*: Inhibition by chitin oligosaccharides. *Infect. Immun.* 48: 720–728.

Lefkowitz, S.S., Gelderman, M.P., Lefkowitz, D.L., Moguilevsky, N., and Bollen, A. (1996). Phagocytosis and intracellular killing of *Candida albicans* by macrophages exposed to myeloperoxidase. *J. Infect. Dis.* 173: 1202–1207.

Lehrer, R.I. and Cline, M.J. (1969). Leukocyte myeloperoxidase deficiency and disseminated candidiasis: the role of myeloperoxidase in resistance to *Candida* infection. *J. Clin. Invest.* 48: 1478–1488.

Lehrer, R.I. and Ganz, T. (1996). Endogenous vertebrate antibiotics. Defensins, protegrins and other cysteine rich antimicrobial peptides. *Ann. NY Acad. Sci.* 797: 228–239.

Leigh, J.E., Steele, C., Wormley, F., and Fidel, P.L. Jr. (2002). Salivary cytokine profiles in the immunocompetent individual with *Candida*-associated denture stomatitis. *Oral Microbiol. Immunol.* 17: 311–314.

Lenander-Lumikari, M. (1992). Inhibition of *Candida albicans* by the Peroxidase/SCN-/H_2O_2 system. *Oral Microbiol. Immunol.* 7: 315–320.

Liljemark, W.F. and Gibbons, R.J. (1973). Suppression of *C. albicans* by human oral streptococci in gnotobiotic mice. *Infect. Immun.* 8: 846–849.

Lo, H.J., Kohler, J.R., DiDomenico, B., Loebenberg, D., Cacciapuoti, A., and Fink, G.R. (1997). Nonfilamentous *C. albicans* mutants are avirulent. *Cell* 90: 939–949.

Lockhart, S.R., Joly, S., Vargas, K., Swails-Wenger, J., Enger, L., and Soll, D.R. (1999). Natural defenses against *Candida* colonization breakdown in the oral cavities of the elderly. *J. Dent. Res.* 78: 857–868.

Lukasser-Vogl, E., Gruber, A., Lass-Florl, C., Eder, A., Hogasen, A.K., Morgan, B.P., Dierich, M.P., and Wurzner, R. (2000). Membrane attack complex formation on yeast as trigger of selective release of terminal complement proteins from human polymorphonuclear leukocytes. *FEMS Immunol. Med. Microbiol.* 28: 15–23.

MacFarlane, T.W. (1975). Defense mechanisms of the mouth, with particular reference to patients with Sjorgren's syndrome. DDS Thesis, *University of Glasgow*, Glasgow.

Majerus, P.M. and Courtois, P.A. (1992). Susceptibility of *Candida albicans* to peroxidase-catalyzed oxidation products of thiocyanate, iodide and bromide. *J. Biol. Buccale.* 20: 241–245.

Marodi, L., Forehand, J.R., and Johnston, R.B. Jr. (1991). Mechanisms of host defense against *Candida* species. II. Biochemical basis for the killing of *Candida* by mononuclear phagocytes. *J. Immunol.* 146: 2790–2794.

Marodi, L., Tournay, C., Kaposzta, R., Johnston, R.B. Jr., and Moguilevsky, N. (1998). Augmentation of human macrophage candidacidal capacity by recombinant human myeloperoxidase and granulocyte-macrophage colony-stimulating factor. *Infect. Immun.* 66: 2750–2754.

McNeely, T.B., Dealy, M., Dripps, D.J., Orenstein, J.M., Eisenberg, S.P., and Wahl, S.M. (1995). Secretory leukocyte protease inhibitor: a human saliva protein exhibiting anti-human immunodeficiency virus 1 activity *in vitro*. *J. Clin. Invest.* 96: 456–464.

Miyauchi, M., Takata, T., Ito, H., Ogawa, I., Kudo, Y., Takekoshi, T., and Nikai, H. (1998). Distribution of macrophage lineage cells in rat gingival tissue after topical application of lipopolysaccharide: An immunohistochemical study using monoclonal antibodies: OX6, ED1 and ED2. *J. Periodontal. Res.* 33: 345–351.

Muller, F., Froland, S.S., Brandtzaeg, P., and Fagerhol, M.K. (1993). Oral candidiasis is associated with low levels of parotid calprotectin in individuals with infection due to human immunodeficiency virus. *Clin. Infect. Dis.* 16: 301–302.

Murthy, A.R., Lehrer, R.I., Harwig, S.S., and Miyasaki, K.T. (1993). In vitro candidastatic properties of the human neutrophil calprotectin complex. *J. Immunol.* 151: 6291–6301.

Myers, T.A., Leigh, J.E., Arribas, A.R., Hager, S., Clark, R., Lilly, E., and Fidel, P.L. Jr. (2003). Immunohistochemical evaluation of T cells in oral lesions from human immunodeficiency virus-positive persons with oropharyngeal candidiasis. *Infect. Immun.* 71: 956–963.

Nguyen, C. and Katner, H.P. (1997). Myeloperoxidase deficiency manifesting as pustular candidal dermatitis. *Clin. Infect. Dis.* 24: 258–260.

Nomanbhoy, F., Steele, C., Yano, J., and Fidel, P.L. Jr. (2002). Vaginal and oral epithelial cell anti-*Candida* activity. *Infect. Immun.* 70: 7081–7088.

O'Daniels, D.M., Larsen, N.M., Reznik, D.A., et al. (2000). Prevalence and risk factors of *Candida dubliniensis* in oral candidasis (OC) among HIV-seropositive patients. In *40th Annual Interscience Conference on Antimicrobial Agents and Chemotherapy*. American Society for Microbiology, September 17–20, 2000, Toronto, p. 382.

Odds, F.C. (1988). *Candida* and candidosis: a review and bibliography. *Bailliere Tindale*, London.

O'Grady, J.F. and Reade, P.C. (1993). Role of thermal trauma in experimental oral mucosal *Candida* infections in rats. *J. Oral Pathol. Med.* 22: 132–137.

Okuda, T., Yasuoka, T., and Oka, N. (1991). Myeloperoxidase deficiency as a predisposing factor for deep mucocutaneous candidiasis: A case report. *J. Oral Maxillofac. Surg.* 49: 183–186.

Olsen, I. and Birkeland, J.M. (1977). Denture stomatitis-yeast occurrence and the pH of saliva and denture plaque. *Scand. J. Dent. Res.* 85: 130–134.

Oppenheim, F.G., Xu, T., McMillian, F.M., Levitz, S.M., Diamond, R.D., Offner, G.D., and Troxler, R.F. (1988). Histatins, a novel family of histidine-rich proteins in human parotid secretion. Isolation, characterization, primary structure, and fungistatic effects on *Candida albicans*. *J. Biol. Chem.* 263: 7472–7477.

Orozco, A.S., Zhou, X., and Filler, S.G. (2000). Mechanisms of the proinflammatory response of endothelial cells to *Candida albicans* infection. *Infect. Immun.* 68: 1134–1141.

Phelan, J.A., Begg, M.D., Lamster, I.B., Gorman, J., Mitchell-Lewis, D., Bucklan, R.D., and el-Sadr, W.M. (1997). Oral candidiasis in HIV infection: predictive value and comparison of findings in injecting drug users and homosexual men. *J. Oral Pathol. Med.* 26: 237–243.

Raj, P.A., Edgerton, M., and Levine, M.J. (1990). Salivary histatin 5: dependence of sequence, chain length, and helical conformation for candidacidal activity. *J. Biol. Chem.* 265: 3898–3905.

Raj, P.A., Marcus, E., and Sukumaran, D.K. (1998). Structure of human salivary histatin 5 in aqueous and nonaqueous solutions. *Biopolymers* 45: 51–67.

Redding, S.W. (2001). The role of yeasts other than *Candida albicans* in oropharyngeal candidiasis. *Curr. Opin. Infect. Dis.* 14: 673–677.

Redding, S.W., Rinaldi, M.G., and Hicks, J.L. (1988). The relationship of oral *Candida tropicalis* infection to systemic candidiasis in a patient with leukemia. *Spec. Care Dentist.* 8: 111–114.

Redding, S.W., Zellars, R.C., Kirkpatrick, W.R., McAtee, R.K., Caceres, M.A., Fothergill, A.W., Lopez-Ribot, J.L., Bailey, C.W., Rinaldi, M.G., and Patterson, T.F. (1999). Epidemiology of oropharyngeal *Candida* colonization and infection in patients receiving radiation for head and neck cancer. *J. Clin. Microbiol.* 37: 3896–3900.

Redding, S.W., Bailey, C.W., Lopez-Ribot, J.L., Kirkpatrick, W.R., Fothergill, A.W., Rinaldi, M.G., and Patterson, T.F. (2001). *Candida dubliniensis* in radiation-induced oropharyngeal candidiasis. *Oral Surg. Oral Med. Oral Pathol. Oral Radiol. Endod.* 91: 659–662.

Redding, S.W., Kirkpatrick, W.R., Coco, B.J., Sadkowski, L., Fothergill, A.W., Rinaldi, M.G., Eng, T.Y., and Patterson, T.F. (2002). *Candida glabrata* oropharyngeal candidiasis in patients receiving radiation treatment for head and neck cancer. *J. Clin. Microbiol.* 40: 1879–1881.

Reichart, P.A., Philipsen, H.P., Schmidt-Westhausen, A., and Samaranayake, L.P. (1995). Pseudomembranous oral candidiasis in HIV infection: ultrastructural findings. *J. Oral Pathol. Med.* 24: 276–281.

Rennie, J.S., Hutcheon, A.W., MacFarlane, T.W., and MacDonald, D.G. (1983). The role of iron deficiency in experimentally-induced oral candidosis in the rat. *J. Med. Microbiol.* 16: 363–369.

Rodriguez-Adrian, L.J., Grazziutti, M.L., Rex, J.H., and Anaissie, E.J. (1998). The potential role of cytokine therapy for fungal infections in patients with cancer: Is recovery from neutropenia all that is needed? *Clin. Infect. Dis.* 26: 1270–1278.

Romagnoli, P., Pimpinelli, N., Mori, M., Reichart, P.A., Eversole, L.R., and Ficarra, G. (1997). Immunocompetent cells in oral candidiasis of HIV-infected patients: An immunohistochemical and electron microscopical study. *Oral Dis.* 3: 99–105.

Rouabhia, M., Ross, G., Page, N., and Chakir, J. (2002). Interleukin-18 and gamma interferon production by oral epithelial cells in response to exposure to *Candida albicans* or lipopolysaccharide stimulation. *Infect. Immun.* 70: 7073–7080.

Samaranayake, L.P. (1986). Nutritional factors and oral candidosis. *J. Oral Pathol.* 15: 61–65.

Samaranayake, L.P. and MacFarlane, T.W. (1990). *Oral Candidosis*. Wright, London.

Samaranayake, Y.H. and Samaranayake, L.P. (2001). Experimental oral candidiasis in animal models. *Clin. Microbiol. Rev.* 14: 398–429.

Samaranayake, L.P., Hamilton, D., and MacFarlane, T.W. (1994). The effect of indigenous bacterial populations on buccal epithelial cells on subsequent microbial adhesion in vitro. *Oral Microbiol. Immunol.* 9: 236–240.

Samaranayake, Y.H., Samaranayake, L.P., Pow, E.H., Beena, V.T., and Yeung, K.W. (2001). Antifungal effects of lysozyme and lactoferrin against genetically similar, sequential *Candida albicans* isolates from a human immunodeficiency virus-infected southern Chinese cohort. *J. Clin. Microbiol.* 39: 3296–3302.

Santarpia, R.P. III, Cho, M.I., and Pollock, J.J. (1990). Parameters affecting the inhibition of *Candida albicans* GDH 2023 and GRI 2773 blastospore viability by purified synthetic salivary histidine-rich polypeptides. *Oral Microbiol. Immunol.* 5: 226–232.

Saville, S.P., Lazzell, A.L., Monteagudo, C., and Lopez-Ribot, J.L. (2003). Engineered control of cell morphology in vivo reveals distinct roles for yeast and filamentous forms of *Candida albicans* during infection. *Eukaryot. Cell* 2: 1053–1060.

Sawaki, K., Mizukawa, N., Yamaai, T., Fukunaga, J., and Sugahara, T. (2002). Immunohistochemical study on expression of alpha-defensin and beta-defensin-2 in human buccal epithelia with candidiasis. *Oral Dis.* 8: 37–41.

Schaller, M., Mailhammer, R., Grassl, G., Sander, C.A., Hube, B., and Korting, H.C. (2002). Infection of human oral epithelia with *Candida* species induces cytokine expression correlated to the degree of virulence. *J. Invest. Dermatol.* 118: 652–657.

Scully, C., el-Kabir, M., and Samaranayake, L.P. (1994). *Candida* and oral candidosis: A review. *Crit. Rev. Oral Biol. Med.* 5: 125–157.

Slots, J. (1992). *Contemporary Oral Microbiology and Immunology*. Mosby, St. Louis, MO.

Sobel, J.D. (1988). Pathogenesis and epidemiology of vulvovaginal candidiasis. *Ann. NY Acad. Sci.* 544: 547–557.

Sohnle, P.G., Collins-Lech, C., and Wiessner, J.H. (1991). The zinc-reversible antimicrobial activity of neutrophil lysates and abscess fluid supernatants. *J. Infect. Dis.* 164: 137–142.

Sohnle, P.G., Hunter, M.J., Hahn, B., and Chazin, W.J. (2000). Zinc-reversible antimicrobial activity of recombinant calprotectin (migration inhibitory factor-related proteins 8 and 14). *J. Infect. Dis.* 182: 1272–1275.

Soukka, T., Tenovuo, J., and Lenander-Lumikari, M. (1992). Fungicidal effect of human lactoferrin against *Candida albicans*. *FEMS Microbiol. Lett.* 69: 223–228.

Squier, C.A. and Finkelstein, M.W. (2003). Oral mucosa. In A. Nanci (ed.), *Ten Cate's Oral Histology*. Mosby, St. Louis, MO.

Steele, C., and Fidel, P.L. Jr. (2002). Cytokine and chemokine production by human oral and vaginal epithelial cells in response to *Candida albicans*. *Infect. Immun.* 70: 577–583.

Steele, C., Leigh, J., Swoboda, R., and Fidel, P.L. Jr. (2000). Growth inhibition of *Candida* by human oral epithelial cells. *J. Infect. Dis.* 182: 1479–1485.

Steele, C., Leigh, J., Swoboda, R., Ozenci, H., and Fidel, P.L. Jr. (2001). Potential role for a carbohydrate moiety in anti-*Candida* activity of human oral epithelial cells. *Infect. Immun.* 69: 7091–7099.

Sweet, S.P., Denbury, A.N., and Challacombe, S.J. (2001). Salivary calprotectin levels are raised in patients with oral candidiasis or Sjogren's syndrome but decreased by HIV infection. *Oral Microbiol. Immunol.* 16: 119–123.

Tanida, T., Ueta, E., Tobiume, A., Hamada, T., Rao, F., and Osaki, T. (2001). Influence of aging on candidal growth and adhesion regulatory agents in saliva. *J. Oral Pathol. Med.* 30: 328–335.

Tomee, J.F., Hiemstra, P.S., Heinzel-Wieland, R., and Kauffman, H.F. (1997). Antileukoprotease: an endogenous protein in the innate mucosal defense against fungi. *J. Infect. Dis.* 176: 740–747.

Tomee, J.F., Koeter, G.H., Hiemstra, P.S., and Kauffman, H.F. (1998). Secretory leukoprotease inhibitor: a native antimicrobial protein presenting a new therapeutic option? *Thorax* 53: 114–116.

Tonetti, M.S., Imboden, M.A., and Lang, N.P. (1998). Neutrophil migration into the gingival sulcus is associated with transepithelial gradients of interleukin-8 and ICAM-1. *J. Periodontol.* 69: 1139–1147.

Ueta, E., Osaki, T., Yoneda, K., and Yamamoto, T. (1993). Functions of salivary polymorphonuclear leukocytes (SPMNs) and peripheral blood polymorphonuclear leukocytes (PPMNs) from healthy individuals and oral cancer patients. *Clin. Immunol. Immunopathol.* 66: 272–278.

Ueta, E., Tanida, T., Doi, S., and Osaki, T. (2000). Regulation of *Candida albicans* growth and adhesion by saliva. *J. Lab. Clin. Med.* 136: 66–73.

Vargas, K.G. and Joly, S. (2002). Carriage frequency, intensity of carriage and strains of oral yeast species vary in the progression to oral candidiasis in human immunodeficiency virus-positive individuals. *J. Clin. Microbiol.* 40: 341–350.

Vazquez, J.A., Hidalgo, J.A., and De Bono, S. (2000). Use of sargramostim (rh-GM-CSF) as adjunctive treatment of fluconazole-refractory oropharyngeal candidiasis in patients with AIDS: A pilot study. *HIV Clin. Trials* 1: 23–29.

Villar, C.C., Kashleva, H., and Dongari-Bagtzoglou, A. (2004). Role of *Candida albicans* polymorphism in the interactions with oral epithelial cells. *Oral Microbiol. Immunol.* 19: 262–269.

Villar, C.C., Kashleva, H., Mitchell, A.P., and Dongari-Bagtzoglou, A. (in press). Invasive phenotype of *C. albicans* affects the host proinflammatory response to infection. *Infect. Immun.*

Voganatsi, A., Panyutich, A., Miyasaki, K.T., and Murthy, R.K. (2001). Mechanism of extracellular release of human neutrophil calprotectin complex. *J. Leukoc. Biol.* 70: 130–134.

Wakabayashi, H., Hiratani, K., Uchida, K., and Yamaguchi, H. (1996). Antifungal spectrum and fungicidal mechanism of an N-terminal peptide of bovine lactoferrin. *J. Infect. Chemother.* 1: 185–189.

Weber, M.L., Abela, A., de Repentigny, L., Garel, L., and Lapointe, N. (1987). Myeloperoxidase deficiency with extensive candidal osteomyelitis of the base of the skull. *Pediatrics* 80: 876–879.

Weinert, M., Grimes, R.M., and Lynch, D.P. (1996). Oral manifestations of HIV infection. *Ann. Intern. Med.* 125: 485–496.

Wilkieson, C., Samaranayake, L.P., MacFarlane, T.W., Lamey, P.J., and MacKenzie, D. (1991). Oral candidosis in the elderly in long term hospital care. *J. Oral Pathol. Med.* 20: 13–16.

Williams, D.W., Potts, A.J., Wilson, M.J., Matthews, J.B., and Lewis, M.A. (1997). Characterisation of the inflammatory cell infiltrate in chronic hyperplastic candidosis of the oral mucosa. *J. Oral Pathol. Med.* 26: 83–89.

Xu, T., Levitz, S.M., Diamond, R.D., and Oppenheim, F.G. (1991). Anticandidal activity of major human salivary histatins. *Infect. Immun.* 59: 2549–2554.

Yamaguchi, H. (1975). Control of dimorphism in *Candida albicans* by zinc: Effect on cell morphology and composition. *J. Gen. Microbiol.* 86: 370–372.

Yano, J.E., Lilly, C., Steele, D., Fortenberry, D., and Fidel, P.L. (in press). Oral and vaginal epithelial cell anti-*Candida* activity is acid labile and does not require live epithelial cells. *Oral Microbiol. Immunol.*

Zunino, S.J. and Hudig, D. (1988). Interactions between human natural killer (NK) lymphocytes and yeast cells: Human NK cells do not kill *Candida albicans*, although *C. albicans* blocks NK lysis of K562 cells. *Infect. Immun.* 56: 564–569.

3

Humoral Factors in the Protection of the Oral Cavity against Candidiasis

Stephen J. Challacombe, Durdana Rahman, Mukesh Mistry, and Julian R. Naglik

1. Introduction

The health of the oral cavity is dependent on the integrity of the mucosa, which normally prevents the penetration of microorganisms as well as macromolecules in the diet and environment that might be antigenic. The oral mucosa is protected by both innate and specific immune factors, and the epithelium itself is capable of responding to microbial challenge. The nature of the epithelial cell responses and the action of

Department of Oral Medicine and Pathology, Guys, Kings and St Thomas Dental Institute, Kings College London, UK.

the cytokines that they produce has been the subject of much recent investigation. The oral mucosa is covered by a mucin layer some 30 μm thick, but the superficial epithelial cells are constantly being desquamated so that attachment and reattachment of potentially pathogenic organisms such as *Candida* is a constant process. The oral mucous membranes are therefore protected by a series of both non-specific innate factors, which include the physical factors, i.e., mucin and the cornification of the epithelial cell layer and thickness of the epithelium as well as the lipid-rich layers within the epithelium that inhibit penetration of macromolecules, and humoral factors derived from both secretions, tissue fluids, and epithelial cells within the cells.

From a specific immunity perspective, the oral mucosa is protected (or damaged) by the secretory (mucosal) immune system and the systemic immune system. Antibodies in the saliva may be stimulated locally or centrally and serum antibodies can reach the mucosal surface via tissue fluids and crevicular fluid. Epithelial cells may respond to cellular immunity, which could also be induced at local or distant sites.

Understanding the mechanisms of protection against oral candidiasis is a particular challenge since not only is there a complexity of host defensive factors, but also several different forms of oral candidiasis, some of which are superficial and some penetrative, and the yeast itself produces both yeast and hyphal forms in different circumstances. *Candida* organisms are found as commensals in approximately 40% of the population (Arendorf and Walker, 1980) and the organism has a predilection for certain epithelial sites and particularly the dorsum of the tongue. In superficial *Candida* infections it might be expected that humoral immunity, especially secretory IgA might play a predominant role. In other forms of *Candida* infection where penetration of the epithelial cells takes place, cell-mediated immunity (CMI) may be expected to be operative in addition to humoral immunity. Both immune cells and *Candida* organisms themselves in hyphal or yeast form may induce an epithelial cytokine response, which may play a further role in protection or damage.

This review will concentrate on humoral factors, both innate and specific, in relation to protection of the oral cavity against candidiasis.

2. Host Factors Predisposing to Oral Candidiasis

Oral candidiasis is a superficial mycosis and can present in a variety of clinical forms. The presence of *Candida* alone is not an indication of disease since yeasts can be found as a commensal in approximately 40% of the population. Candidiasis is essentially a disease of the diseased and reflects as much changes in host defences as increased pathogenicity of the organism. Oral candidiasis has been associated with a variety of predisposing factors and these are summarised in Table 3.1.

3. Classification of Oral *Candida* Infections

Candida species can be found as commensals in the mouths approximately 40% of normal subjects in amounts up to approximately 800 colony forming units (CFU)/ml. There is usually some underlying precipitating factor for oral candidiasis, often an immunodeficiency and in patients with various forms of candidiasis (Table 3.2), salivary counts of greater than 20,000 CFU/ml may be found. Oral candidiasis is a common condition, especially in patients with xerostomia, those taking immunosuppressive drugs, those with other oral diseases, and in patients with HIV infection where approximately 40% may have oral candidiasis. All forms of candidiasis are

Table 3.1. Host Factors Predisposing to Oral Candidiasis

Local
Reduced salivary flow—e.g., Sjogren's syndrome, drugs
Epithelial changes, e.g., lichen planus, leukoplakia
Changes in commensal flora
High carbohydrate diet
Smoking
Systemic
Altered hormone state
Diabetes
Hypothyroidism
Hyperparathyroidism
Adrenal suppression Iron or folate deficiencies
Immunosuppression
Drugs
Immunodeficiencies
Altered polymorph function

strongly associated with smoking. Oral candidiasis is most commonly caused by the yeast *Candida albicans*, and to a far lesser extent by *C. parapsilosis*, *C. tropicalis*, *C. glabrata*, *C. krusei*, *C. pseudotropicalis*, and *C. guilliermondi* (Odds and Webster, 1988). More recently oral candidiasis has been associated with *C. dubliniensis* in HIV-infected individuals (Sullivan et al., 1995), other immunocompromised groups, and in Sjogren's syndrome (Challacombe et al., unpublished).

Acute pseudomembranous candidiasis (thrush, Fig. 3.1A) is a common infection in very young, elderly, or debilitated people. The white plaques are easily removable and contain *Candida* hyphae, spores, epithelial cells, and polymorphs (Fig. 3.1B). The condition is chronic in those with HIV-induced immune deficiency.

Acute atrophic candidiasis (Fig. 3.1C) is also known as antibiotic sore mouth because it frequently occurs during antibiotic therapy. This is a response to the suppression of the normal bacterial flora, and there is a widespread erythematous stomatitis with accompanying depapillation of the tongue.

Chronic atrophic candidiasis (CAC) (Fig. 3.1D) is also known as denture sore mouth and is very common. It presents as a relatively asymptomatic confluent erythema and inflammation of the entire denture-bearing mucosa of the palate. This results

Table 3.2. Classification of Oral Candidiasis

Acute	Acute/chronic	Chronic
Pseudomembranous candidiasis (thrush)	Erythematous candidiasis (HIV-associated)	Hyperplastic candidiasis
		Candida leucoplakia
		Median rhomboid glossitis
Atrophic candidiasis (antibiotic sore tongue/mouth)	Angular cheilitis	Atrophic candidiasis (denture-induced stomatitis)
		Mucocutaneous candidiasis

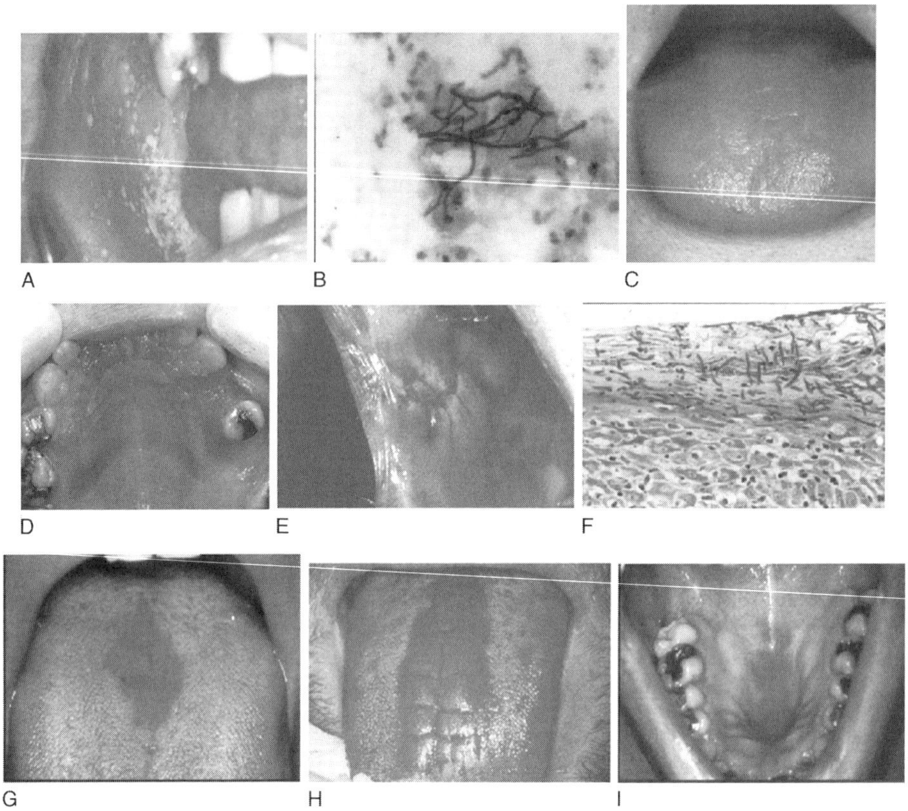

Figure 3.1. (A) *Acute pseudomembranous candidiasis*. Note the white plaques, which consist of hyphae, desquamated epithelial cells, and polymorphonuclear leukocytes. (B) Cytological smear from pseudomembranous candidiasis showing hyphae, desquamated epithelial cells, and polymorphonuclear leukocytes (Periodic acid Shiff stain). (C) *Acute atrophic candidiasis* (antibiotic sore tongue) showing generalised depapillation of the dorsum of the tongue secondary to *Candida* overgrowth. (D) *Chronic atrophic candidiasis*. Chronic atrophic candidiasis in a patient who wears a cobalt chrome partial upper denture. The mid-portion of the palate is of normal color, but the mucosa under the denture is very erythematous. (E) *Chronic hyperplastic candidiasis*. Mixed red and white plaques inside the buccal mucosa in the commissure areas. These are often slightly raised and histologically show hyphal invasion. (F) Section from chronic hyperplastic candidiasis showing invading hypha forms of *Candida* (PAS stain). (G) Median rhomboid glossitis, a form of chronic hyperplastic candidiasis of the tongue, usually found at the junction of the anterior two thirds and posterior third of the tongue. (H) *Erythematous candidiasis*. The central portion of this tongue is very erythematous as well as depapillated. This patient has AIDS. (I) *Erythematous candidiasis*. The central portion of the palate is very erythematous. No white plaques are seen. This patient has AIDS.

from *Candida* colonization of the surface of the denture, usually in patients who wear their prostheses continuously day and night. There is no evidence of invasion by *Candida* hyphae.

Chronic hyperplastic candidiasis (CHC) (Fig. 3.1E) is a speckled or nodular chronic leucoplakia usually found in middle-aged or elderly patients. It is an invasive form of candidiasis with hyphae present often throughout the depth of the epithelium (Fig. 3.1F). There is a significant risk of malignant transformation. One form of CHC, which affects the dorsum of the tongue, is known as median rhomboid glossitis (Fig. 3.1G).

A more recently recognised entity, *erythematous candidiasis*, is often found associated with HIV infection. It presents as areas of erythema in the absence of white plaques (Challacombe, 1991), usually of the tongue (Fig. 3.1H) or palate (Fig. 3.1I).

Angular cheilitis is probably not a condition that occurs in the absence of intraoral increases in *Candida*, which probably acts as the reservoir for infection. There are a number of cofactors such as iron deficiency and inadequate denture construction involved in the pathogenesis of the disease although it is highly likely that the frequently cracked, macerated, thin, moist atrophic epithelium would be a key predisposing factor.

Chronic oral hyperplastic candidiasis may occur as part of *chronic mucocutaneous candidiasis* (CMCC), often with identifiable immunological or endocrine abnormalities as major factors. Endocrine disorders such as hypothyroidism, hypoparathyroidism, and adrenal insufficiency, have a familial incidence and are found in children and young adults, particularly in girls. The most frequently associated endocrine manifestations include idiopathic hyperparathyroidism and hypoadrenocorticism, but candidiasis follows only where there is an immune defect (Kostiala et al., 1979).

Thus there are several different forms of oral candidiasis with a varying preponderance of yeast or hyphal forms, and with or without invasion of the host tissues. It is certainly possible or even likely that immune mechanisms for protection vary with the different clinical forms.

4. General Considerations for Oral Mucosal Immunity to *Candida*

Theoretically, SIgA, serum IgG transudating through the mucosa, and cellular immunity might all play a role in protection of mucosal surfaces against *Candida* infections. Animal models have largely concentrated on systemic candidiasis possibly because of the difficulties in obtaining reproducible and relevant models of mucosal candidiasis.

Evidence suggests a role for CMI, even at mucosal surfaces. Infection with *C. albicans* is an almost universal finding in patients with severe immunodeficiency of the T cell type. It is, however, rarely seen in patients with B cell defects in the absence of concomitant T cell defects. Oral *Candida* infections are found in about 40% of HIV-infected individuals and in over 75% of patients who suffer from the acquired immunodeficiency syndrome (AIDS) (Palmer et al., 1996). Both erythematous and pseudomembranous candidiasis is found, particularly in association with low CD4 counts. However, in IgA-deficient individuals, a markedly increased prevalence of *Candida* infection is apparent, and in patients with CMCC, over 50% have reduced salivary IgA antibodies (Lehner et al., 1972).

In CMCC a wide spectrum of immune abnormalities have been reported, ranging from lowered serum IgM and IgG antibodies to defects in lymphocyte transformation and mitogen stimulation in the most severe types of CMCC (Lehner et al., 1972). It is not clear, however, whether these immune defects are primary to the disease or a consequence of it. Some studies have shown restoration of immune functions once *Candida* has been cleared by antifungal therapy (Valdimarsson et al., 1973).

The observation that only slight alterations in host physiological state can turn a normally harmless commensal yeast into an aggressive pathogen in the immunocompromised host points to the significance of the immune response in protection against *Candida* pathogenicity. At the mucosal level, CMI due to T cells represents the dominant protective response against *C. albicans* with Th1-type responses associated with resistance and Th2-type responses correlating with susceptibility (Romani et al., 1991a,b, 1993). Systemic CMI may play a more important role in oral candidiasis than vaginal candidiasis with local CMI responses, orchestrated by epithelial cells, chemokines, and cytokines being more relevant in the latter (Saavedra et al., 1999; Steele et al., 1999).

Using a germ-free mouse model of oral candidiasis, we have observed that adoptive transfer of mesenteric lymph node (MLN) cells after intragastric (i.g.) immunisation with whole cells of *C. albicans* or *C. glabrata*, and spleen cells after intraperitoneal (i.p.) immunisation, lead to significantly reduced colonisation of *C. albicans* cells in saliva after challenge (Rahman and Challacombe, 1995) though the protective antigens were not identified. $CD8^+$ cells from MLNs, but not $CD4^+$ cells, were responsible for this effect after i.g. immunisation, whereas after i.p. immunisation both $CD8^+$ and $CD4^+$ cells from the spleen were responsible for reduced colonisation of mice. These and other studies (Fidel et al., 1995a,b) indicate the importance of local and systemic CMI in the protection against mucosal candidiasis, though antibodies have also been shown to be protective in experimental vaginitis (De Bernardis et al., 1997).

In early animal studies using the rhesus monkey, the role of cellular immunity in chronic oral candidiasis was suggested since azathioprine-treated monkeys showed a depression of cellular immunity to *Candida* but a normal humoral antibody response. These animals had a prolonged and severe oral mucosal *Candida* infection, suggesting that cellular immunity to *Candida* is of primary importance in host resistance rather than serum antibody (Budtz-Jorgensen, 1973).

Most models since have been in mice and rats, but there appears to be strong evidence for the role of CD4 cells in protection against systemic candidiasis (Romani et al., 1997a–c), as well as an important immunoregulatory role for neutrophils (Romani et al., 1996). The protective immunity seems to be associated with Th1 rather than Th2 responses. It is not clear, however, whether these findings are totally transferable to mucosal surfaces and to all types of oral candidiasis. Intragastric inoculation can lead to intestinal candidiasis and protective Th1 responses but defective IgA production from Peyer's patches (Bistoni et al., 1993). By contrast, oral immunisation and subsequent oral challenge in a murine model have shown the induction of salivary antibodies in the absence of detectable serum antibodies and inhibition of oral colonisation (Rahman and Challacombe, 1995).

A critical role for CMI in the host defence against oral candidiasis is suggested by the observations in a model of chronic oral *C. albicans* infection in immunodeficient mice that lack T lymphocytes (Farah et al., 2002a). Complete resolution of the infection in mice reconstituted with functional $CD4^+$ T cells was found. There was evidence that the transferred $CD4^+$ T cells infiltrated the oral tissues, and presumably exerted their activity there. Additionally, draining lymphocytes isolated from the submandibular and superficial cervical lymph nodes secreted high titres of IL-12, and moderate levels of IFN-γ, suggesting a role for these cytokines in clearance (Farah et al., 2002b). These data also support the role for Th1-type cytokines and protective immunity in the resolution of oral candidiasis in infected mice. However, histology of hyperplastic candidiasis shows microabsecesses of polymorphs suggesting a non-specific role for innate immunity including polymorphonuclear neutrophils (PMNs), epithelial cells, and possibly toll-like receptors (TLRs).

5. Humoral Immunity against Oral Candidiasis

A variety of studies have attempted to address the question of whether antibodies might be protective, in which case they might be expected to be higher in controls than in patients, or whether antibodies might reflect the antigenic load in which case they would be expected to be higher in patients than in controls.

Studies of antibodies in humans in oral candidiasis have used both serum and saliva, with the main objectives of identifying responses in relation to clinical disease or sometimes using antibodies to identify individual genes expressed (Cheng et al., 2003).

A summary of the studies is shown in Table 3.3. With regard to salivary IgA antibodies, they have been found to be raised in patients with CAC (Kantardjiev and Popova, 2002) using immunofluorescence and whole cells and in patients with malignancies (Dorko et al., 2002). However, salivary antibodies were not found to be raised in two groups of HIV-positive subjects using whole cells and enzyme-linked immunosorbent assay (ELISA) (Belazi et al., 2002; Wozniak et al., 2002), while serum IgG antibodies were reduced.

A non-specific role of IgA has been suggested by the finding that in patients who are *Candida* positive, the carriage rate of *Candida* is inversely proportional to the non-specific secretory IgA level whereas serum levels are unrelated (Kurnatowski and Kurnatowska, 1999).

In addition to secreted aspartyl proteinases (Saps), other specific antigens of *Candida* have been examined including heat shock mannoproteins. Antibodies in saliva and in serum have been reported against these mannoproteins in patients with oral or vaginal candidiasis (Ivanyi and Ivanyi, 1990; Swoboda et al., 1993; Polonelli et al., 1994). Kozel et al. (2004) used serum to identify antibodies reactive with *C. albicans* mannan and showed a normal distribution in 34 subjects though no account was taken of *Candida* colonisation. Functionally, however, the anti-mannan IgG did not appear to be needed for opsonophagocytic killing by neutrophils as long as there was normal complement levels in the individuals.

5.1. Saps and Oral Humoral Immunity

The Saps appear to play a major role in virulence by mediating adherence, causing tissue damage, and evading of host immune responses (reviewed by Naglik et al., 2003b). Ten *SAP* genes have been identified that encode a proteinase family between 35 and 50 kDa (Hube, 2000), which include two major subfamilies based on nucleotide acid sequences identity (*SAP1–3* and *4–6*).

The contribution of the Saps to *C. albicans* pathogenesis has been clearly demonstrated using *SAP*-deficient mutants and proteinase inhibitors. These studies demonstrated that different *SAP* genes appear to be essential for mucosal (*SAP1–3*) (Watts et al., 1998; De Bernardis et al., 1999; Schaller et al., 1999) and systemic (*SAP4–6*) (Hube et al., 1997; Sanglard et al., 1997) infections. The Sap isoenzymes appear to have a variety of functions in vivo, which are probably called upon during different stages and types of *C. albicans* infections. There might be an expectation, therefore, that responses against different Saps might be different in mucosal and systemic candidiasis.

Recently, we have analysed *SAP1–8* expression in over 130 subjects with oral and vaginal *C. albicans* infection or asymptomatic carriage (Naglik et al., 1999, 2003a,b). *SAP2* and *SAP5* were the most common

Table 3.3. Serum and Salivary Antibodies to *Candida* in Humans

Diagnosis	Patients	Controls	Antigen	Salivary antibodies	Serum antibodies	Method	Reference
CAC			Whole cells	IgG, IgA raised	IgG raised	IIF	Kantardjiev and Popova (2002)
Cancer	63	–	Whole cells	–	23/63 positive	IIF	Dorko et al. (2002)
CMCC	1	–	Gliadin	–	Positive	ELISA	Garcia et al. (2002)
HIV	34	30	Whole cells	IgA not raised	IgG lower	ELISA	Belazi et al. (2002)
HIV/OPC	68	33	Whole cells	IgA not raised	IgG subclasses not raised	ELISA	Wozniak et al. (2002)
HIV/OC	6	11	SAP1,6	IgA raised	IgG and IgA raised	Immunofluorometric	Drobacheff et al. (2001)
HIV/OC	15	?	SAP 2,6	IgA raised	Related to infection	Immunofluorometric	Millon et al. (2001)
OC	167	?	None	SIgA non-specific low	Serum IgA non-specific normal		Kurnatowski and Kurnatowska (1999)
OPC	Pooled		*Candida* heat shock proteins	Salivary antibodies	Serum antibodies	Western blots	Polonelli et al. (1994) and Swoboda et al. (1993)
CAC/VVC	30	30	HsP 65	40	Serum IgG raised		Ivanyi and Ivanyi (1990)

CAC, chronic atrophic candidiasis; CMCC, chronic mucocutaneous candidiasis; HIV, human immunodeficiency virus; OPC, oropharyngeal candidiasis; OC, oral candidiasis; VVC, vulvovaginal candidiasis; IIF, immunoflourescence; ELISA, enzyme-linked immunosorbent assay.

genes expressed during both infection and carriage, possibly indicating a permanent interaction of these proteinases with host factors at mucosal surfaces. *SAP1*, *SAP3*, *SAP4*, *SAP7*, and *SAP8* expression correlated with oral disease, whereas *SAP1*, *SAP3*, *SAP6*, *SAP7*, and *SAP8* expression correlated with vaginal disease. The results demonstrated that certain *C. albicans SAP* genes are more frequently expressed during active infection compared with carriage and indicate that studies of immunity to Saps in humans should be directed against those proteinases expressed in vivo.

5.2. Host Immune Responses to Saps

Very few studies have investigated the interaction between Saps and the host immune response. While high titres of anti-Sap IgG antibodies have been demonstrated in sera of candidiasis patients (Macdonald and Odds, 1980; Rüchel and Boning, 1983; Rüchel et al., 1988), few detailed studies on mucosal antibody responses, using saliva or vaginal secretions, against the Saps have been performed.

However, recently two reports have addressed this. In a small study of six patients with oral candidiasis and HIV infection, salivary IgA antibodies to Sap1 and Sap6 were found to be raised in patients compared with controls. Serum IgG and IgA antibodies were also raised (Drobacheff et al., 2001). Similarly in a series of 15 patients with oral candidiasis and HIV infection, Millon et al. (2001) found salivary IgA antibodies to Sap2 and Sap6 to be raised and related to infection. These studies are suggestive of both inferences that responses in HIV are not impaired in this regard and that if shown to be specific, Sap1 and Sap6 may be expressed in such infections. Taken overall, the evidence would suggest that oral candidiasis can induce a response to both whole cells of *Candida* and to *Candida* Saps and would not exclude the possibility that such antibodies might subsequently be protective.

Preliminary data from our laboratory have demonstrated strong anti-Sap2 salivary IgA and serum IgG responses in mice after intranasal (i.n.) immunisation, indicating the immunogenic potential of the *C. albicans* proteinases. Furthermore, we have detected anti-Sap2 secretory IgA responses in human saliva of both *Candida* carriers and patients with *C. albicans* infections (Naglik et al., unpublished).

Although Sap2 is known to be immunogenic and can induce antibody responses, the protective potential of Sap antibodies in vivo remains unclear. De Bernardis et al. (1997) showed a protective effect of anti-Sap2 IgA antibodies in experimental vaginitis in rats. This not only demonstrated that Sap2 contributed to vaginal infections and was a target of the host immune response, but also suggested that anti-Sap IgA antibodies could afford protection against *C. albicans* infections at mucosal sites in vivo.

No studies have yet reported the mechanisms of antibody protection or whether other members of the proteinase family can induce protective responses. Key questions remain such as whether Sap-specific antibodies can inhibit proteinase activity and whether passive immunisation could produce a protective or infection-attenuating response? Recently, we assessed the ability of saliva and serum, purified IgG, and Sap2-specific antibodies to inhibit *C. albicans* Sap2 proteinase activity, but found no strong evidence for Sap2 inhibition (Naglik et al., 2005). In addition, Borg et al. (1988) demonstrated that three monoclonal IgM antibodies raised against Sap2 did not inhibit enzyme activity. Furthermore, a *C. albicans* Sap-specific murine IgG monoclonal antibody was mapped to a specific region of Sap2 (Asp77–Gly103) but was also found not to inhibit Sap2 activity (Na et al., 1999). Another study used sera from patients with oral and systemic candidiasis to delineate six Sap2 epitopes, but human recombinant antibodies against two of these epitopes were not protective in a lethal mouse model of candidiasis (Ghadjari et al., 1997).

Identification of SIgA epitopes would arguably be more relevant than IgG or IgM epitopes to *C. albicans* infection at mucosal sites and it is quite conceivable that a cocktail of epitopes from different proteinases may be required before neutralising or protective antibody responses are attained against *C. albicans* infections.

5.3. Functional Aspects of Serum and Salivary Antibodies to *Candida*

There have been many attempts to identify functional activity of serum or salivary antibodies in vitro and in addition some conclusions can be drawn from in vivo models. (Table 3.4) Thus Holmes et al. (2002) showed that while whole saliva promoted the binding of *C. albicans* to epithelial cell lines, human *Candida*-specific IgA antibodies could inhibit the adhesion. These antibodies could be absorbed by both *Candida* or by an anti-IgA. These findings seem to suggest that IgA in the human oral cavity could be functional. This concept is reinforced by the observation that saliva also promotes the adhesion of *C. albicans* to polystyrene and that salivary IgA antibodies inhibited this adhesion (San-Millan et al., 2000) and the mechanism appeared to be blockage of the adhesins in the cell wall. Interestingly, these authors reported that while saliva increased the adhesion of whole cells of *C. albicans* to polystyrene, they inhibited the germinated cells, suggesting that function of antibodies may differentiate between the different forms of *Candida* and thus might be different in the various forms of oral candidiasis. In contrast, Sweet et al. (1995), using human desquamated buccal epithelial cells, showed that binding of *Candida* was inhibited by saliva and that this inhibition did not appear to be related to the antibody content.

There is evidence that antibodies may be capable of anti-*Candida* function without the presence of cells. Thus it has been shown that recombinant anti-idiotypic antibodies representing the internal image of a yeast killer toxin could be microbicidal in vitro against *Candida* (Conti et al., 2002) (Table 3.4). Antibodies have been used in vivo in humans and Tollemar et al. (1999) used a bovine antibody against *Candida* in bone marrow transplant patients. Repeated oral treatment resulted in a reduction of the colonisation in seven out of ten patients.

There is a suggestion that B cells and therefore antibodies may be more protective against systemic candidiasis than oral candidiasis. In a B cell knockout mouse model the mice remained resistant to mucosal infection with *Candida* but significantly more susceptible to systemic candidiasis (Wagner et al., 1996). Oral immunisation with whole cells of *Candida* has been shown to result in increased resistance to oral candidiasis (van Wyk and van der, 1994; Rahman and Challacombe, 1995). While this immunisation has been shown to induce salivary IgA antibodies to *Candida*, protection could not be ascribed to antibodies since adoptive transfer with both CD4 and in some models CD8 cells could result in protection in the recipient (Rahman and Challacombe, 1995).

There seems to be good evidence that at least monoclonal antibodies to *C. albicans* can result in inhibition of adherence to epithelial cells (Moragues et al., 2003) and also inhibition to polystyrene and by analogy with the solid surface of dentures (Rodier et al., 2003). Serum IgG antibodies can also exhibit such inhibition of adherence. This raises the possibility that in CAC naturally occurring IgA antibodies or serum transudate of IgG antibodies could play a role in inhibiting adherence to dentures, though this has not been proven. This type of response may be antigen specific since immunisation with *C. albicans* of mice resulted in antibodies, which were protective and those against the β1–6 glucan were blocking (inhibiting adherence) and protective (Bromuro et al., 2002) (Table 3.4).

5.4. Oral Immunity to *Candida* in HIV Infection

Although patients with HIV infection may have profound systemic cell-mediated immune deficiencies, mucosal immunity appears to be intact until late in the disease process. Thus, Coogan and Challacombe (2000) showed that salivary IgA antibodies to a 65-kDa heat shock protein were raised in HIV-infected patients compared with controls, and with patients with AIDS. These responses were further raised in the presence of candidiasis. Although $CD4^+$ cells are low in number in HIV-positive individuals, $CD8^+$ cells appear to be the main infiltrate in CHC in either HIV-positive or HIV-negative individuals (Myers et al., 2003). Some authors have found no relationship of salivary antibodies with candidiasis in HIV infection (Wozniak et al., 2002) whilst others have shown that antibodies to specific *Candida* antigens such as Saps are related to the amount of colonisation and infection (Millon et al., 2001).

In general, results from HIV suggest that mucosal responses are not impaired until later on in the infection and particularly in AIDS (Challacombe and Sweet, 1997).

5.5. Serum Antibodies—Responses to Oral *Candida* Infection in Humans

Serum antibodies against whole cell or *Candida* antigens can be detected in the sera of most persons, given sensitive enough detection techniques. This probably reflects the fact that *Candida* is a commensal in the mouth and other mucosal surfaces of approximately 40% of the population and also that such antigens are able to stimulate a systemic serum antibody response.

Few studies, however, have attempted to discover whether serum antibodies differ between the four main types of oral *Candida* infections seen in non-immunocompromised individuals. If it is accepted that CAC is

Table 3.4. Mechanisms Reported for Antibody Activity against *Candida*

Action	Substrate	Class	Author
Inhibition of adherence	Hep2 cells	Monoclonal	Moragues et al. (2003)
Inhibition of germination	*Candida* blastospores	Monoclonal	Moragues et al. (2003)
Inhibition of colonisation	Human mouth	Bovine anti-*Candida*	Tollemar et al. (1999)
Inhibition of adherence	Epithelial cells	Salivary IgA antibody	Holmes et al. (2002)
Inhibition of adherence	Polystyrene	Saliva IgA	San-Millan et al. (2000) and Rodier et al. (2003)
Candicidal	*Candida* cells	Monoclonal	Conti et al. (2002) and Moragues et al. (2003)
Opsonisation	PMN and *Candida*	Recombinant human single chain	Wellington et al. (2003)
Fungal clearance	In vivo mouse	IgG	Montagnoli et al. (2003)

predominated by the yeast form and that CHC is dominated by an invasive hyphal form of *Candida*, it might be expected that this would be reflected in serum antibodies against yeast or hyphal-specific antigens. This remains an area to be further studied but it has been reported that serum antibodies to whole cells were higher in CAC than in the CHC group (Lehner, 1970). This would bear repeating.

Antibody responses have been reported against a variety of *Candida* antigens ranging from 18 to 120 kDa and including Saps, phospholipases, and heat shock proteins. There was considerable interest in an antigen of molecular weight of 47 kDa because antibodies against this antigen had seemed to be predictive of recovery from systemic *C. albicans* infection (Matthews et al., 1987). However, this does not seem to be a major antigen in most murine models of mucosal candidiasis.

It is possible for serum antibodies to have a role against mucosal candidiasis in the oral cavity. There is evidence for direct transudation of serum IgG into saliva and this is markedly increased in CAC. In addition, crevicular fluid antibodies derived more directly from serum constitute 1 to 2 ml to the 5–700 ml of saliva per day.

5.6. Salivary IgA Subclass Antibodies to *Candida*

IgA subclass antibodies have been reported in a few studies in patients with CAC. IgA antibodies and IgA1 antibodies were increased in comparison with the controls (Ivanyi and Ivanyi, 1990). However, it is possible that some of this IgA1 antibody might have been derived from inflammation in the oral cavity itself. However, Coogan et al. (1994) showed that in HIV infection IgA1 and IgA2 subclass antibodies against *Candida* were raised in both whole and parotid saliva compared with controls. This suggested that patients with HIV were not significantly immunocompromised when compared with controls and that *Candida* infection could induce subclass responses in these patients. More recently, Wellington et al. (2003) have demonstrated enhanced phagocytosis of *Candida* by polymorphonuclear leucocytes (PMNs) mediated by a recombinant human antibody—single chain. This demonstrates another mechanism that may be operative in vivo, especially considering that PMNs are a major cell type around invading hyphae. It might be expected that if this mechanism was operative in vivo that it would be active against the CHC rather than the CAC type of oral candidiasis.

An interesting development is the derivation of peptides from single chain recombinant and idiotypic antibodies, which retain microbicidal activity (Polonelli et al., 2003). This killer peptide has been used in vivo where in a rat model of vaginal candidiasis local post-challenge administration of KP was efficacious in rapidly ablating infections. It probably acts through its interaction with the β-glucan KT receptor on *C. albicans* but it has not yet been reported as being used in an oral infection. The concept of modelling in vivo activity by using monoclonal antibodies was studied further by Moragues et al. (2003) where a monoclonal raised against the main target of salivary secretory IgA in the cell wall of the *C. albicans* was demonstrated to show three separate anti-*C. albicans* activities: (1) inhibition of adherence to Hep2 cells, (2) inhibition of germination, and (3) direct candicidal activity.

6. Innate Factors against Oral Candidiasis

6.1. Epithelial Cell Factors, TLR etc.

This aspect is covered in more detail elsewhere. However, one of the exciting new areas of immunology has been the recognition that epithelial cells play an active part in innate immunity and that epithelial cells can produce factors interactive with the immune system upon contact with bacteria and other antigens. Some of these factors appear to be microbicidal to *Candida*. For example, Pivarcsi et al. (2003) showed that antimicrobials induced from epithelial cells can kill *Candida*. This appeared to be dependent on the *Candida* induction of TLR2 and TLR4 as well as IL-8 expression. Interestingly antibodies against TLR2 or TLR4 blocked both IL-8 and microbicidal activity. TLRs are a novel protein family that recognise conserved motifs called pathogen-associated molecular patterns (PAMPs), which represent broad groups of microbial pathogens or components (bacteria, fungi, RNA, and DNA). Stimulation of TLRs causes an immediate defensive response, including the production of an array of antimicrobial peptides and proinflammatory cytokines (through NF-κB), and the expression of costimulatory molecules, which are essential for the activation of adaptive immunity. *C. albicans* can induce immunostimulation through mannan or phospholipomannan recognised by TLR4 (Netea et al., 2002).

Induction of TLR and the interactions with *Candida* are reviewed elsewhere, but it is clear that this similar interaction with *Candida* induces soluble factors and that these may play a role in defence of the oral cavity (Netea et al., 2004). It is however established that adherence of *Candida* to epithelial cells, perhaps stimulated by Saps, result in upregulation of TLR2 and TLR4 in epithelial cells (Roeder et al., 2004)

It is now clear that epithelial cells on stimulation with microbes can produce a number of chemokines and cytokines. The biological relevance of these in vivo is not yet clear. Granulocyte-macrophage colony-stimulating factor (GM-CSF) responses of oral epithelial cells to *Candida* have been shown to be dependent on contact and are strain and viability dependent (Dongari-Bagtzoglou and Kashleva, 2003). Interestingly these responses are optimal with hyphae rather than yeast forms. Epithelial cells can have direct anti-*Candida* activity (Nomanbhoy et al., 2002). Such activity appears to require direct contact and is not mediated by soluble factors (Steele et al., 2001). Contact of epithelial cells with *Candida* can have differential expression of cytokines. Whilst IFN-γ is the preferential response of epithelial cells to *C.albicans*, IL-18 expression was downregulated by the presence of the yeasts (Rouabhia et al., 2002).

6.2. Cytokines

In animal models, however, there has been some intensive study of cytokines in relation to oral candidiasis in an attempt to answer questions of their relationship with protection. Farah et al. (2001a), in an irradiated mouse model, showed that CD4 cell depletion led to increased colonisation and infection with *Candida*. This showed that IL-12 from the draining submandibular lymph nodes was higher in these infected animals than in controls, suggesting that IL-12 might have a role in clearance of the fungus. These same authors showed in a slight modification of this model that CD4 or CD8 cell depletion did not affect the severity of oral candidiasis but that depletion of PMNs did (Farah et al., 2001b). Again IL-12 as well as IFN-γ were raised in draining lymph nodes, drawing an inference that the mechanism of action of CD4 was via PMNs. However, Farah et al. (2002b) suggested that TNF-α was best related to the recovery from oral infection or resistance to infection in nude BALB/c mice.

IL-12, IFN-γ, and IL-4 were also shown to be associated with rapid elimination of *C. albicans* in a BALB/c mouse model (Elahi et al., 2000) who also showed that neutralisation of IL-4 with antibody resulted in delayed clearance. This suggests that the T cell response in the local lymph nodes correlates with rapid oral clearance that may be Th0 since both IL-4 and IFN-γ were involved. Knockout mice have given further insight into mechanisms. IFN-γ knockout mice appear to be more susceptible to *Candida* infection (Balish et al., 1998) though these animals also had a poor Th2-antibody response. IL-12 seems to be related to mucosal infection in a number of studies (Elahi et al., 2000; Farah et al., 2001a,b) and overall there is consistency in results that proinflammatory cytokines are produced by oral epithelial cells constitutively and enhanced in contact with *C. albicans*. These include IL-1-α and TNF-α (Steele and Fidel, 2002).

Few studies have examined the cytokine profile in humans. Leigh et al. (2002) showed that in HIV-negative denture wearers with candidiasis there was a mixed Th1/Th2 profile of cytokines in saliva, which was not significantly different from controls. The cytokine pattern suggested Th1 activity. This suggests that saliva might be useful as a fluid to measure upregulation of cytokines, but it remains to be shown whether they are active in this medium. In an earlier study the salivary Th1/Th2-type cytokine profile was evaluated in HIV-positive individuals (Leigh et al., 2001). In contrast to some other studies IL-10 concentrations were the highest in these patients followed by IL-4 and IFN-γ and surprisingly IL-12 was either not detectable or at very low levels. The salivary Th2-type cytokine profile did not appear to be related to the CD4 count. This appears to be the first study to evaluate the Th1/Th2-type cytokine expression in saliva of HIV-positive individuals and confirmed that a constitutive expression of cytokines was present in the whole saliva of healthy individuals. IL-12 levels were particularly high in some controls. The authors concluded that the Th0/Th1-type cytokine profile in HIV-negative individuals is consistent with the association of Th1-type cytokines in immunocompetent individuals reported elsewhere. Overall, these data suggested a Th1-type profile in controls and a Th2-type profile in those with oral candidiasis, and suggested that the Th2-type profile may indicate susceptibility to candidiasis. However, the fact that many HIV-positive individuals with a Th2-type cytokine profile do not have oral candidiasis suggests that other factors such as innate defences may predominate over CMI as the protective mechanism in this group.

6.3. Salivary Histatins

Salivary histatins are a family of basic histidine-rich proteins in which therapeutic potency against oral candidiasis is apparent and thus have promise as therapeutic agents for humans with oral candidiasis. Salivary histatins appear to be particularly active against intact cells rather than hyphae (Edgerton et al., 1998) and appear to bind to a 67-kDa protein in the cell wall. Salivary histatin 5 (Hst5) is a potent toxin for *C. albicans*; it induces non-cytolytic efflux of *Candida* cellular ATP, potassium, and magnesium in the absence of cytolysis without implicating these ion movements in the toxins' fungicidal activity. Potassium is regulated by a TOK-1 gene and this has now been described in *C. albicans* (Baev et al., 2003). However, even in TOK-1 knockouts Hst5 treatment still resulted in substantial killing of *Candida*, demonstrating that the TOK-1 pp channels are not the primary site of Hst5 action.

Biological activity is suggested by the finding that a range of *C. albicans* isolates from the oral cavities of HIV-positive patients were susceptible to Hst5 (Nikawa et al., 2002). However, *C. albicans* isolates from HIV-positive individuals appear to be less sensitive to Hst5 than oral isolates from HIV-negative individuals. Salivary-derived mucin peptide (MUC7) and Hst5 were tested in a vaginal model and not shown to promote significant differences even though they possessed potent in vitro antifungal activity (Intini et al., 2003). This suggests that caution should be expressed in over interpreting in vitro activities to in vivo.

The mechanism of action of Hst5 is not confirmed. Thus Baev et al. (2002) showed that salivary Hst5 resulted in depletion of intracellular ATP and that this led to disruption of the irregulatory circuits for the volume of cells. In other words, that treatment with salivary Hst5 led to pleomorphism of the *Candida* cells. Interestingly, Edgerton et al. (2000) suggested that salivary Hst5 and neutrophil-derived defensin 1 (HNP1) killed *C. albicans* via shared pathways. They showed that HNP1 prevented Hst5 binding to *Candida*-binding protein, suggesting that although these two peptides are functionally distinct that they have overlapping actions.

6.4. Defensins

Defensins are cationic, arginine-rich peptides containing 28 to 44 amino acids. Their molecular weights vary from 3 to 5 kDa. They all share a typical tertiary structure despite differences in primary structure. Defensins have a broad antimicrobial spectrum encompassing not only *Candida* but also Gram-negative and Gram-positive bacteria. They are also chemotactic for monocytes, PMNs, and T cells. The highest density is found in granulocytes where defensins 1–4 may make up 10% of the total protein. HD5 and HD6 are of epithelial origin. HBD-2 is upregulated by TNF-α, IL-1β, and yeasts in keratinocyte cultures (Fellermann and Stange, 2001).

In one immunohistochemical study on expression of HBD-2 in human buccal epithelial cells with candidiasis, Sawaki et al. (2002) showed that HBD-2 signals could be found constitutively in most buccal epithelium but that the signal intensity was upregulated in oral candidiasis. These results were confirmed by Abiko et al. (2002) who also suggested that HBD-2 may play an important role in protection from *C. albicans* infection. Earlier work with HBD-1 showed that it was expressed in tongue epithelium and the expression was related to the *Candida* activity (Shi et al., 1999). It is tempting to suggest that certain defensins may be active in vivo and responsible for natural resistance in humans to oral *Candida* colonisation, but this has yet to be demonstrated.

6.5. Other Soluble Factors

There are additional soluble factors in saliva, which have been shown to have anti-*Candida* activity. Earlier work had reported that lysozyme in parotid saliva was increased in relation to the oral *Candida* load (Yeh et al., 1997) though the pathway of such stimulation was not identified. Statherin mediates a dose-dependent adhesion of *C. albicans* to epithelial cells (Johansson et al., 2000). This adhesion could be inhibited by specific IgG antibodies to statherin, suggesting that antibodies derived from the gingival crevice could be active in vivo. Other workers have suggested that complement factors may have a role in homeostasis of *Candida*. Triebel et al. (2003) showed that in normal sera containing complement factors that Sap activity was reduced, growth of *Candida* was reduced, and phagocytosis was enhanced. However, these results suggest that in vivo these could only be active around the gingival crevice and might explain why this is not a favourite site for *Candida* colonisation.

7. Conclusions

There are several soluble factors that may be active against oral candidiasis in the oral cavity. The major one of these is antibody but anti-*Candida* factors also include defensins, histatins, and cytokines. Analysing protective factors in the oral cavity is challenging since both systemic and mucosal immunity can play a role, and there are several different forms of oral candidiasis where either yeast or hyphal forms predominate, and these infections may be acute or chronic. Review of the literature reveals a common though not universal finding that serum IgG antibodies are raised in different forms of oral candidiasis and there is a majority view that salivary IgA antibodies may also be raised. These studies indicate that the presence of *Candida* in the oral cavity in disease can stimulate a response in both mucosal and systemic humoral systems. The main target antigens in yeast and hyphal forms may be different. Functional aspects of antibodies have largely been examined in vitro. Inhibition of adherence to epithelial cells by both monoclonal IgG and salivary IgA has been demonstrated, as well as inhibition of adherence to polystyrene. Antibody-mediated inhibition of germination of *Candida* and inhibition of colonisation and fungal clearance have also been reported. A further mechanism is candicidal activity demonstrated by monoclonal antibodies but not yet by naturally induced serum or salivary antibodies. In vivo, inhibition of colonisation in humans has been demonstrated as proof of principle by the application of bovine anti-*Candida*, but the role of other mechanisms in vivo remains to be confirmed. Inhibition of Sap activity is an attractive hypothesis and has been reported in vaginal candidiasis though not confirmed to date in oral candidiasis. Thus, there are several different mechanisms whereby antibodies present in saliva or coming into the oral cavity from serum may influence candidiasis and could be protective. However, demonstrating the latter has proved elusive and it is likely that a number of different mechanisms are operative concurrently in any protection of the oral cavity against the various forms of candidiasis.

References

Abiko, Y., Jinbu, Y., Noguchi, T., Nishimura, M., Kusano, K., Amaratunga, P., Shibata, T., and Kaku, T. (2002). Upregulation of human beta-defensin 2 peptide expression in oral lichen planus, leukoplakia and candidiasis an immunohistochemical study. *Pathol. Res. Pract.* 198: 537–542.

Arendorf, T.M. and Walker, D.M. (1980). The prevalence and intra-oral distribution of *Candida albicans* in man. *Arch. Oral Biol.* 25: 1–10.

Baev, D., Li, X.S., Dong, J., Keng, P., and Edgerton, M. (2002). Human salivary histatin 5 causes disordered volume regulation and cell cycle arrest in *Candida albicans. Infect. Immun.* 70: 4777–4784.

Balish, E., Wagner, R.D., Vazquez-Torres, A., Pierson, C., and Warner, T. (1998). Candidiasis in interferon-gamma knockout (IFN-gamma-/-) mice. *J. Infect. Dis.* 78: 478–487.

Belazi, M., Fleva, A., Drakoulakos, D., and Panayiotidou, D. (2002). Salivary IgA and serum IgA and IgG antibodies to *Candida albicans* in HIV-infected subjects. *Int. J. STD AIDS* 13: 373–377.

Bistoni, F., Cenci, E., Mencacci, A., Schiaffella, E., Mosci, P., Puccetti, P., and Romani, L. (1993). Mucosal and systemic T helper cell function after intragastric colonization of adult mice with *Candida albicans. J. Infect. Dis.* 168: 1449–1457.

Borg, M., Watters, D., Reich, B. and Rüchel, R. (1988). Production and characterization of monoclonal antibodies against secretory proteinase of *Candida albicans* CBS 2730. *Zbl. Bakteriol. Hyg. A.* 268: 62–73.

Bromuro, C., Torosantucci, A., Chiani, P., Conti, S., Polonelli, L., and Cassone, A. (2002). Interplay between protective and inhibitory antibodies dictates the outcome of experimentally disseminated candidiasis in recipients of a *Candida albicans* vaccine. *Infect. Immun.* 70: 5462–5470.

Budtz-Jorgensen, E. (1973). Immune response to *Cándida albicans* in monkeys with experimental candidiasis in the palate. *Scand. J. Dent. Res.* 81: 360–371.

Challacombe, S. (1991). Revised classification of HIV-associated oral lesions. *Br. Dent. J.* 170: 305–306.

Challacombe, S.J. and Sweet, S.P. (1997). Salivary and mucosal immune responses to HIV and its co-pathogens. *Oral Dis.* 3 (Suppl. 1): S79–S84.

Cheng, S., Nguyen, M.H., Zhang, Z., Jia, H., Handfield, M., and Clancy, C.J. (2003). Evaluation of the roles of four *Candida albicans* genes in virulence by using gene disruption strains that express URA3 from the native locus. *Infect. Immun.* 71: 6101–6103.

Conti, S., Magliani, W., Arseni, S., Frazzi, R., Salati, A., Ravanetti, L., and Polonelli, L. (2002). Inhibition by yeast killer toxin-like antibodies of oral *Streptococci* adhesion to tooth surfaces in an ex vivo model. *Mol. Med.* 8: 313–317.

Coogan, M.M. and Challacombe, S.J. (2000). Serum and salivary antibodies to a mycobacterial 65-kDa stress protein are elevated in HIV-positive patients and modified by oral candidiasis. *Oral Microbiol. Immunol.* 15: 284–289.

Coogan, M.M., Sweet, S., and Challacombe S.J. (1994). Immunoglobulin A (IgA), IgA1 and IgA2 antibodies to *Candida albicans* in whole and parotid saliva in human immunodeficiency virus (HIV) infection and AIDS. *Infect. Immun.* 62: 892–896.

De Bernardis, F., Boccanera, M., Adriani, D., Spreghini, E., Santoni, G., and Cassone, A. (1997). Protective role of antimannan and anti-aspartyl proteinase antibodies in an experimental model of *Candida albicans* vaginitis in rats. *Infect. Immun.* 65: 3399–3405.

De Bernardis, F., Arancia, S., Morelli, L., Hube, B., Sanglard, D., Schafer, W., and Cassone, A. (1999). Evidence that members of the secretory aspartyl proteinase gene family, in particular SAP2, are virulence factors for *Candida vaginitis. J. Infect. Dis.* 179: 201–208.

Dongari-Bagtzoglou, A. and Kashleva, H. (2003). Granulocyte-macrophage colony-stimulating factor responses of oral epithelial cells to *Candida albicans. Oral Microbiol. Immunol.* 18: 165–170.

Dorko, E., Jenca, A., Pilipcinec, E., and Tkacikova, L. (2002). Detection of anti-*Candida* antibodies by the indirect immunofluorescence assay in patients with cancer in the orofacial region. *Folia Microbiol. (Praha)* 47: 732–736.

Drobacheff, C., Millon, L., Monod, M., Piarroux, R., Robinet, E., Laurent, R., and Meillet, D. (2001). Increased serum and salivary immunoglobulins against *Candida albicans* in HIV-infected patients with oral candidiasis. *Clin. Chem. Lab Med.* 39: 519–526.

Edgerton, M., Koshlukova, S.E., Lo, T.E., Chrzan, B.G., Straubinger, R.M., and Raj, P.A. (1998). Candidacidal activity of salivary histatins. Identification of a histatin 5-binding protein on *Candida albicans. J. Biol. Chem.* 273: 20438–20447.

Edgerton, M., Koshlukova, S.E., Araujo, M.W., Patel, R.C., Dong, J., and Bruenn, J.A. (2000). Salivary histatin 5 and human neutrophil defensin 1 kill *Candida albicans* via shared pathways. *Antimicrob. Agents Chemother.* 44: 3310–3316.

Elahi, S., Pang, G., Clancy, R., and Ashman, R.B. (2000). Cellular and cytokine correlates of mucosal protection in murine model of oral candidiasis. *Infect. Immun.* 68: 5771–5777.

Farah, C.S., Hong, S., Wanasaengsakul, S., Elahi, S., Pang, G., Gotjamanos, T., Seymour, G.J., Clancy, R.L., and Ashman, R.B. (2001a). Irradiation-induced oral candidiasis in an experimental murine model. *Oral Microbiol. Immunol.* 16: 358–363.

Farah, C.S., Elahi, S., Pang, G., Gotjamanos, T., Seymour, G.J., Clancy, R.L., and Ashman, R.B. (2001b). T cells augment monocyte and neutrophil function in host resistance against oropharyngeal candidiasis. *Infect. Immun.* 69: 6110–6118.

Farah, C.S., Elahi, S., Drysdale, K., Pang, G., Gotjamanos, T., Seymour, G.J., Clancy, R.L., and Ashman, R.B. (2002a). Primary role for CD4(+) T lymphocytes in recovery from oropharyngeal candidiasis. *Infect. Immun.* 70: 724–731.

Farah, C.S., Gotjamanos, T., Seymour, G.J., and Ashman, R.B. (2002b). Cytokines in the oral mucosa of mice infected with *Candida albicans. Oral Microbiol. Immunol.* 17: 375–378.

Fellermann, K. and Stange, E.F. (2001) Defensins—innate immunity at the epithelial frontier. *Eur. J. Gastroenterol. Hepatol.* 13: 771–776.

Fidel, P.L. Jr., Lynch, M.E., and Sobel, J.D. (1995a). Circulating CD4 and CD8 T cells have little impact on host defense against experimental vaginal candidiasis. *Infect. Immun.* 63: 2403–2408.

Fidel, P.L. Jr., Lynch, M.E., Conaway, D.H., Tait, L., and Sobel, J.D. (1995b). Mice immunized by primary vaginal *Candida albicans* infection

develop acquired vaginal mucosal immunity. *Infect. Immun.* 63: 547–553.
Garcia, Y.H., Diez, S.G., Aizpun, L.T., and Oliva, N.P. (2002). Antigliadin antibodies associated with chronic mucocutaneous candidiasis. *Pediatr. Dermatol.* 19: 415–418.
Ghadjari, A., Matthews, R.C., and Burnie, J.P. (1997). Epitope mapping *Candida albicans* proteinase (SAP 2). *FEMS Immunol. Med. Microbiol.* 19: 115–123.
Holmes, A.R., Bandara, B.M., and Cannon, R.D. (2002). Saliva promotes *Candida albicans* adherence to human epithelial cells. *J. Dent. Res.* 81: 28–32.
Hube, B. (2000). Extracellular proteinases of human pathogenic fungi. *Contrib. Microbiol.* 5: 126–137.
Hube, B., Sanglard, D., Odds, F.C., Hess, D., Monod, M., Schafer, W., Brown, A.J., and Gow, N.A. (1997). Disruption of each of the secreted asparty1 proteinase genes SAP1, SAP2, and SAP3 of *Candida albicans* attenuates virulence. *Infect. Immun.* 65: 3529–3538.
Intini, G., Aguirre, A., and Bobek, L.A. (2003). Efficacy of human salivary mucin MUC7-derived peptide and histatin 5 in a murine model of candidiasis. *Int. J. Antimicrob. Agents* 22: 594–600.
Ivanyi, L. and Ivanyi, J. (1990). Elevated antibody levels to mycobacterial 65-kDa stress protein in patients with superficial candidiasis. *J. Infect. Dis.* 162: 519–522.
Johansson, I., Bratt, P., Hay, D.I., Schluckebier, S., and Stromberg, N. (2000). Adhesion of *Candida albicans*, but not *Candida krusei*, to salivary statherin and mimicking host molecules. *Oral Microbiol. Immunol.* 15: 112–118.
Kantardjiev, T.V. and Popova, E.V. (2002). Anti-*Candida* antibodies in serum and saliva of patients with denture stomatitis. *Folia Med. (Plovdiv.)* 44: 39–44.
Kostiala, A.A., Jormalainen, S., and Kosunen, T.U. (1979). Detection of experimental bacteremia and fungemia by examination of buffy coat prepared by a micromethod. *Am. J. Clin. Pathol.* 72: 437–443.
Kozel, T.R., MacGill, R.S., Percival, A., and Zhou, Q. (2004). Biological activities of naturally occurring antibodies reactive with *Candida albicans* mannan. *Infect. Immun.* 72: 209–218.
Kurnatowski, P. and Kurnatowska, A.J. (1999). Fungi of *Candida* species in the pharynx and some parameters of humoral and cellular immunity in patients. *Panminerva Med.* 41: 149–151.
Lehner, T. (1970). Serum fluorescent antibody and immunoglobulin estimations in candidosis. *J. Med. Microbiol.* 3: 475–481.
Lehner, T., Wilton, J.M., and Ivanyi, L. (1972). Immunodeficiencies in chronic muco-cutaneous candidosis. *Immunology* 22: 775–787.
Leigh, J.E., Barousse, M., Swoboda, R.K., Myers, T., Hager, S., Wolf, N.A., Cutright, J.L., Thompson, J., Sobel, J.D., and Fidel, P.L. Jr. (2001). *Candida*-specific systemic cell-mediated immune reactivities in human immunodeficiency virus-positive persons with mucosal candidiasis. *J. Infect. Dis.* 183: 277–285.
Leigh, J.E., Steele, C., Wormley, F., and Fidel, P.L. Jr. (2002). Salivary cytokine profiles in the immunocompetent individual with *Candida*-associated denture stomatitis. *Oral Microbiol. Immunol.* 17: 311–314.
Macdonald, F. and Odds, F.C. (1980). Purified *Candida albicans* proteinase in the serological diagnosis of systemic candidosis. *JAMA* 243: 2409–2411.
Matthews, R.C., Burnie, J.P., and Tabaqchali, S. (1987). Isolation of immunodominant antigens from sera of patients with systemic candidiasis and characterization of serological response to *Candida albicans. J. Clin. Microbiol.* 25: 230–237.
Millon, L., Drobacheff, C., Piarroux, R., Monod, M., Reboux, G., Laurent, R., and Meillet, D. (2001). Longitudinal study of anti-*Candida albicans* mucosal immunity against aspartic proteinases in HIV-infected patients. *J. Acquir. Immune Defic. Syndr. 1* 26: 137–144.
Montagnoli, C., Bozza, S., Bacci, A., Gaziano, R., Mosci, P., Morschhauser, J., Pitzurra, L., Kopf, M., Cutler, J., and Romani, L. (2003). A role for antibodies in the generation of memory antifungal immunity. *Eur. J. Immunol.* 33: 1193–1204.
Moragues, M.D., Omaetxebarria, M.J., Elguezabal, N., Sevilla, M.J., Conti, S., Polonelli, L., and Ponton, J. (2003). A monoclonal antibody directed against a *Candida albicans* cell wall mannoprotein exerts three anti-*C. albicans* activities. *Infect. Immun.* 71: 5273–5279.
Myers, T.A., Leigh, J.E., Arribas, A.R., Hager, S., Clark, R., Lilly, E., and Fidel, P.L. Jr. (2003).

Immunohistochemical evaluation of T cells in oral lesions from human immunodeficiency virus-positive persons with oropharyngeal candidiasis. *Infect. Immun.* 71: 956–963.

Na, B.-K., Chung, G.-T., and Song, C.-Y. (1999). Production, characterisation and epitope mapping of a monoclonal antibody against aspartic proteinase of *Candida albicans. Clin. Diag. Lab. Immunol.* 6: 429–433.

Naglik, J.R., Newport, G., White, T.C., Fernandes-Naglik, L.L., Greenspan, J.S., Greenspan, D., Sweet, S.P., Challacombe, S.J., and Agabian, N. (1999). In vivo analysis of secreted aspartyl proteinase expression in human oral candidiasis. *Infect. Immun.* 67: 2482–2490.

Naglik, J.R., Rodgers, C.A., Shirlaw, P.J., Dobbie, J.L., Fernandes-Naglik, L.L., Greenspan, D., Agabian, N., and Challacombe, S.J. (2003a). Differential expression of *Candida albicans* secreted aspartyl proteinase and phospholipase B genes in humans correlates with active oral and vaginal infections. *J. Infect. Dis.* 188: 469–79.

Naglik, J.R., Challacombe, S.J., and Hube, B. (2003b). *Candida albicans* secreted aspartyl proteinases in virulence and pathogenesis. *Microbiol. Mol. Biol. Rev.* 67: 400–428.

Naglik, J.R., Scott, J., Rahman, D., Mistry, M., and Challacombe, S.J. (2005). Serum and saliva antibodies do not inhibit *Candida albicans* Sap2 proteinase activity using a BSA hydrolysis assay. *Med. Mycol.* 43: 73–77.

Netea, M.G., Van der Graaf, C.A., Vonk, A.G., Verschueren, I., Van der Meer, J.W., and Kullberg, B.J. (2002). The role of toll-like receptor (TLR) 2 and TLR4 in the host defense against disseminated candidiasis. *J. Infect. Dis.* 185: 1483–1489.

Netea, M.G., Sutmuller, R., Hermann, C., Van der Graaf, C.A., Van der Meer, J.W., van Krieken, J.H., Hartung, T., Adema, G., and Kullberg, B.J. (2004). Toll-like receptor 2 suppresses immunity against *Candida albicans* through induction of IL-10 and regulatory T cells. *J. Immunol.* 172: 3712–3718.

Nikawa, H., Jin, C., Makihira, S., Hamada, T., and Samaranayake, L.P. (2002). Susceptibility of *Candida albicans* isolates from the oral cavities of HIV-positive patients to histatin-5. *J. Prosthet. Dent.* 88: 263–267.

Nomanbhoy, F., Steele, C., Yano, J., and Fidel, P.L. Jr. (2002). Vaginal and oral epithelial cell anti-*Candida* activity. *Infect. Immun.* 70: 7081–7088.

Odds, F.C. and Webster, C.E. (1988). Effects of azole antifungals in vitro on host/parasite interactions relevant to *Candida* infections. *J. Antimicrob. Chemother.* 22: 473–481.

Palmer, D.A., Boardman, B., and Bauchner, H. (1996). Sixth and eighth graders and acquired immunodeficiency syndrome: the results of focus group analysis. *J. Adolesc. Health* 19: 297–302.

Pivarcsi, A., Bodai, L., Rethi, B., Kenderessy-Szabo, A., Koreck, A., Szell, M., Beer, Z., Bata-Csorgoo, Z., Magocsi, M., Rajnavolgyi, E., Dobozy, A., and Kemeny, L. (2003). Expression and function of toll-like receptors 2 and 4 in human keratinocytes. *Int. Immunol.* 15: 721–730.

Polonelli, L., Gerloni, M., Conti, S., Fisicaro, P., Cantelli, C., Portincasa, P., Almondo, F., Barea, P.L., Hernando, F.L., and Ponton, J. (1994). Heat-shock mannoproteins as targets of secretory IgA in *Candida albicans. J. Infect. Dis.* 69: 1401–1405.

Polonelli, L., Magliani, W., Conti, S., Bracci, L., Lozzi, L., Neri, P., Adriani, D., De Bernardis, F., and Cassone, A. (2003). Therapeutic activity of an engineered synthetic killer antiidiotypic antibody fragment against experimental mucosal and systemic candidiasis. *Infect. Immun.* 71: 6205–6212.

Rahman, D. and Challacombe, S.J. (1995). Oral immunization against mucosal candidiasis in a mouse model. *Adv. Exp. Med. Biol.* 371B: 1663–1666.

Rodier, M.H., Imbert, C., Kauffmann-Lacroix, C., Daniault, G., and Jacquemin, J.L. (2003). Immunoglobulins G could prevent adherence of *Candida albicans* to polystyrene and extracellular matrix components. *J. Med. Microbiol.* 52: 373–377.

Roeder, A., Kirschning, C.J., Rupec, R.A., Schaller, M., and Korting, H.C. (2004). Toll-like receptors and innate antifungal responses. *Trends Microbiol.* 12: 44–49.

Romani, L., Mocci, S., Cenci, E., Rossi, R., Puccetti, P., and Bistoni, F. (1991a). *Candida albicans*-specific Ly-2^{+} lymphocytes with cytolytic activity. *Eur. J. Immunol.* 21: 1567–1570.

Romani, L., Mocci, S., Bietta, C., Lanfaloni, L., Puccetti, P., and Bistoni, F. (1991b). Th1 and

Th2 cytokine secretion patterns in murine candidiasis: association of Th1 responses with acquired resistance. *Infect. Immun.* 59: 4647–4654.
Romani, L., Mencacci, A., Cenci, E., Spaccapelo, R., Mosci, P., Puccetti, P., and Bistoni, F. (1993). CD4+ subset expression in murine candidiasis. Th responses correlate directly with genetically determined susceptibility or vaccine-induced resistance. *J. Immunol.* 150: 925–931.
Romani, L., Mencacci, A., Cenci, E., Puccetti, P., and Bistoni, F. (1996). Neutrophils and the adaptive immune response to *Candida albicans*. *Res. Immunol.* 147: 512–518.
Romani, L., Bistoni, F., and Puccetti, P. (1997a). Initiation of T-helper cell immunity to *Candida albicans* by IL-12: the role of neutrophils. *Chem. Immunol.* 68: 110–135.
Romani, L., Mencacci, A., Cenci, E., Del Sero, G., Bistoni, F., and Puccetti, P. (1997b). An immunoregulatory role for neutrophils in CD4+ T helper subset selection in mice with candidiasis. *J. Immunol.* 158: 2356–2362.
Romani, L., Bistoni, F., and Puccetti, P. (1997c). Initiation of T-helper cell immunity to *Candida albicans* by IL-12: the role of neutrophils. *Chem. Immunol.* 68: 110–135.
Rouabhia, M., Ross, G., Page, N., and Chakir, J. (2002). Interleukin-18 and gamma interferon production by oral epithelial cells in response to exposure to *Candida albicans* or lipopolysaccharide stimulation. *Infect. Immun.* 70: 7073–7080.
Rüchel, R. and Boning, B. (1983). Detection of *Candida* proteinase by enzyme immunoassay and interaction of the enzyme with alpha-2-macroglobulin. *J. Immunol. Meth.* 61: 107–116.
Rüchel, R., Boning-Stutzer, B., and Mari, A. (1988). A synoptical approach to the diagnosis of candidosis, relying on serological antigen and antibody tests, on culture, and on evaluation of clinical data. *Mycoses* 31: 87–106.
Saavedra, M., Taylor, B., Lukacs, N., and Fidel, P.L. Jr. (1999). Local production of chemokines during experimental vaginal candidiasis. *Infect. Immun.* 67: 5820–5826.
Sanglard, D., Hube, B., Monod, M., Odds, F.C., and Gow, N.A. (1997). A triple deletion of the secreted aspartyl proteinase genes SAP4, SAP5, and SAP6 of *Candida albicans* causes attenuated virulence. *Infect. Immun.* 65: 3539–3546.
San-Millan, R., Elguezabal, N., Regulez, P., Moragues, M.D., Quindos, G., and Ponton, J. (2000). Effect of salivary secretory IgA on the adhesion of *Candida albicans* to polystyrene. *Microbiology* 146: 2105–2112.
Sawaki, K., Mizukawa, N., Yamaai, T., Fukunaga, J., and Sugahara, T. (2002). Immunohistochemical study on expression of alpha-defensin and beta-defensin-2 in human buccal epithelia with candidiasis. *Oral Dis.* 8: 37–41.
Schaller, M., Korting, H.C., Schafer, W., Bastert, J., Chen, W., and Hube, B. (1999). Secreted aspartic proteinase (Sap) activity contributes to tissue damage in a model of human oral candidosis. *Mol. Microbiol.* 34: 169–180.
Shi, J., Zhang, G., Wu, H., Ross, C., Blecha, F., and Ganz, T. (1999). Porcine epithelial beta-defensin 1 is expressed in the dorsal tongue at antimicrobial concentrations. *Infect. Immun.* 67: 3121–3127.
Steele, C. and Fidel, P.L. Jr. (2002) Cytokine and chemokine production by human oral and vaginal epithelial cells in response to *Candida albicans*. *Infect. Immun.* 70: 577–583.
Steele, C., Ozenci, H., Luo, W., Scott, M., and Fidel, P.L. Jr. (1999). Growth inhibition of *Candida albicans* by vaginal cells from naive mice. *Med. Mycol.* 37: 251–259.
Steele, C., Leigh, J., Swoboda, R., Ozenci, H., and Fidel, P.L. Jr. (2001). Potential role for a carbohydrate moiety in anti-*Candida* activity of human oral epithelial cells. *Infect. Immun.* 69: 7091–7099.
Sullivan, D.J., Westerneng, T.J., Haynes, K.A., Bennett, D.E., and Coleman, D.C. (1995). *Candida dubliniensis* sp. nov.: phenotypic and molecular characterization of a novel species associated with oral candidosis in HIV-infected individuals. *Microbiology* 141: 1507–1521.
Sweet, S.P., Cookson, S., and Challacombe, S.J. (1995). *Candida albicans* isolates from HIV-infected and AIDS patients exhibit enhanced adherence to epithelial cells. *J. Med. Microbiol.* 43: 452–457.
Swoboda, R., Miyasaki, S., Greenspan, D., and Greenspan, J.S. (1993). Heat-inducible ATP-binding proteins of *Candida albicans* are recognized by sera of infected patients. *J. Gen. Microbiol.* 139: 2995–3003.
Tollemar, J., Gross, N., Dolgiras, N., Jarstrand, C., Ringden, O., and Hammarstrom, L. (1999).

Fungal prophylaxis by reduction of fungal colonization by oral administration of bovine anti-*Candida* antibodies in bone marrow transplant recipients. *Bone Marrow Transplant.* 23: 283–290.

Triebel, T., Grillhosl, B., Kacani, L., Lell, C.P., Fuchs, A., Speth, C., Lass-Florl, C., Steinmann, J., Dierich, M.P., and Wurzner, R. (2003). Importance of the terminal complement components for immune defence against *Candida*. *Int. J. Med. Microbiol.* 292: 527–536.

Valdimarsson, H., Higgs, J.M., Wells, R.S., Yamamura, M., Hobbs, J.R., and Holt, P.J. (1973). Immune abnormalities associated with chronic mucocutaneous candidiasis. *Cell Immunol.* 6: 348–361.

van Wyk, C.W. and van der, B.P. (1994). Retention of acquired resistance to *C. albicans* by mice during short term immunosuppression. *J. Dent. Assoc. S. Afr.* 49: 15–20.

Wagner, R.D, Vazquez, T.A, Jones, C.J, Warner, T., and Balish, E. (1996). B Cell knockout mice are resistant to mucosal and systemic candidiasis of endogenous origin but susceptible to experimental systemic candidiasis. *J. Infect. Dis.* 174: 589–597.

Watts, H.J., Cheah, F.S., Hube, B., Sanglard, D., and Gow, N.A. (1998). Altered adherence in strains of *Candida albicans* harbouring null mutations in secreted aspartic proteinase genes. *FEMS Microbiol. Lett.* 159: 129–135.

Wellington, M., Bliss, J.M., and Haidaris, C.G. (2003). Enhanced phagocytosis of *Candida* species mediated by opsonization with a recombinant human antibody single-chain variable fragment. *Infect. Immun.* 71: 7228–7231.

Wozniak, K.L., Leigh, J.E., Hager, S., Swoboda, R.K., and Fidel, P.L. Jr. (2002). A comprehensive study of *Candida*-specific antibodies in the saliva of human immunodeficiency virus-positive individuals with oropharyngeal candidiasis. *J. Infect. Dis.* 185: 1269–1276.

Yeh, C.K., Dodds, M.W., Zuo, P., and Johnson, D.A. (1997). A population-based study of salivary lysozyme concentrations and candidal counts. *Arch. Oral Biol.* 42: 25–31.

4

Oral Candidiasis: Clinical Manifestations and Cellular Adaptive Host Responses

Robert B. Ashman and Camile S. Farah

School of Dentistry, University of Queensland, Brisbane, Queensland, Australia.

1. Introduction

Many *Candida* species are commensals of the oral mucosa. They are usually innocuous, but when conditions are favorable, they can proliferate and cause disease. *Candida* spp. are readily isolated from various sites within the oral cavity, but simple carriage does not inevitably result in the development of clinical symptoms. Whether the organism remains as a commensal, or proliferates and causes disease, is usually determined by preexisting or concomitant alterations in the integrity of the immune system.

Oral candidiasis is seen most frequently in patients at-risk, such as those suffering from HIV/acquired immunodeficiency syndrome (AIDS), immunosuppression, diabetes, xerostomia, or those wearing dentures (Fotos and Hellstein, 1992); however, clinical observations in these and other patient groups have suggested that these predisposing factors are almost invariably associated with deficiencies in innate and adaptive immune functions that compromise effective host responses against the infection. The seminal observations by Kirkpatrick and colleagues (1971) on children with chronic mucocutaneous candidiasis (CMC) strongly implicated defects in cell-mediated immunity as a major predisposing factor, and the importance of T lymphocytes, and $CD4^+$ cells in particular, has been confirmed by the high incidence of oral candidiasis in HIV-infected individuals whose $CD4^+$ lymphocyte counts are declining.

In this chapter, the epidemiology of the disease, associated risk factors, and clinical features are briefly outlined. This is followed by reviews of the host immune factors relevant to recovery from oral infection in humans and mice, and the discussion concludes with an evaluation of the ways in which these immune mechanisms may relate to the clinical manifestations of the disease.

2. Epidemiology of Oral Candidiasis

2.1. *Candida* Species

Candidiasis is most commonly caused by the yeast *C. albicans*, and to a far lesser extent by *C. glabrata*, *C. krusei*, *C. tropicalis*, *C. pseudotropicalis*, *C. parapsilosis*, and *C. guilliermondi* (Odds, 1988). More recently, oral candidiasis in HIV-positive individuals has been associated with *C. dubliniensis* (Sullivan et al., 1995).

C. albicans is a commensal residing in the oral cavity of the majority of healthy persons (Odds, 1988). It is a dimorphic fungus that can exist both in a yeast phase (blastospore, blastoconidial) and a hyphal (mycelial) phase. Depending on the environmental conditions, they may develop either in the mycelial form, composed of long branching septae or filaments, or as spherical or ovoid yeast cells. In the yeast phase *C. albicans* are from 2–8 to 3–14 μm in size, but hyphae can extend a few hundred micrometers (Saltarelli, 1989). They reproduce by multilateral budding and do not undergo a sexual cycle. Dimorphism is relevant both to the pathogenicity of the yeast and to the clinical problems of diagnosis and treatment (Saltarelli, 1989).

C. albicans is the most common *Candida* species isolated from the oral cavity both in the healthy and the diseased (Samaranayake and MacFarlane, 1990). Symptom-free oral carriage of *Candida* organisms has been recognized for many years, with the reported prevalence ranging from 3% to 48% in clinically normal mouths of healthy adults (Arendorf and Walker, 1980), and 45% to 65% in healthy children (Odds, 1988). The oral carriage of yeasts is higher in hospitalized than ambulant patients, with a median carriage rate of 54.7% for all species and 38.1% for *C. albicans* alone (Wilkieson et al., 1991).

In the past *C. dubliniensis* was probably identified as an atypical strain of *C. albicans*. Although it was initially found to colonize the oral cavity and to be a cause of oropharyngeal candidiasis (OPC) in HIV-positive patients (Sullivan et al., 1995), it has since been found to colonize and infect various other groups (Redding, 2001; Kantarcioglu and Yucel, 2002; Tekeli et al., 2002). Incidence rates for *C. dubliniensis* in oral cultures from adults vary from 3% in asymptomatic HIV-negative individuals to 32% in HIV-positive patients with clinical signs and symptoms of OPC (Coleman et al., 1997; Meiller et al., 1999; Fisher et al., 2001; Giammanco et al., 2002). *C. dubliniensis* has also been detected in pediatric patients (Sano et al., 2000), with one study reporting positive cultures in 11% of HIV-positive pediatric patients (Brown et al., 2000). Mixed infections, especially with *C. albicans*, are common in patients who are positive for oral *C. dubliniensis* (Schorling et al., 2000).

C. glabrata is much less pathogenic than *C. albicans*, but in recent years it has emerged as a significant pathogen in humans. It is currently the second to third leading cause of candidiasis of all kinds and comprises approximately 5% of all *Candida* isolates (Thuraisingam and Denning, 2000). The role of *C. glabrata* in OPC is controversial, and the yeast is mostly seen in cases of systemic candidiasis. *C. glabrata* is commonly isolated along with *C. albicans* when cultured from patients with OPC. *C. glabrata* makes up between 5% and 10% of all oral isolates recovered from HIV positive patients who have OPC (Fidel et al., 1999). OPC can be caused solely by *C. glabrata* (Hoegl et al., 1998), with one study reporting that up to 14% of all oropharyngeal infections were caused by this species (Masia Canuto et al., 2000). It was estimated that approximately 30% of patients over 80 years of age were colonized orally with *C. glabrata* (Lockhart et al., 1999), but the percentage was almost doubled if the patients wore dentures.

OPC caused by *C. tropicalis* has been reported but is relatively rare. Colonization on the other hand is quite common; approximately 6% of yeast isolates other than *C. albicans* in HIV-positive patients are *C. tropicalis* (Cartledge et al., 1999). It is a pathogenic organism, especially in patients receiving chemotherapy for hematologic malignancies, and OPC associated with *C. tropicalis* can cause fungemia in these patients (Redding, 2001).

Oral colonization with *C. krusei* is common, making up approximately 20% of yeasts other than *C. albicans* cultured in HIV-positive patients (Cartledge et al., 1999), but OPC caused by *C. krusei* alone is rare.

2.2. Pathogen Risk Factors

Oral infection with *Candida* is associated with certain pathogenic variables. Adhesion of the yeast to epithelial cell walls, an important first step of infection, is promoted by fungal wall components such as mannose, C3d receptors, mannoprotein, and saccharins (Ghannoum et al., 1986; Brassart et al., 1991; Kanbe et al., 1991). Hydrophobicity (Hazen et al., 1991) and the ability to bind to host fibronectin (Klotz and Smith, 1991) are also important pathogenic mechanisms used by the yeast in the initial stages of infection. Some other factors important in host infection include germ tube formation (Sobel et al., 1984), presence of mycelia (Saltarelli et al., 1975), endotoxins (Cutler et al., 1972), and proteinases (Kwon-Chung et al., 1985).

The family of secreted aspartyl proteinases (SAPs) are considered to be one of the more important of the putative virulence factors of *C. albicans*. Analysis of patients with asymptomatic *Candida* carriage, and those with oral candidiasis, showed that

SAP2 and SAPs 4 to 6 were expressed in both subpopulations, whereas SAP1 and SAP3 were observed only in patients with oral disease (Naglik et al., 1999). More extensive studies (Naglik et al., 2003a) confirmed that SAP2 and SAP5 were the most common genes expressed during both infection and carriage, whereas expression of SAP1, SAP3, SAP4, SAP7, and SAP8 correlated with oral disease. Using an in vitro model, the gene products of SAPs1 to 3, but not SAPs4 to 6, appeared to be predominantly responsible for damage to reconstituted human epithelium (Schaller et al., 1999), although studies with specific SAP mutants suggested that the yeast may have the ability to compensate for the loss of one SAP gene by the upregulation of others.

Interestingly, viable, but not heat-killed *Candida*, was able to induce increased expression of genes coding for a variety of immunologically relevant cytokines and chemokines by epithelial cells (Schaller et al., 2002), and cytokine production correlated with the virulence of the organism. This suggests that the "quality" of the infectious challenge may influence the nature of the immune response elicited. This concept will be considered later, in relation to the different manifestations of oral infection.

2.3. Host Risk Factors

Although the transition from commensalism to disease may be associated with the virulence characteristics of the organism, it is widely accepted that host factors are of paramount importance in the development of the infection. *Candida* species are strictly opportunistic pathogens, which cause disease when the host defenses are defective—hence the designation "disease of the diseased" given to *Candida* infections (Trousseau, 1869).

The local intraoral environmental milieu, such as the presence of prostheses, plays a crucial role in the disease process. Indeed it is the combination of the microbial virulence factors, environmental factors, and host defense factors that determines the ultimate outcome of infection. The major local and systemic factors that predispose humans to candidiasis have been classified as natural, dietary, mechanical, and iatrogenic (Odds, 1988), but only those relevant to immune dysfunction are considered here.

Host defense mechanisms are impaired in patients with malignant disease, particularly as a consequence of chemotherapy and radiotherapy. Longitudinal studies of patients undergoing radiation therapy to the head and neck show significant increases in *Candida* species counts on the tongue surface, in whole saliva, and in dental plaque (Epstein et al., 1984; Samaranayake et al., 1988). Therapeutic interventions can also reduce numbers and impair the function of polymorphonuclear and mononuclear phagocytes, leading to oral candidiasis (Kostiala, 1986).

Chronic hyperplastic candidiasis may occur as part of CMC, often with identifiable immunologic or endocrine abnormalities as major factors. Endocrine disorders such as hypothyroidism, hypoparathyroidism, and adrenal insufficiency, have a familial incidence and are found in children and young adults, particularly in girls. The most frequently associated endocrine manifestations include idiopathic hyperparathyroidism and hypoadrenocorticism, but candidiasis follows only where there is an immune defect (Kostiala et al., 1979).

Fungal infections, particularly atrophic and pseudomembranous candidiasis, are common in patients with HIV infection. The immunodeficiency affecting T helper lymphocytes during HIV infection makes patients with the disease more predisposed to secondary infections, notably opportunistic *Candida* infections. The first patient diagnosed with AIDS presented with oral candidiasis (Gottlieb et al., 1981a), and oral candidiasis was a common feature in patients who eventually developed AIDS (Gottlieb et al.,

1981b). Oral candidiasis occurs in 75% of HIV-positive patients (Palmer et al., 1996) and 92% of patients diagnosed with AIDS had oral candidiasis (McCarthy et al., 1991). Indeed more than 90% of patients who are HIV-positive will develop at least one episode of oral candidiasis during the progression to AIDS. The erythematous variant is most frequently seen in these patients, followed by the pseudomembranous, angular cheilitis, and then hyperplastic candidiasis (Samaranayake and MacFarlane, 1990).

A myriad of immunological abnormalities occur as a consequence of HIV infection, particularly as the disease progresses to AIDS (Fauci, 1993). Monocytes and macrophages express CD4, and HIV can directly infect these cells (Alkhatib et al., 1996). There are also other alterations to mononuclear phagocyte function including alterations in phenotypic marker expression, accessory cell function, chemotaxis, cytokine production, and respiratory burst activity (Ho et al., 1994; Trial et al., 1995; Wahl et al., 1996). Nonetheless, profound $CD4^+$ T cell depletion is the immunological hallmark of AIDS, and is the most likely factor accounting for the increased susceptibility of these patients to opportunistic infections. The role for $CD4^+$ T cells in host resistance against opportunistic fungal infections is supported by the frequent occurrence of fungal infections in patients with idiopathic $CD4^+$ T cell lymphocytopenia, a condition characterized by low $CD4^+$ counts in the absence of HIV infection (Duncan et al., 1993).

Oral candidiasis occurs in association with congenital deficiencies in both innate and adaptive immunity. Chronic recalcitrant mucocutaneous candidiasis is particularly common in patients with DiGeorge's syndrome (Cleveland et al., 1968), a condition characterized by depletion of T cells in the thymus-dependent areas of lymph nodes and in peripheral blood due to thymic hypoplasia. Patients with severe combined immunodeficiency (SCID) syndrome demonstrate multiple defects in cell-mediated immune functions, and frequently suffer from CMC that may disseminate to other tissues (Porter and Scully, 1990). Syndromes that affect innate immunity include hereditary myeloperoxidase (MPO) deficiency, in which the lack of MPO in the granules of polymorphonuclear leukocytes (PMNLs) and macrophages results in impaired killing of *C. albicans* (Lehrer and Cline, 1969; Klebanoff, 1970), and predisposes to recurrent episodes of oral thrush or CMC in these patients (Lehrer and Cline, 1969; Kirkpatrick et al., 1971). Patients with Chediak–Higashi syndrome, an autosomal recessive disease presenting with abnormal neutrophils, neutropenia, and impaired chemotaxis (Wolff, 1972; Oliver and Essner, 1975), also commonly suffer from candidal infections.

3. Clinical Manifestations of Oral Candidiasis

The classification of oral candidiasis has been fraught with difficulties and complications, due to the many manifestations the disease can take and because of the multifaceted etiology of the different conditions involved. Recently, it has been suggested that oral candidiasis can be arranged into two categories based on the distribution of the lesions (Scully et al., 1994): Category I, candidal infections confined to oral and perioral tissues (primary oral candidiasis) and Category II, disorders where oral candidiasis is a manifestation of generalized systemic mucocutaneous candidal infection (secondary oral candidiasis). Category II lesions are divided into subgroups, which take into account CMC and other immune defect disorders such as SCID syndrome, DiGeorge's syndrome, and AIDS.

The following clinical descriptions are based on revised classifications by Samaranayake and Yaacob (1990), Holmstrup and Axell (1990), and Samaranayake (1991).

denture-bearing mucosa, especially under maxillary prostheses (Fig. 4.1c). The patient is usually symptom-free, but may complain of slight soreness and angular cheilitis can be a presenting complaint. Other factors such as bacterial accumulation, reduced salivary protection, and mechanical irritation may be implicated in denture stomatitis, which is present in approximately 50% of complete denture wearers (Budtz-Jorgensen, 1974). Histological examination of the tissues beneath the dentures shows proliferative or degenerative responses (Razek and Shaaban, 1978) with reduced keratinization and thinner epithelium (Watson and MacDonald, 1982). Tissue invasion by *Candida* does not occur as commonly as other forms of oral candidiasis, and relatively little yeast is isolated from the mucosal surface (Budtz-Jorgensen, 1974).

3.5. Angular Cheilitis

Clinically, angular cheilitis presents as sore, erythematous, fissured lesions, affecting the angles of the mouth, and is commonly associated with denture stomatitis (Fig. 4.1d) (Budtz-Jorgensen, 1974). In orofacial granulomatosis, a significant number of patients have angular cheilitis (Samaranayake, 1988), and it may also be seen in AIDS (Samaranayake and Holmstrup, 1989). As mentioned earlier, the condition can be associated with iron deficiency anemia or vitamin B_{12} deficiency (Scully and Cawson, 1998).

3.6. Median Rhomboid Glossitis

Median rhomboid glossitis is characterized by an area of papillary atrophy that is elliptical or rhomboid-like, symmetrically placed and centered at the midline of the tongue, anterior to the circumvallate papillae (Fig. 4.1e) (Walker and Arendorf, 1990). Occasionally, midline glossitis presents with a hyperplastic exophytic or lobulated appearance. Histopathologically, candidal hyphae are seen invading the superficial layers of the parakeratotic epithelium with elongated hyperplastic rete ridges extending into the corium, a PMNL infiltrate occupying the epithelium, and a lymphocyte infiltration in the corium erupting into the bases of the epithelial processes (Walker and Arendorf, 1990).

3.7. Chronic Mucocutaneous Candidiasis

CMC is a term given to a group of heterogeneous disorders that are characterized by persistent superficial candidal infection of the mouth, skin, and nail beds, sometimes producing granulomatous masses over the face and scalp (Fig. 4.1b) (Kirkpatrick et al., 1971; Edwards et al., 1978). The principal clinical features include chronic oral candidiasis, chronic cutaneous candidiasis, and chronic vulvovaginal candidiasis (Chilgren et al., 1967). Oral candidiasis has been observed in more than 90% of all CMC patients (Odds, 1988). The tongue can become enlarged, fissured, and may have hyperplastic nodules on the lateral borders. Painful angular cheilitis is frequent (Porter and Scully, 1990). CMC is associated with a variety of primary immunodeficiencies such as SCID syndrome, Nezelof's syndrome (thymic alymphoplasia), DiGeorge syndrome (congenital thymic aplasia), hyperimmunoglobulin E syndrome, MPO deficiency, and endocrine disorders, especially Addison's disease and hypoparathyroidism (Porter and Scully, 1990, 1993a,b). The oral lesions of CMC have histopathological features similar to those of chronic candidiasis (Cawson and Lehner, 1968), although candidal infection can occasionally spread into the pharynx, larynx, or esophagus, but further visceral involvement is rare (Porter and Scully, 1990).

4. Cellular Adaptive Host Responses

4.1. Clinical Studies

CMC is frequently seen in association with endocrinopathies (Kirkpatrick et al., 1971), but it is generally recognized that the main predisposing factor is a defect in cell-mediated immunity (Kirkpatrick, 1994). These patients can be grouped according to their specific abnormalities in immunological responsiveness (Kirkpatrick, 1989), but there is no *Candida*-specific defect common to all groups. Nevertheless, therapy directed at restoration of cellular immune function generally results in remission, and the demonstrable link between systemic cell-mediated immunity and mucosal defense mechanisms has been crucial in developing an understanding of the pathogenesis of the disease.

The link between CMC, immunodeficiency, and endocrinopathies is now well-recognized, but with the spread of HIV infection and AIDS, and the increasing use of aggressive chemotherapeutic regimens for transplantation and cancer patients, severe oropharyngeal infections are appearing in a much greater variety of clinical contexts. These include situations in which there is a deficiency in cell-mediated immune responses, as well as others in which the dominant feature is neutropenia. These observations suggest that host responses against oral and OPC may involve not only cells of the adaptive immune response, but also phagocytic cells, and other nonspecific innate immune effector mechanisms.

Human epithelial cells from the oral cavity have recently been shown to possess inhibitory activity against both *Candida* yeasts and hyphae (Steele et al., 2000). The anti-*Candida* activity required cell contact, and in these experiments, neither saliva nor culture supernatants alone inhibited *Candida* growth, nor was the epithelial cell activity enhanced in the presence of saliva. Although differential staining showed that the effect of the epithelial cells was candidastatic rather than candidacidal (Nomanbhoy et al., 2002), the phenomenon may be of some biological significance, as epithelial cell anti-*Candida* activity was significantly lower in HIV-positive patients with OPC (Steele et al., 2000). The oral epithelial cells may also act to enhance effector cell activity through the production of cytokines and/or chemokines that increase recruitment of phagocytic cells and stimulate innate immunity.

After challenge with *C. albicans*, primary oral mucosal epithelial cells and oral epithelial cell lines produced interleukin-8 (IL-8) (Dongari-Bagtzoglou and Kashleva, 2003b), and a proportion also produced granulocyte-macrophage colony-stimulating factor (GM-CSF) (Dongari-Bagtzoglou and Kashleva, 2003a). Both responses were dependent on physical contact with viable yeasts and were optimal when the yeast germinated into hyphae. IL-8 secretion was dependent, at least in part, on autocrine production of IL-1α (Dongari-Bagtzoglou and Kashleva, 2003b). In addition, oral fibroblasts have been shown to produce both IL-6 and IL-8 after exposure to *C. albicans* in culture (Dongari-Bagtzoglou et al., 1999). Thus, the oral mucosa may, after infection, produce a cytokine microenvironment that is able to influence the development and maturation of the cell-mediated immune response against the yeast.

It is currently believed that host responses against *C. albicans* are determined predominantly by the relative dominance of Th1-type cytokines that lead to recovery and the development of protection, or Th2-type cytokines, that are associated with susceptibility to infection (Romani, 1999). However, studies in humans have given variable results. Adult patients with chronic oral candidiasis showed significantly lower levels of serum IFN-γ healthy controls (Szkaradkiewicz et al., 1998), but there have been no more recent studies of oral candidiasis in the absence of other infections.

Analysis of salivary cytokine profiles in normal (HIV-negative) individuals showed a Th0/Th1 profile, whereas in HIV-positive individuals, it was of a predominantly Th2-type (Leigh et al., 1998), apparently as a consequence of a reduction in Th1-type rather than an enhancement of Th2-type cytokines. HIV-positive individuals with OPC tended to show a more exaggerated Th2-type salivary cytokine profile, but the relevance of this to the pathogenesis of the *Candida* infection is unclear at present. Both HIV-positive and HIV-negative patients displayed *Candida*-specific lymphocyte proliferative responses, and although skin test reactivity to *C. albicans* antigens in HIV-positive patients with low $CD4^+$ cell counts was reduced compared to controls (Leigh et al., 2001), there were no consistent differences in systemic immune responses that correlated with the development of OPC.

Denture stomatitis is another manifestation of oral infection with *C. albicans*, although the extent of colonization appears to be related to the severity of the inflammation induced by external factors, such as smoking or the wearing of dentures at night (Barbeau et al., 2003). Patients with *Candida*-associated denture stomatitis show impaired responses against antigens of *C. albicans*, as demonstrated by skin test and leukocyte migration inhibition assays (Davenport and Wilton, 1971), and may have overactive suppressor T cells or other lymphocyte/phagocyte defects (Iacopino and Wathen, 1992), indicating that normal immunoregulatory responses can also be impaired.

Nevertheless, analysis of salivary cytokines in HIV-negative individuals either with or without denture stomatitis demonstrated a mixed Th1/Th2 profile (Leigh et al., 2002), with no significant differences between the two groups, indicating that susceptibility to *Candida*-associated denture stomatitis in the immunocompetent patient was not associated with a bias towards production of Th2-type cytokines. In contrast, analysis of serum levels of interleukins and their soluble receptors found significant increases in the concentrations of IL-6 and TNF-α in both patients with dentures, and those with denture stomatitis, compared to normal controls (Pietruski et al., 2000), whereas concentrations of soluble TNF receptor were reduced in these same groups.

Phenotypic analysis by immunohistochemistry and electron microscopy of cells of the oral mucosal immune system present in biopsies of erythematous and pseudomembranous candidiasis in HIV-positive patients has shown that the superficial lamina propria and basal epithelial layer was populated by $CD1a^+$ Langerhans cells, with an infiltration of $CD8^+$ lymphocytes. $CD36^+$ dendritic macrophages and lymphocytes were detected within the submucosa, although $CD4^+$ cells were absent from the infiltrate (Romagnoli et al., 1997). In the pseudomembranous form, $CD14^+$ leukocytes were found in the basal epithelial layer. Langerhans cells were significantly more numerous in erythematous than in pseudomembranous candidiasis. It is clear that oral candidiasis is associated with perturbations in the number and state of differentiation of lymphocytes and dendritic cells, these being more severe in the pseudomembranous than in the erythematous form. These alterations may play a role in the pathogenesis and evolution of the disease (Romagnoli et al., 1997).

Further immunohistochemical evaluation of T cells in both HIV-negative and HIV-positive individuals showed a majority of $CD8^+$ rather than $CD4^+$ cells equally distributed throughout the buccal mucosa in cases where these patients were OPC-negative, irrespective of blood $CD4^+$ cell numbers. In contrast, $CD8^+$ cells in lesions from HIV-positive/OPC-positive persons were present in significantly higher numbers, and concentrated at the lamina propria–epithelium interface, a considerable distance from the *Candida* at the outer epithelium. Dual fluorescence and confocal microscopy confirmed that the majority of $CD8^+$, but not $CD4^+$ cells, were T cells by the presence or absence, respectively, of CD3 on each cell type. These results suggest that $CD8^+$ T cells may be important for oral host defense against OPC, especially when $CD4^+$ T cell numbers are reduced (Myers et al., 2003).

Characterization of the inflammatory cell infiltrate in oral mucosal biopsy material of chronic hyperplastic candidiasis (Williams et al., 1997) showed that T lymphocytes were the dominant cell type, with fewer macrophages and B lymphocytes. Many Ig-containing cells were seen, and although IgG-containing cells predominated, there was a high proportion of IgA-containing cells with few IgM-containing cells. Many neutrophils, together with smaller numbers of T lymphocytes and macrophages, were seen in the epithelium. These authors have suggested that mucosal defense to *Candida* infection involves a cell-mediated reaction in which there is recruitment of macrophages and local production of immunoglobulin with a prominent IgA component.

4.2. Mouse Models

Mucosal candidiasis has been studied in a number of different models—gastrointestinal (GI), vaginal, and oral—and it has perhaps been too readily assumed that results obtained from infection of one particular mucosal site (e.g., the GI tract) can be extrapolated to other manifestations of the disease. It has recently become clear that this is not the case (Fidel, 2002), and that there may be significant differences in the "mix" of adaptive and innate immune responses that mediate responsiveness to *Candida* at the different mucosal sites. Nevertheless, many valuable insights have been obtained by Balish and colleagues using infection of the GI tract, and in the following discussion, attempts will be made to integrate these findings with those from the various oral models.

Models used for the study of oral candidiasis have been of three kinds: those using normal mice (Lacasse et al., 1993; Elahi et al., 2000; Farah et al., 2001a), those using immunodeficient mice (Farah et al., 2002b), and those that involve conditioning by treatment with immunosuppressive drugs (Kamai et al., 2001; Takakura et al., 2003).

4.2.1. Studies in Normal Mice

In general, the study of oral infection in normal mice has sought to identify crucial host variables by comparison of responses in genetically defined inbred mice. In inbred mice, oral candidiasis closely resembles the human disease (Farah et al., 2002b). BALB/c and DBA/2 mice are of the same major histocompatibility complex (MHC) type, but BALB/c is C5-sufficient, whereas DBA/2 is C5-deficient. Although DBA/2 mice were somewhat more prone to infection than BALB/c mice (Chakir et al., 1994), oral infection in both strains resulted in an increase in $MAC\text{-}1^+$ cells and a comparable recruitment of $CD4^+$ and $CD8^+$ T lymphocytes into the mucosal tissue. Thus, in contrast to systemic infection, complement-derived chemotactic factors appear to have little or no effect on inflammatory processes in the oral mucosa. In addition, the number of intraepithelial $CD4^+$ T cells was five- to sevenfold greater in infected animals when compared to control mice (Deslauriers et al., 1995). Using the same mouse strains, Elahi and colleagues (2000) demonstrated significantly higher *Candida* specific proliferation by cells from the draining lymph nodes of BALB/c as compared to DBA/2 mice, after oral infection.

Although these studies in vitro strongly implicated T cells in the host response against oral infection, initial attempts to demonstrate their essential role in host resistance in normal mice by antibody depletion of CD4 or CD8 cells mice were unsuccessful. However, when the head and neck were irradiated, at a dose sufficient to block lymphocyte proliferation, depletion of $CD4^+$, but not $CD8^+$, lymphocytes caused a prolongation of infection and increased the severity of oral lesions (Farah et al., 2001b). This was interpreted as indicating that the immune response in the oral cavity was essentially self-contained, but that $CD4^+$ cells from the systemic circulation had the potential to exert a protective effect. An alternative, but not mutually exclusive explanation, is that irradiation-induced tissue damage favored further proliferation of the yeast. This could place additional demands on the local immune response, resulting in recruitment of $CD4^+$ cells from the peripheral circulation. In the irradiated mice, recovery from infection was associated with production of high levels of IL-12 by lymph node cells, but concentrations of IFN-γ in infected mice were comparable to those in controls.

The importance of T cells and cell-mediated immunity in oral candidiasis has been supported by studies in infectious disease models. Mice infected with the Du5H(G6T2) mixture of mouse leukemia viruses develop a disease (murine AIDS or MAIDS) that exhibits many of the immune abnormalities found in human HIV infection. When these animals were orally colonized with *C. albicans*, approximately 30% developed recurring 2- to 3-week episodes of acute *Candida* proliferation, which were thought to result from virally induced fluctuations in the levels of $CD4^+$ T cells (Deslauriers et al., 1997). Similarly, transgenic mice that expressed HIV type 1 in immune cells (de Repentigny et al., 2002) showed a sustained enhancement of oral burdens of *C. albicans*, penetration by *Candida* hyphae of the stratified squamous epithelium of the oral cavity, and a mononuclear inflammatory cell infiltrate in the mucosa.

These results are generally consistent with those derived from models of orogastric candidiasis. Euthymic mice infected in this manner developed *Candida*-specific lymphoproliferative and delayed-type hypersensitivity (DTH) responses that correlated with the clearance of hyphae from mucosal surfaces (Balish et al., 1990). Conversely, depletion of $CD4^+$ lymphocytes from T cell-sufficient *bg/bg nu/*$^+$ mice using an anti-CD4 monoclonal antibody increased their susceptibility to *Candida* infection of the tongue and esophagus (Cantorna and Balish, 1991), and confirmed that the $CD4^+$ cell population was crucial for protection of mice from orogastric candidiasis, although neither IL-2 nor IFN-γ was essential for an effective host response. In disseminated candidiasis, the different subsets of $CD4^+$ T helper cells, and cytokines produced by them, show a strong correlation with susceptibility and protection from infection (Romani, 1999), and parallels have been drawn between this and GI infection.

For example, BALB/c mice are resistant to systemic challenge with an avirulent isolate of *C. albicans*, and protective host responses are associated with a Th1 cytokine profile (Romani et al., 1993). In contrast, systemic infection of these mice with a virulent isolate causes early mortality, whereas GI colonization with the virulent yeast results in the production of both Th1- and Th2-type cytokines by $CD4^+$ cells from Peyer's patches and mesenteric lymph nodes, and clearance of the yeast from the intestine (Cenci et al., 1995). DBA/2Cr mice develop fatal disseminated candidiasis after intravenous infection with the avirulent strain of *C. albicans* (Romani et al., 1993), but intragastric inoculation with the virulent strain was again associated with the induction of Th1-type cell-mediated immune responses and eventual clearance of the infection (Bistoni et al., 1993).

These data suggest that activation of Th1-type cytokine responses is associated with recovery from orogastric *Candida* infection, but the nature of the effector pathways, and the relevance of the Th2-like response in the "resistant" BALB/c strain, have not yet been resolved.

4.2.2. Studies in Immunodeficient Mice

C. albicans is recognized as an organism that is uniquely adept in exploiting deficiencies in host responsiveness, and significant advances have been made in understanding yeast–host relationships by the use of mutant and genetically modified mice. In humans, cellular immunodeficiency, particularly that associated with HIV infection, substantially increases the risk of mucosal infections with *C. albicans*, and this condition has been modeled by the use of the T cell-deficient "nude" mouse.

Nude mice were shown to be markedly more susceptible to oral infection than euthymic controls (Farah et al., 2002b), and developed a chronic infection. There was extensive hyphal penetration of the oral epithelium, associated with infiltration of PMNLs and the formation of microabscesses. Mice of the CBA/CaH strain that are predisposed to severe tissue pathology (Ashman and Papadimitriou, 1987) acquired a greater fungal burden and developed more severe lesions after oral infection than the "low pathology" BALB/c mice. This is consistent with the regulation of tissue susceptibility by the *Carg1* gene (Ashman, 1998). Established infections in nude mice could be cleared by the adoptive transfer of syngeneic lymphocytes (Farah et al., 2002b), and the protective effect was mediated by the $CD4^+$, but not the $CD8^+$ lymphocyte subset. After reconstitution, IFN-γ and IL-12 were produced by lymphocytes from the cervical and submaxillary lymph nodes of the infected mice, but IL-4 and IL-10 were generally not detected.

Similar conclusions have been drawn from studies of orogastric candidiasis. Nude mice were unable to clear *Candida* from the stomach or the tongue (Balish et al., 1990), and did not develop either DTH or lymphoproliferative responses to *C. albicans* antigens. After intragastric or oral inoculation, both SCID mice, which lack functional T and B cells, and multiply-immunodeficient (*bg/bg, nu/nu*) mice, which are deficient in both T cells and phagocytic cells, develop a persistent GI infection, whereas mice that lack only phagocytic cells (*bg/bg, nu/$^+$*) are able to clear the infection efficiently (Cantorna and Balish, 1990). Transgenic epsilon 26 mice have defects in both natural killer cells and T cells and are highly susceptible to oro-esophageal and gastric candidiasis (Balish et al., 2001), but resistant to acute systemic candidiasis and systemic candidiasis of endogenous origin. Granulocytes were the major effector population responsible for protection against systemic infection (Balish et al., 2001), whereas T cells appeared to be essential for protection against mucosal infection. In contrast, B cell knockout (KO) mice, which lack both functional B cells and antibodies, were as resistant to orogastric candidiasis as immunocompetent controls (Narayanan et al., 1991), further substantiating a convincing case that cell-mediated immunity plays a central role in host protection against mucocutaneous candidiasis.

4.2.3. γ/δ T Cells

The γ/δ subset of T cells represents an important component of the mucosal immune system that has been implicated in the process of host defense against the yeast. In BALB/c and DBA/2 mice, oral infection with *C. albicans* resulted in an expansion of the γ/δ cell population (Chakir et al., 1994; Elahi et al., 2000), although the strains showed different kinetics, with the influx commencing on day 3 in the BALB/c mice, but on day 5 in the DBA/2 strain (Chakir et al., 1994). In both strains, the increase in γ/δ cell numbers was associated with a substantial decrease in the number of viable organisms recovered from the mucosal tissue. Oral colonization of B cell-deficient mice, which have a normal T cell response, increased the number of both α/β and γ/δ T cells in the GI mucosa (Jones-Carson et al.,

1997), and an accumulation of γ/δ T cells in the peritoneal cavity was also observed after intraperitoneal infection of immunocompetent and KO mice with *C. albicans* (Jones-Carson et al., 1995). In vitro, the γ/δ T cells enhanced nitric oxide production and macrophage candidacidal activity, and depletion in vivo abrogated expression of inducible NO synthase in the mucosa and enhanced susceptibility to *Candida* infection. Interestingly, mice lacking both α/β and γ/δ T cells were found to be susceptible to orogastric candidiasis, but not to acute systemic candidiasis (Jones-Carson et al., 2000), patterns of susceptibility that are similar to those seen in nude mice (Ashman et al., 2004).

4.2.4. Role of Cytokines

In systemic candidiasis, the roles of the Th1 and Th2 cytokines as regulators of host immune responses have been well established (Romani, 1999), whereas in oral infection, the identity of the cytokine mediator(s) of host resistance remains elusive and the relationship seems more complex. In general, IL-12 and IFN-γ were the dominant cytokines produced by lymphocytes from the draining lymph nodes of recovering animals (Farah et al., 2001a), but levels of IL-4 and IL-10 did not show any association with recovery from oral infection. TNF-α was the only cytokine that appeared to be unique to infected oral mucosa (Farah et al., 2002a). A comparison of host responses in the relatively resistant BALB/c or infection-prone DBA/2 mice showed that rapid clearance of *C. albicans* from the mucosa of BALB/c mice was associated with an early increase in levels of IL-4, IL-12, and IFN-γ in cells from the cervical lymph nodes, whereas in the infection-prone DBA/2 mice, expression of message for IL-4 was delayed, and the levels secreted were lower (Elahi et al., 2000). In BALB/c mice, monoclonal antibody neutralization of IL-4 increased the fungal burden and delayed the clearance of the yeast. Thus, IL-4 appears to be an important mediator of protection in oral candidiasis. In contrast, IL-12-deficient mice were highly susceptible to primary GI infection and showed an elevated production of IL-4 with a concomitant reduction in IFN-γ (Mencacci et al., 1998). Treatment of mice with GI candidiasis by administration of soluble IL-4 receptor (sIL-4R) accelerated clearance of the yeast from the stomach and stimulated Th1-associated resistance (Puccetti et al., 1994).

It might have been expected that the use of mice in which specific cytokine genes had been genetically deleted would have enabled some of these conflicts to be resolved; however, studies of candidiasis in cytokine KO mice has confused, rather than clarified the issue. In one study, IFN-γ KO mice showed increased susceptibility to both gastric and systemic candidiasis (Balish et al., 1998), whereas another reported no effect on either form of the disease (Qian and Cutler, 1997), and a third found increased mortality of the KO mice, although the increased susceptibility did not correlate with the extent of organ colonization (Kaposzta et al., 1998). Ablation of IL-10 increased resistance against both GI (Del Sero et al., 1999) and systemic (Vazquez-Torres et al., 1999) candidiasis, but deletion of the gene for IL-4 had no effect (Kaposzta et al., 1998). Mice lacking the homologue for the IL-8 receptor showed increased susceptibility to gastric and acute systemic candidiasis (Balish et al., 1999), with a slower influx of polymorphonuclear neutrophils into infected tissues, and a reduction in the candidacidal capacity of these cells.

In contrast, recent studies of oral candidiasis in IFN-γ, IL-4, IL-10, and iNOS KO mice have failed to demonstrate any alteration in the severity or course of the disease (Farah, unpublished data). In TNF-α KO mice, there was an early increase in the fungal burden in the oral cavity, but the duration of the infection was not different from controls. Infection in IL-12 KO mice, however, was similar to that in T cell-deficient nude mice (Farah, unpublished data) in that the fungal burden in the oral cavity increased and the infection became chronic, persisting undiminished for at least 3 months. The precise role of IL-12 as a mediator of host resistance, the anomalous position of IFN-γ, and the importance of IL-4 remain to be resolved. Our failure to identify a particular cytokine or set of cytokines as a crucial link in the effector pathway against the yeast may be due to a redundancy among the cytokines that masks the effect of gene deletion in KO mice; however, it is difficult to evaluate the significance of such functional overlap in vivo. Alternatively, there may exist additional effector pathways; or there may be significant, as yet unidentified, differences between the experimental models. Based on the work undertaken by the authors, a hypothetical pathway for activation of effector cells in oral candidiasis is presented in Fig. 4.2.

4.2.5. Candidacidal Effector Mechanisms

Although T cells have been shown to be essential for recovery from oral candidiasis, neither αβ nor γδ T cells have any candidacidal or candidastatic effect per se. Therefore, other cell types are required for the eradication of the yeasts from the infected mucosa.

Depletion of neutrophils or inactivation of macrophages/monocytes increased the severity of oral infection in BALB/c mice, but had a lesser effect in the CBA/CaH strain (Farah et al., 2001a). Ablation of both cell populations further increased infection in BALB/c mice, but dramatically exacerbated the fungal burden in the CBA/CaH strain. In the absence of activation, *Candida* killing by phagocytic cells (both neutrophils and macrophages) is relatively inefficient, but the candidacidal potential of both cell types is significantly enhanced by exposure to Th1-type cytokines, such as IFN-γ and TNF-α. It thus seems that phagocytic cells play a more dominant role in the susceptible CBA/CaH mice than in the resistant strains, although there was no significant difference in clearance of chronic infections in nude mice of either strain after reconstitution with lymphocytes (Farah et al., 2002b).

Nevertheless, recent studies in nude mice have thrown further light on the critical role of the bone marrow in the determination of tissue susceptibility to infection with *C. albicans* (Ashman and Papadimitriou, 1992). Bone marrow colony formation in vitro was unchanged in immunocompetent mice infected either orally or systemically (Wanasaengsakul and Ashman, 2004); however, it was significantly depressed in chronically infected, "high pathology" CBA/CaH nude mice, compared to BALB/c. Reconstitution of nude mice with T cells significantly increased the colony-forming response in infected BALB/c, but not in infected CBA/CaH mice. These results suggest that T cell-mediated enhancement of phagocytic cell production by the bone marrow may be one effector pathway.

The importance of phagocytic cells in host resistance was confirmed by treatment of SCID mice with cyclophosphamide (Balish et al., 1993). This caused severe neutropenia and impairment of innate immune mechanisms, and enhanced their susceptibility to mucosal candidiasis. Furthermore, impairment of macrophage function in SCID mice by administration of poly(I–C) increased susceptibility to disseminated candidiasis of endogenous (GI tract) origin (Jensen et al., 1992, 1994), but the resistance of immunocompetent controls to mucosal candidiasis was not altered by treatment with poly(I–C) alone. Interference with both macrophage and neutrophil function was necessary to render these mice susceptible to the disease (Jensen et al., 1993).

GI colonization of athymic (Jones-Carson et al., 1995) and SCID (Vazquez-Torres et al., 1995b) mice with *C. albicans*

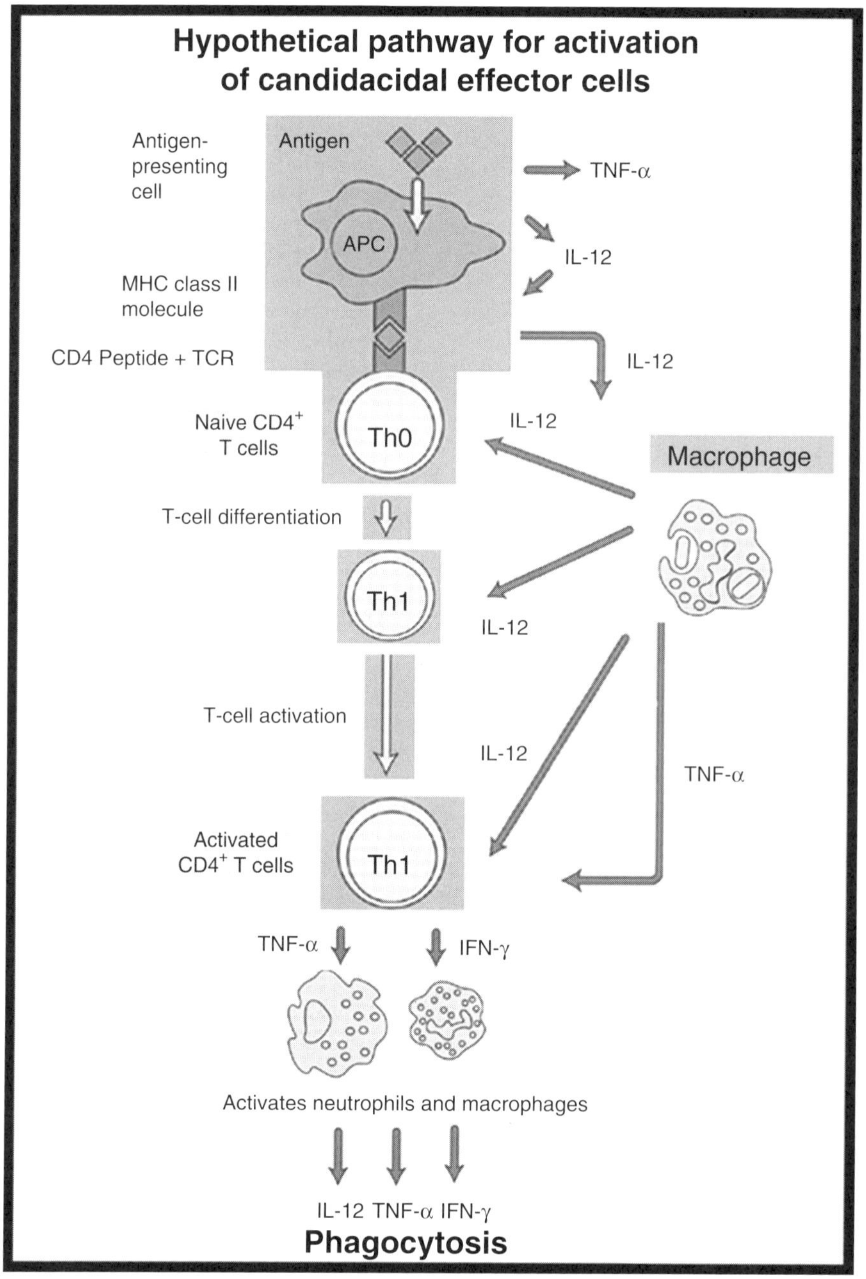

Figure 4.2. Hypothetical pathway for activation of effector cells in oral candidiasis. Stimulation of antigen-presenting cells (APC) by antigen(s) of *Candida* results in the production of TNF-α, which increases recruitment of inflammatory cells, and augments the candidacidal activity of phagocytic cells early in the course of infection. The APCs secrete IL-12, which drives the differentiation of naïve CD4+ T cells, and induces a Th1-type cellular immune response. The Th1 cytokines (IFN-γ and TNF-α) act both separately and synergistically to promote *Candida* killing by both neutrophils and macrophages; while both IL-12 and IFN-γ act on the APC in a feedback loop to enhance their activation.

stimulated the expression of inducible nitric oxide synthase (iNOS) in the gastric and oral mucosa. Inhibition of NO production in SCID mice enhanced their susceptibility to orogastric candidiasis, but in athymic mice, the expression of iNOS was controlled by γ/δ T cells (Jones-Carson et al., 1995) because depletion of these cells not only abrogated the expression of iNOS in the tongue and stomach, but also increased susceptibility to orogastric candidiasis. In contrast, immunocompetent mice did not express iNOS in the orogastric mucosa after they were monoassociated with *C. albicans* and mucosal candidiasis was not exacerbated after treatment with NOS inhibitors (Jones-Carson et al., 1995). However, no direct correlation was demonstrable between nitric oxide production and *Candida* killing (Vazquez-Torres et al., 1995a), suggesting that nitric oxide was candidastatic rather than candidacidal, and was associated with or induced other macrophage candidacidal mechanisms.

In inbred mice, NO was detected in the effector phase of the response against oral infection (Elahi et al., 2001b). Concentrations of NO in the saliva of mice increased after infection and saliva from infected mice inhibited the growth of yeast in vitro. Neutralization of IL-4 in vivo caused a marked reduction of NO levels in saliva (Elahi et al., 2001b), and in cultures of cervical lymph node cells after stimulation with *C. albicans* antigen. Conversely, treatment with NG-monomethyl-L-arginine (MMLA), which inhibits NO synthesis, led to an increase in *C. albicans* in the oral cavity and a concomitant abrogation of expression mRNA for IL-4, but not IFN-γ, in lymphocytes from the draining lymph nodes. Paradoxically, inhibition of IL-4 production was accompanied by an increase in IFN-γ production in susceptible DBA/2 mice (Elahi et al., 2001b), which tends to argue against a strict Th1/Th2 dichotomy as a determinant of resistance and susceptibility in oral candidiasis. However, in a different model, treatment of orally infected mice with aminoguanidine (AG), which inhibits iNOS, had no effect on the magnitude or duration of infection (Farah, unpublished data).

4.2.6. Role of the Infectious Challenge

The above review of results from models of oral and GI candidiasis has identified a number of common themes in mechanisms of host defense, but anomalies still remain. The contrast between the results of Elahi and Farah is of particular interest, as both groups were using the same isolate of the yeast (3630, from the Mycology Reference Laboratory at the Royal North Shore Hospital). After oral infection, DBA/2 mice showed a bimodal pattern of colonization (Chakir et al., 1994), a feature reproduced by Elahi et al. (2000), whereas in the experiments of Farah (Ashman et al., 2003), only a single peak was observed. It seemed probable that the course of oral infection in this mouse strain was influenced by the actual technique used for infection. Elahi et al. (2000) pressed the yeast onto the gums using a small swab, whereas Farah et al. (2001a) introduced a suspension of yeasts into the mouth, without damaging or traumatizing the oral mucosa. Thus, in the former case, microtrauma may have facilitated both deeper penetration of the yeast and the rapid elicitation of protective cell-mediated immune response. When inoculation was atraumatic, adhesion of the yeast to the oral mucosa may have been more difficult to establish, and innate immune mechanisms more directly involved, leading to more effective resistance against initial colonization by the yeasts.

This observation led us to test the hypothesis that there was a gradation in host responses from innate to adaptive immunity, which was determined by the severity of the infectious challenge. Nude mice develop chronic infections after oral challenge with 10^8 yeasts. However, as the doses used for infection were progressively decreased, the magnitude of the fungal burden in the chronically infected mice decreased proportionally, until eventually, the nude mice were able to clear the infection completely (Ashman et al., 2004). Thus, the requirement for CD4+ T cells for clearance of the infection in these mice apparently relates to the immunological deficit that permitted the infection to become established—a situation comparable to the susceptibility to oropharyngeal candidiasis of HIV/AIDS patients. It is noteworthy that in neither the human nor the experimental model is there any systemic dissemination of the mucosal infection, suggesting that innate immunity may also play a major role in the response against systemic disease.

4.2.7. Experimental Immunity and Protection

The genetic background of the mice influences the nature and magnitude of *Candida*-specific memory responses in systemic infection, in that the susceptible CBA/CaH mice tend to show lower cell-mediated immune responses (Ashman, 1990), but greater levels of antibody-mediated protection (Ashman and Papadimitriou, 1988) than the more resistant BALB/c strain. However, following oral infection, *Candida*-specific DTH responses developed in the relatively infection-prone DBA/2, but not in the more resistant BALB/c mice (Chakir et al., 1994). Humoral immune responses were detectable after infection had resolved (Elahi et al., 2000), but levels of serum IgG and salivary IgA antibodies were higher in BALB/c than in DBA/2 mice. In neonatal mice, primary infection of the GI tract primed them for enhanced DTH responses and conferred protection from systemic challenge as adults (Domer, 1988), whereas adult mice infected via the oral cavity, but not intravenously, were protected against a second oral infection (Farah, unpublished data). However, neither serum nor cells from orally or systemically immunized mice, transferred into naive recipients, was able to protect against oral challenge.

5. Prospects for Vaccination

Vaccination against *C. albicans* is a challenge, because of the commensal nature of the organism and because humans are colonized with the yeast in the early postnatal period. A thorough understanding of the mechanisms that confer protective immunity is fundamental to successful vaccine design, particularly in view of the problems inherent in delivering protection to mucosal surfaces. Direct immunization of the oral cavity has been shown to have therapeutic potential in mice (Elahi et al., 2001a). Mice given the oral vaccine had a reduction in colonization associated with increased levels of secretion of IFN-γ and IL-4 from the regional node cells and increased levels of nitric oxide in saliva. The use of mannan–protein conjugates as immunogens has been shown to have potential (Han et al., 1999), but perhaps a more exciting approach is the use of cytokines as adjuvants (Deepe, 1997). Another approach to vaccination against oral *C. albicans* infection has been the use of oral *Lactobacillus acidophilus* (LAVRI-A1) to induce local cytokines and enhance clearance (Elahi et al., 2003). Protective antibodies against *C. albicans*, including a human recombinant mAb specific for *C. albicans* hsp90 (Mycofab), are also being evaluated (Matthews and Burnie, 2001).

Vaccination of the immunocompromised host represents a further challenge, as vaccines that rely on a competent immune system are unlikely to be useful in immunodeficient patients. In these cases, protective antibodies could be more beneficial than cellular immunity because of the longevity of the circulating antibodies. Ultimately though, a vaccine in these patients will not succeed unless it is linked with attempts to restore the integrity of the immune system. This might be done by delivering the vaccine with cytokines that are known to enhance the immune response

(Deepe, 1997), or introducing the vaccine with immunocompetent T or B cells, to promote its immunogenic potential.

6. Conclusion

There is now convincing evidence, both clinical and experimental, that cell-mediated immunity is crucial to host recovery from oral or OPC. This infection, however, appears to demonstrate a gradation between the involvement of the innate and adaptive immune responses, depending on the severity of the challenge. $CD4^+$ lymphocytes are certainly involved in the more severe manifestations of the disease, but the precise pathways through which they interact with the phagocytic effector cells that clear the infection have yet to be completely elucidated. Oral immunization can confer protection, but again, the mechanisms by which this is achieved require further investigation.

Acknowledgments

Research from the authors' laboratory has been supported by grants from the National Health and Medical Research Council of Australia and the Australian Dental Research Foundation.

References

Alkhatib, G., Combadiere, C., Broder, C.C., Feng, Y., Kennedy, P.E., Murphy, P.M., and Berger, E.A. (1996). CC CKR5: A RANTES, MIP-1α, MIP-1β receptor as a fusion cofactor for macrophage-tropic HIV-1. *Science* 272: 1955–1958.

Arendorf, T.M. and Walker, D.M. (1980). The prevalence and intra-oral distribution of *Candida albicans* in man. *Arch. Oral Biol.* 25: 1–10.

Ashman, R.B. (1990). Murine candidiasis: Cell-mediated immune responses correlate directly with susceptibility and resistance to infection. *Immunol. Cell Biol.* 68: 15–20.

Ashman, R.B. (1998). A gene (*Cargl*) that regulates tissue resistance to *Candida albicans* maps to chromosome 14 of the mouse. *Microb. Pathog.* 25: 333–335.

Ashman, R.B. and Papadimitriou, J.M. (1987). Murine candidiasis. Pathogenesis and host responses in genetically distinct inbred mice. *Immunol. Cell Biol.* 65: 163–171.

Ashman, R.B. and Papadimitriou, J.M. (1988). Murine candidiasis: Strain dependence of host responses after immunization. *Immunol. Cell Biol.* 66: 231–237.

Ashman, R.B. and Papadimitriou, J.M. (1992). Genetic resistance to *Candida albicans* infection is conferred by cells derived from the bone marrow. *J. Infect. Dis.* 166: 947–948.

Ashman, R.B., Papadimitriou, J.M., Fulurija, A., Drysdale, K.E., Farah, C.S., Naidoo, O., and Gotjamanos, T. (2003). Role of complement C5 and T lymphocytes in pathogenesis of disseminated and mucosal candidiasis in susceptible DBA/2 mice. *Microb. Pathog.* 34: 103–113.

Ashman, R.B., Farah, C.S., Wanasaengsakul, S., Hu, Y., Pang, G., and Clancy, R.L. (2004). Innate versus adaptive immunity in *Candida albicans* infection. *Immunol. Cell Biol.* 82: 196–204.

Balish, E., Filutowicz, H., and Oberley, T.D. (1990). Correlates of cell-mediated immunity in *Candida albicans*-colonized gnotobiotic mice. *Infect. Immun.* 58: 107–113.

Balish, E., Jensen, J., Warner, T., Brekke, J., and Leonard, B. (1993). Mucosal and disseminated candidiasis in gnotobiotic SCID mice. *J. Med. Vet. Mycol.* 31: 143–154.

Balish, E., Wagner, R.D., Vazquez-Torres, A., Pierson, C., and Warner, T. (1998). Candidiasis in interferon-gamma knockout (IFN-γ -/-) mice. *J. Infect. Dis.* 178: 478–487.

Balish, E., Wagner, R.D., Vazquez-Torres, A., Jones-Carson, J., Pierson, C., and Warner, T. (1999). Mucosal and systemic candidiasis in IL-8rh-/- BALB/c mice. *J. Leukoc. Biol.* 66: 144–150.

Balish, E., Warner, T., Pierson, C.J., Bock, D.M., and Wagner, R.D. (2001). Oroesophageal candidiasis is lethal for transgenic mice with combined natural killer and T-cell defects. *Med. Mycol.* 39: 261–268.

Barbeau, J., Seguin, J., Goulet, J.P., de Koninck, L., Avon, S.L., Lalonde, B., Rompre, P., and Deslauriers, N. (2003). Reassessing the presence of *Candida albicans* in denture-related stomatitis.

Oral Surg. Oral Med. Oral Pathol. Oral Radiol. Endod. 95: 51–59.

Bistoni, F., Cenci, E., Mencacci, A., Schiaffella, E., Mosci, P., Puccetti, P., and Romani, L. (1993). Mucosal and systemic T helper cell function after intragastric colonization of adult mice with *Candida albicans. J. Infect. Dis.* 168: 1449–1457.

Brassart, D., Woltz, A., Golliard, M., and Neeser, J.R. (1991). In vitro inhibition of adhesion of *Candida albicans* clinical isolates to human buccal epithelial cells by Fuc alpha 1–2gal beta-bearing complex carbohydrates. *Infect. Immun.* 59: 1605–1613.

Brown, D.M., Jabra-Rizk, M.A., Falkler, W.A. Jr., Baqui, A.A., and Meiller, T.F. (2000). Identification of *Candida dubliniensis* in a study of HIV-seropositive pediatric dental patients. *Pediatr. Dent.* 22: 234–238.

Budtz-Jorgensen, E. (1974). The significance of *Candida albicans* in denture stomatitis. *Scand. J. Dent. Res.* 82: 151–190.

Cantorna, M.T. and Balish, E. (1990). Mucosal and systemic candidiasis in congenitally immunodeficient mice. *Infect. Immun.* 58: 1093–1100.

Cantorna, M.T. and Balish, E. (1991). Role of $CD4^+$ lymphocytes in resistance to mucosal candidiasis. *Infect. Immun.* 59: 2447–2455.

Cartledge, J.D., Midgley, J., and Gazzard, B.G. (1999). Non-albicans oral candidosis in HIV-positive patients. *J. Antimicrob. Chemother.* 43: 419–422.

Cawson, R.A. and Lehner, T. (1968). Chronic hyperplastic candidiasis-candidal leukoplakia. *Brit. J. Dermatol.* 80: 9–16.

Cenci, E., Mencacci, A., Spaccapelo, R., Tonnetti, L., Mosci, P., Enssle, K.H., Puccetti, P., Romani, L., and Bistoni, F. (1995). T helper cell type 1 (Th1)- and Th2-like responses are present in mice with gastric candidiasis but protective immunity is associated with Th1 development. *J. Infect. Dis.* 171: 1279–1288.

Chakir, J., Cote, L., Coulombe, C., and Deslauriers, N. (1994). Differential pattern of infection and immune response during experimental oral candidiasis in BALB/c and DBA/2 (H-2d) mice. *Oral Microbiol. Immunol.* 9: 88–94.

Chilgren, R.A., Quie, P.G., Meuwissen, H.J., and Hong, R. (1967). Chronic mucocutaneous candidiasis, deficiency of delayed hypersensitivity, and selective local antibody defect. *Lancet* 2: 688–693.

Cleveland, W.W., Fogel, B.J., Brown, W.T., and Kay, H.E. (1968). Foetal thymic transplant in a case of DiGeorge's syndrome. *Lancet* 2: 1211–1214.

Coleman, D., Sullivan, D., Harrington, B., Haynes, K., Henman, M., Shanley, D., Bennett, D., Moran, G., McCreary, C., and O'Neill, L. (1997). Molecular and phenotypic analysis of *Candida dubliniensis*: A recently identified species linked with oral candidosis in HIV-infected and AIDS patients. *Oral Dis.* 3(Suppl, 1): S96–S101.

Cutler, J.E., Friedman, L., and Milner, K.C. (1972). Biological and chemical characterization of toxic substances from *Candida albicans. Infect. Immun.* 6: 616–627.

Daniels, T.E., Schwartz, O., Larsen, V., Dabelsteen, E., and Pindborg, J. (1985). Langerhans cells in candidal leukoplakia. *J. Oral Pathol.* 14: 733–739.

Davenport, J.C. and Wilton, J.M. (1971). Incidence of immediate and delayed hypersensitivity of *Candida albicans* in denture stomatitis. *J. Dent. Res.* 50: 892–896.

de Repentigny, L., Aumont, F., Ripeau, J.S., Fiorillo, M., Kay, D.G., Hanna, Z., and Jolicoeur, P. (2002). Mucosal candidiasis in transgenic mice expressing human immunodeficiency virus type 1. *J. Infect. Dis.* 185: 1103–1114.

Deepe, G.S. Jr. (1997). Prospects for the development of fungal vaccines. *Clin. Microbiol. Rev.* 10: 585–596.

Del Sero, G., Mencacci, A., Cenci, E., d'Ostiani, C.F., Montagnoli, C., Bacci, A., Mosci, P., Kopf, M., and Romani, L. (1999). Antifungal type 1 responses are upregulated in IL-10-deficient mice. *Microbes Infect.* 1: 1169–1180.

Deslauriers, N., Coulombe, C., Carre, B., and Goulet, J.P. (1995). Topical application of a corticosteroid destabilizes the host-parasite relationship in an experimental model of the oral carrier state of *Candida albicans. FEMS Immunol. Med. Microbiol.* 11: 45–55.

Deslauriers, N., Cote, L., Montplaisir, S., and de Repentigny. (1997). Oral carriage of *Candida albicans* in murine AIDS. *Infect. Immun.* 65: 661–667.

Dodd, C.L., Greenspan, D., Katz, M.H., Westenhouse, J.L., Feigal, D.W., and Greenspan, J.S. (1991). Oral candidiasis in HIV infection: pseudomembraneous and erythematous candidiasis show similar rates of progression to AIDS. *AIDS* 5: 1339–1343.

Domer, J.E. (1988). Intragastric colonization of infant mice with *Candida albicans* induces systemic immunity demonstrable upon challenge as adults. *J. Infect. Dis.* 157: 950–958.

Dongari-Bagtzoglou, A. and Kashleva, H. (2003a). Granulocyte-macrophage colony-stimulating factor responses of oral epithelial cells to *Candida albicans. Oral Microbiol. Immunol.* 18: 165–170.

Dongari-Bagtzoglou, A. and Kashleva, H. (2003b). *Candida albicans* triggers interleukin-8 secretion by oral epithelial cells. *Microb. Pathog.* 34: 169–177.

Dongari-Bagtzoglou, A., Wen, K., and Lamster, I.B. (1999). *Candida albicans* triggers interleukin-6 and interleukin-8 responses by oral fibroblasts in vitro. *Oral Microbiol. Immunol.* 14: 364–370.

Duncan, R.A., von Reyn, C.F., Alliegro, G.M., Toossi, Z., Sugar, A.M., and Levitz, S.M. (1993). Idiopathic CD4+ T-lymphocytopenia—four patients with opportunistic infections and no evidence of HIV infection. *N. Engl. J. Med.* 328: 393–398.

Edwards, J.E. Jr., Lehrer, R.I., Stiehm, E.R., Fischer, T.J., and Young, L.S. (1978). Severe candidal infections: Clinical perspective, immune defense mechanisms, and current concepts of therapy. *Ann. Intern. Med.* 89: 91–106.

Elahi, S., Pang, G., Clancy, R., and Ashman, R.B. (2000). Cellular and cytokine correlates of mucosal protection in murine model of oral candidiasis. *Infect. Immun.* 68: 5771–5777.

Elahi, S., Clancy, R., and Pang, G. (2001a). A therapeutic vaccine for mucosal candidiasis. *Vaccine* 19: 2516–2521.

Elahi, S., Pang, G., Ashman, R.B., and Clancy, R. (2001b). Nitric oxide-enhanced resistance to oral candidiasis. *Immunology* 104: 447–454.

Elahi, S., Pang, G., and Clancy, R. (2003). Development of surrogate markers for oral immunisation against *Candida albicans. Vaccine* 21: 671–677.

Epstein, J.B., Truelove, E.L., and Izutzu, K.T. (1984). Oral candidiasis: Pathogenesis and host defense. *Rev. Infect. Dis.* 6: 96–106.

Farah, C.S., Elahi, S., Pang, G., Gotjamanos, T., Seymour, G.J., Clancy, R.L., and Ashman, R.B. (2001a). T cells augment monocyte and neutrophil function in host resistance against oropharyngeal candidiasis. *Infect. Immun.* 69: 6110–6118.

Farah, C.S., Hong, S., Wanasaengsakul, S., Elahi, S., Pang, G., Gotjamanos, T., Seymour, G.J., Clancy, R.L., and Ashman, R.B. (2001b). Irradiation-induced oral candidiasis in an experimental murine model. *Oral Microbiol. Immunol.* 16: 358–363.

Farah, C.S., Elahi, S., Drysdale, K., Pang, G., Gotjamanos, T., Seymour, G.J., Clancy, R.L., and Ashman, R.B. (2002a). Primary role for CD4+ T lymphocytes in recovery from oropharyngeal candidiasis. *Infect. Immun.* 70: 724–731.

Farah, C.S., Gotjamanos, T., Seymour, G.J., and Ashman, R.B. (2002b). Cytokines in the oral mucosa of mice infected with *Candida albicans. Oral Microbiol. Immunol.* 17: 375–378.

Fauci, A.S. (1993). Multifactorial nature of human immunodeficiency virus disease: Implications for therapy. *Science* 262: 1011–1018.

Fidel, P.L. Jr. (2002). Distinct protective host defenses against oral and vaginal candidiasis. *Med. Mycol.* 40: 359–375.

Fidel, P.L. Jr., Vazquez, J.A., and Sobel, J.D. (1999). *Candida glabrata*: Review of epidemiology, pathogenesis, and clinical disease with comparison to *C. albicans. Clin. Microbiol. Rev.* 12: 80–96.

Finlay, I.G. (1986). Oral symptoms and *Candida* in the terminally ill. *Brit. Med. J. (Clin. Res. Ed.)* 292: 592–593.

Fisher, J.M., Basson, N.J., and van Zyl, A. (2001). Identification of *Candida dubliniensis* in a HIV-positive South African population. *S. Afr. Dent. J.* 56: 599–601.

Fotos, P.G. and Hellstein, J.W. (1992). *Candida* and candidosis. Epidemiology, diagnosis and therapeutic management. *Dent. Clin. North Am.* 36: 857–878.

Ghannoum, M.A., Burns, G.R., Elteen, K.A., and Radwan, S.S. (1986). Experimental evidence for the role of lipids in adherence of *Candida* spp. to human buccal epithelial cells. *Infect. Immun.* 54: 189–193.

Giammanco, G.M., Pizzo, G., Pecorella, S., Distefano, S., Pecoraro, V., and Milici, M.E. (2002). Identification of *Candida dubliniensis* among oral yeast isolates from an Italian population of human immunodeficiency virus-infected (HIV+) subjects. *Oral Microbiol. Immunol.* 17: 89–94.

Gottlieb, M.S., Schroff, R., Schanker, H.M., Weisman, J.D., Fan, P.T., Wolf, R.A., and

Saxon, A. (1981a). *Pneumocystis carinii* pneumonia and mucosal candidiasis in previously healthy homosexual men: Evidence of a new acquired cellular immunodeficiency. *N. Engl. J. Med.* 305: 1425–1431.

Gottlieb, M.S., Shanker, H.M., and Fan, P.T. (1981b). *Pneumocystis* pneumonia-Los Angeles. *MMWR Morb. Mortal. Wkly. Rep.* 30: 250–251.

Han, Y., Ulrich, M.A., and Cutler, J.E. (1999). *Candida albicans* mannan extract-protein conjugates induce a protective immune response against experimental candidiasis. *J. Infect. Dis.* 179: 1477–1484.

Hazen, K.C., Brawner, D.L., Riesselman, M.H., Jutila, M.A., and Cutler, J.E. (1991). Differential adherence of hydrophobic and hydrophilic *Candida albicans* yeast cells to mouse tissues. *Infect. Immun.* 59: 907–912.

Ho, W.Z., Cherukuri, R., and Douglas, S.D. (1994). The macrophage and HIV-1. *Immunol. Ser.* 60: 569–587.

Hoegl, L., Thoma-Greber, E., Rocken, M., and Korting, H.C. (1998). Persistent oral candidosis by non-albicans *Candida* strains including *Candida glabrata* in a human immunodeficiency virus-infected patient observed over a period of 6 years. *Mycoses* 41: 335–338.

Holmstrup, P. and Axell, T. (1990). Classification and clinical manifestations of oral yeast infections. *Acta Odontol. Scand.* 48: 57–59.

Iacopino, A.M. and Wathen, W.F. (1992). Oral candidal infection and denture stomatitis: A comprehensive review. *J. Am. Dent. Assoc.* 123: 46–51.

Jensen, J., Vazquez-Torres, A., and Balish, E. (1992). Poly(I.C)-induced interferons enhance susceptibility of SCID mice to systemic candidiasis. *Infect. Immun.* 60: 4549–4557.

Jensen, J., Warner, T., and Balish, E. (1993). Resistance of SCID mice to *Candida albicans* administered intravenously or colonizing the gut: Role of polymorphonuclear leukocytes and macrophages. *J. Infect. Dis.* 167: 912–919.

Jensen, J., Warner, T., and Balish, E. (1994). The role of phagocytic cells in resistance to disseminated candidiasis in granulocytopenic mice. *J. Infect. Dis.* 170: 900–905.

Jones-Carson, J., Vazquez-Torres, A., van der Heyde, H.C., Warner, T., Wagner, R.D., and Balish, E. (1995). γ/δ T cell-induced nitric oxide production enhances resistance to mucosal candidiasis. *Nat. Med.* 1: 552–557.

Jones-Carson, J., Vazquez-Torres, F.A., and Balish, E. (1997). B cell-independent selection of memory T cells after mucosal immunization with *Candida albicans*. *J. Immunol.* 158: 4328–4335.

Jones-Carson, J., Vazquez-Torres, A., Warner, T., and Balish, E. (2000). Disparate requirement for T cells in resistance to mucosal and acute systemic candidiasis. *Infect. Immun.* 68: 2363–2365.

Kamai, Y., Kubota, M., Hosokawa, T., Fukuoka, T., and Filler, S.G. (2001). New model of oropharyngeal candidiasis in mice. *Antimicrob. Agents Chemother.* 45: 3195–3197.

Kanbe, T., Li, R.K., Wadsworth, E., Calderone, R.A., and Cutler, J.E. (1991). Evidence for expression of the C3d receptor of *Candida albicans* in vitro and in vivo obtained by immunofluorescence and immunoelectron microscopy. *Infect. Immun.* 59: 1832–1838.

Kantarcioglu, A.S. and Yucel, A. (2002). The presence of fluconazole-resistant *Candida dubliniensis* strains among *Candida albicans* isolates from immunocompromised or otherwise debilitated HIV-negative Turkish patients. *Rev. Iberoam. Micol.* 19: 44–48.

Kaposzta, R., Tree, P., Marodi, L., and Gordon, S. (1998). Characteristics of invasive candidiasis in gamma interferon- and interleukin-4-deficient mice—role of macrophages in host defence against *Candida albicans*. *Infect. Immun.* 66: 1708–1717.

Kirkpatrick, C.H. (1989). Chronic mucocutaneous candidiasis. *Eur. J. Clin. Microbiol. Infect. Dis.* 8: 448–456.

Kirkpatrick, C.H. (1994). Chronic mucocutaneous candidiasis. *J. Amer. Acad. Dermatol.* 31: S14–S17.

Kirkpatrick, C.H., Rich, R.R., and Bennett, J.E. (1971). Chronic mucocutaneous candidiasis: Model-building in cellular immunity. *Ann. Intern. Med.* 74: 955–978.

Klebanoff, S.J. (1970). Myeloperoxidase: Contribution to the microbicidal activity of intact leukocytes. *Science* 169: 1095–1097.

Klotz, S.A. and Smith, R.L. (1991). A fibronectin receptor on *Candida albicans* mediates adherence of the fungus to extracellular matrix. *J. Infect. Dis.* 163: 604–610.

Kostiala, I. (1986). Acute fungal stomatitis in compromised host. Causative agents, serological findings, topical treatment. *Proc. Finn. Dent. Soc.* 82(Suppl. 7–8): 1–96.

Kostiala, I., Kostiala, A.A., and Kahanpaa, A. (1979). Oral mycoses and their treatment. *Acta Odontol. Scand.* 37: 87–101.

Kwon-Chung, K.J., Lehman, D., Good, C., and Magee, P.T. (1985). Genetic evidence for role of extracellular proteinase in virulence of *Candida albicans. Infect. Immun.* 49: 571–575.

Lacasse, M., Fortier, C., Chakir, J., Cote, L., and Deslauriers, N. (1993). Acquired resistance and persistence of *Candida albicans* following oral candidiasis in the mouse: A model of the carrier state in humans. *Oral Microbiol. Immunol.* 8: 313–318.

Lehner, T. (1967). Oral candidosis. *Dent. Pract. Dent. Rec.* 17: 209–216.

Lehrer, R.I. and Cline, M.J. (1969). Leukocyte myeloperoxidase deficiency and disseminated candidiasis: The role of myeloperoxidase in resistance to *Candida* infection. *J. Clin. Invest.* 48: 1478–1488.

Leigh, J.E., Steele, C., Wormley, F.L. Jr., Luo, W., Clark, R.A., Gallaher, W., and Fidel, P.L. Jr. (1998). Th1/Th2 cytokine expression in saliva of HIV-positive and HIV-negative individuals: A pilot study in HIV-positive individuals with oropharyngeal candidiasis. *J. Acquir. Immune Defic. Syndr. Hum. Retrovirol.* 19: 373–380.

Leigh, J.E., Barousse, M., Swoboda, R.K., Myers, T., Hager, S., Wolf, N.A., Cutright, J.L., Thompson, J., Sobel, J.D., and Fidel, P.L. Jr. (2001). *Candida*-specific systemic cell-mediated immune reactivities in human immunodeficiency virus-positive persons with mucosal candidiasis. *J. Infect. Dis.* 183: 277–285.

Leigh, J.E., Steele, C., Wormley, F., and Fidel, P.L. Jr. (2002). Salivary cytokine profiles in the immunocompetent individual with *Candida*-associated denture stomatitis. *Oral Microbiol. Immunol.* 17: 311–314.

Lockhart, S.R., Joly, S., Vargas, K., Swails-Wenger, J., Enger, L., and Soll, D.R. (1999). Natural defenses against *Candida* colonization breakdown in the oral cavities of the elderly. *J. Dent. Res.* 78: 857–868.

Masia Canuto, M., Gutierrez Rodero, F., Ortiz de la Tabla Ducasse, V., Hernandez Aguado, I., Martin Gonzalez, C., Sanchez Sevillano, A., and Martin Hidalgo, A. (2000). Determinants for the development of oropharyngeal colonization or infection by fluconazole-resistant *Candida* strains in HIV-infected patients. *Eur. J. Clin. Microbiol. Infect. Dis.* 19: 593–601.

Matthews, R. and Burnie, J. (2001). Antifungal antibodies: A new approach to the treatment of systemic candidiasis. *Curr. Opin. Investig. Drugs* 2: 472–476.

McCarthy, G.M., Mackie, I.D., Koval, J., Sandhu, H.S., and Daley, T.D. (1991). Factors associated with increased frequency of HIV-related oral candidiasis. *J. Oral Pathol. Med.* 20: 332–336.

Meiller, T.F., Jabra-Rizk, M.A., Baqui, A., Kelley, J.I., Meeks, V.I., Merz, W.G., and Falkler, W.A. (1999). Oral *Candida dubliniensis* as a clinically important species in HIV-seropositive patients in the United States. *Oral Surg. Oral Med. Oral Pathol. Oral Radiol. Endod.* 88: 573–580.

Mencacci, A., Cenci, E., Del Sero, G., d'Ostiani, C.F., Mosci, P., Trinchieri, G., Adorini, L., and Romani, L. (1998). IL-10 is required for development of protective Th1 responses in IL-12-deficient mice upon *Candida albicans* infection. *J. Immunol.* 161: 6228–6237.

Myers, T.A., Leigh, J.E., Arribas, A.R., Hager, S., Clark, R., Lilly, E., and Fidel, P.L. Jr. (2003). Immunohistochemical evaluation of T cells in oral lesions from human immunodeficiency virus-positive persons with oropharyngeal candidiasis. *Infect. Immun.* 71: 956–963.

Naglik, J.R., Newport, G., White, T.C., Fernandes Naglik, L.L., Greenspan, J.S., Greenspan, D., Sweet, S.P., Challacombe, S.J., and Agabian, N. (1999). In vivo analysis of secreted aspartyl proteinase expression in human oral candidiasis. *Infect. Immun.* 67: 2482–2490.

Naglik, J.R., Challacombe, S.J., and Hube, B. (2003a). *Candida albicans* secreted aspartyl proteinases in virulence and pathogenesis. *Microbiol. Mol. Biol. Rev.* 67: 400–428.

Narayanan, R., Joyce, W.A., and Greenfield, R.A. (1991). Gastrointestinal candidiasis in a murine model of severe combined immunodeficiency syndrome. *Infect. Immun.* 59: 2116–2119

Nomanbhoy, F., Steele, C., Yano, J., and Fidel, P.L. Jr. (2002). Vaginal and oral epithelial cell anti-*Candida* activity. *Infect. Immun.* 70: 7081–7088.

Odds, F.C. (1988). *Candida and Candidosis.* Balliere Tindall, London.

Oliver, C. and Essner, E. (1975). Formation of anomalous lysosomes in monocytes, neutrophils, and eosinophils from bone marrow of mice with Chediak-Higashi syndrome. *Lab. Invest.* 32: 17–27.

Palmer, G.D., Robinson, P.G., Challacombe, S.J., Birnbaum, W., Croser, D., Erridge, P.L.,

Hodgson, T., Lewis, D., McLaren, A., and Zakrzewska, J.M. (1996). Aetiological factors for oral manifestations of HIV. *Oral Dis.* 2: 193–197.

Pietruski, J.K., Pietruska, M.D., Jablonska, E., Sacha, P., Zaremba, M., and Stokowska, W. (2000). Interleukin 6, tumor necrosis factor alpha and their soluble receptors in the blood serum of patients with denture stomatitis and fungal infection. *Arch. Immunol. Ther. Exp. (Warsz)*. 48: 101–105.

Porter, S.R. and Scully, C. (1990). Chronic mucocutaneous candidosis and related syndromes. In L.P. Samaranayake and T.W. MacFarlane (eds), *Oral Candidosis*. Wright, London, pp. 200–211.

Porter, S.R. and Scully, C. (1993a). Orofacial manifestations in primary immunodeficiencies: Polymorphonuclear leukocyte defects. *J. Oral Pathol. Med.* 22: 310–311.

Porter, S.R. and Scully, C. (1993b). Orofacial manifestations in primary immunodeficiencies: T lymphocyte defects. *J. Oral Pathol. Med.* 22: 308–309.

Puccetti, P., Mencacci, A., Cenci, E., Spaccapelo, R., Mosci, P., Enssle, K.-H., Romani, L., and Bistoni, F. (1994). Cure of murine candidiasis by recombinant soluble interleukin-4 receptor. *J. Infect. Dis.* 169: 1325–1331.

Qian, Q.F. and Cutler, J.E. (1997). Gamma interferon is not essential in host defense against disseminated candidiasis in mice. *Infect. Immun.* 65: 1748–1753.

Razek, M.K. and Shaaban, N.A. (1978). Histochemical and histopathologic studies of alveolar mucosa under complete dentures. *J. Prosthet. Dent.* 39: 29–36.

Redding, S.W. (2001). The role of yeasts other than *Candida albicans* in oropharyngeal candidiasis. *Curr. Opin. Infect. Dis.* 14: 673–677.

Romagnoli, P., Pimpinelli, N., Mori, M., Reichart, P.A., Eversole, L.R., and Ficarra, G. (1997). Immunocompetent cells in oral candidiasis of HIV-infected patients: An immunohistochemical and electron microscopical study. *Oral Dis.* 3: 99–105.

Romani, L. (1999). Immunity to *Candida albicans*: Th1, Th2 cells and beyond. *Curr. Opin. Microbiol.* 2: 363–367.

Romani, L., Mencacci, A., Cenci, E., Spaccapelo, R., Mosci, P., Puccetti, P., and Bistoni, F. (1993). $CD4^+$ subset expression in murine candidiasis. Th responses correlate directly with genetically determined susceptibility or vaccine-induced resistance. *J. Immunol.* 150: 925–931.

Saltarelli, C.G. (1989). *Candida albicans. The Pathogenic Fungus*. Hemisphere Publishing, New York.

Saltarelli, C.G., Gentile, K.A., and Mancuso, S.C. (1975). Lethality of *Candida* strains as influenced by the host. *Can. J. Microbiol.* 21: 648–654.

Samaranayake, L.P. (1988). Oral candidosis: Predisposing factors and pathogenesis. In D.D. Derrick (ed.), *Dental Annual 1989*. Wright, Bristol, pp. 219–235.

Samaranayake, L.P. (1991). Superficial oral fungal infections. *Curr. Opin. Dent.* 1: 415–422.

Samaranayake, L.P. and Holmstrup, P. (1989). Oral candidiasis and human immunodeficiency virus infection. *J. Oral Pathol. Med.* 18: 554–564.

Samaranayake, L.P. and MacFarlane, T.W. (1990). *Oral Candidosis*. Wright, London.

Samaranayake, L.P. and Yaacob, H.B. (1990). Classification of oral candidosis. In L.P. Samaranayake and T.W. MacFarlane (eds), *Oral Candidosis*. Wright, London, pp. 124–155.

Samaranayake, L.P., Robertson, A.G., MacFarlane, T.W., Hunter, I.P., MacFarlane, G., Soutar, D.S., and Ferguson, M.M. (1988). The effect of chlorhexidine and benzydamine mouthwashes on mucositis induced by therapeutic irradiation. *Clin. Radiol.* 39: 291–294.

Sano, A., Vilela, M.M., Takahashi, I., Fukushima, K., Takizawa, K., da Silva, M.T., Uno, J., Nishimura, K., and Miyaji, M. (2000). Isolation of *Candida dubliniensis* from the oral cavity of an HIV-positive child in Brazil. *Nippon Ishinkin Gakkai Zasshi*. 41: 177–181.

Schaller, M., Korting, H.C., Schafer, W., Bastert, J., Chen, W., and Hube, B. (1999). Secreted aspartic proteinase (Sap) activity contributes to tissue damage in a model of human oral candidosis. *Mol. Microbiol.* 34: 169–180.

Schaller, M., Mailhammer, R., Grassl, G., Sander, C.A., Hube, B., and Korting, H.C. (2002). Infection of human oral epithelia with *Candida* species induces cytokine expression correlated to the degree of virulence. *J. Invest. Dermatol.* 118: 652–657.

Schorling, S.R., Kortinga, H.C., Froschb, M., and Muhlschlegel, F.A. (2000). The role of *Candida dubliniensis* in oral candidiasis in human immunodeficiency virus-infected individuals. *Crit. Rev. Microbiol.* 26: 59–68.

Scully, C. and Cawson, R.A. (1998). *Medical Problems in Dentistry*. Butterworth-Heinemann, Oxford.

Scully, C., el-Kabir, M., and Samaranayake, L.P. (1994). *Candida* and oral candidosis: A review. *Crit. Rev. Oral Biol. Med.* 5: 125–157.

Sobel, J.D., Muller, G., and Buckley, H.R. (1984). Critical role of germ tube formation in the pathogenesis of candidal vaginitis. *Infect. Immun.* 44: 576–580.

Steele, C., Leigh, J., Swoboda, R., and Fidel, P.L. Jr. (2000). Growth inhibition of *Candida* by human oral epithelial cells. *J. Infect. Dis.* 182: 1479–1485.

Sullivan, D.J., Westerneng, T.J., Haynes, K.A., Bennett, D.E., and Coleman, D.C. (1995). *Candida dubliniensis* sp. Nov.: Phenotypic and molecular characterization of a novel species associated with oral candidosis in HIV-infected individuals. *Microbiology* 141: 1507–1521.

Szkaradkiewicz, A., Szponar, E., Krzeminska-Jaskowiak, E., and Tulecka, T. (1998). Serum interferon-gamma (IFN-γ) in chronic oral candidosis. *Med. Mycol.* 36: 269–273.

Takakura, N., Sato, Y., Ishibashi, H., Oshima, H., Uchida, K., Yamaguchi, H., and Abe, S. (2003). A novel murine model of oral candidiasis with local symptoms characteristic of oral thrush. *Microbiol. Immunol.* 47: 321–326.

Tekeli, A., Dolapci, I., Cesur, S., Tekeli, E., and Icli, F. (2002). *Candida dubliniensis* studies and isolation of *Candida* types in oropharyngeal specimens from oncologic patients. *Mikrobiyol. Bul.* 36: 57–63.

Thuraisingam, A.I. and Denning, D.W. (2000). *Candida glabrata* oesophagitis in a patient without HIV infection. *Eur. J. Clin. Microbiol. Infect. Dis.* 19: 561–562.

Trial, J., Birdsall, H.H., Hallum, J.A., Crane, M.L., Rodriguez-Barradas, M.C., de Jong, A.L., Krishnan, B., Lacke, C.E., Figdor, C.G., and Rossen, R.D. (1995). Phenotypic and functional changes in peripheral blood monocytes during progression of human immunodeficiency virus infection. Effects of soluble immune complexes, cytokines, subcellular particulates from apoptotic cells, and HIV-1-encoded proteins on monocytes phagocytic function, oxidative burst, transendothelial migration, and cell surface phenotype. *J. Clin. Invest.* 95: 1690–1701.

Trousseau, U. (1869). *Lectures on Clinical Medicine Delivered at the Hotel-Dieu Paris*. New Syndenham Society, London.

Vazquez-Torres, A., Jones-Carson, J., and Balish, E. (1995a). Nitric oxide production does not directly increase macrophage candidacidal activity. *Infect. Immun.* 63: 1142–1144.

Vazquez-Torres, A., Jones-Carson, J., Warner, T., and Balish, E. (1995b). Nitric oxide enhances resistance of SCID mice to mucosal candidiasis. *J. Infect. Dis.* 172: 192–198.

Vazquez-Torres, A., Jones-Carson, J., Wagner, R.D., Warner, T., and Balish, E. (1999). Early resistance of interleukin-10 knockout mice to acute systemic candidiasis. *Infect. Immun.* 67: 670–674.

Wahl, S.M., Orenstein, J.M., and Smith, P.D. (1996). Macrophage function in HIV-1 infection. In S. Gupta (ed.), *Immunology of HIV Infection*. Plenum Press, New York, pp. 303–336.

Walker, D.M. and Arendorf, T.M. (1990). Candidal leukoplakia, chronic multifocal candidosis and median rhomboid glossitis. In L.P. Samaranayake and T.W. MacFarlane (eds), *Oral Candidosis*. Wright, London, pp. 184–211.

Wanasaengsakul, S. and Ashman, R.B. (2004). Bone marrow colony-formation in vitro after infection of genetically defined inbred mice with *Candida albicans*. *Microb. Pathog.* 36: 211–217.

Watson, I.B. and MacDonald, D.G. (1982). Oral mucosa and complete dentures. *J. Prosthet. Dent.* 47: 133–140.

Wilkieson, C., Samaranayake, L.P., MacFarlane, T.W., Lamey, P.J., and MacKenzie, D. (1991). Oral candidosis in the elderly in long term hospital care. *J. Oral Pathol. Med.* 20: 13–16.

Williams, D.W., Potts, A.J., Wilson, M.J., Matthews, J.B., and Lewis, M.A. (1997). Characterisation of the inflammatory cell infiltrate in chronic hyperplastic candidosis of the oral mucosa. *J. Oral Pathol. Med.* 26: 83–89.

Wolff, S.M. (1972). The Chediak-Higashi syndrome: Studies of host defenses. *Ann. Intern. Med.* 76: 293–306.

5

The Innate and Adaptive Immune Response to Pulmonary *Histoplasma capsulatum* Infection

George S. Deepe, Jr.

University of Cincinnati College of Medicine, Cincinnati, OH.

1. Introduction

The dimorphic fungus, *Histoplasma capsulatum*, is a facultative intracellular pathogen that is endemic to many regions of the Americas including the midwestern and southeastern United States, Central, and South America. *H. capsulatum* is found in the soil as mycelia that contain both macro- and microconidia. The preferred niche is bird or bat guano that is decayed, has an acidic pH, and a high nitrogen content. The fungus exists best in temperate climates that are not arid (Deepe, 2000).

Infection of humans and other mammals with *H. capsulatum* appears to be largely a consequence of chance. Upon disruption of soil, mycelial fragments and microconidia are inhaled and reach terminal bronchioles and alveolar spaces where they initiate the infectious process. Upon exposure to a temperature of 37°C, the mycelial and microconidia convert to the yeast phase, which is the form that is largely responsible for the clinical and pathological manifestations of histoplasmosis. The progression of the infectious process requires intracellular growth of the yeast form until cell-mediated immunity is activated. Once this arm of the immune system is engaged, replication of the organism is arrested, and eventually the fungal burden is decreased. It is likely that much of the growth inhibition transpires within granulomas, the pathological hallmark of a successful cell-mediated immune response. Yeast phase cells are entrapped within granulomas, but they apparently are not entirely eliminated from tissues. A proportion of the infecting inoculum remains viable within tissues for years. Thus, the organism can establish a dormant or persistent state in the human host (Deepe, 2000).

Active infection has a multitude of clinical manifestations. Acute pulmonary infection often presents as an influenza-like illness that spontaneously resolves. In this form, multiple rheumatologic manifestation may be apparent (Rosenthal et al., 1983). In those with preexisting lung disease such as emphysema, a chronic cavitary disease can develop (Goodwin et al., 1976, 1981). At the other end of the clinical spectrum is progressive disseminated histoplasmosis in which multiple organ systems, both visceral and lymphoid, are involved. This form of histoplasmosis is ultimately fatal if not clinically suspected and detected (Goodwin et al., 1980). Disseminated disease is usually observed in those whose immune systems are impaired from infections such as human immunodeficiency virus (HIV) or from pharmacologic agents including corticosteroids, cyclosporine, and cyclophosphamide (Wheat et al., 1982; Wheat and Small, 1984). The most grave clinical manifestation of disseminated infection is one with high fever, encephalopathy, and disseminated intravascular coagulation. Prompt antifungal treatment is necessary for a successful outcome. In the following chapter, the innate and adaptive elements of the host response to this fungus will be reviewed. The mechanisms that are required for the generation of protective immunity and those that subvert the protective immune response will be detailed. Figure 5.1 illustrates the major constituents of the innate and adaptive immunity to this fungus.

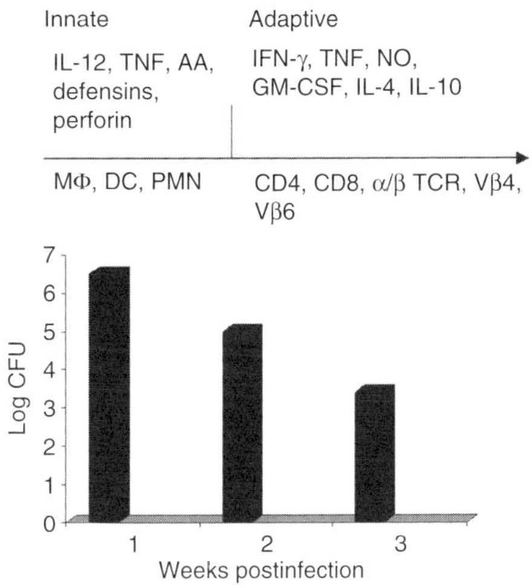

Figure 5.1. Summary of critical elements in host defenses to *H. capsulatum*. Bar graph illustrates the typical course of the burden of infection in a visceral organ, and the chronology of innate and adaptive immunity. NO, nitric oxide; AA, arachidonic acid metabolites.

2. Innate Immunity

The innate arm of immunity, present in many multicellular forms of life, is composed of a limited repertoire of receptors that are encoded within the germline. These receptors distinguish self from nonself and have evolved to respond to products of invading microbes. This branch is critically important in the initial confrontation with *H. capsulatum* since subversion of the innate immune system obviates the generation of an effective adaptive immune response.

2.1. Cellular Constituents of Innate Immunity

2.1.1. The Contact between H. capsulatum and Phagocytes

H. capsulatum morphotypes are principally engulfed by three cell types, neutrophils, immature dendritic cells, and monocytes/macrophages (MΦ) (Bullock and Wright, 1987; Newman et al., 1990, 1993, 2000; Schnur and Newman, 1990; Brummer et al., 1991; Eissenberg et al., 1991; Kurita et al., 1991a,b; Couto et al., 1994; Medeiros et al., 1999, 2002; Gildea et al., 2001). The point of contact is a pivotal feature of this interaction since it establishes the subsequent fate of the organisms within phagocytes. In fact, the fate of intracellular yeasts differs among the effector cell populations (Fig. 5.2).

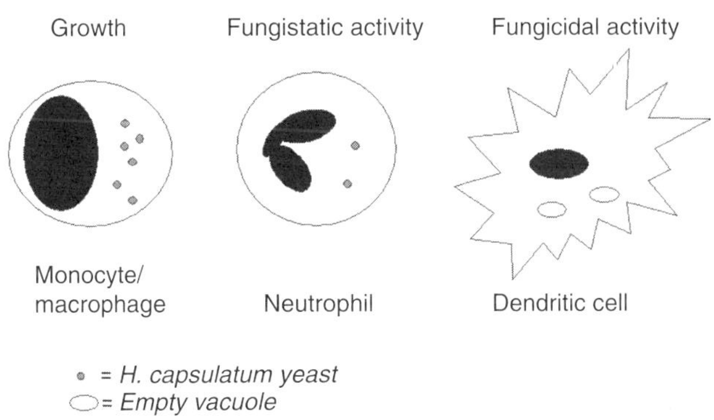

Figure 5.2. Fate of *H. capsulatum* in effector cell populations. The organism replicates in MΦ, growth is inhibited within neutrophils, and dendritic cells kill the organism.

Unopsonized *H. capsulatum* yeasts and conidia bind to the CD11/CD18 family of adhesin-promoting receptors on both monocytes/MΦ and neutrophils (Bullock and Wright, 1987). Attachment to this family of receptors provides a conduit for gaining access to the intracellular compartment of these phagocytes. A major ligand for this contact appears to be surface-expressed heat shock protein (hsp) 60 (Long et al., 2003). This molecule, which is typically found within the cytoplasm, decorates the surface of yeasts as small clusters of protein rather than a uniform, circumferential distribution. The topology suggests that there are limited numbers of hsp 60 molecules for engagement.

One issue to be resolved is to understand the means by which a cytosolic protein gains access to the surface. One possibility is that hsp 60 is shed from yeasts and attaches to the surface. This scenario would be similar to that found for the surface antigen, BAD1, of *Blastomyces dermatitidis*. This protein is released into the extracellular milieu and reattaches to chitin within the cell wall of this fungus (Brandhorst and Klein, 2000). Alternatively, *H. capsulatum* hsp 60 may be transported to the surface although a classical signal peptide has not been identified. Nevertheless, there is precedent for the surface expression of hsp 60. *Bordetella pertussis* and *Legionella pneumophila* both express this molecule on the surface (Hoffman et al., 1990; Burns et al., 1992).

Yeasts attach to the surface of immature dendritic cells. Despite the expression of the CD11/CD18 family on this cell population (McCarthy et al., 1997), yeasts predominantly, if not exclusively, bind to the very late antigen (VLA)-5 molecule (Gildea et al., 2001). The ligand on *H. capsulatum* that engages this receptor does not seem to be hsp 60. The finding that yeast cells engage a different receptor on dendritic cells than MΦ might account for the disparate fate of this fungal element within the two populations of cells.

2.1.2. Intracellular Fate of the Fungus in Cells of Innate Host Defenses

2.1.2.1. Neutrophils Human and murine neutrophils phagocytose unopsonized *H. capsulatum* yeast, but fungistasis by this phagocytic population requires incubation with either heat labile (complement) or heat stable (antibody) serum opsonins (Brummer et al., 1991; Kurita et al., 1991a,b; Newman et al., 1993). Although engulfment of yeast cells triggers a respiratory burst, the products of this reaction are not responsible for the fungistatic effect. Cells from subjects with chronic granulomatous disease, an inherited trait in which the respiratory burst can not be generated, exert fungistasis (Newman et al., 1993).

The contribution of neutrophils to human host defenses in vivo remain to be elucidated. Elimination of neutrophils from mice in a primary infection converts a nonlethal infection into one that is lethal (Zhou et al., 1998). Since these cells are capable of elaborating cytokines such as interleukin (IL)-12 and tumor necrosis factor (TNF)-α (Romani et al., 1997; Maatta et al., 1998), it may be possible that the death of the animals is caused as much by the loss of the cytokine release as the absence of cells that exert fungistatic activity.

2.1.2.2. Dendritic Cells This cell population is crucial in the interaction between host and pathogen. Dendritic cells are the most potent antigen-presenting cell population and are key to directing the immune response towards a T helper (Th)1 or a Th2 (Palucka and Banchereau, 1999). Human dendritic cells derived from monocytes cultured in the presence of granulocyte-macrophage colony-stimulating factor (GM-CSF) and IL-4 ingest and rapidly kill *H. capsulatum* yeast (Gildea et al., 2001). Degradation of yeasts can be observed within this cell population within 2 h of incubation. By 24 h, dendritic cells contain many empty vacuoles that once harbored these yeasts. The prompt response by dendritic cells against yeasts suggests that a preformed molecule or molecules express fungicidal activity.

2.1.2.3. Monocytes and MΦ In contrast to neutrophils and dendritic cells, intracellular residence of yeast or conidia within monocytes or MΦ does not result in the death of fungal elements. Conidia germinate and yeast cells replicate within monocytes or MΦ (Kimberlin et al., 1981; Bullock and Wright, 1987). Thus, these two cell populations provide a safe haven for the fungus to thrive and replicate.

Monocytes and MΦ accommodate actively growing yeast cells and cannot halt intracellular replication unless they have been activated (Wu-Hsieh and Howard, 1984). The presence of these cells is, however, essential for survival of the host. Functional impairment of these populations in mice by injection of silica markedly enhances susceptibility to infection (Von Behren et al., 1983a,b), and pretreatment with polyvinylpyrrolidine reverses this effect (Von Behren et al., 1983a,b). Dysfunctional phagocytic cells most likely lead to disease exacerbation by their inability to (1) phagocytose the fungus and (2) generate mediators that are important in host defenses (e.g., nitric oxide or TNF-α), or both.

Yeasts possess a number of potential mechanisms to elude the plethora of potential killing mechanisms of activated MΦ. Yeasts survive an oxidative burst generated by plastic-adherent MΦ from humans. Therefore, this organism must produce molecules that blunt the action of reactive oxygen intermediates. One such candidate is catalase although other scavengers of oxidative metabolites may be generated (Howard, 1983). In contrast to the findings with human MΦ, *H. capsulatum* inhibits the oxidative burst by murine MΦ (Eissenberg and Goldman, 1987; Wolf et al., 1987).

The organism may promote intracellular survival within MΦ by inhibiting apoptosis. Human phagocytes that have ingested yeasts are more resistant to apoptosis-inducing stimuli (Medeiros et al., 2002). This suppression is associated with a decrement in the expression of CD11b on the surface of cells. By inhibiting apoptosis, the fungus may lengthen the time of its existence with this phagocytic population.

Another instrument that phagocytes utilize to combat invasion by infectious agents is to fuse a phagosome with a lysosome. This process produces a vacuole that contains acidic proteinases whose enzymatic activity can digest the cell membrane and cell wall of pathogens upon acidification of the compartment. Pathogens can avoid the destructive properties of this compartment by inhibiting fusion, escaping from the vacuole, or by coexisting in it. *H. capsulatum* yeasts are found within phagolysosomes in the murine MΦ line, P388D1 (Eissenberg et al., 1988). Yeast cells contained within the phagolysosomes of this MΦ line alkalinize the pH to between 6 and 6.5 (Eissenberg et al., 1993). This value represents a delicate balance between survival and death. A pH of 6 to 6.5 is sufficiently acidic to permit yeast cells to remove iron from transferrin, one of the major iron-binding proteins. Iron is essential for yeast cell growth whether in vitro or in vivo (Sutcliffe et al., 1980; Howard, 1999; Woods, 2003). The pH of 6 to 6.5 blunts the biological activity of the acid proteinases found within phagolysosomes.

The importance of pH regulation and iron acquisition is supported by additional data analyzing human MΦ exposed to chloroquine, a weak base. Treatment of *H. capsulatum*-infected MΦ with this biochemical results in the death of yeasts whereas chloroquine does not alter yeast growth in a cell-free system (Newman et al., 1994). The fungicidal action of chloroquine-treated MΦ was reversed by exposure to iron nitriloacetate, a form of iron that can be utilized at any pH, but not by apotransferrin.

Iron limitation is a key element in host defenses expressed by MΦ.

In contrast to the findings in P388D1 cells, *H. capsulatum* yeast cells appear to thwart phagolysosomal fusion in human MΦ or in another murine MΦ cell line RAW264.7 (Newman et al., 1997; Strasser et al., 1999). This action is another survival strategy since inhibition prevents the yeast from entering one of the most hostile environments for a pathogen. In the RAW MΦ, yeasts actively diminish the accretion in phagosomes of vacuolar ATPase, a membrane-bound enzyme that generates and maintains an acidic pH within the phagosomal and endosomal pathways (Strasser et al., 1999). By suppressing the accumulation of this enzyme, a highly acidic pH (<6) cannot be produced. Consequently, acid proteinases are not active and growth of yeasts can proceed unabated.

Although particular cytokines activate the antimicrobial properties of MΦ (discussed below in adaptive immunity), they are not the only stimuli. Interestingly, human MΦ that are adhered to gelled type I collagen are fungistatic against *H. capsulatum* (Newman et al., 1997). This inhibitory activity requires that the collagen matrix develop a lattice since adherence of MΦ to nongelled collagen does not transform the cells into expressing antifungal properties. The effect is specific for collagen since other extracellular matrix proteins including fibronectin, vitronectin, and laminin do not induce an antifungal effect. Exposure of the bound MΦ to several cytokines including IL-3, GM-CSF, TNF-α, interferon (IFN)-γ, or MΦ (M)-CSF does not increase fungistasis. Thus, the formation of a three-dimensional complex is the signal that activates MΦ. When compared to plastic-adherent MΦ, the collagen-adherent MΦ manifest a marked increase in phagolysosomal fusion. These data may seem paradoxical since prior data suggest that this fungus can survive within a phagolysosome. However, the confluence of many phagolysosomes may overwhelm the defenses of *H. capsulatum*.

The findings describing the interaction of *H. capsulatum* with yeast cells or conidia with human monocytes or MΦ are performed nearly exclusively with cells from healthy individuals. *H. capsulatum* can act as an opportunistic pathogen, and as described above, disseminated histoplasmosis often develops in immunosuppressed individuals including those harboring the HIV whose $CD4^+$ T cell count is less than 100 cells/μl (Wheat and Small, 1984). HIV infects not only T cells but also MΦ and can perturb the function of the latter population. MΦ from HIV-infected individuals phagocytize fewer yeast than cells from those who are HIV seronegative, and the explanation is that fewer unopsonized yeast bind to the surface of MΦ from HIV-infected individuals (Chaturvedi et al., 1995; Chaturvedi and Newman, 1997). Phagocytosis is not altered, but rather binding is. Another finding of note in these studies is that the generation time of *H. capsulatum* in MΦ form HIV-infected subjects is more accelerated as compared to controls (Chaturvedi and Newman, 1997). Although a doubling time has not been reported, incorporation of ^{3}H-leucine by yeasts in MΦ from HIV-infected subjects substantially exceeds that in HIV seronegative subjects.

Mononuclear cells from HIV-infected subjects may have a number of immunological perturbations to account for these findings. If MΦ from healthy subjects are infected in vitro with a MΦ-tropic strain of HIV the findings are similar to those described above. Fewer yeasts are bound and ingested by HIV-infected MΦ in vitro. This decrement is a result of the HIV envelope glycoprotein, gp120, which interferes with binding to the CD11/CD18 family (Chaturvedi and Newman, 1997). Although fewer yeasts were ingested by MΦ from HIV-infected subjects, once inside, yeasts replicate more rapidly. The accelerated intracellular growth observed in MΦ from HIV-positive individuals appears to be the result of a serum factor that is yet to be identified (Chaturvedi and Newman, 1997). The more vigorous growth of yeasts within MΦ from HIV-infected individuals may account, in part, for the rapid progression of disease.

In contrast to the effector role that MΦ play in containing this fungal infection, these cells from infected mice or humans can suppress T cell-dependent responses (Stobo et al., 1976; Artz and Bullock, 1979a,b). In mice infected intravenously with *H. capsulatum* yeasts, a nylon-wool adherent population of splenic MΦ depresses T cell-dependent antibody production in vitro (Nickerson et al., 1981; Watson and Bullock, 1982). The nonspecific suppressive activity of these cells directly correlates with the fungal burden in the spleens. Similarly, a population of suppressor MΦ from the peripheral blood of humans with disseminated histoplasmosis depresses the proliferative response to a mitogenic stimulus (Stobo et al., 1976).

2.1.2.4. Natural Killer (NK) Cells There is little evidence that these cells play much of a role in controlling infection. Beige mice that possess defective NK cell activity are no more susceptible to infection than wild-type controls (Patino et al., 1987). The effect of these cells may not be apparent in an immunocompetent host since T cells appear to be the dominant force in host's ability to eliminate the fungus. In altered states of immunity, the influence of NK cells may be uncovered. *H. capsulatum* is a fatal infection in severe combined immunodeficiency mice that lack both T and B cells. Immunity can be improved by administration of IL-12. This treatment boosts the production of IFN-γ most likely by NK cells (Zhou et al., 1997). Thus, this cell population can enhance the protective immune response, but under conditions in which the dominant cell populations involved in protective immunity are absent or dysfunctional.

2.2. Acellular Constituents of Innate Immunity

2.2.1. Cytokines

Among the cytokines that are important in innate defenses, IL-12 is perhaps the key cytokine known to induce the differentiation of T cells into a Th1 phenotype (Seder and Paul, 1994). The induction of a Th1 response is a necessity for host survival to *H. capsulatum* (Wu-Hsieh, 1989; Allendoerfer and Deepe, 1997; Allendoerfer et al., 1997; Zhou et al., 1997; Clemons et al., 2000). IL-12 can be generated by MΦ, dendritic cells, neutrophils, and B cells in response to a variety of stimuli (Heufler et al., 1996; Trinchieri and Gerosa, 1996).

In vivo, transcripts for IL-12 are detected in the lungs of *H. capsulatum*-infected mice as early as day 3 after intranasal challenge (Cain and Deepe, 1998). Neutralization of IL-12 at the time of yeast challenge or the genetic absence of this cytokine in mice converts a nonlethal infection into a lethal one (Zhou et al., 1995; Allendoerfer et al., 1997). The absence of IL-12 in vivo is not only associated with a failure to generate IFN-γ but also nitric oxide whose production requires the presence of the latter cytokine (Zhou et al., 1995, Allendoerfer et al., 1997). Interestingly, mice deficient in IL-12 or IFN-γ or both, manifest an exuberant influx of neutrophils in the lungs (Cain and Deepe, 2000). The influx of cells indicates that the signals driving cellular migration are intact. Although neutrophils can inhibit the growth of *H. capsulatum* yeasts, the presence of massive numbers of these cells is obviously ineffective in elimination of this fungus in mice-deficient IL-12 and/or IFN-γ.

The inimical effects accompanying IL-12 neutralization can be mitigated by treatment of mice with monoclonal antibody (mAb) to IL-4 (Allendoerfer et al., 1997). Inhibiting the biological activity of this cytokine in the absence of IL-12 most likely restores the balance between IFN-γ and IL-4. The necessity of the host for IL-12 is dictated by the time at which it is lost during the infection. Neutralization of IL-12 beginning at the time of infection or 3 days postinfection renders mice highly susceptible to a pulmonary challenge with *H. capsulatum* yeasts. Interdiction at day 5 postinfection with mAb to IL-12 does not alter survival (Allendoerfer et al., 1997). By day 5 of infection, the Th1 phenotype has differentiated sufficiently to be independent of IL-12. This freedom from a reliance on IL-12 coincides with the production of IFN-γ (Allendoerfer et al., 1997; Cain and Deepe, 1998).

Reduction in endogenous IL-12 alters the character of the inflammatory response to *H. capsulatum*. Mice administered mAb to IL-12 and infected with this fungus manifest a decrease in the number of T cells in lungs and an increase in the number of neutrophils (Cain and Deepe, 2000). Neutralization of IL-12 increases the number of $CD80^+$ cells, but decreases the number of $CD86^+$ cells and class II major histocompatibility complex $(MHC)^+$ cells. The importance of these perturbations remains speculative, but the decrease in $CD86^+$ cells class II MHC^+ may contribute to the poor host resistance mechanisms in IL-12 deficient mice.

The source for IL-12 production in murine or human infection with *H. capsulatum* has not been defined. MΦ appear to be an unlikely source since signaling through one of the major receptors for unopsonized *H. capsulatum* yeasts, CD11b, inhibits production of IL-12. One mechanism by which ligation of CD11b impairs IL-12 production is by interfering with IFN-γ-mediated tyrosine phosphorylation (Marth and Kelsall, 1997). Dendritic cells, on the other hand, are a likely candidate. The reason is that yeasts mainly, if not exclusively, engage VLA-5, and signaling through this receptor may prompt IL-12 generation. This supposition requires experimental validation.

TNF-α is another cytokine of the innate immune system that is critically important in host defenses (Smith et al., 1990; Wu-Hsieh et al., 1992; Allendoerfer and Deepe, 1998; Zhou et al., 1998; Allendoerfer et al., 1999). In response to infection with *H. capsulatum*, there is a brisk and rapid production of TNF-α in lungs (Smith et al., 1990). The levels peak within 24 h of infection and decline steeply thereafter. Neutralization of TNF-α markedly increases susceptibility to primary pulmonary and systemic infection in mice (Smith et al., 1990; Wu-Hsieh et al., 1992; Allendoerfer and Deepe, 1998; Zhou et al., 1998). The reasons for the failure of the immune response to control infection when TNF-α is absent have not been completely defined. Several explanations have been excluded. For example, production of IFN-γ in TNF-α-neutralized mice remains vigorous (Allendoerfer and Deepe, 1998). This cytokine does not directly stimulate anti-*Histoplasma* activity of MΦ (Newman et al., 1991; Allendoerfer and Deepe, 1998). Moreover the absence of TNF-α does not alter the architecture of the inflammatory response or the number of several cell populations including neutrophils, MΦ, $CD4^+$, and $CD8^+$ cells in lungs (Allendoerfer and Deepe, 1998). These results contrast with other experimental systems in which the presence of TNF-α is key in the migration of inflammatory cells into tissues and in the development of granulomas (Kindler et al., 1989; Huffnagle et al., 1996).

One mechanism to explain the profound alteration in host response in TNF-α-deficient mice is the lack of nitric oxide production, but that may not be the sole reason (Allendoerfer and Deepe, 1998). Since this cytokine exerts multiple biological activities, it is, in fact, quite likely that its absence affects more than just nitric oxide production. Other facets of the protective immune response in TNF-α-deficient mice that require examination are the integrity of T cell-mediated immunity and the role of apoptosis.

Signaling by TNF-α is transduced by two receptors, TNF receptor (R) 1 and 2 (Beutler and Cerami, 1989; Feldmann and Maini, 2001). The genetic absence of TNFR1 and 2 in mice is associated with a progressive infection in response to an otherwise nonlethal inoculum (2×10^6) of *H. capsulatum* yeasts although the two knockout groups manifest differences in susceptibility when various inocula are used. TNFR1$^{-/-}$ mice succumb when as few as 10^3 yeasts are inoculated intranasally whereas TNFR2$^{-/-}$ mice resist up to 10^5 yeasts. The perturbations in immunity also differ between the two groups. TNFR1$^{-/-}$ mice manifest a marked impairment in the inflammatory response to this fungus. Cellular infiltration in the lungs is markedly diminished compared to wild-type controls or to TNFR2$^{-/-}$ mice. In contrast, the absence of TNFR2 is accompanied by a marked decrement in IFN-γ generation, and treatment with recombinant murine IFN-γ restores protective immunity (Allendoerfer and Deepe, 2000). In both groups of mice, generation of nitric oxide is not impaired when compared to controls. The findings listed above contrast with those found in mice whose endogenous TNF-α has been neutralized. To reiterate, these mice are able to mount a vigorous inflammatory response, production of IFN-γ is similar to that of infected controls, and nitric oxide generation is markedly diminished (Allendoerfer and Deepe, 2000). These results suggest that nitric oxide generation is dependent on the engagement of both receptors. Furthermore, there are pronounced differences in the immunological response to *H. capsulatum* in mice lacking the cytokine or the receptor for the cytokine. Even though the biological effect may be similar, in this case inhibiting the biological action of TNF-α, the mechanisms involved in the ineffectiveness of a protective immune response differ.

2.2.2. Collectins

The collectins are a family of proteins that contain a collagen-like region that is responsible for its trimeric structure and a C-type lectin domain that binds to complex carbohydrates on the surface of microbes. Among the collectin family are the surfactant proteins (SP)-A and D. Surfactant proteins line the interface between air and liquid of the lung, and they are important in lung homeostasis. In addition, they are one of the earliest host resistance mechanisms to inhaled pathogens. SP-A and SP-D are hydrophilic and are homologous to the serum opsonin, mannose-binding protein A (McCormack and Whitsett, 2002). One of the primary mechanisms by which the collectins mediate host defenses is to induce aggregation of pathogenic microbes and to opsonize microbes (McCormack and Whitsett, 2002). Evidence has emerged that SP-A and SP-D manifest direct antimicrobial properties. Each of the surfactant proteins directly kills several strains of *Escherichia coli* as well as other Gram negatives (Wu et al., 2003). SP-A and SP-D also express potent anti-*Histoplasma* activity. Incubation of yeast cells with either of these surfactant proteins results in marked fungicidal activity. Exposure of yeasts to either of these proteins results in substantial release of intracellular contents, and this effect is Ca^{2+}-dependent. It appears, therefore, that both SP-A and SP-D alter the integrity of the cell wall and perhaps the cell membrane, resulting in an efflux of intracellular contents. If yeasts are ingested by MΦ and then exposed to surfactant proteins, the fungicidal effect is not observed. The most likely explanation is that only a fraction of the surfactant protein is taken up by MΦ

(McCormack et al., 2003). This finding supports the concept that intracellular residence with this particular cell population provides a sanctuary from host defenses, in this case surfactant proteins.

2.2.3. Antimicrobial Effector Molecules from Phagocytes

The principal mediators within neutrophils that restrict yeast growth are found in azurophil granules (Newman et al., 1993, 2000). The cationic peptides, defensins, contribute to the anti-*Histoplasma* properties of human, but not murine, neutrophils since the latter do not contain these peptides (Eisenhauer and Lehrer, 1992; Couto et al., 1994; Newman et al., 2000). Other candidates for the activity within azurophilic granules are bactericidal permeability-increasing protein and cathepsin G (Newman et al., 2000). Lysozyme and elastase are only weakly active whereas azurocidin and proteinase 3 manifest no antifungal effect (Newman et al., 2000).

2.2.4. Prostaglandins and Leukotrienes

Ingestion of heat-killed *H. capsulatum* by murine MΦ stimulates both prostaglandin E2 and leukotriene C4 production albeit less than that of cells exposed to zymosan (Wolf et al., 1992). IFN-γ priming of *H. capsulatum*-infected MΦ augments only the release of prostaglandin E2 (Wolf et al., 1992). The in vivo significance of production of these arachidonic acid metabolites remains unclear. Prostaglandin E2 can suppress cellular immunity, and it may be one means by which the fungus blunts the activation of an effective cellular immune response. Nonviable *H. capsulatum* yeasts suppress the activity of protein kinase C in MΦ membranes, and this effect may dampen the generation of the oxidative burst since this enzyme is central in the formation of oxidative intermediates. Thus, the absence of an oxidative burst in murine MΦ may be attributed to modulation of protein kinase C activity.

Leukotrienes are known to promote the migration of both neutrophils and MΦ into tissues (Medeiros et al., 1999). Infection with *H. capsulatum* is associated with an early neutrophilic influx followed by MΦ into tissues. The migration of these cells is inhibited by administration of a specific inhibitor of leukotriene synthesis, MK886. These results suggest that leukotrienes are one of the mediators in the generation of inflammation (Medeiros et al., 1999).

2.2.5. Perforin

Another of the cytokine-independent mediators of host control of *H. capsulatum* is perforin. This molecule, expressed by $CD8^+$ T cells, causes lysis of target cells (Young et al., 1989). Mice deficient in this molecule are highly susceptible to a nonlethal primary, but not secondary, challenge with *H. capsulatum*. Perforin knockout mice can be immunized and establish immunological memory, but they lack the ability to resist a primary infection at least at certain inocula sizes (Zhou et al., 2001).

The absence of perforin, however, does not alter the protective function of $CD8^+$ T cells since transfer of this population from *H. capsulatum*-immunized perforin knockout mice confers protection to IFN-γ knockout mice. $CD8^+$ T cells appear to function in both perforin-dependent and -independent manner (Zhou et al., 2001). Perforin is essential for the development of a Th1 response in mice infected with *H. capsulatum* whereas this is not true for mice infected with two other intracellular pathogens, *Mycobacterium tuberculosis* and *Toxoplasma gondii* (Cooper et al., 1997; Denkers et al., 1997; Canaday et al., 2001). In those experimental models, the organisms are efficiently eliminated in the absence of perforin. It is likely that perforin is required for optimal production of IFN-γ and/or TNF-α since either one of these is key in mediating primary immunity.

3. Adaptive Immunity

In contrast to the limited plasticity of the cellular receptors involved in innate immunity, those that mediate adaptive immunity are vastly more plastic in their repertoire. As an example, T cells bear up to 10^{15} (mice) to 10^{21} (humans) different T cell receptors (TCR) as a result of genetic rearrangements (Davis, 1990). This diversity enables T cells to confront and respond to the multitude of antigens that are present in nature. In the following section, the elements of the adaptive immune response that are for controlling histoplasmosis will be discussed.

3.1. Cellular Constituents of Adaptive Immunity

3.1.1. T cells

3.1.1.1. Primary Infection α/β TCR$^+$ cells are required for controlling primary infection with *H. capsulatum* (Allendoerfer et al., 1999). Among the two major subsets, CD4$^+$ and CD8$^+$ cells, the former are the more influential in host resistance (Gomez et al., 1988; Deepe, 1994; Allendoerfer et al., 1999). The absence of CD4$^+$ T cells in mice converts a nonlethal challenge of yeasts into a lethal one irrespective of the route of infection (Gomez et al., 1988; Allendoerfer et al., 1999). As a corollary, the risk of developing histoplasmosis in humans infected with HIV can be stratified by the number of CD4$^+$ cells; they are at much greater risk for progressive, disseminated histoplasmosis if the CD4$^+$ cells is less than 100/μl (Wheat et al., 1990). The susceptibility of mice lacking CD4$^+$ cells is most likely caused by poor production of IFN-γ (Zhou et al., 1998; Allendoerfer et al., 1999). Mice depleted of this cell population manifest depressed levels of this cytokine, which is essential for survival. CD8$^+$ cells, on the other hand, are necessary for optimal elimination, but their absence does not transform a nonlethal infection into one that compromises survival (Allendoerfer et al., 1999). This finding is true for mice that genetically lack CD8$^+$ cells or those whose cells have been eliminated by administration of complement-fixing mAb (Deepe, 1994). The mechanism(s) underlying altered susceptibility in CD8$^+$-deficient mice have not been identified. Elimination of these cells does not modify production of cytokines known to be involved in the generation of protective immunity including IFN-γ, TNF-α, or GM-CSF (Zhou et al., 1998; Allendoerfer et al., 1999).

Collectively, the results indicate that there is a gradation in the functional importance of each of these T cell subpopulations in host control; CD4$^+$ cells are necessary for host survival whereas CD8$^+$ cells provide assistance in clearance of the fungus. By contrast, B cells appear to be dispensable. The burden of infection in mice deficient in mature B cells is quite similar to that of B cell sufficient animals (Allendoerfer et al., 1999).

Under certain experimental conditions, CD8$^+$ T cells may dampen immunity. In mice infected with *H. capsulatum* and a MΦ and endothelial variant clone (13) of lymphocytic choriomeningitis virus (LCMV), there is a sharp decrement in the number of CD4$^+$ T cells and B cells and a failure to control the fungus. CD8$^+$ T cells are responsible for this change since their removal restores not only the presence of CD4$^+$ T cells and B cells, but also the efficacy of the protective immune response (Wu-Hsieh et al., 2001). In this model, CD8$^+$ T cells subserve as an immunosuppressive activity. This finding recalls earlier studies in murine models of disseminated histoplasmosis induced by intravenous injection of yeasts in which $CD8^+$ T cells from actively infected mice suppress T cell-dependent functions in vitro (Nickerson et al., 1981; Watson et al., 1983). The action of these cells is dependent upon a soluble protein or glycoprotein (Deepe et al., 1984).

The organization of the clonal T cell response in lungs of C57BL/6 mice reveals a bias in TCR usage. Among the families expressing the variable region of the β chain (Vβ), $V\beta 4^+$ cells are expanded on days 7 to 14 postinfection, which is the period when T cell-mediated immunity is activated. The amplification of this family is oligoclonal, as determined by sequencing the complementarity determining region 3 (CDR3) of the TCR. This finding suggests that a limited set of epitopes drives the increase in cell number. This elevation has a functional correlate. Depletion of $V\beta 4^+$ cells impairs clearance of the fungus in lungs. Unlike the elimination of $CD4^+$ cells in which the animals die, the absence of $V\beta 4^+$ cells does not lead to a progressive, unrelenting infection. Rather, mice lacking this population manifest a delayed clearance of organisms (Gomez et al., 1998).

3.1.1.2. Secondary Infection Upon exposure to *H. capsulatum*, mice develop a protective immune response in which a subsequent challenge with the fungus results in a more rapid clearance as compared to primary infection (Allendoerfer et al., 1999). In mice with a prior exposure to *H. capsulatum*, the elimination of $CD4^+$ cells blunts the clearance when compared to controls, but eventually yeasts are eliminated. Depletion of $CD8^+$ cells does not alter handling of the infectious process (Allendoerfer et al., 1999). When both subsets are eliminated, the infection progresses to death. Surprisingly, the lungs of mice that lack both $CD4^+$ and $CD8^+$ cells can contain the burden whereas the number of yeasts in lymphoid tissue escalates dramatically, that is up to ~4 $\log_{10}$ colony-forming units (Allendoerfer et al., 1999). Thus, in the absence of the major subsets of T cells, lungs, but not spleens, of immunized mice are capable of controlling infection. The demise of the animals is a consequence of uncontrolled fungal growth in lymphoid tissue, not visceral organs. Similar findings are manifest in B cell deficient mice (Allendoerfer et al., 1999).

One mechanism to explain the difference between lymphoid organs and lungs is production of the cytokine, TNF-α (Allendoerfer et al., 1999). In the model of secondary infection, elimination of $CD4^+$ cells or $CD4^+$ and $CD8^+$ cells markedly diminishes generation of IFN-γ (Allendoerfer et al., 1999). Yet, the course of infection is vastly different between the two groups of mice. Deficiency of $CD4^+$ cells moderately delays clearance of the fungus from the lungs and spleens whereas the absence of $CD4^+$ and $CD8^+$ cells leads to a containment of the infection in lungs but not spleens. Thus, there appears to be little influence of IFN-γ in this form of the infection. On the other hand, TNF-α is a critically important cytokine in handling of yeasts in $CD4^+$- and $CD8^+$-deficient mice. Lung cells from mice lacking both T cell subset and/or B cells are capable of generating TNF-α, but splenocytes are not. Lung production of TNF-α in secondary infection is independent of the presence of T and B cells whereas the spleen requires the presence of both $CD4^+$ and $CD8^+$ cells (Allendoerfer et al., 1999).

There is a shift in the Vβ repertoire in the lungs between primary and secondary *H. capsulatum* infection. Instead of the elevation in $V\beta 4^+$ cells, the $V\beta 6^+$ family is elevated (Gomez et al., 2001). This shift differs from what has been described in mice infected with *Listeria monocytogenes* (Busch et al., 1998). The $V\beta 6^+$ cells are oligoclonal. Elimination of this population, but not the $V\beta 4^+$ family, produces only a modest impairment in host defenses to this fungus. Interestingly, depletion of both $V\beta 4^+$ and

Vβ6+ cells is accompanied by a much more dramatic difference in handling the fungal burden (Gomez et al., 2001). The loss of these two-cell populations markedly impairs clearance. These results suggest that the absence of an elevation in cell number does not necessarily exclude their functional importance.

3.2. Acellular Constituents of Adaptive Immunity

3.2.1. Cytokines

3.2.1.1. Primary Infection The evolution of the adaptive immune response to *H. capsulatum* is critically dependent on the production of several cytokines including IFN-γ, GM-CSF, TNF-α, and IL-12 (Smith et al., 1990; Wu-Hsieh et al., 1992; Zhou et al., 1995, 1997, 1998; Allendoerfer and Deepe, 1997, 1998; Allendoerfer et al., 1997; Deepe et al., 1999; Clemons et al., 2000). The influence of the last two factors on primary infection has been discussed in the context of innate immunity. It is obvious from these data that the effect of IL-12 is largely if not exclusively dependent on its ability to drive production of IFN-γ (Zhou et al., 1995, 1997; Allendoerfer et al., 1997). Following intranasal inoculation of yeasts, IFN-γ production can be detected by day 5, peaks on day 7, and begins to decline thereafter (Cain and Deepe, 1998). The principal source of IFN-γ is CD4+ cells although generation of this cytokine can be detected in both CD8+ and NK cells (Cain and Deepe, 1998).

The absence of IFN-γ renders mice highly susceptible to infection (Allendoerfer et al., 1997; Zhou et al., 1997, 1998). Two disturbances in immunity are associated with this deficiency. First, an imbalance in the levels of IL-4 and IFN-γ exists. IL-4 becomes the dominant cytokine and it subverts the generation of an adaptive response. Second, a deficiency in IFN-γ impairs release of nitric oxide, a critical constituent of host defenses to primary infection with *H. capsulatum* (Zhou et al., 1998). The deficiency in IFN-γ, however, does not impact the production of TNF-α or GM-CSF, two cytokines that mediate host resistance.

The means by which IFN-γ contribute to the adaptive immune response have been defined partially. The principal focus of studies has been the MΦ. This cytokine is a known activator of MΦ function (Boehm et al., 1997), and this assertion is true, at least in part for *H. capsulatum*. Peritoneal murine MΦ incubated with IFN-γ are activated to inhibit the growth of *H. capsulatum* yeasts, but it does not appear that exposure to it leads to killing (Wu-Hsieh and Howard, 1984; Wu-Hsieh et al., 1987, 1992). Activation of murine splenic MΦ requires a priming signal, such as lipopolysaccharide, in addition to IFN-γ (Lane et al., 1993). This cytokine in the presence or absence of lipopolysaccharide fails to activate murine alveolar MΦ (Allendoerfer et al., 1999). Similarly, human monocyte-derived MΦ are not activated by IFN-γ to express anti-*Histoplasma* activity (Fleischmann et al., 1990; Newman et al., 1991). Thus, anti-*Histoplasma* activity of IFN-γ is dependent on the source of MΦ.

Two mechanisms have been proferred to explain the growth inhibitory properties of IFN-γ. Stimulation of peritoneal murine MΦ by this cytokine limits acquisition of iron by diminishing the number of transferrin receptors on the surface of cells. This modulation restricts access to extracellular iron. Exposure to IFN-γ results in the production of nitric oxide that also appears to be responsible for the growth inhibitory properties of this cell population as blocking the production of this reactive nitrogen intermediate restores intracellular growth (Lane et al., 1991). The effect of nitric oxide on the growth of intracellular *H. capsulatum* is mediated by the formation of metal–nitric oxide complexes, specifically iron–nitric oxide. This event removes the metal from being acquired by yeast (Lane et al., 1991, 1994; Bogdan, 2001).

The generation of an efficacious adaptive immune response is also dependent on endogenous GM-CSF. It is requisite for host survival. Neutralization of this cytokine is associated with marked perturbations in the release of a number of soluble mediators in lungs of mice infected with *H. capsulatum* and is associated with a loss of host resistance (Deepe et al., 1999). Neutralization of GM-CSF produces two insults to the protective immune response that ultimately converts a nonlethal challenge of yeasts to a lethal one, but modulation of the character of the inflammatory response is not one of them. Levels of IFN-γ, TNF-α, and nitric oxide, the three mediators required for protection, are depressed compared to lungs from infected controls. The decrement in nitric oxide release may be explained not only by impaired synthesis of IFN-γ and/or TNF-α, but also by a deficiency of GM-CSF, since this cytokine can stimulate nitric oxide production (Hill et al., 1993, 1995; Blau et al., 1997). In addition to the decreases in "protective" mediators, levels of IL-4 and IL-10, two cytokines that may cause disease exacerbation are greater than infected controls. This finding has biological importance since neutralization of either one restores the capacity of GM-CSF-neutralized mice to resist infection. The myriad of subversions in mediator release accompanying inhibition of endogenous GM-CSF activity indicates the existence of a network of cytokine interactions that are interconnected with GM-CSF.

GM-CSF and M-CSF activate murine or human MΦ to express anti-*Histoplasma* activity in vitro. Administration recombinant M-CSF or GM-CSF to mice produces a marked enhancement in the *ex vivo* anti-*Histoplasma* activity by phagocytes (Brummer and Stevens, 1994; Deepe and Gibbons, 2000). For M-CSF, this action is abrogated by blocking the generation of nitric oxide. For human MΦ, M-CSF induces killing of yeasts in a short-term assay (2 h) and fungistasis in a long-term assay (24 h). The effect observed in the short-term assay was dependent on superoxide generation. Neither superoxide, nitric oxide, nor hydrogen peroxide could be implicated in the fungistasis detected in the long-term assay (Brummer and Stevens, 1994).

Two cytokines, IL-4 and IL-10, often are associated with exacerbation of infection with intracellular pathogens (Villard et al., 1995; Suzuki et al., 1996; Launois et al., 1997; Murphy et al., 1998; Himmelrich et al., 2000; Belkaid et al., 2001; Moore et al., 2001; Belkaid, 2003). Regarding the former cytokine, there is both indirect and direct evidence for its role as a mediator that enhances the burden of *H. capsulatum*. Mice infected with a lethal challenge of yeasts are rescued by treatment with mAb to IL-4 (Zhou et al., 1995). Likewise, administration of mAb to IL-4 improves survival of mice deficient in IL-12 and IFN-γ (Allendoerfer et al., 1997). More direct evidence for the inimical effects of IL-4 arises from studies using IL-4 lung transgenic mice in which the IL-4 gene is overexpressed exclusively in the lungs. In these mice, a challenge with *H. capsulatum* results in a higher fungal burden in lungs but not spleens and is not observed until the cellular immune response has been activated (≥7 days postinfection). The whole body and lung levels of IFN-γ and TNF-α are not diminished in the presence of high levels of IL-4. Remarkably the levels of IFN-γ in lungs are considerably higher in the IL-4 lung transgenic mice than wild type. The high levels of IL-4 in the lungs do not subvert the capacity of the host to generate two of the principal cytokines involved in host protection. An additional approach to understanding the role of IL-4 on host defenses to this fungus is to induce IL-4 using an allergen. Mice exposed to *Ascaris* pseudocoelomic fluid develop a Th2 response in lungs dominated by production of IL-4. In such mice, the fungal burden in lungs is higher than controls

(Gildea et al., 2003). Excess production of endogenous IL-4 modulates protective immunity but does not inhibit the generation of a Th1 response. This latter result has clinical implications especially for those with asthma in which a Th2 response dominates in the lungs. It is possible that such individuals may be more susceptible to infection with *H. capsulatum* should they come in contact with the organism.

IL-10 is a potent anti-inflammatory mediator that modulates the adaptive immune response (Moore et al., 2001). In many models of infectious diseases, the absence of IL-10 is associated with enhanced protective immunity (Moore et al., 2001). In IL-10 knockout mice, the clearance of *H. capsulatum* is accelerated but not until the second week of infection which is the time at which T cell-mediated immunity is activated (Deepe and Gibbons, 2003). IL-10 knockout mice infected with *H. capsulatum* manifest higher levels of IFN-γ in lungs and this alteration may explain the heightened efficiency of clearance. These results strongly suggest that IL-10 does not contribute to the innate immune response; rather it is key in the adaptive immune response.

The ameliorative effect associated with the absence of IL-10 can be breached by neutralization of TNF-α or IFN-γ, but not GM-CSF (Deepe and Gibbons, 2003). Treatment of IL-10 knockout mice with mAb to TNF-α or IFN-γ transforms a nonlethal infection into a lethal one. The failure of treatment with mAb to GM-CSF to subvert the protective immune response contrasts sharply with the results found in wild-type mice. In IL-10 knockout mice, the cellular character of the inflammatory response in lungs is not strikingly different than wild-type infected controls. However, the inflammatory cell infiltrate in TNF-α-neutralized mice manifest a decrease in the number of $CD8^+$ T cells in lungs whereas in knockout animals given mAb to IFN-γ there is a pronounced increase in the number of neutrophils and MΦ (Deepe and Gibbons, 2003). Since $CD8^+$ T cells influence host resistance, a decrement in this population may contribute to the impaired immunity in IL-10 knockout mice administered mAb to TNF-α. Despite the influx of neutrophils and MΦ in IFN-γ-neutralized mice, the protective response is ineffective. Hence, TNF-α and IFN-γ are required for the expression of protective immunity even in the absence of IL-10.

IL-2 is a Th1 cytokine that is important in T cell growth and cellular immunity (Smith, 1992). Splenocytes from mice with disseminated histoplasmosis manifest a deficiency in IL-2 during the height of the infection. As the burden wanes, there is recovery of IL-2 generation (Watson et al., 1985). As an extension of these studies, IL-2 treatment of immunocompetent mice with disseminated histoplasmosis improves the depression of T cell-dependent responses but does not alter the fungal burden (Deepe et al., 1986). This dissociation suggests that the immunodepression induced by this fungus is not responsible for or does not contribute to the severity of infection.

3.2.1.2. Secondary Infection TNF-α is at present the principal mediator of protection in secondary infection. Neutralization of this cytokine is associated with progressive infection and eventual death of mice (Allendoerfer and Deepe, 1998; Zhou et al., 1998). IFN-γ appears to be dispensable for secondary infection although one communication reports that IFN-γ knockout mice challenged with *H. capsulatum* succumb to a rechallenge (Allendoerfer et al., 1997). But the weight of the evidence favors the concept that IFN-γ is not a major contributor to control of secondary infection. The mechanism by which the absence of TNF-α modulates protective immunity in secondary infection differs from that found in primary histoplasmosis. In the latter, treatment with mAb to TNF-α is associated with a decrement in nitric oxide production. In secondary infection, no modulation of nitric oxide is observed; rather, there is a dramatic increase in the levels of IL-4 and IL-10 in lungs. The elevation of these cytokines appear to mediate the inimical effects of TNF-α neutralization since administration of mAb to both IL-4 and IL-10, but not either alone, restores the protective immune response (Allendoerfer and Deepe, 1998). Thus, the dysregulation in immunity associated with a deficiency in TNF-α can be corrected by neutralizing the activity of cytokines known to depress immunity.

The loss of the protective immune response that is manifest in TNF-α-neutralized mice can be mimicked by blockade of TNFR1 (Allendoerfer and Deepe, 2000). In mice in which signaling through TNFR1 is blocked, there is a dramatic loss of protection against secondary infection and a marked and broad impairment in the inflammatory response that probably accounts, in part, for the poor host response.

Treatment with mAb to GM-CSF inhibits the efficacy of the protective immune response to secondary histoplasmosis (Deepe et al., 1999). The mechanism for this impaired immunity has not yet been defined. TNF-α and IFN-γ levels are similar to controls, and IL-4 and IL-10 are not different than controls. The inflammatory response does not differ between the two groups. These results contrast with those in primary infection in which several cytokine perturbations are evident in GM-CSF-deficient mice.

As in primary infection, the absence of IL-10 is associated with a more rapid and efficient elimination of *H. capsulatum* yeasts (Deepe and Gibbons, 2003). In secondary infection, the lungs of IL-10 knockout mice exhibit elevated levels of TNF-α and IL-4. Despite the increase in the latter cytokine, the net result is a more vigorous protective immune response in the knockout animals. The integrity of the protective immune response in these animals can be disrupted by administration of mAb to TNF-α, leading to the demise of the animals. TNF-α-neutralized mice manifest depressed numbers of $CD8^+$ T cells in lungs and slightly increased IL-4 levels, both of which may contribute to the impairment in protective immunity.

The accelerated clearance of *H. capsulatum* in IL-10 knockout mice during secondary infection appears not to be a consequence of an enhanced number of memory T cells resident in lungs or spleens 8 weeks after immunization with viable yeasts. Rather, the protective effect is mediated by T cells from immunized IL-10 knockout animals and is more robust than that of T cells from wild-type mice. Thus, fewer T cells from IL-10 knockout mice are required to induce a protective response than those from wild-type.

3.2.2. Antibody

The role of B cells in the adaptive immune response remains largely an enigma. The absence of B cells does not dramatically alter the host response to this fungus in primary or secondary infection. Removal of T cells in B cell-deficient mice also does not uncover any influence of B cells in host defenses. Past experiments also failed to prove any role for antibodies when immune serum from *H. capsulatum*-immunized mice was transferred into naive recipients (Rowley and Huber, 1956). One report indicates that antibodies may be used as immunotherapy to this fungus under certain conditions (Nosanchuk et al., 2003). An IgM mAb to the surface of yeast cells recognizes a histone-like protein. If this mAb is given to mice prior to infection, it ameliorates the course of infection modestly and is associated with a reduction in inflammation and fungal burden. Protection was associated with increases in IL-4, IL-6, and IFN-γ although the significance of this finding is unknown. The salutary effect of the mAb is more pronounced in mice that receive a suboptimal amount of amphotericin B (Nosanchuk et al., 2003). There appears to be an interaction between the mAb and the antifungal agent, which is known to modulate production of cytokines and to signal through Toll-like receptor 2 (Sau et al., 2003). In vitro, mAb-opsonized, but not unopsonized, organisms are killed by a MΦ line J774.16.

3.2.3. CD40 Ligand

The interaction between CD40 and CD40 ligand (CD40L) is thought to be critical in mediating an effective adaptive immune response. Early studies with CD40L knockout mice established that failure of engagement between these two surface molecules often resulted in poor T cell stimulation, impaired IFN-γ production, and a bias to Th2 (Xu et al., 1994; Stuber et al., 1996; Grewal and Flavell, 1997; Lee et al., 2002). Extension to a model of leishmaniasis reveals that the absence of this interaction leads to a progressive infection (Campbell et al., 1996). Moreover, humans who possess a defect in the CD40L gene, otherwise known as the hyper-IgM syndrome, are known to be susceptible to several opportunistic infections (Winkelstein et al., 2003). Infection of CD40L knockout mice with *H. capsulatum* surprisingly results in a strong Th1 response as determined by IFN-γ and nitric oxide production and by the ability of knockout mice to handle the infection identical to that of wild-type (Zhou and Seder, 1998; Wheat et al., 2002). The lack of Th1 immunity observed in CD40L knockout mice infected with *Leishmania* contrasts sharply with the robust response observed in *Histoplasma*-infected animals. The underlying reasons for these differences are not well understood. One explanation that has been preferred is that production of IL-12 by MΦ or dendritic cells in response to *Leishmania* is dependent on the presence of CD40L, whereas this is not the case for *H. capsulatum*. Another postulate is that production of IFN-γ in response to *Leishmania* is strictly reliant upon $CD4^+$ cells and CD40–CD40L interactions. On the other hand, in murine histoplasmosis, NK cells and $CD8^+$ cells in addition to $CD4^+$ cells can generate IFN-γ, thus providing the host salvage pathways for synthesis and release of this Th1 cytokine (Cain and Deepe, 1998; Zhou et al., 1998).

4. Vaccine-induced Immunity

Elucidation of the cellular and molecular requirements for a potential immunogen is critical to the development of highly efficacious and useful vaccines. Without uncovering the immunologic underpinnings of a vaccine, failures cannot be understood, and more efficacious vaccines will not be generated. In this context, this section will discuss the innate and adaptive response to a protective immunogen from *H. capsulatum*.

Over the years, several candidates for a vaccine to *H. capsulatum* have been described. The use of viable yeasts, ribosomes, killed mycelia, and an ethylenediamine extract of yeasts have been reported to confer protection (Salvin, 1956; Garcia and Howard, 1971; Tewari et al., 1977; Medoff et al., 1986; Gomez et al., 1991a,b). More recently, single protein species isolated from the yeast phase of the fungus have been demonstrated to mediate protective immunity. Hsp 60, the H antigen, and an 80-kDa antigen that is recognized by mAb to hsp 70 induce a protective immune response to this fungus (Gomez et al., 1991a,b, 1992, 1995; Deepe and Gibbons, 2001). On the other hand, hsp 70 does not confer a protective immune response (Allendoerfer et al., 1996). Among the protective antigens, the best studied has been hsp 60 and will be the focus of the discussion.

Hsp 60 is a major target of the cellular and humoral response to many pathogenic microbes including *M. tuberculosis*, *M. leprae*, *Chlamydia trachomatis*, *L. pneumophila*, and *Paracoccidioides brasiliensis* (Hoffman et al., 1990; Morrison, 1991; Kong et al., 1993; Izacc et al., 2001; Lewthwaite et al., 2001). Hsp 60 has been utilized as a vaccine for *M. tuberculosis*, *L. pneumophila*, and *Yersinia pestis* (Blander and Horwitz, 1993; Noll et al., 1994; Autenrieth et al., 1995; Noll and Autenrieth, 1996; Tascon et al., 1996). Likewise, recombinant or native hsp 60 from *H. capsulatum* mediate protection against both sublethal and lethal challenges with yeasts in several strains of mice (Gomez et al., 1995). The protective effect of recombinant hsp 60 is confined to a single domain that spans amino acids 172 to 443. This region, termed F3, protects mice against nonlethal and lethal challenges (Deepe et al., 1996).

4.1. Molecular Requirements

Vaccination with recombinant hsp 60 induces the production of several cytokines including IL-12, IL-10, and IFN-γ (Deepe and Gibbons, 2002a,b). The inability of hsp 70 to induce IL-12 and a robust IFN-γ response may be one explanation for the lack of protective efficacy. The factors necessary for vaccine efficacy in the afferent limb of immunity are IL-12, IFN-γ, and IL-10 (Fig. 5.3). The former two but not the latter is required for protection in the efferent limb (Deepe and Gibbons, 2002a,b).

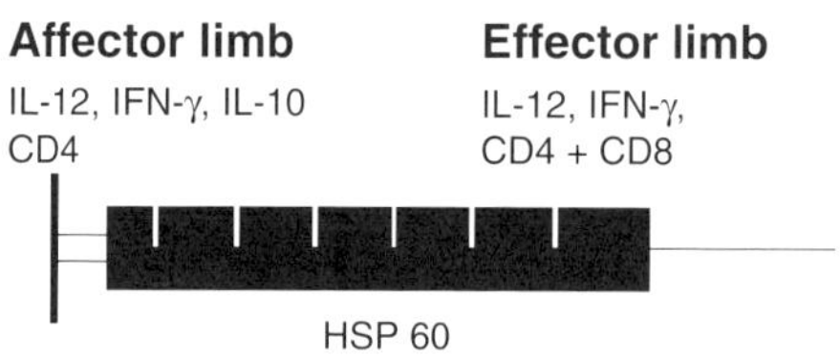

Figure 5.3. Summary of the acellular and cellular elements involved in vaccination-induced immunity. All information is based on the response to heat shock protein 60.

Perhaps the most surprising finding is the upregulation in IL-10 and the reliance of the afferent arm for this cytokine. The preponderance of data would suggest that the absence of this cytokine might enhance vaccine-associated immunity not dampen it. The anti-inflammatory properties of this cytokine probably do not explain its effect on the efficacy of hsp 60. Rather, this cytokine is known to promote the production of IFN-γ, TNF-α, and GM-CSF when given with IL-12 or IL-18 (Cai et al., 1999). One possibility is that IL-10 modulates the production of IFN-γ in response to hsp 60.

4.2. Cellular Requirements

$CD4^+$ cells must be present during the afferent phase of hsp 60-induced protection. If they are eliminated, the protective effect is abolished. In contrast, the absence of either $CD4^+$ or $CD8^+$ cells during the efferent phase does not completely eliminate protection. However, removal of both cell populations does. The principal mechanism by which elimination of $CD4^+$ cells contributes to the lack of efficacy of hsp 60 is by sharply reducing IFN-γ production (Deepe and Gibbons, 2002a,b).

Vaccination with recombinant hsp 60 produces a strong bias in the TCR usage; the vast majority of T cells that recognize this protein express $V\beta 8.1/8.2$. Analysis by sequencing TCR gene indicates that the response within this $V\beta$ family is oligoclonal. $V\beta 4^+$ cells emerge as the dominant population when $V\beta 8.1/8.2^+$ cells are depleted during vaccination (Scheckelhoff and Deepe, 2002). The $V\beta 8.1/8.2^+$ cells are required for protective efficacy since their elimination abolishes the efficacy of recombinant hsp 60. Moreover, the findings indicate that despite the emergence of $V\beta 4^+$ cells as the dominant population in $V\beta 8.1/8.2$-depleted mice, the former are unable to engender a protective response. Extended analysis of the Vβ8.1/8.2 family reveals that approximately 50% of this population is Th1 and among those cells, approximately 50% of those react to the protective fragment, F3. The identification of responsiveness to this fragment is key to the protective activity of the Vβ8.1/8.2$^+$ cells since a Th1 Vβ8.1/8.2$^+$ clone that reacts with F3 transfers protection to TCR α/β and IFN-γ knockout mice. This effect is not observed if a Th1 Vβ8.1/8.2$^+$ clone that is F3 nonresponsive is transferred (Scheckelhoff and Deepe, 2002). The mere fact that a cell is Th1 is not sufficient for protection.

Although Vβ8.1/8.2$^+$ cells are the dominant population in response to hsp 60, they constitute a minor population following vaccination with F3. T cells from F3-immunized mice are principally Vβ6$^+$ and express a limited heterogeneity in terms of CDR3 usage. Like the Vβ8.1/8.2$^+$ cells, the Vβ6$^+$ cells are necessary for vaccine efficacy in both sublethal and lethal challenges. The majority of Vβ6$^+$ cells are Th1, but Th2-expressing cells not only fail to confer protection, but also exacerbate the severity of infection (Deepe and Gibbons, 2002a,b). Collectively, the results with recombinant hsp 60 and F3 suggest that protection mediated by these cells is restricted to small populations whose absence exerts a profound effect on the protective utility of these antigens. The findings also may be one explanation for the failure of a vaccine. The absence of a single TCR family produces a large gap in vaccine efficacy.

5. Summary

In this chapter, the rapidly increasing information regarding the innate and adaptive response to this pathogenic fungus has been reviewed. A summary of the requirements is presented herein, and the principal elements of innate and adaptive immunity are illustrated in Fig. 5.4. The cellular elements that are key in the innate response include dendritic cells, neutrophils, and MΦ. The fate of yeast within each of these cell populations differs. Dendritic cells rapidly kill yeasts, neutrophils exhibit fungistatic activity, and in resting MΦ, the fungus replicates. Thus, the latter population appears to serve as a safe haven for the fungus. Activation of MΦ by several cytokines, IFN-γ in mice, GM-CSF, M-CSF, and IL-3 in humans results in growth arrest in these phagocytes. The differences in the fate of yeasts in dendritic cells compared to MΦ may be explained in part by the binding and ingestion of the organism through CD11/CD18 on the latter and VLA-5 on the former.

Several cytokines of the innate system are crucial for the generation of a protective immune response. IL-12 is essential in the generation of IFN-γ and consequently the Th1 response. TNF-α and GM-CSF also are key cytokines in the generation of a protective immune response. IFN-γ, TNF-α, and GM-CSF regulate the protective immune response in part by inducing the production of nitric oxide, a necessary molecule in the elimination of the fungus during primary infection. In addition, GM-CSF also appears to regulate the production of IFN-γ and TNF-α. IL-4 and IL-10 both appear to inhibit full expression of a robust Th1 response in the innate response.

The adaptive immune response is activated following the first week or so following nonlethal infection with this fungus. CD4$^+$ T cells are the dominant mediators of resistance in primary infection although CD8$^+$ cells do contribute to the expression of an optimal protective response. The preeminence of CD4$^+$ cells is not as apparent in secondary infection. Activation of an effective T cell-mediated immune response most likely requires upregulation in IFN-γ, TNF-α, and GM-CSF but not IL-4, IL-10, or CD40L expression, Distinct subsets of T cells influence the protective immune response—Vβ4$^+$ cells in primary and Vβ6$^+$

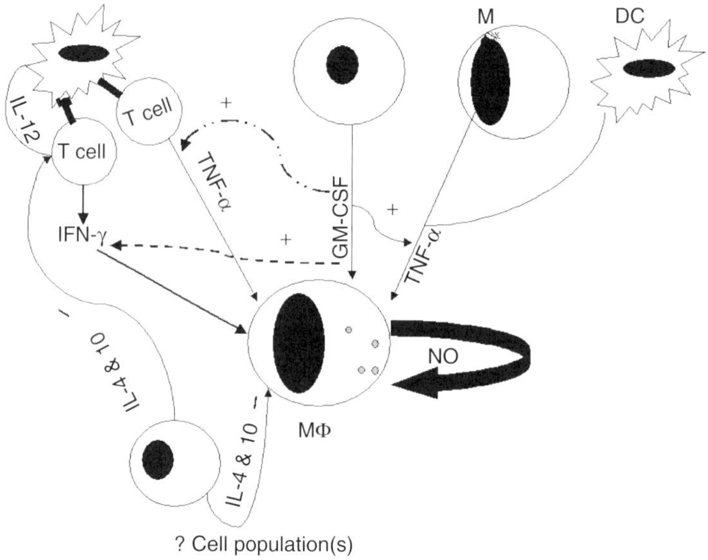

Figure 5.4. The complex nature of the protective immune response to *H. capsulatum*. IL-12, IFN-γ, TNF-α, and GM-CSF modulate the protective immune response to this fungus. GM-CSF is known to regulate production of IFN-γ and TNF-α is a positive manner, that is generation of both of these cytokines is dependent on GM-CSF. On the other hand, IL-4 and IL-10 both inhibit cellular immunity at the level of T cells and MΦ. DC, dendritic cells; +, increases; –, inhibition, ?, cell population or populations not identified.

and Vβ4+ in secondary histoplasmosis. Among the cytokines, TNF-α is absolutely necessary for control of both primary and secondary infections. Neither IL-12, IFN-γ, nor GM-CSF is essential for host control of secondary infection. Thus, once the adaptive immune response has evolved only TNF-α is absolutely required for control of the organism.

The chapter should be viewed only as a starting point rather than a conclusion. The complexities of the host-*Histoplasma* interaction require a great deal of investigation as new host response elements are discovered. Much of what we have learned has been performed on immunocompetent mice and humans. The challenges are to understand the failures in immunologic responsiveness in the immunosuppressed host in order that we may design more aggressive therapies for such individuals in whom the course of infection is often more virulent.

References

Allendoerfer, R. and Deepe, G.S. Jr. (1997). Intrapulmonary response to *Histoplasma capsulatum* in gamma interferon knockout mice. *Infect. Immun.* 65: 2564–2569.

Allendoerfer, R. and Deepe, G.S. Jr. (1998). Blockade of endogenous TNF-α exacerbates primary and secondary pulmonary histoplasmosis. *J. Immunol.* 160: 6072–6082.

Allendoerfer, R. and Deepe, G.S. Jr. (2000). Regulation of infection with *Histoplasma capsulatum* by TNFR1and -2. *J. Immunol.* 165: 2657–2664.

Allendoerfer, R., Maresca, B., and Deepe, G.S. Jr. (1996). Cellular immune responses to recombinant heat shock protein 70 from *Histoplasma capsulatum*. *Infect. Immun.* 64: 4123–4128.

Allendoerfer, R., Biovin, G.P., and Deepe, G.S. Jr. (1997). Modulation of immune responses in murine pulmonary histoplasmosis. *J. Infect. Dis.* 175: 905–914.

Allendoerfer, R., Brunner, G.D., and Deepe, G.S. Jr. (1999). Complex requirements for nascent and memory immunity in pulmonary histoplasmosis. *J. Immunol.* 162: 7389–7396.

Artz, R.P. and Bullock, W.E. (1979a). Immunoregulatory responses in experimental disseminated histoplasmosis: Lymphoid organ histopathology and serological studies. *Infect. Immun.* 23: 884–892.

Artz, R.P. and Bullock, W.E. (1979b). Immunoregulatory responses in experimental disseminated histoplasmosis: Depression of T-cell-dependent and T-effector responses by activation of splenic suppressor cells. *Infect. Immun.* 23: 893–902.

Autenrieth, I.B., Noll, A., Roggenkamp, A., and Heesemann, J. (1995). Heat-shock-protein-specific alpha-beta T cells mediate protection against *Yersinia enterocolitica*. *Contrib. Microbiol. Immunol.* 13: 199–202.

Belkaid, Y. (2003). The role of $CD4^{+}CD25^{+}$ regulatory T cells in *Leishmania* infection. *Expert Opin. Biol. Ther.* 3: 875–885.

Belkaid, Y., Hoffmann, K.F., Mendez, S., Kamhawi, S., Udey, M.C., Wynn, T.A., and Sacks, D.L. (2001). The role of interleukin (IL)-10 in the persistence of *Leishmania major* in the skin after healing and the therapeutic potential of anti-IL-10 receptor antibody for sterile cure. *J. Exp. Med.* 194: 1497–1506.

Beutler, B. and Cerami, A. (1989). The biology of cachectin/TNF—a primary mediator of the host response. *Annu. Rev. Immunol.* 7: 625–655.

Blander, S.J. and Horwitz, M.A. (1993). Major cytoplasmic membrane protein of *Legionella pneumophila*, a genus common antigen and member of the hsp 60 family of heat shock proteins, induces protective immunity in a guinea pig model of Legionnaires' disease. *J. Clin. Invest.* 91: 717–723.

Blau, H., Riklis, S., Van Iwaarden, J.F., McCormack, F.X., and Kalina, M. (1997). Nitric oxide production by rat alveolar macrophages can be modulated in vitro by surfactant protein A. *Am. J. Physiol.* 272: L1198–L1204.

Boehm, U., Klamp, T., Groot, M., Howard, J.C. (1997). Cellular responses to interferon-γ. *Ann. Rev. Immunol.* 15: 745–795.

Bogdan, C. (2001). Nitric oxide and the immune response. *Nat. Immunol.* 2: 907–916.

Brandhorst, T. and Klein, B. (2000). Cell wall biogenesis of *Blastomyces dermatitidis*. Evidence for a novel mechanism of cell surface localization of a virulence-associated adhesin via extracellular release and reassociation with cell wall chitin. *J. Biol. Chem.* 275: 7925–7934.

Brummer, E. and Stevens, D.A. (1994). Effect of macrophage colony-stimulating factor (M-CSF) on macrophage morphology, phagocytosis, and intracellular multiplication of *Histoplasma capsulatum*. *Int. J. Immunopharmacol.* 16: 171–176.

Brummer, E., Kurita, N., Yosihida, S., Nishimura, K., and Miyaji, M. (1991). Fungistatic activity of human neutrophils against *Histoplasma capsulatum*: Correlation with phagocytosis. *J. Infect. Dis.* 164: 158–162.

Bullock, W.E. and Wright, S.D. (1987). Role of the adherence-promoting receptors, CR3, LFA-1, and p150,95, in binding of *Histoplasma capsulatum* by human macrophages. *J. Exp. Med.* 165: 195–210.

Burns, D.L., Kessel, M., Arciniega, J.L., Karpas, A., and Gould-Kostka, J. (1992). Immunochemical localization of a region of chaperonin-60 important for productive interaction with chaperonin-10. *J. Biol. Chem.* 267: 25632–25635.

Busch, D.H., Pilip, I., and Pamer, E.G. (1998). Evolution of a complex T cell receptor repertoire during primary and recall bacterial infection. *J. Exp. Med.* 188: 61–70.

Cai, G., Kastelein, R.A., and Hunter, C.A. (1999). IL-10 enhances NK cell proliferation, cytotoxicity and production of IFN-γ when combined with IL-18. *Eur. J. Immunol.* 29: 2658–2665.

Cain, J. and Deepe G.S. Jr. (1998). Evolution of the primary immune response to *Histoplasma capsulatum* in murine lung. *Infect. Immun.* 66: 1473–1481.

Cain, J. and Deepe G.S. Jr. (2000). Interleukin-12 neutralization alters lung inflammation and leukocyte expression of CD80, CD86, and major histocompatibility complex class II in mice infected with *Histoplasma capsulatum*. *Infect. Immun.* 68: 2069–2076.

Campbell, K.A., Ovendale, P.J., Kennedy, M.K., Fanslow, W.C., Reed, S.G., and Maliszewski, C.R. (1996). CD40 ligand is required for protective cell-mediated immunity to *Leishmania major*. *Immunity* 4: 283–289.

Canaday, D.H., Wilkinson, R.J., Li, Q., Harding, C.V., Silver, R.F., and Boom, W.H. (2001). $CD4^{+}$ and $CD8^{+}$ T cells kill intracellular *Mycobacterium tuberculosis* by a perforin and

Fas/Fas ligand-independent mechanism. *J. Immunol.* 167: 2734–2742.

Chaturvedi, S. and Newman, S.L. (1997). Modulation of the effector function of human macrophages for *Histoplasma capsulatum* by HIV-1. Role of the envelope glycoprotein gp120. *J. Clin. Invest.* 100: 1465–1474.

Chaturvedi, S., Frame, P., and Newman, S.L. (1995). Macrophages from human immunodeficiency virus-positive persons are defective in host defense against *Histoplasma capsulatum*. *J. Infect. Dis.* 171: 320–327.

Clemons, K.V., Darbonne, W.C., Curnutte, J.T., Sobel, R.A., and Stevens, D.A. (2000). Experimental histoplasmosis in mice treated with anti-murine interferon-γ antibody and in interferon-γ gene knockout mice. *Microbes Infect.* 2: 997–1001.

Cooper, A.M., D'Souza, C., Frank, A.A., and Orme, I.M. (1997). The course of *Mycobacterium tuberculosis* infection in the lungs of mice lacking expression of either perforin- or granzyme-mediated cytolytic mechanisms. *Infect. Immun.* 65: 1317–1320.

Couto, M.A., Liu, L., Lehrer, R.I., and Ganz, T. (1994). Inhibition of intracellular *Histoplasma capsulatum* replication by murine macrophages that produce human defensin. *Infect. Immun.* 62: 2375–2378.

Davis, M.M. (1990). T cell receptor gene diversity and selection. *Annu. Rev. Biochem.* 59:475–496.

Deepe, G.S. Jr. (1994). Role of $CD8^+$ T cells in host resistance to systemic infection with *Histoplasma capsulatum* in mice. *J. Immunol.* 152: 3491–3500.

Deepe, G.S. Jr. (2000). *Histoplasma capsulatum*. In G.L. Mandell, R. Dolin, and J.E. Bennett (eds), *Principles and Practice of Infectious Diseases*, Vol. 2. Churchill Livingstone, Philadelphia, pp. 2718–2732.

Deepe, G.S. Jr. and Gibbons, R. (2000). Recombinant murine granulocyte-macrophage colony-stimulating factor modulates the course of pulmonary histoplasmosis in immunocompetent and immunodeficient mice. *Antimicrob. Agents Chemother.* 44: 3328–3336.

Deepe, G.S. Jr. and Gibbons, R. (2001). Protective efficacy of H antigen from *Histoplasma capsulatum* in a murine model of pulmonary histoplasmosis. *Infect. Immun.* 69: 3128–3134.

Deepe, G.S. Jr. and Gibbons, R.S. (2002a). Cellular and molecular regulation of vaccination with heat shock protein 60 from *Histoplasma capsulatum*. *Infect. Immun.* 70: 3759–3767.

Deepe, G.S. Jr. and Gibbons, R.S. (2002b). Functional properties of the T cell receptor repertoire in responding to the protective domain of heat-shock protein 60 from *Histoplasma capsulatum*. *J. Infect. Dis.* 186: 815–822.

Deepe, G.S., Jr. and Gibbons, R.S. (2003). Protective and memory immunity to *Histoplasma capsulatum* in the absence of IL-10. *J. Immunol.* 171: 5353–5362.

Deepe, G.S. Jr., Watson, S.R., and Bullock, W.E. (1984). Cellular origins and target cells of immunoregulatory factors in mice with disseminated histoplasmosis. *J. Immunol.* 132: 2064–2071.

Deepe, G.S. Jr., Taylor, C.L., Harris, J.E., and Bullock, W.E. (1986). Modulation of cellular immune responses in mice with disseminated histoplasmosis by recombinant interleukin-2. *Infect. Immun.* 53: 6–12.

Deepe, G.S. Jr., Gibbons, R., Brunner, G.D., and Gomez, F.J. (1996). A protective domain of heat-shock protein 60 from *Histoplasma capsulatum*. *J. Infect. Dis.* 174: 828–834.

Deepe, G.S. Jr., Gibbons, R., and Woodward, E. (1999). Neutralization of endogenous granulocyte-macrophage colony-stimulating factor subverts the protective immune response to *Histoplasma capsulatum*. *J. Immunol.* 163: 4985–4993.

Denkers, E.Y., Yap, G., Scharton-Kersten, T., Charest, H., Butcher, B.A., Caspar, P., Heiny, S., and Sher, A. (1997). Perforin-mediated cytolysis plays a limited role in host resistance to *Toxoplasma gondii*. *J. Immunol.* 159: 1903–1908.

Eisenhauer, P.B. and Lehrer, R.I. (1992). Mouse neutrophils lack defensins. *Infect. Immun.* 60: 3446–3447.

Eissenberg, L.G. and Goldman, W.E. (1987). *Histoplasma capsulatum* fails to trigger release of superoxide from macrophages. *Infect. Immun.* 55: 29–34.

Eissenberg, L.G., Schlesinger, P.H., and Goldman, W.E. (1988). Phagosome–lysosome fusion in P388D1 macrophages infected with *Histoplasma capsulatum*. *J. Leukoc. Biol.* 43: 483–491.

Eissenberg, L.G., West, J.L., Woods, J.P., and Goldman, W.E. (1991). Infection of P388D1 macrophages and respiratory epithelial cells by *Histoplasma capsulatum*: Selection of avirulent variants and their potential role in persistent histoplasmosis. *Infect. Immun.* 59: 1639–1646.

Eissenberg, L.G., Goldman, W.E., and Schlesinger, P.H. (1993). *Histoplasma capsulatum* modulates the acidification of phagolysosomes. *J. Exp. Med.* 177: 1605–1611.

Feldmann, M. and Maini, R.N. (2001). Anti-TNF-α therapy of rheumatoid arthritis: What have we learned? *Annu. Rev. Immunol.* 19: 163–196.

Fleischmann, J., Wu-Hsieh, B., and Howard, D.H. (1990). The intracellular fate of *Histoplasma capsulatum* in human macrophages is unaffected by recombinant human interferon-γ. *J. Infect. Dis.* 161: 143–145.

Garcia, J.P. and Howard, D.H. (1971). Characterization of antigens from the yeast phase of *Histoplasma capsulatum*. *Infect. Immun.* 4: 116–125.

Gildea, L.A., Morris, R.E., and Newman, S.L. (2001). *Histoplasma capsulatum* yeasts are phagocytosed via very late antigen-5, killed, and processed for antigen presentation by human dendritic cells. *J. Immunol.* 166: 1049–1056.

Gildea, L.A., Gibbons, R., Finkelman, F.D., and Deepe, G.S. Jr. (2003). Overexpression of interleukin-4 in lungs of mice impairs elimination of *Histoplasma capsulatum*. *Infect. Immun.* 71: 3787–3793.

Gomez, A.M., Bullock, W.E., Taylor, C.L., and Deepe, G.S. Jr. (1988). Role of L3T4$^+$ T cells in host defense against *Histoplasma capsulatum*. *Infect. Immun.* 56: 1685–1691.

Gomez, A.M., Rhodes, J.C., and Deepe, G.S. Jr. (1991a). Antigenicity and immunogenicity of an extract from the cell wall and cell membrane of *Histoplasma capsulatum* yeast cells. *Infect. Immun.* 59: 330–336.

Gomez, F.J., Gomez, A.M., and Deepe, G.S. Jr. (1991b). Protective efficacy of a 62-kilodalton antigen, HIS-62, from the cell wall and cell membrane of *Histoplasma capsulatum* yeast cells. *Infect. Immun.* 59: 4459–4464.

Gomez, F.J., Gomez, A.M., and Deepe, G.S. Jr. (1992). An 80-kilodalton antigen from *Histoplasma capsulatum* that has homology to heat shock protein 70 induces cell-mediated immune responses and protection in mice. *Infect. Immun.* 60: 2565–2571.

Gomez, F.J., Allendoerfer, R., and Deepe, G.S. Jr. (1995). Vaccination with recombinant heat shock protein 60 from *Histoplasma capsulatum* protects mice against pulmonary histoplasmosis. *Infect. Immun.* 63: 2587–2595.

Gomez, F.J., Cain, J.A., Gibbons, R., Allendoerfer, R., and Deepe, G.S. Jr. (1998). V$\beta4^+$ T cells promote clearance of infection in murine pulmonary histoplasmosis. *J. Clin. Invest.* 102: 984–995.

Gomez, F.J., Woodward, E.O., Pilcher-Roberts, R., Gibbons, R.S., and Deepe, G.S. Jr. (2001). V$\beta6^+$ and V$\beta4^+$ T cells exert cooperative activity in clearance of secondary infection with *Histoplasma capsulatum*. *J. Immunol.* 166: 2855–2862.

Goodwin, R.A. Jr., Owens, F.T., Snell, J.D., Hubbard, W.W., Buchanan, R.D., Terry, R.T., and Des Prez, R.M. (1976). Chronic pulmonary histoplasmosis. *Medicine (Baltimore)* 55: 413–452.

Goodwin, R.A. Jr., Shapiro, J.L., Thurman, G.H., Thurman, S.S., and Des Prez, R.M. (1980). Disseminated histoplasmosis: Clinical and pathologic correlations. *Medicine (Baltimore)* 59: 1–33.

Goodwin, R.A., Loyd, J.E., and Des Prez, R.M. (1981). Histoplasmosis in normal hosts. *Medicine (Baltimore)* 60: 231–266.

Grewal, I.S. and Flavell, R.A. (1997). The CD40 ligand. At the center of the immune universe? *Immunol. Res.* 16: 59–70.

Heufler, C., Koch, F., Stanzl, U., Topar, G., Wysocka, M., Trinchieri, G., Enk, A., Steinman, R.M., Romani, N., and Schuler, G. (1996). Interleukin-12 is produced by dendritic cells and mediates T helper 1 development as well as interferon-γ production by T helper 1 cells. *Eur. J. Immunol.* 26: 659–668.

Hill, A.D., Redmond, H.P., Austin, O.M., Grace, P.A., and Bouchier-Hayes, D. (1993). Granulocyte-macrophage colony-stimulating factor inhibits tumour growth. *Br. J. Surg.* 80: 1543–1546.

Hill, A.D., Naama, H., Shou, J., Calvano, S.E., and Daly, J.M. (1995). Antimicrobial effects of granulocyte-macrophage colony-stimulating factor in protein-energy malnutrition. *Arch. Surg.* 130: 1273–1277.

Himmelrich, H., Launois, P., Maillard, I., Biedermann, T., Tacchini-Cottier, F., Locksley, R.M., Rocken, M., and Louis, J.A. (2000). In

BALB/c mice, IL-4 production during the initial phase of infection with *Leishmania major* is necessary and sufficient to instruct Th2 cell development resulting in progressive disease. *J. Immunol.* 164: 4819–4825.

Hoffman, P.S., Houston, L., and Butler, C.A. (1990). *Legionella pneumophila* htpAB heat shock operon: nucleotide sequence and expression of the 60-kilodalton antigen in *L. pneumophila*-infected HeLa cells. *Infect. Immun.* 58: 3380–3387.

Howard, D.H. (1983). Studies on the catalase of *Histoplasma capsulatum*. *Infect. Immun.* 39: 1161–1166.

Howard, D.H. (1999). Acquisition, transport, and storage of iron by pathogenic fungi. *Clin. Microbiol. Rev.* 12: 394–404.

Huffnagle, G.B., Toews, G.B., Burdick, M.D., Boyd, M.B., McAllister, K.S., McDonald, R.A., Kunkel, S.L., and Strieter, R.M. (1996). Afferent phase production of TNF-α is required for the development of protective T cell immunity to *Cryptococcus neoformans*. *J. Immunol.* 157: 4529–4536.

Izacc, S.M., Gomez, F.J., Jesuino, R.S., Fonseca, C.A., Felipe, M.S., Deepe, G.S., and Soares, C.M. (2001). Molecular cloning, characterization and expression of the heat shock protein 60 gene from the human pathogenic fungus *Paracoccidioides brasiliensis*. *Med. Mycol.* 39: 445–455.

Kimberlin, C.L., Hariri, A.R., Hempel, H.O., and Goodman, N.L. (1981). Interactions between *Histoplasma capsulatum* and macrophages from normal and treated mice: Comparison of the mycelial and yeast phases in alveolar and peritoneal macrophages. *Infect. Immun.* 34: 6–10.

Kindler, V., Sappino, A.P., Grau, G.E., Piguet, P.F., and Vassalli, P. (1989). The inducing role of tumor necrosis factor in the development of bactericidal granulomas during BCG infection. *Cell* 56: 731–740.

Kong, T.H., Coates, A.R., Butcher, P.D., Hickman, C.J., and Shinnick, T.M. (1993). *Mycobacterium tuberculosis* expresses two chaperonin-60 homologs. *Proc. Natl. Acad. Sci. USA* 90: 2608–2612.

Kurita, N., Brummer, E., Yoshida, S., Nishimura, K., and Miyaji, M. (1991a). Antifungal activity of murine polymorphonuclear neutrophils against *Histoplasma capsulatum*. *J. Med. Vet. Mycol.* 29: 133–143.

Kurita, N., Terao, K., Brummer, E., Ito, E., Nishimura, K., and Miyaji, M. (1991b). Resistance of *Histoplasma capsulatum* to killing by human neutrophils. Evasion of oxidative burst and lysosomal-fusion products. *Mycopathologia* 115: 207–213.

Lane, T.E., Wu-Hsieh, B.A., and Howard, D.H. (1991). Iron limitation and the gamma interferon-mediated antihistoplasma state of murine macrophages. *Infect. Immun.* 59: 2274–2278.

Lane, T.E., Wu-Hsieh, B.A., and Howard, D.H. (1993). Gamma interferon cooperates with lipopolysaccharide to activate mouse splenic macrophages to an antihistoplasma state. *Infect. Immun.* 61: 1468–1473.

Lane, T.E., Wu-Hsieh, B.A., and Howard, D.H. (1994). Antihistoplasma effect of activated mouse splenic macrophages involves production of reactive nitrogen intermediates. *Infect. Immun.* 62: 1940–1945.

Launois, P., Maillard, I., Pingel, S., Swihart, K.G., Xenarios, I., Acha-Orbea, H., Diggelmann, H., Locksley, R.M., MacDonald, H.R., and Louis, J.A. (1997). IL-4 rapidly produced by Vβ 4 Vα 8 $CD4^+$ T cells instructs Th2 development and susceptibility to *Leishmania major* in BALB/c mice. *Immunity* 6: 541–549.

Lee, B.O., Haynes, L., Eaton, S.M., Swain, S.L., and Randall, T.D. (2002). The biological outcome of CD40 signaling is dependent on the duration of CD40 ligand expression: Reciprocal regulation by interleukin (IL)-4 and IL-12. *J. Exp. Med.* 196: 693–704.

Lewthwaite, J.C., Coates, A.R., Tormay, P., Singh, M., Mascagni, P., Poole, S., Roberts, M., Sharp, L., and Henderson, B. (2001). *Mycobacterium tuberculosis* chaperonin 60.1 is a more potent cytokine stimulator than chaperonin 60.2 (Hsp 65) and contains a CD14-binding domain. *Infect. Immun.* 69: 7349–7355.

Long, K.H., Gomez, F.J., Morris, R.E., and Newman, S.L. (2003). Identification of heat shock protein 60 as the ligand on *Histoplasma capsulatum* that mediates binding to CD18 receptors on human macrophages. *J. Immunol.* 170: 487–494.

Maatta, J.A., Sjoholm, U.R., Nygardas, P.T., Salmi, A.A., and Hinkkanen, A.E. (1998). Neutrophils secreting tumor necrosis factor-α infiltrate the central nervous system of BALB/c mice with experimental autoimmune encephalomyelitis. *J. Neuroimmunol.* 90: 162–175.

Marth, T. and Kelsall, B.L. (1997). Regulation of interleukin-12 by complement receptor 3 signaling. *J. Exp. Med.* 185: 1987–1995.

McCarthy, D.A., Macey, M.G., Bedford, P.A., Knight, S.C., Dumonde, D.C., and Brown, K.A. (1997). Adhesion molecules are upregulated on dendritic cells isolated from human blood. *Immunology* 92: 244–251.

McCormack, F.X. and Whitsett, J.A. (2002). The pulmonary collectins, SP-A and SP-D, orchestrate innate immunity in the lung. *J. Clin. Invest.* 109: 707–712.

McCormack, F.X., Gibbons, R., Ward, S.R., Kuzmenko, A., Wu, H., and Deepe, G.S. Jr. (2003). Macrophage-independent fungicidal action of the pulmonary collectins. *J. Biol. Chem.* 278: 36250–36256.

Medeiros, A.I., Silva, C.L., Malheiro, A., Maffei, C.M., and Faccioli, L.H. (1999). Leukotrienes are involved in leukocyte recruitment induced by live *Histoplasma capsulatum* or by the beta-glucan present in their cell wall. *Br. J. Pharmacol.* 128: 1529–1537.

Medeiros, A.I., Bonato, V.L., Malheiro, A., Dias, A.R., Silva, C.L., and Faccioli, L.H. (2002). *Histoplasma capsulatum* inhibits apoptosis and Mac-1 expression in leucocytes. *Scand. J. Immunol.* 56: 392–398.

Medoff, G., Sacco, M., Maresca, B., Schlessinger, D., Painter, A., Kobayashi, G.S., and Carratu, L. (1986). Irreversible block of the mycelial-to-yeast phase transition of *Histoplasma capsulatum*. *Science* 231: 476–479.

Moore, K.W., de Waal Malefyt, R., Coffman, R.L., and O'Garra, A. (2001). Interleukin-10 and the interleukin-10 receptor. *Annu. Rev. Immunol.* 19: 683–765.

Morrison, R.P. (1991). Chlamydial hsp60 and the immunopathogenesis of chlamydial disease. *Semin. Immunol.* 3: 25–33.

Murphy, J.W., Bistoni, F., Deepe, G.S., Blackstock, R.A., Buchanan, K., Ashman, R.B., Romani, L., Mencacci, A., Cenci, E., Fe d'Ostiani, C., Del Sero, G., Calich, V.L., and Kashino, S.S. (1998). Type 1 and type 2 cytokines: From basic science to fungal infections. *Med. Mycol.* 36: 109–118.

Newman, S.L., Bucher, C., Rhodes, J., and Bullock, W.E. (1990). Phagocytosis of *Histoplasma capsulatum* yeasts and microconidia by human cultured macrophages and alveolar macrophages. Cellular cytoskeleton requirement for attachment and ingestion. *J. Clin. Invest.* 85: 223–230.

Newman, S.L., Gootee, L., Bucher, C., and Bullock, W.E. (1991). Inhibition of intracellular growth of *Histoplasma capsulatum* yeast cells by cytokine-activated human monocytes and macrophages. *Infect. Immun.* 59: 737–741.

Newman, S.L., Gootee, L., and Gabay, J.E. (1993). Human neutrophil-mediated fungistasis against *Histoplasma capsulatum*. Localization of fungistatic activity to the azurophil granules. *J. Clin. Invest.* 92: 624–631.

Newman, S.L., Gootee, L., Brunner, G., and Deepe, G.S. Jr. (1994). Chloroquine induces human macrophage killing of *Histoplasma capsulatum* by limiting the availability of intracellular iron and is therapeutic in a murine model of histoplasmosis. *J. Clin. Invest.* 93: 1422–1429.

Newman, S.L., Gootee, L., Kidd, C., Ciraolo, G.M., and Morris, R. (1997). Activation of human macrophage fungistatic activity against *Histoplasma capsulatum* upon adherence to type 1 collagen matrices. *J. Immunol.* 158: 1779–1786.

Newman, S.L., Gootee, L., Gabay, J.E., and Selsted, M.E. (2000). Identification of constituents of human neutrophil azurophil granules that mediate fungistasis against *Histoplasma capsulatum*. *Infect. Immun.* 68: 5668–5672.

Nickerson, D.A., Havens, R.A., and Bullock, W.E. (1981). Immunoregulation in disseminated histoplasmosis: Characterization of splenic suppressor cell populations. *Cell. Immunol.* 60: 287–297.

Noll, A. and Autenrieth, I.B. (1996). Immunity against *Yersinia enterocolitica* by vaccination with Yersinia HSP60 immunostimulating complexes or Yersinia HSP60 plus interleukin-12. *Infect. Immun.* 64: 2955–2961.

Noll, A., Roggenkamp, A., Heesemann, J., and Autenrieth, I.B. (1994). Protective role for heat shock protein-reactive alpha beta T cells in murine yersiniosis. *Infect. Immun.* 62: 2784–2791.

Nosanchuk, J.D., Steenbergen, J.N., Shi, L., Deepe, G.S. Jr., and Casadevall, A. (2003). Antibodies to a cell surface histone-like protein protect against *Histoplasma capsulatum*. *J. Clin. Invest.* 112: 1164–1175.

Palucka, K. and Banchereau, J. (1999). Linking innate and adaptive immunity. *Nat. Med.* 5: 868–870.

Patino, M.M., Williams, D., Ahrens, J., and Graybill, J.R. (1987). Experimental histoplasmosis in the beige mouse. *J. Leukoc. Biol.* 41: 228–235.

Romani, L., Mencacci, A., Cenci, E., Spaccapelo, R., Del Sero, G., Nicoletti, I., Trinchieri, G., Bistoni, F., and Puccetti, P. (1997). Neutrophil production of IL-12 and IL-10 in candidiasis and efficacy of IL-12 therapy in neutropenic mice. *J. Immunol.* 158: 5349–5356.

Rosenthal, J., Brandt, K.D., Wheat, L.J., and Slama, T.G. (1983). Rheumatologic manifestations of histoplasmosis in the recent Indianapolis epidemic. *Arthritis Rheum.* 26: 1065–1070.

Rowley, D.A. and Huber, M. (1956). Growth of *Histoplasma capsulatum* in normal, superinfected, and immunized mice. *J. Immunol.* 77: 15–23.

Salvin, S.B. (1956). Immunization of mice against *Histoplasma capsulatum. Public Health Monogr.* 70: 107–109.

Sau, K., Mambula, S.S., Latz, E., Henneke, P., Golenbock, D.T., and Levitz, S.M. (2003). The antifungal drug amphotericin B promotes inflammatory cytokine release by a toll-like receptor- and CD14-dependent mechanism. *J. Biol. Chem.* 278: 37561–37568.

Scheckelhoff, M. and Deepe, G.S. Jr. (2002). The protective immune response to heat shock protein 60 of *Histoplasma capsulatum* is mediated by a subset of Vß8.1/8.2$^+$ T cells. *J. Immunol.* 169: 5818–5826.

Schnur, R.A. and Newman, S.L. (1990). The respiratory burst response to *Histoplasma capsulatum* by human neutrophils. Evidence for intracellular trapping of superoxide anion. *J. Immunol.* 144: 4765–4772.

Seder, R. and Paul, W. (1994). Acquisition of lymphokine-producing phenotype CD4$^+$ T cells. *Annu. Rev. Immunol.* 12: 635–674.

Smith, K.A. (1992). Interleukin-2. *Curr. Opin. Immunol.* 4: 271–276.

Smith, J.G., Magee, D.M., Williams, D.M., and Graybill, J.R. (1990). Tumor necrosis factor-alpha plays a role in host defense against *Histoplasma capsulatum. J. Infect. Dis.* 162: 1349–1353.

Stobo, J.D., Paul, S., Van Scoy, R.E., and Hermans, P.E. (1976). Suppressor thymus-derived lymphocytes in fungal infection. *J. Clin. Invest.* 57: 319–328.

Strasser, J.E., Newman, S.L., Ciraolo, G.M., Morris, R.E., Howell, M.L., and Dean, G.E. (1999). Regulation of the macrophage vacuolar ATPase and phagosome–lysosome fusion by *Histoplasma capsulatum. J. Immunol.* 162: 6148–6154.

Stuber, E., Strober, W., and Neurath, M. (1996). Blocking the CD40L–CD40 interaction in vivo specifically prevents the priming of T helper 1 cells through the inhibition of interleukin 12 secretion. *J. Exp. Med.* 183: 693–698.

Sutcliffe, M.C., Savage, A.M., and Alford, R.H. (1980). Transferrin-dependent growth inhibition of yeast-phase *Histoplasma capsulatum* by human serum and lymph. *J. Infect. Dis.* 142: 209–219.

Suzuki, Y., Yang, Q., Yang, S., Nguyen, N., Lim, S., Liesenfeld, O., Kojima, T., and Remington, J.S. (1996). IL-4 is protective against development of toxoplasmic encephalitis. *J. Immunol.* 157: 2564–2569.

Tascon, R.E., Colston, M.J., Ragno, S., Stavropoulos, E., Gregory, D., and Lowrie, D.B. (1996). Vaccination against tuberculosis by DNA injection. *Nat. Med.* 2: 888–892.

Tewari, R.P., Sharma, D., Solotorovsky, M., Lafemina, R., and Balint, J. (1977). Adoptive transfer of immunity from mice immunized with ribosomes or live yeast cells of *Histoplasma capsulatum. Infect. Immun.* 15: 789–795.

Trinchieri, G. and Gerosa, F. (1996). Immunoregulation by interleukin-12. *J. Leukoc. Biol.* 59: 505–511.

Villard, O., Candolfi, E., Despringre, J.L., Derouin, F., Marcellin, L., Viville, S., and Kien, T. (1995). Protective effect of low doses of an anti-IL-4 monoclonal antibody in a murine model of acute toxoplasmosis. *Parasite Immunol.* 17: 233–236.

Von Behren, L.A., Chaudhary, S., Khardori, N., Rabinovich, S., Shu, M.D., and Tewari, R.P. (1983a). Effect of silica on the susceptibility of mice to experimental histoplasmosis. *J. Reticuloendothel. Soc.* 34: 99–111.

Von Behren, L.A., Chaudhary, S., Rabinovich, S., Shu, M.D., and Tewari, R.P. (1983b). Protective effect of poly-2-vinylpyridine-N-oxide on susceptibility of silica-treated mice to experimental histoplasmosis. *Infect. Immun.* 42: 818–823.

Watson, S.R. and Bullock, W.E. (1982). Immunoregulation in disseminated histoplasmosis: Characterization of the surface phenotype of splenic suppressor T lymphocytes. *Infect. Immun.* 37: 940–945.

Watson, S.R., Miller, T.B., Redington, T.J., and Bullock, W.E. (1983). Immunoregulation in experimental disseminated histoplasmosis: Flow microfluorometry (FMF) studies of the Thy and Lyt phenotypes of T lymphocytes from infected mice. *J. Immunol.* 131: 984–990.

Watson, S.R., Schmitt, S.K., Hendricks, D.E., and Bullock, W.E. (1985). Immunoregulation in disseminated murine histoplasmosis: Disturbances in the production of interleukins 1 and 2. *J. Immunol.* 135: 3487–3493.

Wheat, L.J. and Small, C.B. (1984). Disseminated histoplasmosis in the acquired immune deficiency syndrome. *Arch. Intern. Med.* 144: 2147–2149.

Wheat, L.J., Slama, T.G., Norton, J.A., Kohler, R.B., Eitzen, H.E., French, M.L., and Sathapatayavongs, B. (1982). Risk factors for disseminated or fatal histoplasmosis. Analysis of a large urban outbreak. *Ann. Int. Med.* 96: 159–163.

Wheat, L.J., Connolly-Stringfield, P.A., Baker, R.L., Curfman, M.F., Eads, M.E., Israel, K.S., Norris, S.A., Webb, D.H., and Zeckel, M.L. (1990). Disseminated histoplasmosis in the acquired immune deficiency syndrome: Clinical findings, diagnosis and treatment, and review of the literature. *Medicine (Baltimore)* 69: 361–374.

Wheat, L.J., Durkin, M., Schnizlein-Bick, C., Bassey, E., Kohler, S., Connolly, P., Goldberg, J., Garringer, T., Brizendine, E., and Thomas, E.K. (2002). Effect of CD40 ligand on the course of murine histoplasmosis. *Med. Mycol.* 40: 501–505.

Winkelstein, J.A., Marino, M.C., Ochs, H., Fuleihan, R., Scholl, P.R., Geha, R., Stiehm, E.R., and Conley, M.E. (2003). The X-linked hyper-IgM syndrome: Clinical and immunologic features of 79 patients. *Medicine (Baltimore)* 82: 373–384.

Wolf, J.E., Kerchberger, V., Kobayashi, G.S., and Little, J.R. (1987). Modulation of the macrophage oxidative burst by *Histoplasma capsulatum*. *J. Immunol.* 138: 582–586.

Wolf, J.E., Massof, S.E., and Peters, S.P. (1992). Alterations in murine macrophage arachidonic acid metabolism following ingestion of nonviable *Histoplasma capsulatum*. *Infect. Immun.* 60: 2559–2564.

Woods, J.P. (2003). Knocking on the right door and making a comfortable home: *Histoplasma capsulatum* intracellular pathogenesis. *Curr. Opin. Microbiol.* 6: 327–331.

Wu, H., Kuzmenko, A., Wan, S., Schaffer, L., Weiss, A., Fisher, J.H., Kim, K.S., and McCormack, F.X. (2003). Surfactant proteins A and D inhibit the growth of Gram-negative bacteria by increasing membrane permeability. *J. Clin. Invest.* 111: 1589–1602.

Wu-Hsieh, B. (1989). Relative susceptibilities of inbred mouse strains C57BL/6 and A/J to infection with *Histoplasma capsulatum*. *Infect. Immun.* 57: 3788–3792.

Wu-Hsieh, B.A., Howard, D.H. (1987). Inhibition of intracellular growth of *Histoplasma capsulatum* by recombinant murine interferon gamma. *Infect. Immun.* 55: 1014–1016.

Wu-Hsieh, B. and Howard, D.H. (1984). Inhibition of growth of *Histoplasma capsulatum* by lymphokine-stimulated macrophages. *J. Immunol.* 132: 2593–2597.

Wu-Hsieh, B.A., Lee, G.S., Franco, M., and Hofman, F.M. (1992). Early activation of splenic macrophages by tumor necrosis factor alpha is important in determining the outcome of experimental histoplasmosis in mice. *Infect. Immun.* 60: 4230–4238.

Wu-Hsieh, B.A., Whitmire, J.K., de Fries, R., Lin, J.S., Matloubian, M., and Ahmed, R. (2001). Distinct CD8 T cell functions mediate susceptibility to histoplasmosis during chronic viral infection. *J. Immunol.* 167: 4566–4573.

Xu, J., Foy, T.M., Laman, J.D., Elliott, E.A., Dunn, J.J., Waldschmidt, T.J., Elsemore, J., Noelle, R.J., and Flavell, R.A. (1994). Mice deficient for the CD40 ligand. *Immunity* 1: 423–431.

Young, L.H., Klavinskis, L.S., Oldstone, M.B., and Young, J.D. (1989). In vivo expression of perforin by $CD8^+$ lymphocytes during an acute viral infection. *J. Exp. Med.* 169: 2159–2171.

Zhou, P. and Seder, R.A. (1998). CD40 ligand is not essential for induction of type 1 cytokine responses or protective immunity after primary or secondary infection with *Histoplasma capsulatum*. *J. Exp. Med.* 187: 1315–1324.

Zhou, P., Sieve, M.C., Bennett, J., Kwon-Chung, K.J., Tewari, R.P., Gazzinelli, R.T., Sher, A., and Seder, R.A. (1995). IL-12 prevents mortality in mice infected with *Histoplasma capsulatum* through induction of IFN-gamma. *J. Immunol.* 155: 785–795.

Zhou, P., Sieve, M.C., Tewari, R.P., and Seder, R.A. (1997). Interleukin-12 modulates the protective immune response in SCID mice infected with *Histoplasma capsulatum*. *Infect. Immun.* 65: 936–942.

Zhou, P., Miller, G., and Seder, R.A. (1998). Factors involved in regulating primary and secondary immunity to infection with *Histoplasma capsulatum*: TNF-α plays a critical role in maintaining secondary immunity in the absence of IFN-gamma. *J. Immunol.* 160: 1359–1368.

Zhou, P., Freidag, B.L., Caldwell, C.C., and Seder, R.A. (2001). Perforin is required for primary immunity to *Histoplasma capsulatum*. *J. Immunol.* 166: 1968–1974.

6

Lung Immunity to *Blastomyces dermatitidis* Infection

Marcel Wüthrich[1] and Bruce S. Klein[1–4]

Departments of Pediatrics[1], Internal Medicine[2], and Medical Microbiology and Immunology[3], the Comprehensive Cancer Center[4], University of Wisconsin Medical School, University of Wisconsin Hospital and Clinics, Madison, WI, 53792.

1. Introduction

The dimorphic fungus *Blastomyces dermatitidis* inhabits moist acidic soil along the Mississippi and Ohio River valleys (Klein et al., 1986). Upon inhalation of conidia or mycelial fragments, it converts to the yeast form within the alveolar spaces and establishes infection. *B. dermatitidis* produces a progressive pulmonary and disseminated infection and is one of the principal systemic mycoses of humans and animals worldwide. The infection may remain pulmonary or may disseminate to other sites such as the skin, bone, or genitourinary tract (Bradsher, 1996). Both pulmonary and disseminated blastomycosis can be fatal. Infections that go undiagnosed or untreated often progress and become fatal even in immunocompetent hosts. The progressive nature of many clinical *B. dermatitidis* infections distinguishes blastomycosis from several other related mycoses such as histoplasmosis, coccidioidomycosis, and paracoccidioidomycosis, which more often occur as self-limited infections. A murine model of *B. dermatitidis* infection has been developed that resembles clinical features of pulmonary blastomycosis in people (Harvey et al., 1978; Wüthrich et al., 1998). Administration of *B. dermatitidis* via the respiratory route, with as few as 10–100 virulent yeast, leads to chronic, progressive pneumonia, which consumes mice within several weeks of infection (Brandhorst et al., 1999). Thus, even a small number of *B. dermatitidis* yeast cannot be resolved by an immunocompetent host. In this chapter, we review aspects of innate and acquired immunity against *B. dermatitidis* infection, and explore some of the molecular determinants that make this agent such a formidable foe for these elements of host immunity.

2. Innate Immunity in the Lungs to *B. dermatitidis* Infection

2.1. Cellular Resistance by Alveolar Macrophages and Polymorphonuclear Neutrophils (PMNs)

Alveolar macrophages are the first line of defense against inhaled microbes, including *B. dermatitidis*. However, alveolar macrophages from normal persons and naïve mice are only modestly capable of ingesting and killing *B. dermatitidis* yeasts. After 72 h of in vitro coincubation of yeasts with pulmonary alveolar macrophages from normal persons, only 12–18% of the cells had ingested the yeast, and the population of yeast had surprisingly increased by 52% over the starting inoculum (Bradsher et al., 1987). In coculture assays with murine alveolar macrophages from normal animals and yeasts, only 0–5% of the yeasts were killed after 4 h (Brummer and Stevens, 1987; Brummer et al., 1988). One explanation for the seemingly modest fungicidal activity of alveolar macrophages for *B. dermatitidis* might relate to the correspondingly modest respiratory burst the fungus triggers in alveolar macrophages. Under optimal conditions in which monolayers of murine alveolar macrophages are challenged with *B. dermatitidis* conidia, the particles elicit a respiratory burst (measured by O_2^- production) only 25–31% of that seen with the potent stimulus of zymosan, and the suboptimal response is independent of fungal strain (Sugar and Field, 1987a). Similar trends were found when *B. dermatitidis* yeast strains were evaluated in this assay system (Sugar and Field, 1987b).

Upon a naturally acquired infection by conidia of *B. dermatitidis* or an experimental pulmonary challenge with yeast in mice, mononuclear phagocytes, predominantly PMNs influx into the site of infection and form characteristic pyogranulomatous lesions. Human PMNs phagocytize infective conidia rapidly and efficiently. In vitro, under conditions in which PMNs and conidia were cocultured at a ratio of 10:1, PMNs phagocytized 83% of the particles in 1 h and 90% in 2 h. However, PMNs killed conidia more slowly and incompletely; after 1 h only 18% of conidia were killed and after 3 h the maximum, 50% were killed. The phagocytosis and killing of *B. dermatitidis* conidia by PMNs is accomplished mainly by oxidative mechanisms. By 20 min of coincubation of conidia with human PMNs, phagocytes have produced peak values of oxidative burst chemicals that are approximately 70% of the positive control values produced by zymosan, a potent trigger of oxidative metabolism (Drutz and Frey, 1985).

The yeasts of *B. dermatitidis* are considerably more difficult for PMNs to phagocytize and kill than conidia, regardless of the strain size. Drutz and Frey (1985) found that an average of only 18% of the yeasts of six strains were killed when PMNs and yeasts were coincubated for 2 h at the optimal ratio of 10 PMNs per yeast. Upon exposure to *B. dermatitidis* yeasts, PMNs display a rapid and pronounced oxidative burst as measured by chemiluminescence response (Sixbey et al., 1979; Drutz and Frey, 1985; Schaffner et al., 1986), although this is smaller than the oxidative burst that follows exposure to conidia. Further, yeasts are 50 times more resistant than conidia to the lethal effects of H_2O_2 (Schaffner et al., 1986). For most yeasts of *B. dermatitidis*, the mechanisms of killing by PMNs may be similar to that described by Diamond et al. (Diamond and Krzesicki, 1978; Diamond et al., 1978) for filamentous fungi: an extracellular process whereby the PMNs attach directly to yeast cells and empty granule contents into the extracellular space.

The relative ease with which nonspecific phagocytes dispense with *B. dermatitidis* conidia and, conversely, the relative difficulty that these cells have in ingesting and killing yeasts in the absence of immune activation suggest that the dimorphism of *B. dermatitidis* confers a selective advantage with regard to pathogenicity. On one hand, the extreme susceptibility of conidia to the gamut of nonspecific defense mechanisms may in part explain the relative rarity of blastomycosis as a clinically apparent problem. On the other hand, resistance of the yeast form explains why the organism is a primary fungal pathogen in the normal host, in contrast to opportunistic fungal pathogens that require compromised host defenses to establish infection and disease.

2.2. BAD1 Expression is Restricted to the Pathogenic Yeast form of *B. dermatitidis*

Conversion to the yeast phase appears to offer the organism protection from host immune defenses (Drutz and Frey, 1985; Sugar and Picard, 1991). *B. dermatitidis* conidia are more sensitive than yeast to the killing mechanisms of neutrophils, monocytes, and macrophages. It is possible that induction of phase-specific factors enhance survival of yeast within the host. Despite their potential roles in pathogenesis, few yeast phase-specific genes have been identified, and little is known about their roles in virulence.

BAD1 was identified from the yeast phase of *B. dermatitidis* using patient antisera (Klein et al., 1993). This highly immunogenic 120-kDa protein localizes to the cell wall and is also found in in vitro culture supernatants (Klein et al., 1992; Klein and Newman, 1996). The central portion of the protein consists of a 24-amino-acid repeat showing homology to invasin, a protein from *Yersinia* spp. involved in mediating binding to and uptake by host M cells (Klein et al., 1993; Hogan et al., 1995). This tandem repeat region has been shown to be sufficient for binding to cell surface receptors CD11b/CD18 (CR3) and CD14 on human macrophages (Newman et al., 1995). Expression of BAD1 is restricted to the yeast phase and controlled transcriptionally by a mechanism that appears to be shared with at least one other systemic dimorphic fungus, *Histoplasma capsulatum*, suggesting that elements of this pathogenetically crucial process may be conserved (Rooney et al., 2001).

2.3. BAD1 Adhesin is Indispensable for Pathogenicity of *B. dermatitidis*

Despite the worldwide occurrence and growing incidence of fungal infections, little is known about the factors that account for their pathogenicity. In many cases, pathogenicity can be attributed to the ability of fungi and other microbes to adhere to target tissues, but the lack of tractable genetic systems in systemic dimorphic fungi has severely limited our understanding of the responsible products. We have recently developed the ability to genetically manipulate *B. dermatitidis* using DNA-mediated gene transfer (Hogan and Klein, 1997). This transformation system opened the way toward targeting genes, creating knockout strains, and formally testing the role of candidate factors such as BAD1 in adherence and virulence of *B. dermatitidis*.

Targeted disruption of the BAD1 locus in two independent strains abolished BAD1 expression and resulted in impaired binding and entry of yeasts into macrophages, and loss of adherence to lung tissue. Each of these properties was fully restored after reconstitution of BAD1 by means of gene transfer (Brandhorst et al., 1999). This study confirmed and extended prior observations by demonstrating that BAD1 is necessary for binding of the yeast to macrophages in vitro, as well as to lung tissue *ex vivo*. Wild-type yeast bound avidly, in a time-dependent manner, whereas knockout yeasts were impaired profoundly in their binding, and binding was largely restored in the BAD1-reconstituted strain. In addition, cells that bound poorly did not enter macrophages, as evidenced by low ingestion indices during the course of the incubation. These observations suggest that BAD1 serves as the principal ligand mediating attachment of yeast to macrophages and host tissue, and the other ligands play a lesser role.

The isogenic strains were also used to address the role of BAD1 in virulence. BAD1 is indispensable for the pathogenicity of *B. dermatitidis* (Brandhorst et al., 1999). Knocking out BAD1 in wild-type strain 26199 rendered these yeast unable to establish a lethal pulmonary infection, even when administered at 100 times the minimal lethal inoculum. Similar results were observed after knocking out BAD1 in a second strain, 60915, further strengthening our conclusions about the importance of BAD1. Analyses of organ load and distribution of infection showed that wild-type yeast grew steadily in the lung and increased sharply in number by 7–14 days after infection. Although the number of knockout yeast that entered the lung was comparable to that of the wild-type yeast immediately after infection, the number of knockout yeast in the lung remained low throughout the observation period. After primary lung infection, wild-type yeast also disseminated to liver and spleen, whereas knockout yeast did not disseminate. This could reflect the ability of wild-type yeast to enter macrophages and disseminate while inside them, or possibly a burden of yeast beyond the lung's capacity. On histological examination, the pulmonary alveoli of mice infected with the wild-type were obliterated with inflammation and yeast, whereas the lungs of mice that received the knockout appeared mostly normal, except for focal well-formed granulomas with small numbers of sequestered organisms.

2.4. Evidence for Non-Adhesive Pathogenic Mechanisms of BAD1 on *B. dermatitidis*

Mechanisms that underlie the virulence-promoting effect of BAD1 have been partially elucidated. According to the results described above, adherence seems to be one of them. Yeast that lack BAD1 bind poorly to the lung ex vivo and to macrophages in vitro (Brandhorst et al., 1999). These findings imply that knockout yeasts are unable to establish infection in the lower respiratory tract because they bind poorly to structures in the airway or alveoli. Nonadherent yeast might be more easily dislodged from the lung, or when lacking the capacity to enter inactivated lung macrophages, more readily recognized and killed by effector cells.

Recent results point to additional defects in *B. dermatitidis* yeast mutated at the BAD1 locus. Following i.v. inoculation of *B. dermatitidis* yeast into mice, wild-type yeast multiplied rapidly in the lung, killing the mice, whereas BAD1 knockout yeast multiplied poorly (B. Klein, M. Wüthrich, T. Brandhorst, and B. Finkel-Jimenez, manuscript in preparation). This finding implies that BAD1 knockout yeasts are defective in pathogenicity even when the route of infection does not require airway or alveolar adherence. This residual defect neither impairs cell-wall integrity of the yeast, nor does it render the yeast more susceptible to phagocyte killing. Instead, immune deviation may be an additional attribute of BAD1 and provide an explanation. Histologic staining of lung sections demonstrates mature granulomas with only small numbers of sequestered yeast in mice that received the knockout, as compared with disorganized granulomas overrun by yeast in mice that received the wild-type (Brandhorst et al., 1999). Similarly, the number and distribution of hematopoietic cells in the lung lesions show corresponding differences. Lungs of knockout-infected mice contain relatively more $CD3^+$ T cells and fewer neutrophils, whereas the lungs of wild-type infected mice demonstrate the opposite. Thus, the profile of inflammatory response is heavily influenced by the presence of BAD1.

2.5. BAD1 Modulates Innate Immune Response to *B. dermatitidis* Infection in the Lung

Based on above findings, we hypothesized that BAD1 modulates innate host immunity early in the course of infection and thereby facilitates establishment of *B. dermatitidis* in the lung. Many diverse microbes escape host elimination by modulation of host immunity (Galan and Collmer, 1999). We demonstrated that BAD1 interferes with host immunity by blocking production of a key proinflammatory cytokine, TNF-α (Finkel-Jimenez et al., 2001). TNF-α is produced chiefly by mononuclear phagocytes and plays a prominent role in host defense against microbes. It has pleotropic immunoregulatory effects including synergizing with IL-12 to increase the production of IFN-γ by NK cells, synergizing with IFN-γ to enhance microbicidal activity of macrophages through NO-dependent mechanisms, and facilitating maturation of the adaptive immune response (Pasparakis et al., 1996; Allendoerfer and Deepe, 1998).

TNF-α contributes to host defense against *B. dermatitidis* infection. Neutralization of TNF-α led to a tenfold elevation in the number of organisms in the lung 1 week after infection. The effect of neutralization was most pronounced in mice infected with the BAD1 knockout; such mice survive over 6 months, whereas mice infected with the wild-type succumb in 14 days (Brandhorst et al., 2003). In mice depleted of TNF-α numbers of colony-forming units (CFUs) for the knockout at 7 days postinfection increased to that normally seen only with the wild-type yeast. Hence, interference with early TNF-α production or function impairs control of pulmonary infection with *B. dermatitidis*.

It is noteworthy, in view of an established role of TNF-α in host defense, that virulent *B. dermatitidis* yeast block the production of TNF-α (Finkel-Jimenez et al., 2001). In comparing the behavior of virulent wild-type yeast with that of BAD1 knockout yeast, we found marked differences between these two strains in evoking TNF-α production in different experimental systems. Mice infected with the knockout had severalfold more TNF-α in alveolar lavage fluid than did mice infected with the virulent strain. In vitro coculture of lung cells with each of the two strains, respectively, confirmed sharp differences in lung TNF-α production (Fig. 6.1A). Furthermore, although the knockout strain evoked robust production of TNF-α in peritoneal macrophages and neutrophils over the entire time-course of in vitro coculture, the virulent wild-type strain initially stimulated a small amount TNF-α production, but then downregulated production. Lastly, the stimulatory phenotype of the knockout could be abolished by the addition of wild-type yeast, demonstrating active downregulation of TNF-α by virulent *B. dermatitidis*.

Multiple lines of evidence demonstrate that BAD1 on wild-type yeast is responsible for blocking production of TNF-α (Finkel-Jimenez et al., 2001). First and most obvious is the fact that the strains used in this study are isogenic, differing only in the expression of BAD1 (Brandhorst et al., 1999). Second, the coating of stimulatory knockout yeast with BAD1, or addition of purified BAD1 into wells with knockout yeast, reversed the effect on immune cells from stimulatory to inhibitory (Fig. 6.1B). Despite these observations, it remained possible that BAD1 through its adhesive property could bind the yeast and phagocyte together, yet on apposition, a second or additional factor could deliver a downregulatory signal to the cell.

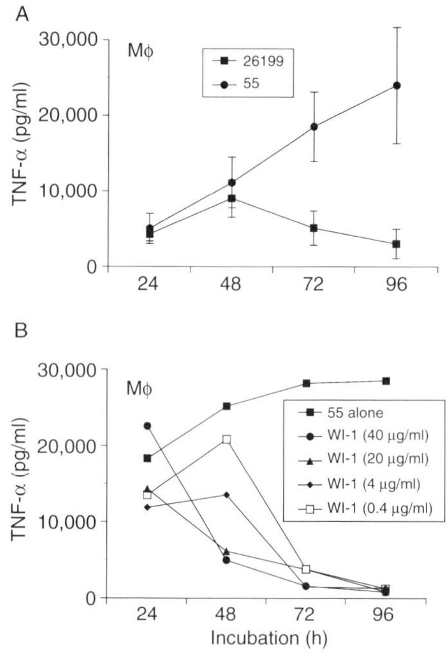

Figure 6.1. BAD1 blocks TNF-α production by phagocytes. Panel A, Isogenic BAD1 plus and minus strains (ATCC 26199 and knockout strain #55) were cocultured in vitro with peritoneal macrophages, and TNF-α levels measured at serial time-points postincubation (denoted on *x*-axis from 24 to 96 h). Wild-type strain 26199 blocks TNF-α production and knockout strain #55 stimulates TNF-α. Panel B, soluble purified BAD1 was added in vitro to wells where knockout strain #55 induced TNF-α production by macrophages. BAD1 blocked TNF-α production in a concentration-dependent manner. Note that BAD1 had previously been named WI-1. Adapted with permission from Finkel-Jimenez, B., Wüthrich, M., Brandhorst, T., and Klein, B.S. (2001). The WI-1 adhesin blocks phagocyte TNF-alpha production, imparting pathogenicity on *Blastomyces dermatitidis*. *J. Immunol.* 166: 2665–2673.

However, soluble, purified BAD1 was shown to inhibit *Saccharomyces cerevisiae*-induced production of TNF-α by phagocytes even though BAD1 is unable to bind the surface of that yeast. Hence, it would appear that BAD1 itself downregulates TNF-α production by phagocytes.

The biological significance of TNF-α downregulation by wild-type yeast was investigated using a gene therapy approach. We reasoned from in vitro data and alveolar lavage fluid analysis that mice infected with wild-type yeast might have insufficient TNF-α levels in vivo at the site of infection, which could be restored via gene therapy. We restored lung TNF-α levels in vivo early in the course of infection with *B. dermatitidis*, using gene therapy. This approach resulted in local pulmonary production of rTNF-α, a significant reduction in the progression of lung infection with wild-type yeast, and correspondingly elevated levels of TNF-α in vivo compared with infected control mice that received control adenovirus expressing *LacZ*. These observations indicate that restoration of TNF-α in infected mice circumvented a pathogenic mechanism of *B. dermatitidis* yeast.

2.6. BAD1 Suppresses Host TNF-α Production through TGF-β-dependent and -independent Mechanisms

Because TNF-α suppression is important in understanding the pathogenesis of this and other infectious diseases, we explored the mechanism(s) responsible for BAD1 inhibition of TNF-α production. We postulated that BAD1 could act directly on the phagocyte by inducing toxicity, apoptosis, or a signaling pathway that shuts off TNF-α production, or alternatively, act indirectly by inducing release of inhibitory product(s) that act in autocrine and paracrine fashions. Such mechanisms are not mutually exclusive.

We demonstrated a mechanism that entails BAD1 induction of TGF-β, which in turn sharply suppresses TNF-α production by phagocytes (Finkel-Jimenez et al., 2002) (Fig. 6.2). We suspected a suppressive mechanism involving a soluble inhibitor from results of a mixing experiment (Finkel-Jimenez et al., 2001). Stimulatory BAD1 knockout yeasts (10^6 cells) were mixed with wild-type yeast (10^3 cells) and added to wells containing 10^6 phagocytes (E:T ratio of 1000:1 with respect to wild-type yeast). Hence, in theory, wild-type yeast in wells interacted with only 1 in

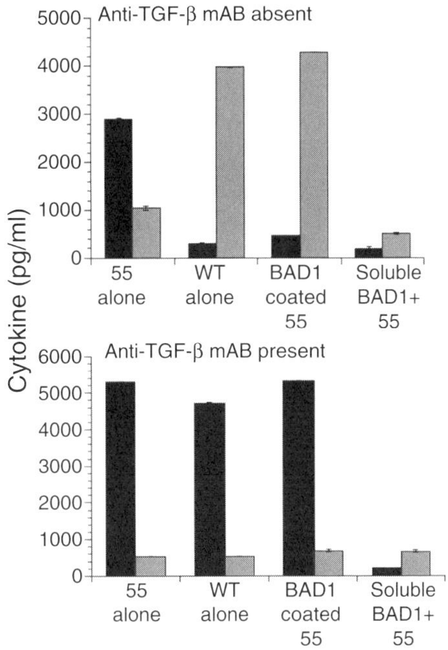

Figure 6.2. BAD1 suppresses TNF-α via TGF-β-dependent and -independent mechanisms. Isogenic BAD1 plus and minus strains (wild-type ATCC strain 26199 and BAD1 knockout #55) or BAD1-coated knockout yeasts were cocultured in vitro with peritoneal macrophages and levels of TNF-α (black bars) and TGF-β (grey bars) quantified after 24–48 h. Wild-type yeast or BAD1-coated knockout yeast induced TGF-β and suppressed TNF-α. Soluble BAD1 failed to induce TGF-β, but nevertheless suppressed TNF-α. Anti-TGF-β neutralized the product and restored TNF-α suppressed by yeast cell surface BAD1. Anti-TGF-β failed to restore TNF-α suppressed in response to soluble BAD1. Thus, surface BAD1 suppresses TNF-α in a TGF-β dependent manner, and soluble BAD1 suppresses TNF-α in a TGF-β independent manner. Adapted with permission from Finkel-Jimenez, B., Wüthrich, M., and Klein, B.S. (2002). BAD1, an essential virulence factor of *Blastomyces dermatitidis*, suppresses host TNF-alpha production through TGF-beta-dependent and -independent mechanisms. *J. Immunol.* 168: 5746–5755.

1000 phagocytes. Despite this, wild-type yeast eliminated TNF-α production in the wells. This result is consistent with release of a factor(s) into medium that modulates activity of all cells in the well, even though wild-type yeast interact with only a small proportion. Our data indicate that phagocytes respond to BAD1 on wild-type yeast by releasing a soluble factor(s) that downregulate TNF-α, and at least one such factor is TGF-β (Finkel-Jimenez et al., 2002). First, conditioned supernatant prepared from wild-type yeast inhibited production of TNF-α in response to BAD1 knockout yeast, whereas control supernatants had little effect. Second, the amount of TGF-β in these supernatants correlated with their ability to inhibit TNF-α production. Third, removal of TGF-β activity in the supernatant reversed its inhibitory effects. Fourth, addition of neutralizing anti-TGF-β mAb to wells with inhibitory wild-type yeast and phagocytes reversed suppression of TNF-α production. Last, addition of rTGF-β to wells with stimulatory BAD1 knockout yeast suppressed production of TNF-α in response to this strain. These results together demonstrate that wild-type yeast, and presumably surface BAD1, downregulates TNF-α production in response to *B. dermatitidis* by inducing TGF-β release from macrophages and neutrophils.

To test whether BAD1 induced TGF-β promotes disease progression and evasion of immunity; we investigated this possibility in an experimental model of pulmonary blastomycosis. We observed that levels of TGF-β in alveolar fluid collected during the first 3 weeks of infection were severalfold higher in response to wild-type yeast compared with BAD1 knockout yeast. However, mAb neutralization of TGF-β did not influence the course of blastomycosis in mice that were infected with wild-type yeast. Neutralization did reduce TGF-β levels in alveolar lavage fluid; however TNF-α levels appeared to be uninfluenced, and, in fact, the TNF-α levels remained far below those detected in the lungs of mice infected with the BAD1 knockout. These findings suggested to us that TGF-β may not be solely responsible for suppressed TNF-α levels in vivo, and that there may be a more complex regulatory mechanism between BAD1 and TFN-α, which encompasses factors in addition to TGF-β.

Our in vitro data demonstrate that, although cell surface-bound BAD1 suppresses TNF-α in a TGF-β-dependent manner, soluble BAD1 conversely suppresses TNF-α in a manner that is independent of TGF-β (Finkel-Jimenez et al., 2002) (Fig. 6.2). We showed that soluble BAD1 sharply suppressed the production of TNF-α by neutrophils and macrophages in response to stimulatory knockout yeast, but TGF-β levels were not elevated, nor did TGF-β neutralization reverse the suppression (as it did when cell surface BAD1 was responsible for suppression). Hence, soluble BAD1 suppression of TNF-α could explain why TGF-β neutralization in vivo neither restored TNF-α levels nor ameliorated disease progression. In support of this concept, we found soluble BAD1 in lung alveolar lavage fluids during the course of infection. The BAD1 concentrations detected in vivo were able to fully suppress TNF-α production in vitro independent of TGF-β and thus potentially account for in vivo observations.

2.7. Adhesive Property of BAD1 is Dispensable for Pathogenicity of *B. dermatitidis*

During cell wall biogenesis, BAD1 is released extracellularly before binding back to the yeast cell surface (Brandhorst and Klein, 2000). Postrelease reassociation with the yeast surface is a surprisingly simple method by which the BAD1 adhesin might evenly coat cell surfaces. The fact that cell-associated and soluble forms of the BAD1 protein exist side-by-side does raise the question of whether one form is predominantly responsible for the observed contribution to *B. dermatitidis* virulence.

We recently reported that binding of yeast to host cells through yeast surface-bound BAD1 is unexpectedly dispensable in the requisite role of BAD1 in pathogenesis (Brandhorst et al., 2003). Deletion of the C-terminal epidermal growth factor (EGF)-like domain profoundly affected BAD1 function, leading to nonassociation with yeast, extracellular accumulation, and impaired yeast adherence to macrophages. Despite the absence of ΔC term-protein on cell surfaces and impaired binding of these strains to macrophages, the defects had no discernible impact on pathogenicity of *B. dermatitidis* in vivo. Stringent outcome measures of both survival and lung CFU in infected mice demonstrated that the C-terminal truncation of BAD1 did not impair progression of pulmonary blastomycosis. We acknowledge that BAD1-mediated adhesion could play its part earlier in the natural progression of blastomycosis, when, presumably, small numbers of organisms (<100) enter a host intranasally in the form of spores. The sizable inoculum of yeast instilled intratracheally could diminish the requirement for BAD1 adherence to tissues during the early phases of infection when the natural response of the lung is geared towards physical ejection of infectious particles.

The ΔC term strains (and protein) retained the ability to suppress TNF-α production by phagocytes in vitro, which might explain how they maintained pathogenicity in vivo. To test this, we also measured TNF-α levels in vivo in the pulmonary compartment after infection with ΔC term strains. During the initial 72 h of infection when lung CFUs were comparable for the strains tested, TNF-α levels were several-fold lower with wild-type yeast and ΔC term yeast compared with BAD1-null strain #55. Given the evidence accumulated in cytokine profiles, survival curves, and binding studies, it seems reasonable to propose that BAD1 exerts its effect on virulence largely by deviating the host immune response.

3. Acquired Immunity in the Lungs to *B. dermatitidis* Infection

3.1. Role of Antibody to Host Resistance

There is little evidence that humoral immunity contributes significantly to host defense against *B. dermatitidis* (Wüthrich and Klein, 2000), although passive transfer of monoclonal antibodies (mAbs) have been shown to ameliorate the course of experimental cryptococcal, candidal, and *Pneumocystis* infections (Dromer et al., 1987, 1989; Gigliotti and Hughes, 1988; Sanford et al., 1990; Dromer and Charreire, 1991; Mukherjee et al., 1992, 1993a,b, 1994a,b; Polonelli et al., 1994; Cassone et al., 1995). Natural infection in humans (Klein and Jones, 1990) and dogs (Klein et al., 2000) with *B. dermatitidis* elicits strong antibody responses to the surface adhesin BAD1. The antibodies are directed chiefly against the adhesive domain, a 25-amino acid repeat. Tandem-repeat-specific mAbs were studied for their opsonic activity in vitro and their capacity to adoptively transfer protection in murine experimental blastomycosis (Wüthrich and Klein, 2000). mAbs to BAD1 enhanced binding and entry of *B. dermatitidis* yeasts into J774.16 macrophages but did not enhance killing or growth inhibition of the yeast. Passive transfer of eight mAbs to BAD1 into three different inbred strains of mice also did not improve the course of experimental infection and sometimes worsened it. μ-Deficient mice were more resistant to experimental blastomycosis than were intact littermates, and passive transfer of the mAbs or their Fab fragments into these mice did not protect them against experimental infection. Thus, antibody to BAD1 does not appear to improve the outcome of murine blastomycosis and may enhance the infection.

3.2. Cell-Mediated Immunity—Delayed-type-Hypersensitivity—T cells and their Products Correlate with Resistance

Efficient resistance to a respiratory challenge may require immunological activation of alveolar macrophages, the first line of defense against inhaled microbes, including *B. dermatitidis*. Indeed, human alveolar macrophages of immune individuals ingest and inhibit the growth of *B. dermatitidis* yeast significantly better than cells of nonimmune persons. The killing of yeasts by murine alveolar macrophages is augmented from 0% to 25% by coincubating the cells with the supernatant of concanavalin A-stimulated splenocytes of 1000 U/ml of IFN-γ (Brummer and Stevens, 1987). Interestingly, antibody to IFN-γ abrogated the effect of the splenocyte supernatant. This suggests that IFN-γ accounts for most or all of the supernatant's immune augmentation. When mice were treated i.p. with 4×10^5 units of recombinant IFN-γ, their pulmonary macrophages showed enhanced killing of *B. dermatitidis* yeast (38%, compared to 5% for cells of control mice) (Brummer et al., 1988).

Mice immunized with either viable or merthiolate-killed yeast demonstrated peak responses of delayed-type hypersensitivity (DTH) that coincided temporally with maximal resistance to a lethal challenge with live *B. dermatitidis* given intranasally (Morozumi et al., 1982), intraperitoneally (Spencer and Cozad, 1973), and intravenously (Cozad and Chang, 1980). This functional capability could be transferred passively to naïve mice by spleen cells of immunized mice, but not by serum (Scillian et al., 1974). These results indicate that the maturation of cell-mediated immunity is a vital aspect of host resistance to the infection.

3.3. Development of Attenuated *B. dermatitidis* for Vaccination

It was discovered that targeted disruption of BAD1 abolishes pathogenicity of *B. dermatitidis* (Brandhorst et al., 1999). In an experimental model of murine pulmonary infection that entails an intratracheal infection with yeast, all mice that were infected with the wild-type strain ATCC 26199 died of pneumonia within 2–4 weeks of infection, whereas all mice infected with a *bad1*-null mutant survived over an extended period of 6–12 months. Re-expression of BAD1 in *trans* in the null mutant restored virulence. Hence these studies fulfilled Koch's molecular postulate for defining BAD1 as an essential virulence factor (Falkow, 1988). The work offered an early example of genetic proof of a virulence factor by gene targeting in systemic dimorphic fungi.

Administration of viable yeast of this attenuated strain vaccinates against lethal pulmonary experimental infection due to isogenic and nonisogenic strains from diverse geographic regions (Wüthrich et al., 2000). This recombinant attenuated vaccine induces DTH and polarized type 1 cytokine responses, which are linked with resistance. Immunization subcutaneously or by the multiple routes, intranasal, subcutaneous, and intravenous, prompts strong DTH, whereas immunization intranasally yields marginal DTH (Fig. 6.3A). Immunization subcutaneously or by the combined route reduces lung CFU by between two and three logs versus controls (Fig. 6.3B). Immunization intranasally reduces lung CFU marginally, but significantly versus controls. In survival studies, 80% of mice immunized subcutaneously and 50% immunized by the combined route survive and most of the survivors demonstrate evidence of sterilizing immunity in the lung (Fig. 6.3C). Thus, vaccine-induced protection in the lung is most effective when the BAD1 null vaccine strain is administered

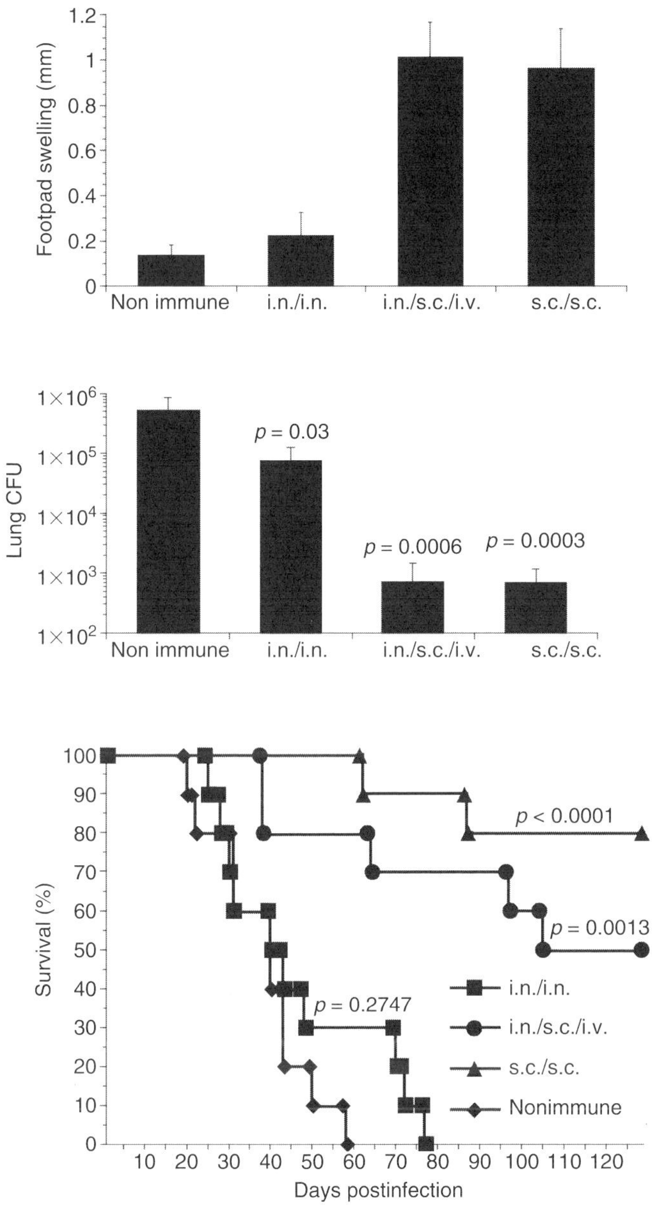

Figure 6.3. Acquired resistance to blastomycosis after vaccination with a recombinant, live, attenuated strain of *B. dermatitidis*. Panel A, DTH responses. C57BL/6 mice received two injections of strain #55 yeast either intranasally (i.n.) or subcutaneously (s.c.), or three injections by multiple routes, i.n., s.c., and intravenously (i.v.), with each injection spaced 2 weeks apart. After immunization, groups of four mice were injected with 10^5 dead yeast of strain #55 into one footpad or PBS into the other. Footpad swelling was measured 24 h later. Error bars are standard errors of the mean (SEM).

Figure 6.3. ***Cont'd*** Panel B, burden of lung infection. Two weeks after immunization, groups of 10 mice were infected i.n. with 10^4 26199 wild-type yeast. Three weeks later, mice were analyzed for lung CFU. Geometric means of CFUs were calculated. Error bars are SEM. *p*-Values are for comparison of each immunized group versus nonimmune controls. Panel C, Survival after infection. Groups of 10 C57BL/6 mice were infected as in panel B and monitored for survival over 128 days. *p*-Values are for comparison of each immunized group versus nonimmune mice. Reprinted with permission from Wüthrich, M., Filutowicz, H.I., and Klein, B.S. (2000). Mutation of the WI-1 gene yields an attenuated *Blastomyces dermatitidis* strain that induces host resistance. *J. Clin. Invest.* 106: 1381–1389.

subcutaneously, but protective efficacy in the lung is minimal when the vaccine is delivered at the site of natural infection.

The parental, wild-type strain ATCC 26199 was not suitable for vaccination. It disseminated from the skin injection site to the lung where infection progressed. Morozumi et al. (1982) reported that subcutaneous administration of live ATCC 26199 yeast protected mice against pulmonary blastomycosis. In contrast to our study, those authors reported that ATCC 26199 yeast injected subcutaneously into each of two sites was cleared by 4 weeks after injection. The discrepancy between their findings and ours might be explained by recent findings about spontaneous variation of ATCC strain 26199. Mutants of 26199 have arisen spontaneously by serial passage in vitro: ATCC 60915 is an attenuated mutant (Brass et al., 1982), and ATCC 60916 is avirulent (Morrison and Stevens, 1991). Phenotypic alterations recently documented in these mutants include partial or complete loss of surface α-(1,3)-glucan (Hogan and Klein, 1994), and changes in the amount of surface and secreted BAD1 (Klein et al., 1994). To guard against loss of pathogenicity in *B. dermatitidis*, including strain 26199, we monitor virulence in mice and measure surface α-(1,3)-glucan and BAD1 routinely during passage. The wild-type strain 26199 used for vaccination by Morozumi et al. (1982) could have mutated spontaneously and lost virulence, which would have escaped attention since phenotypes associated with loss of virulence had not been delineated at that time. It should be emphasized that spontaneous attenuated mutants of dimorphic fungi are often unstable and frequently revert to the virulence phenotype after passage in serum in vitro or animals (Hogan et al., 1996). This fact underscores the importance of using genetically defined and stable mutations for attenuated vaccine strains of dimorphic fungi, rather than spontaneous, uncharacterized mutants. Parenthetically, spontaneous variation does not account for loss of virulence of recombinant strain #55. Resupply of BAD1 in *trans* restores pathogenicity to strain #55, which establishes that loss of BAD1, not another defect, is responsible for loss of virulence (Brandhorst et al., 1999).

Additional attributes make the recombinant, attenuated strain #55 a promising vaccine and source of protective antigens. Vaccination induced substantial resistance: lung CFU 2 to 3 weeks postinfection was reduced by three or more logs, a majority of immunized mice survived a lethal challenge, and most surviving mice had sterilizing immunity. Importantly, vaccinated mice resisted a challenge with both the isogenic wild-type strain and nonisogenic strains from various geographical regions. Thus, vaccine strain #55 shares immunodominant, protective antigen(s) with nonisogenic strains of *B. dermatitidis*. A cell/wall/membrane (CW/M) antigen from the vaccine strain also induces polarized and protective immune responses. Thus, by mutating a pathogenetic locus in a dimorphic fungus, an attenuated vaccine strain was created and was used to elucidate fungal and host elements required for vaccine immunity.

3.4. Elucidation of the Mechanisms of Vaccine Immunity

We explored the mechanisms by which the vaccine above induces immunity (Wüthrich et al., 2002). To elucidate the elements required for vaccine resistance we have used knockout mice, depleted cellular subsets, and neutralized products from vaccinated mice during the expression phase of immunity. For example, to define cell population(s) responsible for vaccine resistance, we vaccinated athymic, nude (nu/nu) mice, TCR-$\alpha^{-/-}$ mice, μ-chain-deficient, and wild-type mice. Vaccinated nude mice and TCR-$\alpha^{-/-}$ mice were unable to resist lethal pulmonary infection with virulent wild-type yeast. In contrast, vaccinated μ-chain-deficient mice and their wild-type littermates resisted reinfection; 80–90% had sterilizing immunity. Thus, αβ-TCR$^+$ T cells are required for vaccine immunity.

To define the role of αβ T cell subsets in vaccine immunity, we depleted CD4 and CD8 T cells alone or together during the expression phase, which we defined as the period after infection. CD4-depleted mice had 100-fold more lung CFU than rat IgG-treated controls, and died 32±2 days after infection; controls all appeared healthy 50 days after infection when the experiment was terminated. In contrast, mice depleted of CD8 cells did not differ significantly from rat IgG-treated controls, as measured by lung CFU and survival. CD4 and CD8 double-depleted animals had 18-fold more lung CFU and a shorter mean survival (25±1 days) than did CD4-depleted mice, and they were as vulnerable as unvaccinated mice. Thus, CD4 cells are chiefly responsible for vaccine resistance in immune-competent hosts; CD8 cells contribute if CD4 cells are absent.

During these studies, we found unexpected plasticity in how the immune system defends against fungi. For example, when we neutralized type 1 cytokines IFN-γ and TNF-α during the expression phase, we significantly impaired vaccine immunity in immunocompetent mice. In contrast, in knockout mice lacking either of these cytokines, we induced levels of vaccine resistance as high as that in wild-type mice (Fig. 6.4A, B). In these immunodeficient mice, other cytokines compensated—TNF-α in IFN-$\gamma^{-/-}$ mice, and granulocyte-macrophage colony-stimulating factor (GM-CSF) in TNF-$\alpha^{-/-}$ mice—during the induction phase of vaccine immunity. These findings raised the possibility that residual elements of immunity in immunodeficient hosts could be educated during the induction phase of immunity to compensate

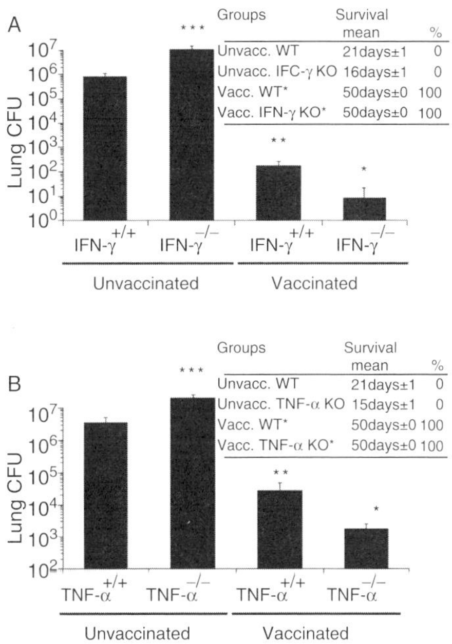

Figure 6.4. IFN-γ and TNF-α are dispensable in vaccine immunity. A and B, knockout and wild-type mice were analyzed for lung CFU 2 weeks after infection or followed for survival. Lung CFU±SEM and survival time ± SEM are shown. %, percent alive 50 days postinfection. *, $p<0.007$ versus unvaccinated controls; **, $p<0.012$ versus vaccinated transgenic mice; ***, $p<0.005$ versus unvaccinated wild-type mice. Reprinted with permission from *J. Immunol.* 2002; 169: 6969–6976.

for elements that were instrumental in vaccine resistance in immunocompetent hosts. We tested this concept by investigating whether CD4 T cells were essential or dispensable in vaccine immunity to pathogenic fungi.

3.5. CD4 T Cells are Dispensable in Vaccine Immunity against *B. dermatitidis* and *H. capsulatum* in Immuno-Deficient Hosts, and CD8 T Cells Compensate

Depletion of T cell subsets during the period of vaccination (defined as the induction phase of vaccine immunity) and throughout the period postinfection gave striking results (Wüthrich et al., 2003). Mice depleted of either CD4 or CD8 T cells acquired levels of vaccine immunity similar to that of rat IgG-treated controls, as assessed by lung CFU analysis (Fig. 6.5A). Animals depleted of both CD4 and CD8 T cells were as susceptible as unvaccinated controls. Thus, T cells are required for vaccine immunity, but CD4 T cells appear to be dispensable when absent during induction of vaccine immunity. CD8 T cells are essential in a CD4 T cell-deficient host.

Survival analysis of CD4-depleted wild-type animals supported the above results and indicated that lung CFU data are a reliable predictor of survival. Mice depleted of CD4 T cells during induction and expression of vaccine immunity survived significantly longer than unvaccinated mice (mean, 123±11 days vs. 23±2 days; $p<0.0001$). At 75 days postinfection, all of the unvaccinated mice were dead, whereas 80% of the CD4 T cell-depleted mice were still alive. Ultimately, 35% of CD4-depleted mice survived a lethal challenge with virulent, wild-type yeast over a prolonged period of 200 days postinfection; all of the survivors had no detectable CFU in their lungs (detection limit of 5 CFU), indicating that they had acquired sterilizing immunity in their lungs. In comparison, 100% of vaccinated, non-T cell-depleted mice survived the lethal challenge and cleared the infection. Thus, in the absence of CD4 T cells, vaccination greatly prolonged survival and a significant proportion of those animals survived and acquired sterilizing immunity.

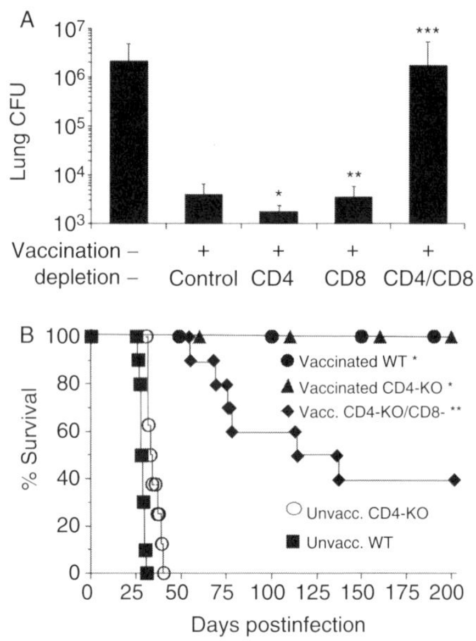

Figure 6.5. Role of CD4 and CD8 T cells during induction of vaccine immunity. (A) Lung CFU. Vaccinated mice were depleted of T cells during vaccination and *B. dermatitidis* infection. *, $p = 0.1983$ versus IgG control; **, $p = 0.9825$ versus control; ***, $p = 0.7$ versus unvaccinated mice. (B) Survival of vaccinated, $CD4^{-/-}$ mice and wild-type mice. Vaccinated $CD4^{-/-}$/CD8-mice were depleted of CD8 cells after vaccination and through *B. dermatitidis* infection. *, $p < 0.0001$ versus unvaccinated mice; **, $p = 0.008$ versus vaccinated $CD4^{-/-}$ mice.

Vaccine immunity evoked in the absence of CD4 cells was durable and persisted for at least 8 weeks postvaccination. CD4-depleted mice that were rested for 8 weeks after vaccination (but maintained CD4-deficient) remained highly resistant to lethal infection. Six out of ten CD4-depleted vac-

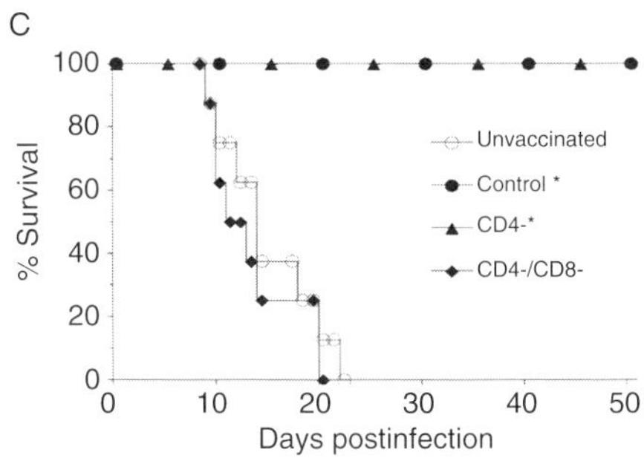

Figure 6.5. *Cont'd* (C) CD8 T cells mediate vaccine immunity to *H. capsulatum*. Anti-CD4-/anti-CD8 denotes vaccinated CD4-depleted mice, depleted of CD8 T cells after vaccination and through infection. *, $p < 0.0002$ versus unvaccinated mice or anti-CD4-/anti-CD8 treated mice. Reprinted with permission from *J. Exp. Med.* 2003; 197: 1405–1416.

cinated mice acquired sterilizing immunity and the remaining four mice had 20–200 lung CFU 25 days postinfection. In contrast, unvaccinated mice appeared moribund with a lung burden of $5.2 \pm 2.9 \times 10^6$ CFU at this time-point. All vaccinated wild-type mice had cleared the infection. Thus, resting of vaccinated CD4-depleted mice indicated durable immunity and even greater resistance to infection.

3.5.1. CD4$^{-/-}$ Mice Acquire Robust Vaccine Immunity

Because depletion of CD4 cells might not be complete, and residual cells could provide sufficient help for other effector cells, we investigated vaccine immunity in CD4$^{-/-}$ mice. Remarkably, all vaccinated CD4 T cell-knockout mice survived an extended period postinfection (Fig. 6.5B); nine out of 11 had in fact acquired sterilizing immunity, and the other two had low numbers of CFU in their lungs (200 and 280 CFU). Survival data generated with class II-knockout mice were similar to those reported for CD4-depleted wild-type mice. Thus, the results obtained using mice congenitally deficient in CD4 cells support the data using CD4 cell depletion and the notion that CD4 T cells are dispensable.

3.5.2. CD4 T Cells are Dispensable in Vaccine Immunity to H. capsulatum

We sought to determine whether our observations could be extended to other pathogenic fungi. We addressed this in an experimental model of pulmonary histoplasmosis, a frequent cause of life-threatening, opportunistic infection in AIDS patients and others with compromised immunity. All the mice that had been vaccinated in either the presence or absence of CD4 T cells survived lethal pulmonary challenge with a wild-type virulent strain G217B, and acquired sterilizing immunity by 50 days postinfection (detection limit of 200 CFU) (Fig. 6.5C) (Wüthrich et al., 2003). In contrast, unvaccinated mice and CD4 T cell-depleted mice that were depleted of CD8 T cells after infection died within 10 to 20 days postinfection. Thus, vaccine resistance also can be raised against pulmonary histoplasmosis in the absence of CD4 T cells.

3.5.3. CD8 T Cells are Required during the Efferent Phase of Vaccine Immunity

Studies above showed that CD8 T cells must be present during vaccine induction when CD4 T cells are absent, but they did not address whether CD8 T cells are required and responsible for immunity during the expression or efferent phase. To determine if CD8 T cells serve as effectors during the efferent phase, we used two approaches. First, mice in whom CD4 T cells were depleted during the induction and expression phases of vaccine immunity were depleted of CD8 T cells upon infection and afterward. Elimination of CD8 T cells after infection reduced resistance to 150-fold, compared to controls depleted only of CD4 T cells. In blastomycosis, elimination of CD8 T cells after infection also reduced mean survival from 200 ± 0 days to 49 ± 5 days (p = 0.007) in vaccinated CD4 knockout mice (Fig. 6.5B), and from 123 ± 11 days to 49 ± 5 days ($p < 0.0001$) in vaccinated CD4-depleted wild-type mice. Corresponding survival rates in the two respective groups went from 100% to 40% at 200 days postinfection, and from 80% to 0% at 75 days postinfection. Similarly, in histoplasmosis, vaccine immunity in CD4-depleted mice depended exclusively on CD8 T cells. Depletion of CD8 cells in these mice reduced survival from 100% to 0% (58).

In the second approach, we adoptively transferred immune CD8 T cells that had been elicited in wild-type mice in the absence of CD4 T cells (58). *Blastomyces* immune CD8 T cells lowered lung CFU 10- to 15-fold vs. HEL-CD8 T cells or no T cells, respectively. Resistance also was adoptively transferred by *Blastomyces*-immune CD8 T cells in a dose-dependent manner, using cell numbers from 10^6 to 2×10^7.

Taken together, our findings indicate that, when CD4 T cells are absent, CD8 T cells are required during the induction phase and participate as effectors during the efferent phase of vaccine immunity against pulmonary *B. dermatitidis* and *H. capsulatum* infection.

3.5.4. Mechanisms of CD8 T Cell Action

We postulated that CD8 T cells mediate vaccine effector functions in three distinct or overlapping ways. First, by production of type 1 cytokines, second by release of cytotoxic granule containing perforin, granulysin, or related molecules, and lastly, by an unconventional mechanism that involves class I major histocompatibility complex (MHC)-independent, direct binding of T cells to yeast, followed by one or more of the effector functions noted above. We observed that type 1 cytokines IFN-γ, TNF-α, and GM-CSF are instrumental in CD8 vaccine immunity (Wüthrich et al., 2003). First, lung cytokine levels (transcript and protein) correlated directly with the influx of CD8 cells into this organ following infection in vaccinated CD4-depleted mice. Second, on intracellular cytokine staining, these lung CD8 T cells selectively expressed these products. Lastly, in functional studies, neutralization of these cytokines significantly impaired CD8 cell vaccine immunity (Wüthrich et al., 2003). In contrast, perforin$^{-/-}$ mice depleted of CD4 cells acquired vaccine immunity as well as wild-type mice. Thus, perforin is dispensable in CD8 vaccine immunity. Nevertheless, perforin or other cytotoxic molecules could still contribute to CD8 effector mechanisms, and we have found that in vitro stimulation of in vivo primed CD8 cells enhances expression of cytotoxic granule products (granzyme B) in the cells. Lastly, we found that CD8 cells require class I MHC for vaccine immunity (see below; Wüthrich et al., 2003), in contrast to studies of *Cryptococcus neoformans* and *Candida albicans* (Levitz et al., 1995), where T cells exert direct antifungal effector functions in the absence of MHC.

These results establish the significant role and function of CD8 cells in vaccine immunity to fungi in immune-deficient hosts. The findings raise questions that must be answered to fully understand the mechanisms that are operative. Among the questions are: What cell(s) and processing pathway(s) cross-prime and -present exogenous fungal antigens on class I MHC during CD8 vaccine immunity, and in particular, how do they do so in the absence of CD4 T cell help.

3.6. Investigating Cross-presentation and -priming of CD8 T Cells by Dendritic Cells

An enigma is how CD8 cells become activated during infections with *B. dermatitidis*, a predominantly extracellular pathogen, and with *H. capsulatum*, an intracellular pathogen that resides in the phagolysosome with no demonstrated access to the cytosol. Because of the reported precedent of direct antifungal activity of T cells (Levitz et al., 1995), we explored the requirement for MHC class I. Adoptively transferred CD8 T cells protected wild-type mice, but not $\beta 2m^{-/-}$ mice lacking class I. Thus, CD8 immunity against *B. dermatitidis* requires MHC class I for antigen presentation and protection. These results suggest that exogenous fungal antigens are being processed for cross-presentation and -priming of class I restricted CD8 cells as part of vaccine immunity to these fungi. We have begun to study the cellular and molecular mechanisms that govern this physiologically relevant aspect of immunity to fungi.

Bone marrow-derived APC harbor a unique pathway for MHC I presentation of exogenous antigens. This pathway permits cross-presentation of pathogen or pathogen-infected cells and priming of cytotoxic T lymphocytes (CTL) responses against microbial infections. All three bone marrow-derived APC (i.e., macrophages, DC, and B cells) have been reported to present class I-restricted, exogenously derived antigens in vitro. In vivo, however, CD8 cross-priming persists in the absence of B cells (Shen et al., 2003). Moreover, only DC are able to induce naïve CTL to respond by cross-priming (Ronchetti et al., 1999); presumably because DC are best able to supply the necessary costimulatory signals. Recently, it was shown formally that DCs were responsible for in vivo priming of CD8 T cells by exogenous microbial antigens. Using a novel diphtheria toxin-based system that allows the inducible, short-term ablation of DC in vivo Jung et al. (2002) showed that DC are required to cross-prime CD8 precursors in vivo in experimental models of infection with *Listeria monocytogenes* and *Plasmodium yoelii*. For these reasons, we have focused on DC to investigate the cellular and molecular mechanisms behind cross-presentation of exogenous fungal antigen for priming antifungal CD8 cells that confer vaccine immunity.

We have tested the ability of primary DC to serve as APC. We used CD8 T cells from *Blastomyces*-vaccinated, CD4-deficient mice as responders in in vitro antigen presentation assays. Two weeks after mice were vaccinated (Wüthrich et al., 2003), lymph nodes and spleens were removed, and CD8 cells purified (>95% purity) using magnetic beads. DC and other types of APC (plus yeast stimuli) were tested for stimulation of these responders. DC evoked robust CD8 T cell responses, when live yeast were used as the stimulus, whereas soluble antigen failed to trigger a robust type 1 cytokine T cell response, as measured by IFN-γ and GM-CSF production in vitro using in vivo elicited CD8 T cells as responders.

Future work will explore the requirements for processing and presentation of antigens to CD8 T cells. Priming of naïve CD8 T cells by DC typically involves antigen degradation by cytosolic proteosomes, delivery of peptides by TAP into the ER, and binding of class I MHC. T cells must recognize antigen–MHC complexes and also receive a second signal, for example, through B7-CD28 "costimulation." CD4 helper T cells license DC for antigen presentation and B7 costimulation through the interaction of CD40L on the T cell and CD40 on the DC. There are notable exceptions to this rule (Kundig et al., 1996; Whitmire et al., 1996; Hamilton et al., 2001; Shedlock et al., 2003). We have already shown that CD4 T cells are dispensable for CD8 T cell immunity. We postulate that CD40–CD40L interactions also will be dispensable when vaccine immunity against *B. dermatitidis* and *H. capsulatum* is mediated by CD8 cells. In support of this idea, *B. dermatitidis* and *H. capsulatum* yeast alone represent a sufficient inflammatory stimulus that can directly induce maturation of DC and license them for antigen presentation (unpublished observations). We monitored DC using two of three well-established phenotypes for maturation (Reis e Sousa et al., 1999): (1) surface expression of B7-1, B7-2, and MHC class II and CD40 (⇑ with maturation); (2) TNF-α, IL-1-β, and IL-12 production (⇑ with maturation); and (3) endocytosis of particles (⇓ with maturation). Culture of DC with *B. dermatitidis* or *H. capsulatum* yeast enhanced maturation of the cells, as measured by the first two parameters. We postulate that pattern recognition receptors, particularly TLR, are pivotal in maturation of DC when conventional mechanisms of CD8 priming are absent in immune-deficient hosts.

4. Summary and Future Prospects

B. dermatitidis produces a primary progressive pneumonia in immune-competent hosts, but can also behave as an opportunistic pathogen. The primary pathogenic potential of this fungus is unusual among the systemic dimorphic fungi, where infections are often asymptomatic or mild and self-limited. Although conidia of the fungus are sensitive to phagocytosis and killing by mononuclear and polymorphonuclear leukocytes, conversion to the yeast enhances resistance of *B. dermatitidis* to these cellular defenses. A reason for enhanced pathogenicity of the yeast is expression of BAD1, which is a major virulence factor expressed during the transition. BAD1 impairs activity of phagocytes against the yeast, blunts proinflammatory cytokine responses, and shapes the quality of adaptive immunity. Targeted deletion of BAD1 abolishes pathogenicity of the fungus and has led to the development of a live-attenuated vaccine strain, which is effective in a murine model and under study in field trials in dogs. Creation of this strain has made possible investigation into the mechanisms of protective immunity. Resistance in healthy hosts depends on T cells rather than B cells and antibody, and $CD4^+$ T cells that produces type 1 cytokine (TNF-α, IFN-γ, and GM-CSF) are crucial in the expression of vaccine immunity. In immune-deficient hosts, there is sufficient redundancy of the immune system so that loss of these cytokines can be compensated. Even the loss of type 1 cytokine-producing $CD4^+$ T cells can be compensated by $CD8^+$ T cells during the induction of vaccine immunity. Hence, vaccines may induce resistance even in patients with impaired immunity, suggesting that vaccines can be developed for immune-deficient hosts. Understanding antigen processing and presentation mechanisms and development of memory immunity under these unusual circumstances will allow rational design of safe, effective vaccines that harness natural or unnatural lung immunity against *B. dermatitidis* and other fungal pathogens.

References

Allendoerfer, R. and Deepe, G.S. Jr. (1998). Blockade of endogenous TNF-alpha exacerbates primary and secondary pulmonary histoplasmosis by differential mechanisms. *J. Immunol.* 160: 6072–6082.

Bradsher, R.W. (1996). Histoplasmosis and blastomycosis. *Clin. Infect. Dis.* 22(Suppl. 2): S102–S111.

Bradsher, R.W., Balk, R.A., and Jacobs, R.F. (1987). Growth inhibition of *Blastomyces dermatitidis* in alveolar and peripheral macrophages from patients with blastomycosis. *Am. Rev. Respir. Dis.* 135: 412–417.

Brandhorst, T. and Klein, B. (2000). Cell wall biogenesis of *Blastomyces dermatitidis*. Evidence for a novel mechanism of cell surface localization of a virulence-associated adhesin via extracellular release and reassociation with cell wall chitin. *J. Biol. Chem.* 275: 7925–7934.

Brandhorst, T.T., Wüthrich, M., Warner, T., and Klein, B. (1999). Targeted gene disruption reveals an adhesin indispensable for pathogenicity of *Blastomyces dermatitidis*. *J. Exp. Med.* 189: 1207–1216.

Brandhorst, T., Wüthrich, M., Finkel-Jimenez, B., and Klein, B. (2003). A C-terminal EGF-like domain governs BAD1 localization to the yeast surface and fungal adherence to phagocytes, but is dispensable in immune modulation and pathogenicity of *Blastomyces dermatitidis*. *Mol. Microbiol.* 48: 53–65.

Brass, C., Volkmann, C.M., Philpott, D.E., Klein, H.P., Halde, C.J., and Stevens, D.A. (1982). Spontaneous mutant of *Blastomyces dermatitidis* attenuated in virulence for mice. *Sabouraudia* 20: 145–158.

Brummer, E. and Stevens, D.A. (1987). Activation of pulmonary macrophages for fungicidal activity by gamma-interferon or lymphokines. *Clin. Exp. Immunol.* 70: 520–528.

Brummer, E., Hanson, L.H., Restrepo, A., and Stevens, D.A. (1988). In vivo and in vitro activation of pulmonary macrophages by IFN-gamma for enhanced killing of *Paracoccidioides brasiliensis* or *Blastomyces dermatitidis. J. Immunol.* 140: 2786–2789.

Cassone, A., Boccanera, M., Adriani, D., Santoni, G., and De Bernardis, F. (1995). Rats clearing a vaginal infection by *Candida albicans* acquire specific, antibody-mediated resistance to vaginal reinfection. *Infect. Immun.* 63: 2619–2624.

Cozad, G.C. and Chang, C.T. (1980). Cell-mediated immunoprotection in blastomycosis. *Infect. Immun.* 28: 398–403.

Diamond, R.D. and Krzesicki, R. (1978). Mechanisms of attachment of neutrophils to *Candida albicans* pseudohyphae in the absence of serum, and of subsequent damage to pseudohyphae by microbicidal processes of neutrophils in vitro. *J. Clin. Invest.* 61: 360–369.

Diamond, R.D., Krzesicki, R., and Jao, W. (1978). Damage to pseudohyphal forms of *Candida albicans* by neutrophils in the absence of serum in vitro. *J. Clin. Invest.* 61: 349–359.

Dromer, F. and Charreire, J. (1991). Improved amphotericin B activity by a monoclonal anti-*Cryptococcus neoformans* antibody: Study during murine cryptococcosis and mechanisms of action. *J. Infect. Dis.* 163: 1114–1120.

Dromer, F., Charreire, J., Contrepois, A., Carbon, C., and Yeni, P. (1987). Protection of mice against experimental cryptococcosis by anti-*Cryptococcus neoformans* monoclonal antibody. *Infect. Immun.* 55: 749–752.

Dromer, F., Perronne, C., Barge, J., Vilde, J.L., and Yeni, P. (1989). Role of IgG and complement component C5 in the initial course of experimental cryptococcosis. *Clin. Exp. Immunol.* 78: 412–417.

Drutz, D.J. and Frey, C.L. (1985). Intracellular and extracellular defenses of human phagocytes against *Blastomyces dermatitidis* conidia and yeasts. *J. Lab. Clin. Med.* 105: 737–750.

Falkow, S. (1988). Molecular Koch's postulates applied to microbial pathogenicity. *Rev. Infect. Dis.* 10(Suppl. 2): S274–S276.

Finkel-Jimenez, B., Wüthrich, M., Brandhorst, T., and Klein, B.S. (2001). The WI-1 adhesin blocks phagocyte TNF-alpha production, imparting pathogenicity on *Blastomyces dermatitidis. J. Immunol.* 166: 2665–2673.

Finkel-Jimenez, B., Wüthrich, M., and Klein, B.S. (2002). BAD1, an essential virulence factor of *Blastomyces dermatitidis*, suppresses host TNF-alpha production through TGF-beta-dependent and -independent mechanisms. *J. Immunol.* 168: 5746–5755.

Galan, J.E. and Collmer, A. (1999). Type III secretion machines: Bacterial devices for protein delivery into host cells. *Science* 284: 1322–1328.

Gigliotti, F. and Hughes, W.T. (1988). Passive immunoprophylaxis with specific monoclonal antibody confers partial protection against *Pneumocystis carinii pneumonitis* in animal models. *J. Clin. Invest.* 81: 1666–1668.

Hamilton, S.E., Tvinnereim, A.R., and Harty, J.T. (2001). *Listeria monocytogenes* infection overcomes the requirement for CD40 ligand in exogenous antigen presentation to $CD8(^{+})$ T cells. *J. Immunol.* 167: 5603–5609.

Harvey, R.P., Schmid, E.S., Carrington, C.C., and Stevens, D.A. (1978). Mouse model of pulmonary blastomycosis: Utility, simplicity, and quantitative parameters. *Am. Rev. Respir. Dis.* 117: 695–703.

Hogan, L.H. and Klein, B.S. (1994). Altered expression of surface alpha-1,3-glucan in genetically related strains of *Blastomyces dermatitidis* that differ in virulence. *Infect. Immun.* 62: 3543–3546.

Hogan, L.H. and Klein, B.S. (1997). Transforming DNA integrates at multiple sites in the dimorphic fungal pathogen *Blastomyces dermatitidis. Gene* 186: 219–226.

Hogan, L.H., Josvai, S., and Klein, B.S. (1995). Genomic cloning, characterization, and functional analysis of the major surface adhesin WI-1 on *Blastomyces dermatitidis* yeasts. *J. Biol. Chem.* 270: 30725–30732.

Hogan, L.H., Klein, B.S., and Levitz, S.M. (1996). Virulence factors of medically important fungi. *Clin. Microbiol. Rev.* 9: 469–488.

Jung, S., Unutmaz, D., Wong, P., Sano, G., De los Santos, K., Sparwasser, T., Wu, S., Vuthoori, S., Ko, K., Zavala, F., Pamer, E.G., Littman, D.R., and Lang, R.A. (2002). In vivo depletion of

CD11c(+) dendritic cells abrogates priming of CD8(+) T cells by exogenous cell-associated antigens. *Immunity* 17: 211–220.

Klein, B.S. and Jones, J.M. (1990). Isolation, purification, and radiolabeling of a novel 120-kDa surface protein on *Blastomyces dermatitidis* yeasts to detect antibody in infected patients. *J. Clin. Invest.* 85: 152–161.

Klein, B.S. and Newman, S.L. (1996). Role of cell-surface molecules of *Blastomyces dermatitidis* in host-pathogen interactions. *Trends Microbiol.* 4: 246–251.

Klein, B.S., Vergeront, J.M., and Davis, J.P. (1986). Epidemiologic aspects of blastomycosis, the enigmatic systemic mycosis. *Sem. Respir. Infect.* 1: 29–39.

Klein, B.S., Sondel, P.M., and Jones, J.M. (1992). WI-1, a novel 120-kilodalton surface protein on *Blastomyces dermatitidis* yeast cells, is a target antigen of cell-mediated immunity in human blastomycosis. *Infect. Immun.* 60: 4291–4300.

Klein, B.S., Hogan, L.H., and Jones, J.M. (1993). Immunologic recognition of a 25-amino acid repeat arrayed in tandem on a major antigen of *Blastomyces dermatitidis. J. Clin. Invest.* 92: 330–337.

Klein, B.S., Chaturvedi, S., Hogan, L.H., Jones, J.M., and Newman, S.L. (1994). Altered expression of surface protein WI-1 in genetically related strains of *Blastomyces dermatitidis* that differ in virulence regulates recognition of yeasts by human macrophages. *Infect. Immun.* 62: 3536–3542.

Klein, B.S., Squires, R.A., Lloyd, J.K., Ruge, D.R., and Legendre, A.M. (2000). Canine antibody response to *Blastomyces dermatitidis* WI-1 antigen. *Am. J. Vet. Res.* 61: 554–558.

Kundig, T.M., Shahinian, A., Kawai, K., Mittrucker, H.W., Sebzda, E., Bachmann, M.F., Mak, T.W., and Ohashi, P.S. (1996). Duration of TCR stimulation determines costimulatory requirement of T cells. *Immunity* 5: 41–52.

Levitz, S.M., Mathews, H.L., and Murphy, J.W. (1995). Direct antimicrobial activity of T cells. *Immunol. Today* 16: 387–391.

Morozumi, P.A., Brummer, E., and Stevens, D.A. (1982). Protection against pulmonary blastomycosis: Correlation with cellular and humoral immunity in mice after subcutaneous nonlethal infection. *Infect. Immun.* 37: 670–678.

Morrison, C.J. and Stevens, D.A. (1991). Mechanisms of fungal pathogenicity: Correlation of virulence in vivo, susceptibility to killing by polymorphonuclear neutrophils in vitro, and neutrophil superoxide anion induction among *Blastomyces dermatitidis* isolates. *Infect. Immun.* 59: 2744–2749.

Mukherjee, J., Scharff, M.D., and Casadevall, A. (1992). Protective murine monoclonal antibodies to *Cryptococcus neoformans. Infect. Immun.* 60: 4534–4541.

Mukherjee, J., Casadevall, A., and Scharff, M.D. (1993a). Molecular characterization of the humoral responses to *Cryptococcus neoformans* infection and glucuronoxylomannan-tetanus toxoid conjugate immunization. *J. Exp. Med.* 177: 1105–1116.

Mukherjee, J., Pirofski, L.A., Scharff, M.D., and Casadevall, A. (1993b). Antibody-mediated protection in mice with lethal intracerebral *Cryptococcus neoformans* infection. *Proc. Natl. Acad. Sci. USA* 90: 3636–3640.

Mukherjee, J., Scharff, M.D., and Casadevall, A. (1994a). *Cryptococcus neoformans* infection can elicit protective antibodies in mice. *Can. J. Microbiol.* 40: 888–892.

Mukherjee, S., Lee, S., Mukherjee, J., Scharff, M.D., and Casadevall, A. (1994b). Monoclonal antibodies to *Cryptococcus neoformans* capsular polysaccharide modify the course of intravenous infection in mice. *Infect. Immun.* 62: 1079–1088.

Newman, S.L., Chaturvedi, S., and Klein, B.S. (1995). The WI-1 antigen of *Blastomyces dermatitidis* yeasts mediates binding to human macrophage CD11b/CD18 (CR3) and CD14. *J. Immunol.* 154: 753–761.

Pasparakis, M., Alexopoulou, L., Douni, E., and Kollias, G. (1996). Tumour necrosis factors in immune regulation: Everything that's interesting is . . . new! *Cytokine Growth Factor Rev.* 7:223–229.

Polonelli, L., De Bernardis, F., Conti, S., Boccanera, M., Gerloni, M., Morace, G., Magliani, W., Chezzi, C., and Cassone, A. (1994). Idiotypic intravaginal vaccination to protect against candidal vaginitis by secretory, yeast killer toxin-like anti-idiotypic antibodies. *J. Immunol.* 152: 3175–3182.

Reis e Sousa, C., Sher, A., and Kaye, P. (1999). The role of dendritic cells in the induction and regulation of immunity to microbial infection. *Curr. Opin. Immunol.* 11: 392–399.

Ronchetti, A., Rovere, P., Iezzi, G., Galati, G., Heltai, S., Protti, M.P., Garancini, M.P., Manfredi, A.A., Rugarli, C., and Bellone, M. (1999). Immunogenicity of apoptotic cells in vivo: Role of antigen load, antigen-presenting cells, and cytokines. *J. Immunol.* 163: 130–136.

Rooney, P.J., Sullivan, T.D., and Klein, B.S. (2001). Selective expression of the virulence factor BAD1 upon morphogenesis to the pathogenic yeast form of *Blastomyces dermatitidis*: Evidence for transcriptional regulation by a conserved mechanism. *Mol. Microbiol.* 39: 875–889.

Sanford, J.E., Lupan, D.M., Schlageter, A.M., and Kozel, T.R. (1990). Passive immunization against *Cryptococcus neoformans* with an isotype-switch family of monoclonal antibodies reactive with cryptococcal polysaccharide. *Infect. Immun.* 58: 1919–1923.

Schaffner, A., Davis, C.E., Schaffner, T., Markert, M., Douglas, H., and Braude, A.I. (1986). In vitro susceptibility of fungi to killing by neutrophil granulocytes discriminates between primary pathogenicity and opportunism. *J. Clin. Invest.* 78: 511–524.

Scillian, J.J., Cozad, G.C., and Spencer, H.D. (1974). Passive transfer of delayed hypersensitivity to *Blastomyces dermatitidis* between mice. *Infect. Immun.* 10: 705–711.

Shedlock, D.J., Whitmire, J.K., Tan, J., MacDonald, A.S., Ahmed, R., and Shen, H. (2003). Role of CD4 T cell help and costimulation in CD8 T cell responses during *Listeria monocytogenes* infection. *J. Immunol.* 170: 2053–2063.

Shen, H., Whitmire, J.K., Fan, X., Shedlock, D.J., Kaech, S.M., and Ahmed, R. (2003). A specific role for B cells in the generation of CD8 T cell memory by recombinant *Listeria monocytogenes*. *J. Immunol.* 170: 1443–1451.

Sixbey, J.W., Fields, B.T., Sun, C.N., Clark, R.A., and Nolan, C.M. (1979). Interactions between human granulocytes and *Blastomyces dermatitidis*. *Infect. Immun.* 23: 41–44.

Spencer, H.D. and Cozad, G.C. (1973). Role of delayed hypersensitivity in blastomycosis of mice. *Infect. Immun.* 7: 329–334.

Sugar, A. and Field, K. (1987a). Production of superoxide (O_2^-) by *Blastomyces dermatitidis* conidia and murine bronchoalveolar macrophages stimulated with conidia. *Clin. Res.* 35: 493A.

Sugar, A. and Field, K. (1987b). Production of superoxide (O_2^-) by *Blastomyces dermatitidis* (Bd) yeast forms and challenged murine bronchoalveolar macrophages (BAM). *Abstr. Annu. Meet. ASM* F45: 396.

Sugar, A.M. and Picard, M. (1991). Macrophage- and oxidant-mediated inhibition of the ability of live *Blastomyces dermatitidis* conidia to transform to the pathogenic yeast phase: Implications for the pathogenesis of dimorphic fungal infections. *J. Infect. Dis.* 163: 371–375.

Whitmire, J.K., Slifka, M.K., Grewal, I.S., Flavell, R.A., and Ahmed, R. (1996). CD40 ligand-deficient mice generate a normal primary cytotoxic T-lymphocyte response but a defective humoral response to a viral infection. *J. Virol.* 70: 8375–8381.

Wüthrich, M. and Klein, B.S. (2000). Investigation of anti-WI-1 adhesin antibody-mediated protection in experimental pulmonary blastomycosis. *J. Infect. Dis.* 181: 1720–1728.

Wüthrich, M., Chang, W.L., and Klein, B.S. (1998). Immunogenicity and protective efficacy of the WI-1 adhesin of *Blastomyces dermatitidis*. *Infect. Immun.* 66: 5443–5449.

Wüthrich, M., Filutowicz, H.I., and Klein, B.S. (2000). Mutation of the WI-1 gene yields an attenuated *Blastomyces dermatitidis* strain that induces host resistance. *J. Clin. Invest.* 106: 1381–1389.

Wüthrich, M., Filutowicz, H.I., Warner, T., and Klein, B.S. (2002). Requisite elements in vaccine immunity to *Blastomyces dermatitidis*: Plasticity uncovers vaccine potential in immune-deficient hosts. *J. Immunol.* 169: 6969–6976.

Wuthrich, M., Filutowicz, H.I., Warner, T., Deepe, G.S. Jr., and Klein, B.S. (2003). Vaccine immunity to pathogenic fungi overcomes the requirement for CD4 help in exogenous antigen presentation to CD8[+] T cells: Implications for vaccine development in immune-deficient hosts. *J. Exp. Med.* 197: 1405–1416.

7

Innate Immunity in the Lungs to Cryptococcal Infection

Kazuyoshi Kawakami

Department of Microbiology and Immunology, School of Health Sciences, Faculty of Medicine, Tohoku University, Sendai, Japan.

1. Introduction

Humans breathe about 10,000 liters of air per day. Therefore, the airway is always exposed to infectious agents, such as bacteria, fungi, and viruses, and environmental hazards, including cigarette smoke, pollutants, and allergens. To protect against these harmful stresses, highly sophisticated immune systems are developed in the lung. These systems are largely divided into two distinct categories: innate and acquired immunity. The former consists of humoral antimicrobial molecules, complements, phagocytic cells, such as neutrophils and alveolar macrophages, and other innate immune cells, including dendritic cells (DCs), natural killer (NK) cells, NKT cells, antigen receptor γδ-bearing T (γδ T) cells, and B1-B cells. On the other hand, acquired immunity is characterized by antigen-specific cell-mediated and antibody-mediated immune responses. Recent development in research of the innate immune system includes the identification of Toll-like receptors (TLRs) that specifically recognize various microbial components called pathogen-associated molecular patterns (PAMPs), such as lipopolysaccharide (LPS), peptidoglycan, lipoarabinomannan (LAM), and lipopeptides. In addition, other cell surface molecules recognizing PAMPs have been identified, which include receptors for complement components, mannose, and β-glucan. These discoveries accelerate the understanding of innate immune mechanisms operating against infectious pathogens.

Cryptococcus neoformans is a yeast-like fungal pathogen with a thick polysaccharide capsule. Infection takes place by inhaling the desiccated yeast cells into the lungs. The organisms reach the subpleural area to establish the primary lesions. In normal hosts, the infection is usually self-limiting, since host defense mechanisms can eliminate the infection. In contrast, in immunocompromised patients with impaired cell-mediated immunity, the infection is not limited to the primary site of infection; it frequently disseminates to the central nervous system, which is often associated with a high mortality in these patients. Disseminated infection of this fungal microbe to the brain has attracted attention as a serious problem, particularly with the increased number of patients with acquired immunodeficiency syndrome (AIDS).

The host defense against *C. neoformans* is critically regulated by cell-mediated immunity (Lim and Murphy, 1980), and $CD4^+$ T cells play a central role in eradicating this infection (Mody et al., 1990; Hill and Harmsen, 1991; Huffnagle et al., 1991). The balance between type-1 helper T (Th1) and Th2 cytokines markedly influences the outcome of infection; the predominant synthesis of Th1 cytokines over Th2 protects mice from infection, whereas infection is exacerbated under a Th2-dominant condition (Kawakami et al., 1997; Koguchi and Kawakami, 2002). Mice depleted of Th1-type cytokines (e.g., IFN-γ and TNF-α) are highly susceptible to cryptococcal infection (Huffnagle et al., 1996; Kawakami et al., 1996), while the infection is less severe in mice lacking Th2 cytokines (e.g., IL-4 and IL-10) than control mice (Decken et al., 1998; Blackstock et al., 1999). Differentiation of naïve helper T cells into Th1 cells absolutely requires the presence of IL-12 (Trinchieri, 1995), and this response is strongly potentiated by IL-18 (Robinson et al., 1997). In recent investigations (Decken et al., 1998: Kawakami et al., 2000a), targeted disruption of the gene for IL-12 or IL-18 resulted in attenuated host resistance and Th1 response to *C. neoformans*, indicating the role of these cytokines in the development of host protective response.

In this chapter, recent research developments in innate immune defense against cryptococcal infection in the respiratory system are highlighted with particular emphasis on the role of innate immune lymphocytes, such as NKT cells and $\gamma\delta$ T cells, based on our data using a murine model of pulmonary cryptococcal infection.

2. General Characteristics of Host Defense in the Lung

Host defense mechanisms against infectious microbial pathogens develop in the upper and lower respiratory tracts. Initially, anatomical and mechanical host defense systems trap large-sized particles in the inhaled air. These systems include nasal hairs, nasopharyngeal channels, glottis, and highly divided branches of bronchi. The particles are caught by the mucous blanket lining the bronchial surface that contains viscid glycoproteins called mucins and cleared by ciliary movement and coughing up to the oropharynx. In contrast, small-sized particles less than 5 μm in diameter, including most infectious pathogens, reach the alveolar spaces where they can cause pulmonary infection. *C. neoformans* in the inhaled air from environment is usually in an acapsular form, the size of which is 1 to 5 μm in diameter (Powell et al., 1972), suggesting the ability of this fungal pathogen to penetrate into the terminal air spaces. In order to keep lung sterility, additional host defense mechanisms are found in these areas, which are largely divided into two categories: innate and acquired host defense systems. The former consists of humoral components, including antimicrobial proteins and complements, phagocytic cells like neutrophils and macrophages, dendritic cells, and innate immune lymphocytes, while the latter is associated with antibody-mediated and cell-mediated immune responses. Furthermore, in the airway, specific mucosal immune systems composed of nasal-associated lymphoid tissue (NALT) and bronchus-associated lymphoid tissue (BALT) play important roles as the mucosal barriers in the acquired phase of host defense (Pabst, 1992; Wu and Russell, 1997).

3. Humoral Components Operate in Innate Host Defense

In the respiratory tract, many antimicrobial molecules are secreted by various immune and non-immune cells, which include lysozyme, fibronectin, lactoferin, transferin, defensins, cathelicidin, collectins, and complements (Zhang et al., 2000). I will discuss here the role of defensins, collectins, and complements in conjunction with host defense against cryptococcal infection.

3.1. Defensins

Defensins are antimicrobial cationic peptides of a small molecular weight (2 to 6 kDa) that contain six cysteines and three intramolecular disulfide bonds. Based on their size and pattern of disulfide bonds, these molecules are largely classified into two categories, α- and β-defensins (Lehrer et al., 1993). In human, so far eight defensins have been identified, including six α-defensins [human defensins (HD)-1 to 6] and two β-defensins [human β-defensins (HBD)-1 and 2]. HD-1, -2, -3, and -4 constitute 30 to 50% of the total protein in azurophilic granules of neutrophils and are also released from these cells into the airway lining fluids, while

HBD-1 and -2 are synthesized by the airway epithelial cells (Zhang et al., 2000). Defensins exert a broad-spectrum antimicrobial activity by permeabilizing the membrane of microorganisms, including bacteria, fungi, and viruses (Lehrer et al., 1993; Zhang et al., 2000). *C. neoformans* is directly killed by α-defensin from rabbit and rhesus macaque in a dose-dependent manner (Alcouloumre et al., 1993; Tang et al., 1999).

In addition, recent studies have identified a variety of immunomodulatory roles for defensins (Yang et al., 2002; Ganz, 2003). These include the activation of complement system, induction of IL-8 production by epithelial cells, augmentation of expression of adhesion molecules on neutrophils and their adhesion responses, induction of chemotaxis of leukocytes, and enhancement of proliferation and cytokine production of $CD4^+$ T cells. Thus, defensins may be involved in the innate and acquired phase host defense against cryptococcal infection through their immunoregulatory as well as antimicrobial activities.

3.2. Collectins

Collectins, collagenous C-type lectins, are oligomeric proteins composed of carbohydrate-recognition domains (CRDs) attached to collagenous regions and recognize PAMPs through calcium-dependent binding to mannose-specific carbohydrates (Clark et al., 2000). In addition to mannose-binding lectin (MBL) and conglutinin in plasma, the surfactant protein A and D (SP-A and SP-D), present in the surface layer of alveolar spaces, belong to the collectin superfamily. SP-A and SP-D bind a variety of infectious pathogens including Gram-positive and -negative bacteria, mycobacteria, fungi, and viruses, mainly via their CRD domains (Clark et al., 2000; McCormack and Whitsett, 2002). Such binding results in enhanced phagocytosis of microorganisms by alveolar macrophages and neutrophils (McCormack and Whitsett, 2002). SP-A binds to both acapsular and encapsulated forms of *C. neoformans* in a concentration-dependent manner, although three-fold better binding is observed with the acapsular form. Despite this feature, SP-A fails to function as an opsonin in the phagocytosis of this fungal pathogen by macrophages (Walenkamp et al., 1999). On the other hand, SP-D binds to the acapsular form, but either does not bind to the encapsulated form of *C. neoformans*, or does bind to a lesser extent. In contrast to SP-A, SP-D causes aggregation of acapsular yeast cells, which may stimulate their removal by enhancing the mucociliary clearance (Schelenz et al., 1995; van de Wetering et al., 2004).

3.3. Complement

The complement system is activated via three distinct pathways: classical, alternative, and lectin pathways. Whereas the activation of the classical pathway occurs from C1q subcomponent only in the presence of antigen–antibody complex, the alternative pathway is directly activated by interaction of C3 component with microbial surfaces and does not require the existence of antibody for its activation. The activation of recently identified lectin pathway is initiated by the binding of MBL with a structure similar to that of C1q, to carbohydrate (Fujita, 2002). The activated components of the complement pathways play various roles in the host defense. The deposition of C3b and iC3b fragments on the surface of microorganisms facilitates their phagocytosis by neutrophils and macrophages through interaction with complement receptor type 1 (CR1) and type 3 (CR3), respectively. In addition, C3a and C5a fragments initiate the inflammatory responses by attracting the recruitment of neutrophils into the sites of inflammation.

C. neoformans is a potent activator of the complement system. Previous studies showed that encapsulated *C. neoformans* directly activates the alternative pathway, which results in the deposition of C3 fragments on the capsular surface of this fungal microbe (Kozel et al., 1989, et al 1991). Similar deposition was detected on the surface of encapsulated cryptococci derived from the infected tissues in mice (Truelsen et al., 1992). In non-immune hosts, this pathway is considered dominant at the innate phase of infection, although the classical pathway may be triggered through binding to naturally occurring antibodies to the cell wall polysaccharide components. In contrast, further studies will be required for understanding the contribution of lectin pathway.

Early studies showed that fresh serum enhanced the engulfment of *C. neoformans* by phagocytes, and that such activity was lost by heating at 56°C (Mitchell and Friedman, 1972; Diamond et al., 1974; Davies et al., 1982). The opsonic potential of serum was attributed to the activation of complement system in in vitro experiments showing the blocking by treatment with antibodies specific for complement receptors (Levitz and Tabuni, 1991; Collins and Bancroft, 1992). The importance of the complement system in the host defense to cryptococcal infection was also documented in vivo in animals depleted of C3 by treatment with cobra venom factor or neutralizing antibody. These animals died of this infection earlier than did untreated animals (Graybill and Ahrens, 1981; Cross et al., 1997). Similar results are reported using congenitally C5-deficient mice, which were associated with increased susceptibility to the infection and with attenuated recruitment of neutrophils (Rhodes, 1985; Lovchik and Lipscomb, 1993). Thus, the complement system appears to play an important role in the innate phase resistance against cryptococcal infection by operating as opsonins and chemotactic factors in the lung.

4. Recognition of Cryptococcus

4.1. Nonopsonic Phagocytosis

Upon entry into alveolar spaces, *C. neoformans* are first recognized and then phagocytosed by macrophages. In this process, complement acts as opsonins via interaction with particular receptors, such as CR1, CR3, and CR4 (Levitz and Tabuni, 1991; Collins and Bancroft, 1992). Recently, however, nonopsonic phagocytosis by macrophages has been reported by several investigators. In earlier studies, the ingestion of acapsular *C. neoformans* was thought to be independent of complement, as indicated by the failure of anti-CR3 mAb to inhibit this response and efficient phagocytosis without prior opsonization (Cross and Bancroft, 1995). For nonopsonic engulfment of cryptococci, several cell surface receptors on phagocytic cells appear to be involved. CR3 mediates nonopsonic binding of *Mycobacterium tuberculosis* via a binding site distinct from the complement-binding site, which leads to the entrance of this bacterium into macrophages (Cywes et al., 1996). In the case of *C. neoformans*, a direct interaction between glucuronoxylomannan (GXM) and CR3 may facilitate phagocytosis by macrophages (Zaragoza et al., 2003). In previous investigations, receptors for mannose and β-glucan were suggested to mediate nonopsonic ingestion of the acapsular strain of *C. neoformans* and synthesis of proinflammatory cytokines by macrophages (Cross and Bancroft, 1995). Mannose receptor is also likely to participate in the phagocytosis of this fungal microbe for antigen presentation to T cells by dendritic cells (Syme et al., 2002). Recently, dendritic cell-specific ICAM-3-grabbing nonintegrin (DC-SIGN) and Dectin-1 have been identified as the receptors for mannose and β-glucan, respectively (Feinberg et al., 2001; Brown et al., 2002), which are found to act in the nonopsonic recognition of *Candida albicans* and zymosan by macrophages (Cambi et al., 2003; Taylor et al., 2004). The role of these receptors in phagocytosis of cryptococci remains to be elucidated.

4.2. Toll-like Receptors (TLRs)

The TLRs are evolutionally conserved from *Drosophila* to mammalian. *Drosophila* Toll are originally discovered as molecules that deliver signals for the expression of antifungal peptides (Lemaitre et al., 1996). TLRs are expressed on macrophages and dendritic cells and involved in the recognition of PAMPs from various infectious pathogens, followed by signaling to nuclei via NFκB and MAP-kinases for the expression of cytokines and cell surface molecules (Akira et al., 2001; Takeda et al., 2003). TLR2 is activated by peptidoglycan, bacterial lipoproteins, and mycobacterial lipoarabinomannan, TLR3 by double-stranded RNA, TLR4 by LPS, TLR5 by flagellin, and TLR9 by bacterial CpG-DNA (Takeda et al., 2003). Upon ingestion by macrophages, *C. neoformans* secrete polysaccharides, including GXM, galactoxylomannan and mannoproteins, into phagosomes, in which various sets of TLRs are expressed. Recently, GXM was shown to interact with TLR4 and to activate NFκB in phagocytic cells, although such interaction did not result in the activation of MAP-kinases and production of TNF-α (Shohaml et al., 2001). Thus, further effort is still required to uncover the contribution of these receptors in the innate immune response against this fungal microbe.

5. Innate Cellular Host Defense

In addition to activation of the cellular response, the invading pathogens also activate the humoral components of the innate immune mechanisms. In the airways, alveolar-resident macrophages, which permanently reside in the alveolar spaces, first encounter these pathogens, followed by recruitment of other cellular components including phagocytic cells and innate immune lymphocytes. Here, I discuss the role of alveolar macrophages, neutrophils, and dendritic cells (DCs) in the local host defense against pulmonary cryptococcal infection.

5.1. Alveolar Macrophages

In the lung, alveolar macrophages (AMϕ) play a key role in the local host defense mechanism by exerting both phagocytic and immunoregulatory functions. After invading the terminal respiratory tract, AMϕ phagocytize infectious pathogens opsonized by complement fragments through complement receptors (CR1, CR3, and CR4). The microorganisms are also recognized via interaction with other PAMP receptors present on the surface of AMϕ. AMϕ express TLR2, TLR4, DC-SIGN, and Dectin-1 (Soilleux et al., 2002; Oshikawa and Sugiyama, 2003; Steele et al., 2004), all of which are considered important in the recognition of fungal PAMPs (Shohaml et al., 2001; Cambi et al., 2003; Steele et al., 2004; Roeder et al., 2004; Taylor et al., 2004). Following such recognition, AMϕ release proinflammatory cytokines and chemokines and express co-stimulatory molecules, which results in the recruitment of neutrophils, macrophages, DCs, and innate immune lymphocytes, from the peripheral circulation into alveolar spaces and in the activation of these inflammatory cells.

In vitro studies indicate that AMϕ can phagocytize, kill, and present antigens in *C. neoformans* infection. AMϕ efficiently phagocytize the fungal microorganisms opsonized by serum (Bulmer and Tacker, 1975). The fungicidal activity against encapsulated *C. neoformans* in unstimulated human AMϕ is limited compared with other natural effector cells, peripheral blood monocytes, and neutrophils, although the acapsular strain is killed to a higher degree (Vecchiarelli et al., 1994a). Cryptococcus-laden AMϕ show a potent antigen-presenting activity to $CD4^+$ T cells in context of HLA class II DR molecules, as indicated by their proliferative response and IFN-γ production (Vecchiarelli et al., 1994b). In addition, culture of AMϕ with this fungal microbe causes the production of proinflammatory cytokines, including IL-1β, TNF-α, IL-6, IL-12, and IL-18, and chemokines, such as monocyte chemoattractant protein-1 (MCP-1) (Vecchiarelli et al., 1994b; Li and Mitchell, 1997; He et al., 2003; our unpublished data), which may contribute to the regulation of host immune responses that takes place in the bronchoalveolar spaces. Interestingly, these activities in human AMϕ are down-regulated by encapsulation of *C. neoformans* (Vecchiarelli et al., 1994b). In contrast, the in vivo role of AMϕ in the local protection against pulmonary cryptococcosis remains to be fully understood, although earlier investigations demonstrated that depletion of macrophages by systemic administration of silica markedly decreased the host resistance to cryptococcal infection (Monga, 1981).

Thus, AMϕ play a key role in the initiation of host protective response against *C. neoformans* at the gateway of the airway tract. In addition to the phagocytic and fungicidal functions, AMϕ exert immunoregulatory activities through the production of various proinflammatory cytokines and chemokines, which could provide a great influence on the quality of subsequent immune responses, recruitment of innate immune cells, and the activation and development of acquired immune responses.

5.2. Neutrophils

Although the development of cryptococcosis is not clinically associated with neutropenia, neutrophils are highly active in engulfing and killing *C. neoformans* in vitro (Miller and Mitchell, 1991). Neutrophils are thought to contribute to the innate defenses against cryptococcosis, particularly early in the course of infection before the development of acquired immune responses. In animal models, an influx of neutrophils into tissues is observed soon after cryptococcal challenge and is associated with rapid, but partial, clearance of the organisms (Gadebusch and Johnson, 1966; Perfect et al., 1980). Neutrophilia caused by administration of cyclophosphamide is associated with exacerbation of this infection, although the same treatment also affects lymphocyte function (Graybill and Mitchell, 1978). In mouse models of cryptococcosis, boosting neutrophil-mediated host defenses by administration of granulocyte colony-stimulating factor (G-CSF) resulted in reduced brain tissue burden and prolonged survival of mice treated with fluconazole (Graybill et al., 1977). In human, neutrophils are frequently found in pathology specimens taken from patients with cryptococcosis (Baker and Haugen, 1955; Lee et al., 1996).

Recently, accumulating evidence highlights the immunoregulatory role of neutrophils in the host defense against infectious pathogens. In pulmonary infection with *Legionella pneumophila*, neutrophils play an important role in protection through polarizing the immune response toward a Th1-dominant condition (Tateda et al., 2001). Similarly, neutropenic mice are more susceptible to *M. tuberculosis* infection than mice bearing normal counts of neutrophils, which is associated with reduced expression of IFN-γ and iNOS (Pedrosa et al., 2000). Interestingly, Mednick and co-workers (2003) reported opposite results, indicating the enhanced survival of mice infected with a lethal dose of *C. neoformans* probably by coordinating inflammatory responses via modulation of cytokine synthesis in the lung.

In our previous studies, accumulation of neutrophils was not associated with protective host responses against lethal pulmonary infection with *C. neoformans* (Kawakami, 1999). The infected mice showed little or no expression of CC- and ELR^- CXC-chemokines that attract lymphocytes and macrophages, but ELR^+ CXC-chemokines that recruit neutrophils. These observations were consistent with poor infiltration of mononuclear leukocytes, but accumulation of neutrophils at the site of infection. Administration of IL-12 that rescued mice from lethal infection polarized the chemokine and cellular inflammatory responses toward the preferential accumulation of lymphocytes and macrophages, but not of neutrophils. These findings may provide evidence arguing against the protective role of neutrophils in infection with *C. neoformans*.

Thus, the contribution of neutrophils to the host defense against cryptococcal infection remains controversial. However, any such role is not likely pronounced according to the previous observations reported.

5.3. Dendritic Cells

DC is an efficient antigen-presenting cell for naïve T lymphocytes. Immature DCs that develop from $CD34^+$ progenitors in the bone marrow are characterized by their ability to capture antigens by endocytosis and phagocytosis. After capturing antigens, DCs undergo maturation that is associated with the expression of processed antigens in context of MHC class II and upregulation of co-stimulatory molecules, such as CD40, CD80, and CD86, expressed on their surface (Banchereau et al., 2000). During these changes, DCs migrate from the infected tissues into the T cell area of draining lymph nodes, where they encounter naïve antigen-specific $CD4^+$ T cells (Guermonprez et al., 2002). DCs have an important role in determining the profile of cytokine production by T cells, i.e., Th1 or Th2 cells. In human, monocyte-derived DCs seem to promote the differentiation of Th1 cells by producing IL-12, while Th2 cells are likely induced by plasmacytoid-derived DCs (Moser and Murphy, 2000). DCs express many receptors for PAMPs, including TLRs, mannose receptors, and β-glucan receptors. Interaction of these receptors with the PAMPs leads to the production of proinflammatory cytokines and increased expression of co-stimulatory molecules by DCs. IL-12 and IL-18 released from these cells strongly promote the production of IFN-γ by innate immune lymphocytes, such as NK, NKT, and γδ T cells, as well as the differentiation of Th1 cells (Trinchieri, 1995; Robinson et al., 1997; Okamura et al., 1998; Qureshi et al., 1999; Baxevanis et al., 2003).

The cell-mediated immune responses are essential for the host defense against cryptococcal infection. The involvement of DCs in the development of cell-mediated immunity against this fungal microbe is not well understood. Bauman and co-workers (2000) examined the kinetics of DC accumulation in the draining lymph nodes after subcutaneous immunization with cryptococcal antigens. The protective anticryptococcal immune responses are associated with preferential accumulation of myeloid DCs in the draining lymph nodes, while lymphoid DC is the major subset in the unprotected mice. Accumulation of DCs in the lymph nodes is regulated by TNF-α (Bauman et al., 2003). In our unpublished data, DCs, identified as cells expressing both CD11c and class II MHC molecules, migrate into paratracheal lymph nodes after pulmonary infection with *C. neoformans*, although further investigation is required for understanding the role of these cells in the local host defense in the lung.

6. Innate Immune Lymphocytes

C. neoformans show the features of intracellular parasitism within phagocyte cells, as is well known in *M. tuberculosis*, *Listeria monocytogenes*, and *Salmonella typhimurium* (Feldmesser et al., 2001). Because such pathogens resist the killing mechanisms, phagocytes fail to eradicate them without any activation. The innate immune lymphocytes, such as NK, NKT, and γδ T cells, can enhance their killing activity through the production of IFN-γ, although the overall potential is not sufficient for complete eradication of the infection, which needs more potent protective mechanisms by developing subsequent acquired immune responses. Based on this property, the innate immune lymphocytes have been recognized merely as a "temporary protector" until the acquired immune response is established. However, recent investigations disagree with this concept. In this respect, accumulating evidences suggest that innate immune lymphocytes are the cells that determine the quality of acquired immune responses (Horwitz et al., 1999; Nishimura et al., 2000; Schaible and Kaufmann, 2000). Thus, the early host protective responses mediated by these cells is more than a "temporary protector" before development of acquired immunity.

6.1. NK Cells

NK cells play a role in the innate cellular host defense mechanisms to eliminate virus-infected cells and tumor cells (Trinchieri, 1989). NK cells express their killing activity through a non-phagocytic mechanism, which is mediated by several killing molecules including perforin and granzyme B (Kagi et al., 1996). In host defense against infectious pathogens, NK cells regulate the innate defense mechanisms through the production of cytokines such as IFN-γ (Dunn and North, 1991; Laskay et al., 1993; Scharton and Scott, 1993). This process operates especially in the early phase of infection before the establishment of a specific immune response mediated by T cells, through the enhancement of the antimicrobial activity of phagocytic cells. IL-12 and IL-18 potentiate the tumoricidal activity as well as production of IFN-γ by NK cells and act synergistically when these cytokines are administered in combination (Okamura et al., 1995, 1998; Trinchieri, 1995; Zhang et al., 1997; Hyodo et al., 1999).

Earlier studies also indicated the role of NK cells in eliminating *C. neoformans* from the host. In a series of studies, Murphy and co-workers demonstrated that NK cells inhibited the growth of fungal microorganisms by directly binding to them (Murphy and MacDaniel, 1982; Nabavi and Murphy, 1985; Hidore and Murphy, 1989; Hidrore et al., 1990, et al 1991a, et al b; Murphy et al., 1991, et al 1993). Other studies by various investigators indicated that mice defective in NK cell activity were more susceptible to intravenous challenge with *C. neoformans* than control animals (Hidore and Murphy, 1986; Lipscomb et al., 1991; Scharton and Scott, 1993). These early observations emphasized the role of NK cells in eliminating *C. neoformans* from infected organs through a direct fungicidal activity. In contrast, our studies showed that SCID mouse-derived splenic NK cells, which were stimulated with a combination of IL-12 and IL-18, did not show any direct cryptococcocidal effect, although the production of IFN-γ and cytolytic activity to NK-sensitive tumor cells were markedly induced by the same treatment. NK cells rather upregulated the nitric oxide (NO)-mediated antifungal activity against *C. neoformans* through the production of IFN-γ (Kawakami et al., 2000b). Thus, NK cells contribute to the host defense against cryptococcal infection by regulating the immune response as well as by directly killing this fungal microbe.

The in vivo role of NK cells, which form approximately 5 to 6% of the lymphocyte population in lung (Kawakami et al., 2001a), in the local host defense against cryptococcal infection in airway tissues remains to be fully understood. In earlier studies, lung infection was not aggravated in mice depleted of NK cells by administration of anti-NK1.1 mAb (Lipscomb et al., 1987), although the same treatment deleted not only NK cells but also NKT cells. However, NK cells appear to be the source of IFN-γ to control *C. neoformans* infection in mice receiving a combined treatment with IL-12 and IL-18 (Qureshi et al., 1999) or in mice with a genetic disruption of IL-12p40 gene (Kawakami et al., 2000a). In contrast, IFN-γ production and host protection from cryptococcal infection caused by administration of unmethylated synthetic DNA-containing CpG-motif do not involve NK cells (our unpublished data). Thus, the in vivo role of NK cells in anticryptococcal host response appears to vary in different settings; further studies will be necessary to better understand this role.

6.2. NKT Cells

6.2.1. Characteristics

NKT cell is a unique T cell subset sharing some features with NK cells. Originally, this population was identified as a lymphocyte subset that expresses both T cell receptor (TCR) αβ and NK1.1 or NKR-P1 (CD161) in mice (Godfrey et al., 2000; Taniguchi and Nakayama, 2000). Specific characteristics of this cell type include highly limited repertoire with an invariant Vα chain consisting of Vα14-Jα18 (formerly Jα281) gene segment and highly skewed Vβ chains, Vβ8.2, 7, and 2 in mice and with Vα24Jα18 and Vβ11 in human. Accordingly, these cells are called invariant (*i*)NKT cells. The mouse *i*NKT cells are either $CD4^+$ or double negative (DN) and usually do not express CD8, while $CD8^+$ subset can be found in human. The development of *i*NKT cells is dependent on the non-classical MHC class I molecule CD1d, which is composed of non-polymorphic heavy chain and β2 microglobulin because this population disappears in CD1d gene-disrupted (CD1d-KO) mice. The glycosphingolipid, α-galactosylceramide (α-GalCer) that was originally discovered in marine sponge as a novel anticancer agent, is recognized by *i*NKT cells in context with CD1d, which results in their strong activation. These cells are found in large numbers in the liver, thymus, and bone marrow and in small numbers in the spleen and lungs.

6.2.2. Role in Host Defense to Infection

NKT cells contribute to development of both Th1 and Th2 responses under different experimental conditions (Lehuen et al., 1998; Carnaud et al., 1999; Cui et al., 1999; Singh et al., 1999). Although the significance of NKT cells in infectious diseases remains to be fully elucidated, to date there are several published studies on this issue. Three roles are identified for these cells in host defense against infectious pathogens. First, the clinical course of *M. tuberculosis* and *Salmonella choleraesuis* infection is not much affected by manipulations designed to suppress the activity of NKT cells (Behar et al., 1999; Ishigami et al., 1999). Second, infection with *Listeria monocytogenes* or *Toxoplasma gondii* is rather improved by the similar manipulations (Szalay et al., 1999; Nakano et al., 2001). Finally, mice lacking NKT cells are more susceptible to infection caused by *Leishmania major*, *Pseudomonas aeruginosa*, *Streptococcus pneumoniae*, *Borrelia burgdorferi*, and *Plasmodium yoelii* than control mice (Ishikawa et al., 2000; Kumar et al., 2000; Mannoor et al., 2001; Nieuwnhuis et al., 2002; Kawakami et al., 2003). Thus, the role of NKT cells seems different among infectious pathogens.

6.2.3. Accumulation of iNKT Cells in Lung after Cryptococcal Infection

Recently, we reported the increase of NKT cells in lungs after intratracheal infection with *C. neoformans* (Kawakami et al., 2001a). Inflammatory leukocytes obtained from the homogenates of infected lungs were stained with anti-TCRαβ and -NK1.1 mAbs to discriminate conventional T, NK, and NKT cells. The proportions of conventional T, NK, and NKT cells, as indicated by $TCR\alpha\beta^+NK1.1^-$, $TCR\alpha\beta^-NK1.1^+$, and $TCR\alpha\beta^+NK1.1^+$ cells, respectively, started to increase on day 1, reached peak values on day 6 and then decreased on day 10 post-infection. Interestingly, NKT cells most profoundly increased at the infected sites among these cells. We further defined the dynamics of *i*NKT cells bearing $V\alpha14^+$ TCR in the infected lungs by detecting cells bound to either anti-Vα14 mAb or α-GalCer-loaded CD1d tetramer. Similar kinetics was observed in this particular subset of NKT cells using both strategies for detection. Thus, $V\alpha14^+$ NKT cells as well as conventional T and NK cells were found to increase in the lungs after intratracheal infection with *C. neoformans*.

Migration of inflammatory leukocytes from the peripheral circulation to the site of infection is critically regulated by a variety of chemokines, which are classified into two major subgroups, CXC- and CC-chemokines, based on the arrangement of two N-terminal cysteine residues (Rossi and Zlotnik, 2000). ELR^+ CXC-chemokines, including IL-8, are neutrophil-mediated inflammatory responses, while ELR^- CXC-chemokines (e.g., IP-10 and

Mig) and CC-chemokines (e.g., MCP-1, MIP-1α, -1β, and RANTES) predominantly attract lymphocytes and macrophages. Many investigators have reported that resting or activated NK cells are attracted to the site of infection by many chemokines, including MCP-2, -3, MIP-1α, RANTES, IP-10, and lymphotactin, under various conditions (Allavena et al., 1994; Maghazachi et al., 1994, 1997; Taub et al., 1995; Giancarlo et al., 1996; Loetscher et al., 1996 et al). In contrast, MIP-2 was the only chemokine known to function in trafficking NKT cells until MCP-1 was identified as a chemoattractant for these cells (Faunce et al., 2001). In MCP-1KO mice, accumulation of NKT cells in lungs was not observed after infection with *C. neoformans* (Kawakami et al., 2001a). Consistent with these data, MCP-1 production preceded the kinetics of NKT cell-mediated inflammatory responses. Thus, NKT cell trafficking into the fungus-infected sites involves at least in part the production of MCP-1, although other chemokines may contribute, as observed in NK cells.

6.2.4. Role of iNKT cells in Th1 Response and Host Defense to Cryptococcal Infection

A remarkable feature of NKT cells is the expeditious and abundant production of IFN-γ and IL-4 upon stimulation via their antigen receptors (Godfrey et al., 2000; Taniguchi and Nakayama, 2000). Accumulating evidence suggests that NKT cells are involved in the regulation of Th1 and Th2 cell development. On the other hand, host defense against cryptococcal infection is critically regulated by the balance between Th1- and Th2-mediated immune responses (Kawakami et al., 1997; Koguchi and Kawakami, 2002). These findings suggest that NKT cells may affect the host immune responses and protection against infection with this fungal microorganism. In our study (Kawakami et al., 2001), the Th1-mediated immune responses, as indicated by antigen-specific IFN-γ production by T cells and delayed-type hypersensitivity reaction, were significantly ameliorated in Jα18-KO mice lacking *i*NKT cells, compared with control wild-type mice. In contrast, Th2 cytokine synthesis was not altered in these mice. Furthermore, the clearance of fungal microorganisms from the infected sites was significantly delayed in Jα18-KO mice, compared with control mice. These findings demonstrate that *i*NKT cells function not only in the innate immune phase but also in bridging the establishment of Th1-mediated acquired immune responses, which leads to host protection against cryptococcal infection.

6.2.5. Induction of Th1 Response and Protection against Cryptococcal Infection by Ligand-Specific Activation of iNKT Cells

*i*NKT cells recognize α-GalCer by their antigen receptors in the context of CD1d molecules expressed on DCs (Kawano et al., 1997; Godfrey et al., 2000; Taniguchi and Nakayama, 2000). Such engagement causes prompt secretion of both IFN-γ and IL-4 by these cells and emergence of their cytolytic activity against tumor cells. Toura et al. (1999) indicated that administration of DCs pulsed with α-GalCer induced potent antitumor activity through specific activation of *i*NKT cells, and resulted in the complete suppression of melanoma metastasis in the liver.

In infectious diseases, Gonzalez-Aseguinolaza et al. (2000) were the first group to demonstrate the effectiveness of α-GalCer treatment in improving the clinical course of murine malaria. The development of liver stage, but not blood stage, malaria was strongly inhibited via induction of IFN-γ synthesis by α-GalCer. The same group recently revealed that co-administration of α-GalCer potentiated the protective effect against this infection caused by immunization with irradiated malaria parasite (Gonzalez-Aseguinolaza et al., 2002). Our group observed similar effects for this treatment in a murine model of cryptococcal infection (Kawakami et al., 2001b). Administration of α-GalCer strongly enhanced the production of IFN-γ by NK and Th1 cells and significantly reduced the number of live colonies of *C. neoformans* in the infected organs, compared with vehicle treatment. These effects were not detected in Jα18-KO mice, indicating the involvement of *i*NKT cells. IFN-γ production induced by α-GalCer was totally mediated by IL-12, but not IL-18 (Kawakami et al., 2001c). The protective effects by the ligand-specific activation of *i*NKT cells against *P. aeruginosa* and *M. tuberculosis* are recently reported by other investigators (Chackerian et al., 2002; Nieuwenhuis et al., 2002), although their contribution to the host defense against the latter infection is not clearly defined (Behar et al., 1999). These observations suggest that α-GalCer can be a promising immunotherapeutic agent for the treatment of certain intractable infectious diseases including cryptococcal meningitis in immunodeficient patients.

6.3. γδ T cells

In addition to conventional T cells bearing TCRαβ, a distinct subset of T cells expressing novel antigen receptors consisting of γ and δ chains, designated as γδ T cells, was discovered approximately 20 years ago (Hayday, 2000). In sharp contrast to αβ T cells, which are the major population in lymphoid tissues such as lymph node and spleen, γδ T cells are preferentially localized in non-lymphoid tissues, including epidermis, where they are known as dendritic epidermal T cells (DETC), and mucosal/epithelial tissues, such as intestine, lung, tongue, mammary, uterine, and vaginal epithelia, although some cells exist in lymphoid tissues. Such characteristic localization suggests the role of these cells in first line host defense against infectious agents and other antigens.

6.3.1. Natural Ligands

The number of V gene segments of γδ T cells that determine their diversity is very limited when compared with that of αβ T cells. In addition, particular subsets are localized in the defined anatomical areas and at different developmental stages. Based on these features, the diversity of antigen recognition by γδ T cells is assumed to be limited in contrast to αβ T cells that recognize broad spectrum of antigens (Hayday, 2000; Lahn, 2000). Previous investigations have identified a variety of antigens recognized by these cells from microbial products. Human Vγ9/Vδ2^{+} γδ T cells react with low molecular weight nonproteinaceous antigens, such as prenyl pyrophosphate and nucleotide triphosphate from *M. tuberculosis* and alkylamine from *Proteus morganii*, in non-MHC-restricted manner (Tanaka et al., 1995; Bukowski et al., 1999). In addition, protein antigens can be ligands for the activation of γδ T cells. Human Vγ9/Vδ2^{+} γδ T cells recognize tetanus toxoid in the context of MHC class II molecules (Holoshitz et al., 1992). Mycobacterial heat-shock proteins stimulate both human and mouse γδ T cells (O'Brien et al., 1989, 1992; Born et al., 1990et al). However, no ligand of these cells has so far been identified from fungal microorganisms, including *C. neoformans*.

6.3.2. Regulatory Role in Host Defense to Cryptococcal Infection

In our recent study, we investigated the role of γδ T cells in the development of Th1 response and the host defense against pulmonary infection with *C. neoformans* using a mouse model of pulmonary cryptococcosis (Uezu et al., 2004). γδ T cells rapidly increased in a similar kinetics as observed in

NK and NKT cells. Although the precise mechanism remains to be elucidated, such increase of γδ T cells in the infected lungs was likely to take place in a manner different from that of NK and NKT cells. Accumulation of NK and NKT cells in lungs after cryptococcal infection was markedly reduced in MCP-1KO mice, while such reduction was not found in γδ T cells. At present, the precise mechanism of γδ T cell recruitment remains to be clarified.

Interestingly, clearance of *C. neoformans* in lungs was enhanced in mice lacking γδ T cells, induced by administration of a specific antibody or targeted disruption of Cδ gene. Such increased host defense was associated with the promoted differentiation of Th1 cells and increased production of IFN-γ. These observations suggest the suppressive role of γδ T cells in the host defense against cryptococcal infection. This is in a sharp contrast to the role of NKT cells, which contribute significantly to the development of Th1-type immune response and host resistance to this infection (Kawakami et al., 2001a). Earlier investigations reported anti-inflammatory γδ T cells that produced Th2 cytokines and TGF-β (Wesch et al., 2001; Nagaeva et al., 2002). These observations suggest that these cytokines mediate the down-regulatory effect observed in our study. This speculation was supported by our recent data showing low production of TGF-β in the lungs of Cδ-KO mice totally lacking γδ T cells at earlier phase of cryptococcal infection, although the synthesis of Th2 cytokines, IL-4 and IL-10, was not much different from control mice. In this regard, TGF-β is known to suppress the host defense to infectious pathogens (Hirsch et al., 1997; Letterio and Roberts, 1998; Li et al., 1999; Reed, 1999). Furthermore, other investigations revealed that γδ T cells down-regulate the host defense against infection caused by *L. monocytogenes*, *S. choleraesuis*, and *C. albicans* (Emoto et al., 1995; O'Brien et al., 2000; Wormley et al., 2001). Thus, our study suggests that γδ T cells may suppress the host defense to pulmonary infection with *C. neoformans* via a TGF-β-mediated mechanism.

6.4. Regulation of Host Defense against Cryptococcal Infection by NKT and γδ T Cells

The distinct roles of *i*NKT and γδ T cells in the host resistance against cryptococcal infection suggest that these innate immune lymphocytes co-regulate Th1-mediated response for induction of a moderate host defense. γδ T cells may act to keep the balance of Th1–Th2 response in a proper manner by suppressing the exaggerated Th1 response caused by NKT cells, as speculated in Fig. 7.1. In pulmonary infection with *C. neoformans*, the number of both NKT and γδ T cells in the paratracheal lymph nodes increases in parallel with that of DCs (our unpublished data), which could be consistent with the above hypothesis. Interestingly, in toxoplasmal infection, γδ T cells appear to play a protective role in the host defense by promoting Th1-mediated immune response, while NKT cells are likely to suppress these responses (Hisaeda et al., 1995). This is in sharp contrast to the findings in cryptococcal infection. Although the precise mechanism of such difference remains to be clarified, the role of NKT and γδ T cells in the host protective response seems to vary from one microbe to another.

7. Concluding Remarks

Acquired immunity, an antigen-specific host defense mechanism, had been the central dogma of previous studies on immunological response to infection. Recently, however, the role of innate immune mechanisms, mediated by soluble antimicrobial components, complements, phagocytes, and innate immune lymphocytes, have garnered much attention by many investigators and the biological significance of these cellular components is being

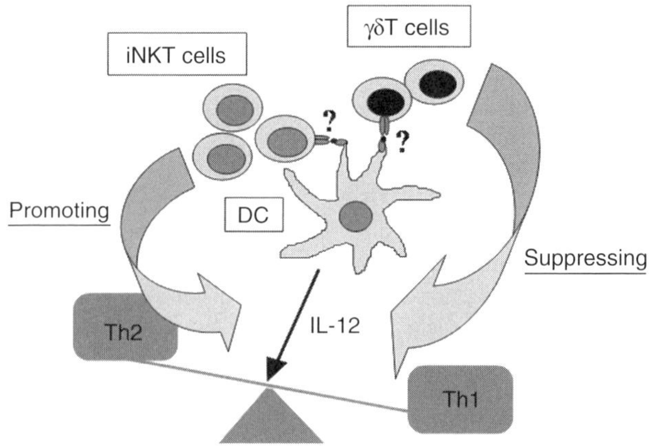

Figure 7.1. *Regulation of Th1–Th2 cytokine balance by iNKT and γδ T cells in cryptococcal infection.* Host defense to cryptococcal infection is critically regulated by Th1–Th2 cytokine balance. The predominant synthesis of Th1 cytokines over Th2 protects mice from infection, whereas infection is exacerbated under a Th2-dominant condition. *i*NKT cells regulate this balance to promote the host protection, whereas γδ T cells counter-regulate this process. Thus, these innate immune lymphocytes may act to keep the host defense in a proper manner, although the mechanism of their activation remains to be elucidated.

extensively explored. Furthermore, the discovery of PAMP receptors has accelerated research in this area. In the host immune response to infectious pathogens, as demonstrated in our series of investigations on cryptococcal infection, the important roles of innate immunity in respiratory tissues, mediated especially by NKT and γδ T cells, have been unveiled. Furthermore, the results of several studies support the involvement of these particular lymphocyte subsets in determining the balance of Th1–Th2 immune responses. Thus, both NKT and γδ T cells seem to participate in bridging early host protection, by innate immune mechanism, to antigen-specific acquired immune responses in pulmonary cryptococcosis.

References

Akira, S., Takeda, K., and Kaisho, T. (2001). Toll-like receptors: critical proteins linking innate and acquired immunity. *Nat. Immunol.* 2: 675–680.

Alcouloumre, M.S., Ghannoum, M.A., Ibrahim, A.S., Selsted, M.E., and Edwards, J.E. Jr. (1993). Fungicidal properties of defensin NP-1 and activity against *Cryptococcus neoformans* in vitro. *Antimicrob. Agents Chemother.* 37: 2628–2632.

Allavena, P., Bianchi, G., Zhou, D., van Damme, J., Jilek, P., Sozzani, S., and Mantovani, A. (1994). Induction of natural killer cell migration by monocyte chemotactic protein-1: -2 and -3. *Eur. J. Immunol.* 24: 3233–3236.

Baker, R.D. and Haugen, R.K. (1955). Tissue changes and tissue diagnosis in cryptococcosis: A study of 26 cases. *Am. J. Clin. Pathol.* 25: 14–24.

Banchereau, J., Briere, F., Caux, C., Davoust, J., Lebecque, S., Liu, Y.J., Pulendran, B., and Palucka K. (2000). Immunobiology of dendritic cells. *Annu. Rev. Immunol.* 18: 767–811.

Bauman, S.K., Nichols, K.L., and Murphy, J.W. (2000). Dendritic cells in the induction of protective and nonprotective anticryptococcal cell-mediated immune responses. *J. Immunol.* 165: 158–167.

Bauman, S.K., Huffnagle, G.B., and Murphy, J.W. (2003). Effects of tumor necrosis factor alpha on dendritic cell accumulation in lymph nodes draining the immunization site and the impact on the anticryptococcal cell-mediated immune response. *Infect. Immun.* 71: 68–74.

Baxevanis, C.N., Gritzapis, A.D., and Papamichail, M. (2003). In vivo antitumor activity of NKT cells activated by the combination of IL-12 and IL-18. *J. Immunol.* 171: 2953–2959.

Blackstock, R., Buchanan, K.L., Adesina, A.M., and Murphy, J.W. (1999). Differential regulation of immune responses by highly and weakly virulent *Cryptococcus neoformans* isolates. *Infect. Immun.* 67: 3601–3609.

Born, W., Hall, L., Dallas, A., Boymel, J., Shinnick, T., Young, D., Brennan, P., and O'Brien, R. (1990). Recognition of a peptide antigen by heat shock-reactive gamma delta T lymphocytes. *Science* 249: 67–69.

Brown, G.D., Taylor, P.R., Reid, D.M., Willment, J.A., Williams, D.L., Martinez-Pomares, L., Wong, S.Y., and Gordon, S. (2002). Dectin-1 is a major beta-glucan receptor on macrophages. *J. Exp. Med.* 196: 407–412.

Bukowski, J.F., Morita, C.T., and Brenner, M.B. (1999). Human gamma delta T cells recognize alkylamines derived from microbes, edible plants, and tea: Implications for innate immunity. *Immunity* 11: 57–65.

Bulmer, G.S. and Tacker, J.R. (1975). Phagocytosis of *Cryptococcus neoformans* by alveolar macrophages. *Infect. Immun.* 11: 73–79.

Cambi, A., Gijzen, K., de Vries, J.M., Torensma, R., Joosten, B., Adema, G.J., Netea, M.G., Kullberg, B.J., Romani, L., and Figdor, C.G. (2003). The C-type lectin DC-SIGN (CD209) is an antigen-uptake receptor for *Candida albicans* on dendritic cells. *Eur. J. Immunol.* 33: 532–538.

Carnaud, C., Lee, D., Donnars, O., Park, S.H., Beavis, A., Koezuka, Y., and Bendelac, A. (1999). Cross-talk between cells of the innate immune system: NKT cells rapidly activate NK cells. *J. Immunol.* 163: 4647–4650.

Chackerian, A., Alt, J., Perera, V., and Behar, S.M. (2002). Activation of NKT cells protects mice from tuberculosis. *Infect. Immun.* 70: 6302–6309.

Clark, H.W., Reid, K.B., and Sim, R.B. (2000). Collectins and innate immunity in the lung. *Microbes Infect.* 2: 273–278.

Collins, H.L. and Bancroft, G.J. (1992). Cytokine enhancement of complement-dependent phagocytosis by macrophages: Synergy of tumor necrosis factor-alpha and granulocyte-macrophage colony-stimulating factor for phagocytosis of *Cryptococcus neoformans*. *Eur. J. Immunol.* 22: 1447–1454.

Cross, C.E. and Bancroft, G.J. (1995). Ingestion of acapsular *Cryptococcus neoformans* occurs via mannose and beta-glucan receptors, resulting in cytokine production and increased phagocytosis of the encapsulated form. *Infect. Immun.* 63: 2604–2611.

Cross, C.E., Collins, H.L., and Bancroft, G.J. (1997). CR3-dependent phagocytosis by murine macrophages: Different cytokines regulate ingestion of a defined CR3 ligand and complement-opsonized *Cryptococcus neoformans*. *Immunology* 91: 289–296.

Cui, J., Watanabe, N., Kawano, T., Yamashita, M., Kamata, T., Shimizu, C., Kimura, M., Shimizu, E., Oike, J., Koseki, H., Tanaka, Y., Taniguchi, M., and Nakayama, T. (1999). Inhibition of T helper cell type 2 cell differentiation and immunoglobulin E response by ligand-activated Vα14 natural killer cells. *J. Exp. Med.* 190: 783–792.

Cywes, C., Godenir, N.L., Hoppe, H.C., Scholle, R.R., Steyn, L.M., Kirsch, R.E., and Ehlers, M.R. (1996). Nonopsonic binding of *Mycobacterium tuberculosis* to human complement receptor type 3 expressed in Chinese hamster ovary cells. *Infect. Immun.* 64: 5373–5383.

Davies, S.F., Clifford, D.P., Hoidal, J.R., and Repine, J.E. (1982). Opsonic requirements for the uptake of *Cryptococcus neoformans* by human polymorphonuclear leukocytes and monocytes. *J. Infect. Dis.* 145: 870–874.

Decken, K., Kohler, G., Palmer-Lehmann, K., Wunderlin, A., Mattner, F., Magram, J., Gately, M.K., and Alber, G. (1998). Interleukin-12 is essential for a protective Th1 response in mice infected with *Cryptococcus neoformans*. *Infect. Immun.* 66: 4994–5000.

Diamond, R.D., May, J.E., Kane, M.A., Frank, M.M., and Bennett, J.E. (1974). The role of the classical and alternate complement pathways in host defenses against *Cryptococcus neoformans* infection. *J. Immunol.* 112: 2260–2270.

Dunn, P.L. and North, R.J. (1991). Early gamma interferon production by natural killer cells is important in defense against murine listeriosis. *Infect. Immun.* 59: 2892–2900.

Emoto, M., Nishimura, H., Sakai, T., Hiromatsu, K., Gomi, H., Itohara, S., and Yoshikai, Y. (1995). Mice deficient in gamma delta T cells are resistant to lethal infection with *Salmonella choleraesuis*. *Infect. Immun.* 63: 3736–3738.

Faunce, D.E., Sonoda, K., and Stein-Streilein, J. (2001). MIP-2 recruits NKT cells to the spleen during tolerance induction. *J. Immunol.* 166: 313–321.

Feinberg, H., Mitchell, D.A., Drickamer, K., and Weis, W.I. (2001). Structural basis for selective recognition of oligosaccharides by DC-SIGN and DC-SIGNR. *Science* 294: 2163–2166.

Feldmesser, M., Tucker, S., and Casadevall, A. (2001). Intracellular parasitism of macrophages by *Cryptococcus neoformans*. *Trends Microbiol.* 9: 273–278.

Fujita, T. (2002). Evolution of the lectin-complement pathway and its role in innate immunity. *Nat. Rev. Immunol.* 2: 346–353.

Gadebusch, H.H. and Johnson, A.G. (1966). Natural host resistance to infection with *Cryptococcus neoformans*. IV. The effect of some cationic proteins on the experimental disease. *J. Infect. Dis.* 116: 551–565.

Ganz, T. (2003). Defensins: Antimicrobial peptides of innate immunity. *Nat. Rev. Immunol.* 3: 710–720.

Giancarlo, B., Silvano, S., Albert, Z., Mantovani, A., and Allavena, P. (1996). Migratory response of human natural killer cells to lymphotactin. *Eur. J. Immunol.* 26: 3238–3241.

Godfrey, D.I., Hammond, K.J.L., Poulton, L.D., Smyth, M.J., and Baxter, A.G. (2000). NKT cells: Facts, functions and fallacies. *Immunol. Today* 21: 573–583.

Gonzalez-Aseguinolaza, G., de Oliveira, C., Tomsaka, M., Hong, S., Bruna-Romero, O., Nakayama, T., Taniguchi, M., Bendelac, A., van Kaer, L., Koezuka, Y., and Tsuji, M. (2000). α-Galactosylceramide-activated Vα14 natural killer T cells mediate protection against murine malaria. *Proc. Natl. Acad. Sci. USA* 97: 8461–8466.

Gonzalez-Aseguinolaza, G., Van Kaer, L., Bergmann, C. C., Wilson, J. M., Schmieg, J., Kronenberg, M., Nakayama, T., Taniguchi, M., Koezuka, Y., and Tsuji, M. (2002). Natural killer T cell ligand alpha-galactosylceramide enhances protective immunity induced by malaria vaccines. *J. Exp. Med.* 195: 617–624.

Graybill, J.R. and Ahrens, J. (1981). Immunization and complement interaction in host defense against murine Cryptococcosis. *J. Reticuloendothel. Soc.* 30: 347–357.

Graybill, J.R. and Mitchell, L. (1978). Cyclophosphamide effects on murine cryptococcosis. *Infect. Immun.* 21: 674–677.

Graybill, J.R., Bocanegra, R., Lambros, C., and Luther, M.F. (1977). Granulocyte colony stimulating factor therapy of experimental cryptococcal meningitis. *J. Med. Vet. Mycol.* 35: 243–247.

Guermonprez, P., Valladeau, J., Zitvogel, L., Thery, C., and Amigorena, S. (2002). Antigen presentation and T cell stimulation by dendritic cells. *Annu. Rev. Immunol.* 20: 621–667.

Hayday, A.C. (2000). Gamma/delta cells: A right time and a right place for a conserved third way of protection. *Annu. Rev. Immunol.* 18: 975–1026.

He, W., Casadevall, A., Lee, S.C., and Goldman, D.L. (2003). Phagocytic activity and monocyte chemotactic protein expression by pulmonary macrophages in persistent pulmonary cryptococcosis. *Infect. Immun.* 71: 930–936.

Hidore, M.R. and Murphy, J.W. (1986). Natural cellular resistance of beige mice against *Cryptococcus neoformans*. *J. Immunol.* 137: 3624–3631.

Hidore, M.R. and Murphy, J.W. (1989). Murine natural killer cell interactions with a fungal target, *Cryptococcus neoformans*. *Infect. Immun.* 57: 1990–1997.

Hidore, M.R., Nabavi, N., Reynolds, C.W., Henkart, P.A., and Murphy, J.W. (1990). Cytoplasmic components of natural killer cells limit the growth of *Cryptococcus neoformans*. *J. Leukoc. Biol.* 48: 15–26.

Hidore, M.R., Mislan, T.W., and Murphy, J.W. (1991a). Responses of murine natural killer cells to binding of the fungal target *Cryptococcus neoformans*. *Infect. Immun.* 59: 1489–1499.

Hidore, M.R., Nabavi, N., Sonleitner, F., and Murphy, J.W. (1991b). Murine natural killer cells are fungicidal to *Cryptococcus neoformans*. *Infect. Immun.* 59: 1747–1754.

Hill, J.O. and Harmsen, A.G. (1991). Intrapulmonary growth and dissemination of an avirulent strain of *Cryptococcus neoformans* in mice depleted of $CD4^+$ or $CD8^+$ T cells. *J. Exp. Med.* 173: 755–758.

Hirsch, C.S., Ellner, J.J., Blinkhorn, R., and Toossi, Z. (1997). In vitro restoration of T cell responses in tuberculosis and augmentation of monocyte effector function against *Mycobacterium tuberculosis* by natural inhibitors of transforming growth factor beta. *Proc. Natl. Acad. Sci. USA* 94: 3926–3931.

Hisaeda, H., Nagasawa, H., Maeda, K., Maekawa, Y., Ishikawa, H., Ito, Y., Good, R.A., and Himeno, K. (1995). Gamma delta T cells play an important role in hsp65 expression and in acquiring protective immune responses against infection with *Toxoplasma gondii*. *J. Immunol.* 155: 244–251.

Holoshitz, J., Vila, L.M., Keroack, B.J., McKinley, D.R., and Bayne, N.K. (1992). Dual antigenic recognition by cloned human gamma delta T cells. *J. Clin. Invest.* 89: 308–314.

Horwitz, D.A., Gray, J.D., and Ohtsuka, K. (1999). Role of NK cells and TGF-beta in the regulation of T-cell-dependent antibody production in health and autoimmune disease. *Microbes Infect.* 1: 1305–1311.

Huffnagle, G.B., Yates, J.L., and Lipscomb, M.F. (1991). Immunity to a pulmonary *Cryptococcus neoformans* infection requires both CD4+ and CD8+ T cells. *J. Exp. Med.* 173: 793–800.

Huffnagle, G.B., Toews, G.B., Burdick, M.D., Boyd, M.B., McAllister, K.S., McDonald, R.A., Kunkel, S.L., and Strieter, R.M. (1996). Afferent phase production of TNF-alpha is required for the development of protective T cell immunity to *Cryptococcus neoformans*. *J. Immunol.* 157: 4529–4536.

Hyodo, Y., Matsui, K., Hayashi, N., Tsutsui, H., Kashiwamura, S., Yamauchi, H., Hiroishi, K., Takeda, K., Tagawa, Y., Iwakura, Y., Kayagaki, N., Kurimoto, M., Okamura, H., Hada, T., Yagita, H., Akira, S., Nakanishi, K., and Higashino, K. (1999). IL-18 up-regulates perforin-mediated NK activity without increasing perforin messenger RNA expression by binding to constitutively expressed IL-18 receptor. *J. Immunol.* 162: 1662–1668.

Ishigami, M., Nishimura, H., Naiki, Y., Yoshioka, K., Kawano, T., Tanaka, Y., Taniguchi, M., Kakumu, S., and Yoshikai, Y. (1999). The roles of intrahepatic Vα14+ NK1.1+ T cells for liver injury induced by *Salmonella* infection in mice. *Hepatology* 29: 1799–1808.

Ishikawa, H., Hisaeda, H., Taniguchi, M., Nakayama, T., Sakai, T., Maekawa, Y., Nakano, Y., Zhang, M., Zhang, T., Nishitani, M., Takashima, M., and Himeno, K. (2000). CD4+ Vα14 NKT cells play a crucial role in an early stage of protective immunity against infection with *Leishmania major*. *Int. Immunol.* 12: 1267–1274.

Kagi, D., Ledermann, B., Burki, K., Zinkernagel, R.M., and Hengartner, H. (1996). Molecular mechanisms of lymphocyte-mediated cytotoxicity and their role in immunological protection and pathogenesis in vivo. *Ann. Rev. Immunol.* 14: 207–232.

Kawakami, K., Tohyama, M., Teruya, K., Kudeken, N., Xie, Q., and Saito, A. (1996). Contribution of interferon-gamma in protecting mice during pulmonary and disseminated infection with *Cryptococcus neoformans*. *FEMS Immunol. Med. Microbiol.* 13: 123–130.

Kawakami, K., Tohyama, M., Qifeng, X., and Saito, A. (1997). Expression of cytokines and inducible nitric oxide synthase mRNA in the lungs of mice infected with *Cryptococcus neoformans*: Effects of interleukin-12. *Infect. Immun.* 65: 1307–1312.

Kawakami, K., Shibuya, K., Qureshi, M.H., Zhang, T., Koguchi, Y., Tohyama, M., Xie, Q., Naoe, S., and Saito, A. (1999). Chemokine responses and accumulation of inflammatory cells in the lungs of mice infected with highly virulent *Cryptococcus neoformans*: effects of interleukin-12. *FEMS Immunol. Med. Microbiol.* 25: 391–402.

Kawakami, K., Koguchi, Y., Qureshi, M.H., Miyazato, A., Yara, S., Kinjo, Y., Iwakura, Y., Takeda, K., Akira, S., Kurimoto, M., and Saito, A. (2000a). IL-18 contributes to host resistance against infection with *Cryptococcus neoformans* in mice with defective IL-12 synthesis through induction of IFN-gamma production by NK cells. *J. Immunol.* 165: 941–947.

Kawakami, K., Koguchi, Y., Qureshi, M.H., Yara, S., Kinjo, Y., Uezu, K., and Saito, A. (2000b). NK cells eliminate *Cryptococcus neoformans* by potentiating the fungicidal activity of macrophages rather than by directly killing them upon stimulation with IL-12 and IL-18. *Microbiol. Immunol.* 44: 1043–1050.

Kawakami, K., Kinjo, Y., Uezu, K., Yara, S., Miyagi, K., Koguchi, Y., Nakayama, T., Taniguchi, M., and Saito, A. (2001a). Monocyte chemoattractant protein-1-dependent increase of Valpha 14 NKT cells in lungs and their roles in Th1 response and host defense in cryptococcal infection. *J. Immunol.* 167: 6525–6532.

Kawakami, K., Kinjo, Y., Yara, S., Koguchi, Y., Uezu, K., Nakayama, T., Taniguchi, M., and Saito, A. (2001b). Activation of Valpha14(+) natural killer T cells by alpha-galactosylceramide results in development of Th1 response and local host resistance in mice infected with *Cryptococcus neoformans*. *Infect. Immun.* 69: 213–220.

Kawakami, K., Kinjo, Y., Yara, S., Uezu, K., Koguchi, Y., Tohyama, M., Azuma, M., Takeda, K., Akira, S., and Saito, A. (2001c). Enhanced gamma interferon production through activation of Valpha14(+) natural killer T cells by alpha-galactosylceramide in interleukin-18-deficient mice with systemic cryptococcosis. *Infect. Immun.* 69: 6643–6650.

Kawakami, K., Yamamoto, N., Kinjo, Y., Miyagi, K., Nakasone, C., Uezu, K., Kinjo, T., Nakayama, T., Taniguchi, M., and Saito, A. (2003). Critical role of Valpha14+ natural killer T cells in the innate phase of host protection against *Streptococcus pneumoniae* infection. *Eur. J. Immunol.* 33: 3322–3330.

Kawano, T., Cui, J., Koezuka, Y., Toura, I., Kaneko, Y., Motoki, K., Ueno, H., Nakagawa, R., Sato, H., Kondo, E., Koseki, H., and Taniguchi, M. (1997).

CD1d-restricted and TCR-mediated activation of Vα14 NKT cells by glycosylceramides. *Science* 278: 1626–1629.

Koguchi, Y. and Kawakami, K. (2002). Cryptococcal infection and Th1–Th2 cytokine balance. *Int. Rev. Immunol.* 21: 423–438.

Kozel, T.R., Wilson, M.A., Pfrommer, G.S., and Schlageter, A.M. (1989). Activation and binding of opsonic fragments of C3 on encapsulated *Cryptococcus neoformans* by using an alternative complement pathway reconstituted from six isolated proteins. *Infect. Immun.* 57: 1922–1927.

Kozel, T.R., Wilson, M.A., and Murphy, J.W. (1991). Early events in initiation of alternative complement pathway activation by the capsule of *Cryptococcus neoformans*. *Infect. Immun.* 59: 3101–3110.

Kumar, H., Belperron, A., Barthold, S.W., and Bockenstedt, L.K. (2000). CD1d deficiency impairs murine host defense against the spirochete, *Borrelia burgdorferi*. *J. Immunol.* 165: 4797–4801.

Lahn, M. (2000). The role of gamma/delta T cells in the airways. *J. Mol. Med.* 78: 409–425.

Laskay, T., Rolinghoff, M., and Solbach, W. (1993). Natural killer cells participate in the early defense against *Leishmania major* infection in mice. *Eur. J. Immunol.* 23: 2237–2241.

Lee, S.C., Dickson, D.W., and Casadevall, A. (1996). Pathology of cryptococcal meningoencephalitis: Analysis of 27 patients with pathogenetic implications. *Hum. Pathol.* 27: 839–847.

Lehrer, R.I., Lichtenstein, A.K., and Ganz, T. (1993). Defensins: Antimicrobial and cytotoxic peptides of mammalian cells. *Annu. Rev. Immunol.* 11: 105–128.

Lehuen, A., Lantz, O., Beaudoin, L., Laloux, V., Carnaud, C., Bendelac, A., Bach, J.F., and Monteiro, R.C. (1998). Overexpression of natural killer T cells protects Valpha14-Jalpha281 transgenic nonobese diabetic mice against diabetes. *J. Exp. Med.* 188: 1831–1839.

Lemaitre, B., Nicolas, E., Michaut, L., Reichhart, J.M., and Hoffmann, J.A. (1996). The dorsoventral regulatory gene cassette spatzle/Toll/cactus controls the potent antifungal response in *Drosophila* adults. *Cell* 86: 973–983.

Letterio, J.J. and Roberts, A.B. (1998). Regulation of immune responses by TGF-beta. *Annu. Rev. Immunol.* 16: 137–161.

Levitz, S.M. and Tabuni, A. (1991). Binding of *Cryptococcus neoformans* by human cultured macrophages. Requirements for multiple complement receptors and actin. *J. Clin. Invest.* 87: 528–535.

Li, R.K. and Mitchell, T.G. (1997). Induction of interleukin-6 mRNA in rat alveolar macrophages by in vitro exposure to both *Cryptococcus neoformans* and anti-*C. neoformans* antiserum. *J. Med. Vet. Mycol.* 35: 327–334.

Li, J., Hunter, C.A., and Farrell, J.P. (1999). Anti-TGF-beta treatment promotes rapid healing of *Leishmania major* infection in mice by enhancing in vivo nitric oxide production. *J. Immunol.* 162: 974–979.

Lim, T.S. and Murphy, J.W. (1980). Transfer of immunity to cryptococcosis by T-enriched splenic lymphocytes from *Cryptococcus neoformans*-sensitized mice. *Infect. Immun.* 30: 5–11.

Lipscomb, M.F., Alvarellos, T., Toews, G.B., Tompkins, R., Evans, Z., Koo, G., and Kumar, V. (1987). Role of natural killer cells in resistance to *Cryptococcus neoformans* infections in mice. *Am. J. Pathol.* 128: 354–361.

Lipscomb, M.F., Alvarellos, T., Toews, G.B., Tompkins, R., Evans, Z., Koo, G., and Kumar, V. (1991). Role of natural killer cells in resistance to *Cryptococcus neoformans* infections in mice. *Am. J. Pathol.* 128: 354–361.

Loetscher, P., Seitz, M., Clark-Lewis, I., Baggiolini, M., and Moser, B. (1996). Activation of NK cells by CC chemokines. Chemotaxis, Ca^{2+} mobilization, and enzyme release. *J. Immunol.* 156: 322–327.

Lovchik, J.A. and Lipscomb, M.F. (1993). Role for C5 and neutrophils in the pulmonary intravascular clearance of circulating *Cryptococcus neoformans*. *Am. J. Respir. Cell. Mol. Biol.* 9: 617–627.

Maghazachi, A.A., Al-Aoukaty, A., and Schall, T.J. (1994). C–C chemokine induce the chemotaxis of NK and IL-2-activated NK cells. Role for G-proteins. *J. Immunol.* 153: 4969–4977.

Maghazachi, A.A., Skalhegg, B.S., Rolstad, B., and Al-Aoukaty, A. (1997). Interferon-inducible protei-10 and lymphotactin induce the chemotaxis and mobilization of intracellular calcium in natural killer cells through pertussis toxin-sensitive and -insensitive heterotrimeric G-proteins. *FASEB J.* 11: 765–774.

Mannoor, M.K., Weerasinfhe, A., Halder, R.C., Reza, S., Morshed, M., Ariyasinghe, A., Watanabe, H., Sekikawa, H., and Abo, T. (2001). Resistance to malarial infection is achieved by the cooperation of $NK1.1^+$ and $NK1.1^-$ subsets of intermediate TCR cells which are constituents of innate immunity. *Cell. Immunol.* 211: 96–104.

McCormack, F.X. and Whitsett, J.A. (2002). The pulmonary collectins, SP-A and SP-D, orchestrate innate immunity in the lung. *J. Clin. Invest.* 109: 707–712.

Mednick, A.J., Feldmesser, M., Rivera, J., and Casadevall, A. (2003). Neutropenia alters lung cytokine production in mice and reduces their susceptibility to pulmonary cryptococcosis. *Eur. J. Immunol.* 33: 1744–1753.

Miller, M.F. and Mitchell, T.G. (1991). Killing of *Cryptococcus neoformans* strains by human neutrophils and monocytes. *Infect. Immun.* 59: 24–28.

Mitchell, T.G. and Friedman, L. (1972). In vitro phagocytosis and intracellular fate of variously encapsulated strains of *Cryptococcus neoformans*. *Infect. Immun.* 5: 491–498.

Mody, C.H., Lipscomb, M.F., Street, N.E., and Toews, G.B. (1990). Depletion of $CD4^+$ ($L3T4^+$) lymphocytes in vivo impairs murine host defense to *Cryptococcus neoformans*. *J. Immunol.* 144: 1472–1477.

Monga, D.P. (1981). Role of macrophages in resistance of mice to experimental cryptococcosis. *Infect. Immun.* 32: 975–978.

Moser, M. and Murphy, K.M. (2000). Dendritic cell regulation of TH1–TH2 development. *Nat. Immunol.* 1: 199–205.

Murphy, J.W. and MacDaniel, D.O. (1982). In vitro reactivity of natural killer (NK) cells on *Cryptococcus neoformans*. *J. Immunol.* 128: 1577–1583.

Murphy, J.W., Hidore, M.R., and Nabavi, N. (1991). Binding interactions of murine natural killer cells with the fungal target *Cryptococcus neoformans*. *Infect. Immun.* 59: 1476–1488.

Murphy, J.W., Hidore, M.R., and Wong, S.C. (1993). Direct interactions of human lymphocytes with the yeast-like organism, *Cryptococcus neoformans*. *J. Clin. Invest.* 91: 1553–1566.

Nabavi, N. and Murphy, J.W. (1985). In vitro binding of natural killer cells to *Cryptococcus neoformans* targets. *Infect. Immun.* 50: 50–57.

Nagaeva, O., Jonsson, L., and Mincheva-Nilsson, L. (2002). Dominant IL-10 and TGF-beta mRNA expression in gamma delta T cells of human early pregnancy decidua suggests immunoregulatory potential. *Am. J. Reprod. Immunol.* 48: 9–17.

Nakano, Y., Hisaeda, H., Sakai, T., Zhang, M., Maekawa, Y., Zhang, T., and Himeno, K. (2001). Role of innate immune cells in protection against *Toxoplasma gondii* at inflamed site. *J. Med. Invest.* 48: 73–80.

Nishimura, T., Kitamura, H., Iwakabe, K., Yahata, T., Ohta, A., Sato, M., Takeda, K., Okumura, K., van Kaer, L., Kawano, T., Taniguchi, M., Nakui, M., Sekimoto, M., and Koda, T. (2000). The interface between innate and acquired immunity: Glycolipid antigen presentation by CD1d-expressing dendritic cells to NKT cells induces the differentiation of antigen-specific cytotoxic T lymphocytes. *Int. Immunol.* 12: 987–994.

O'Brien, R.L., Happ, M.P., Dallas, A., Palmer, E., Kubo, R., and Born, W.K. (1989). Stimulation of a major subset of lymphocytes expressing T cell receptor gamma delta by an antigen derived from *Mycobacterium tuberculosis*. *Cell* 57: 667–674.

O'Brien, R.L., Fu, Y.X., Cranfill, R., Dallas, A., Ellis, C., Reardon, C., Lang, J., Carding, S.R., Kubo, R., and Born, W. (1992). Heat shock protein Hsp60-reactive gamma delta cells: A large, diversified T-lymphocyte subset with highly focused specificity. *Proc. Natl. Acad. Sci. USA* 89: 4348–4352.

O'Brien, R.L., Yin, X., Huber, S.A., Ikuta, K., and Born, W.K. (2000). Depletion of a gamma delta T cell subset can increase host resistance to a bacterial infection. *J. Immunol.* 165: 6472–6479.

Okamura, H., Tsutsui, H., Komatsu, T., Yutsudo, M., Hakura, A., Tanimoto, T., Torigoe, K., Okura, T., Nukada, Y., Hattori, K., Akita, K., Namba, M., Tanabe, F., Konishi, K., Fukuda, S., and Kurimoto, M. (1995). Cloning of a new cytokine that induces IFN-gamma production by T cells. *Nature* 378: 88–91.

Okamura, H., Tsutsui, H., Kashiwamura, S., Yoshimoto, T., and Nakanishi, K. (1998). Interleukin-18: A novel cytokine that augments both innate and acquired immunity. *Adv. Immunol.* 70: 281–312.

Oshikawa, K. and Sugiyama, Y. (2003). Gene expression of Toll-like receptors and associated molecules induced by inflammatory stimuli in the primary alveolar macrophage. *Biochem. Biophys. Res. Commun.* 305: 649–655.

Pabst, R. (1992). Is BALT a major component of the human lung immune system? *Immunol. Today* 13: 119–122.

Pedrosa, J., Saunders, B.M., Appelberg, R., Orme, I.M., Silva, M.T., and Cooper, A.M. (2000). Neutrophils play a protective nonphagocytic role in systemic *Mycobacterium tuberculosis* infection of mice. *Infect. Immun.* 68: 577–583.

Perfect, J.R., Lang, S.D., and Durack, D.T. (1980). Chronic cryptococcal meningitis: A new experimental model in rabbits. *Am. J. Pathol.* 101: 177–194.

Powell, K.E., Dahl, B.A., Weeks, R.J., and Tosh, F.E. (1972). Airborne *Cryptococcus neoformans*:

Particles from pigeon excreta compatible with alveolar deposition. *J. Infect. Dis.* 125: 412–415.

Qureshi, M.H., Zhang, T., Koguchi, Y., Nakashima, K., Okamura, H., Kurimoto, M., and Kawakami, K. (1999). Combined effects of IL-12 and IL-18 on the clinical course and local cytokine production in murine pulmonary infection with *Cryptococcus neoformans*. *Eur. J. Immunol.* 29: 643–649.

Reed, S.G. (1999). TGF-beta in infections and infectious diseases. *Microbes Infect.* 1: 1313–1325.

Rhodes, J.C. (1985). Contribution of complement component C5 to the pathogenesis of experimental murine cryptococcosis. *Sabouraudia* 23: 225–234.

Robinson, D., Shibuya, K., Mui, A., Zonin, F., Murphy, E., Sana, T., Hartley, S.B., Menon, S., Kastelein, R., Bazan, F., and O'Garra, A. (1997). IGIF does not drive Th1 development but synergizes with IL-12 for interferon-gamma production and activates IRAK and NFkappaB. *Immunity* 7: 571–581.

Rossi, D. and Zlotnik, A. (2000). The biology of chemokines and their receptors. *Annu. Rev. Immunol.* 217: 217–242.

Schaible, U.E. and Kaufmann, S.H. (2000). CD1 molecules and CD1-dependent T cells in bacterial infections: A link from innate to acquired immunity? *Semin. Immunol.* 12: 527–535.

Scharton, T.M. and Scott, P. (1993). Natural killer cells are a source of interferon gamma that drives differentiation of $CD4^+$ T cell subsets and induces early resistance to *Leishmania major* in mice. *J. Exp. Med.* 178: 567–577.

Schelenz, S., Malhotra, R., Sim, R.B., Holmskov, U., and Bancroft, G.J. (1995). Binding of host collectins to the pathogenic yeast *Cryptococcus neoformans*: human surfactant protein D acts as an agglutinin for acapsular yeast cells. *Infect. Immun.* 63: 3360–3366.

Shellito, J.E. and Kolls, J.K. (2003). Alveolar macrophage-mediated killing of *Pneumocystis carinii* f. sp. muris involves molecular recognition by the Dectin-1 beta-glucan receptor. *J. Exp. Med.* 198: 1677–1688.

Shohaml, S., Huang, C., Chen, J.M., Golenbock, D.T., and Levitz, S.M. (2001). Toll-like receptor 4 mediates intracellular signaling without TNF-alpha release in response to *Cryptococcus neoformans* polysaccharide capsule. *J. Immunol.* 166: 4620–4626.

Singh, N., Hong, S., Scherer, D.C., Serizawa, I., Burdin, N., Kronenberg, M., Koezuka, Y., and van Kaer, L. (1999). Activation of NK T cells by CD1d and α-galactosylceramide directs conventional T cells to the acquisition of a Th2 phenotype. *J. Immunol.* 163: 2373–2377.

Soilleux, E.J., Morris, L.S., Leslie, G., Chehimi, J., Luo, Q., Levroney, E., Trowsdale, J., Montaner, L.J., Doms, R.W., Weissman, D., Coleman, N., and Lee, B. (2002). Constitutive and induced expression of DC-SIGN on dendritic cell and macrophage subpopulations in situ and in vitro. *J. Leukoc. Biol.* 71: 445–457.

Steele, C., Marrero, L., Swain, S., Harmsen, A.G., Zheng, M., Brown, G.D., Gordon, S., Roeder, A., Kirschning, C.J., Rupec, R.A., Schaller, M., and Korting, H.C. (2004). Toll-like receptors and innate antifungal responses. *Trends Microbiol.* 12: 44–49.

Syme, R.M., Spurrell, J.C., Amankwah, E.K., Green, F.H., and Mody, C.H. (2002). Primary dendritic cells phagocytose *Cryptococcus neoformans* via mannose receptors and Fcgamma receptor II for presentation to T lymphocytes. *Infect. Immun.* 70: 5972–5981.

Szalay, G., Ladel, C.H., Blum, C., Brossay, L., Kronenberg, M., and Kaufmann, S.H.E. (1999). Anti-CD1 monoclonal antibody treatment reverses the production patterns of TGF-β2 and Th1 cytokines and ameliorates listeriosis in mice. *J. Immunol.* 162: 6955–6958.

Takeda, K., Kaisho, T., and Akira, S. (2003). Toll-like receptors. *Annu. Rev. Immunol.* 21: 335–376.

Tanaka, Y., Morita, C.T., Tanaka, Y., Nieves, E., Brenner, M.B., and Bloom, B.R. (1995). Natural and synthetic non-peptide antigens recognized by human gamma delta T cells. *Nature* 375: 155–158.

Tang, Y.Q., Yuan, J., Miller, C.J., and Selsted, M.E. (1999). Isolation, characterization, cDNA cloning, and antimicrobial properties of two distinct subfamilies of alpha-defensins from rhesus macaque leukocytes. *Infect. Immun.* 67: 6139–6144.

Taniguchi, M. and Nakayama, T. (2000). Recognition and function of Vα14NKT cells. *Semin. Immunol.* 12: 543–550.

Tateda, K., Moore, T.A., Deng, J.C., Newstead, M.W., Zeng, X., Matsukawa, A., Swanson, M.S., Yamaguchi, K., and Standiford, T.J. (2001). Early recruitment of neutrophils determines subsequent T1/T2 host responses in a murine model of *Legionella pneumophila* pneumonia. *J. Immunol.* 166: 3355–3361.

Taub, D.D., Sayers, T.J., Carter, C.R., and Ortaldo, J.R. (1995). Alpha and beta chemokines induce NK cell migration and enhance NK-mediated cytolysis. *J. Immunol.* 155: 3877–3888.

Taylor, P.R., Brown, G.D., Herre, J., Williams, D.L., Willment, J.A., and Gordon, S. (2004). The role of SIGNR1 and the beta-glucan receptor (Dectin-1) in the nonopsonic recognition of yeast by specific macrophages. *J. Immunol.* 172: 1157–1162.

Toura, I., Kawano, T., Akutsu, Y., Nakayama, T., Ochiai, T., and Taniguchi, M. (1999). Inhibition of experimental tumor metastasis by dendritic cells pulsed with α-galactosylceramide. *J. Immunol.* 163: 2387–2391.

Trinchieri, G. (1989). Biology of natural killer cells. *Adv. Immunol.* 47: 187–376.

Trinchieri, G. (1995). Interleukin-12: A proinflammatory cytokine with immunoregulatory functions that bridge innate resistance and antigen-specific adaptive immunity. *Annu. Rev. Immunol.* 13: 251–276.

Truelsen, K., Young, T., and Kozel, T.R. (1992). In vivo complement activation and binding of C3 to encapsulated *Cryptococcus neoformans*. *Infect. Immun.* 60: 3937–3939.

Uezu, K., Kawakami, K., Miyagi, K., Kinjo, Y., Kinjo, T., Ishikawa, H., and Saito, A. (2004). Accumulation of gamma-delta T cells in the lungs and their regulatory roles in Th1 response and host defense against pulmonary infection with *Cryptococcus neoformans*. *J. Immunol.* in press.

van de Wetering, J.K., Coenjaerts, F.E., Vaandrager, A.B., van Golde, L.M., and Batenburg, J.J. (2004). Aggregation of *Cryptococcus neoformans* by surfactant protein D is inhibited by its capsular component glucuronoxylomannan. *Infect. Immun.* 72: 145–153.

Vecchiarelli, A., Pietrella, D., Dottorini, M., Monari, C., Retini, C., Todisco, T., and Bistoni, F. (1994a). Encapsulation of *Cryptococcus neoformans* regulates fungicidal activity and the antigen presentation process in human alveolar macrophages. *Clin. Exp. Immunol.* 98: 217–223.

Vecchiarelli, A., Dottorini, M., Pietrella, D., Monari, C., Retini, C., Todisco, T., and Bistoni, F. (1994b). Role of human alveolar macrophages as antigen-presenting cells in *Cryptococcus neoformans* infection. *Am. J. Respir. Cell. Mol. Biol.* 11: 130–137.

Walenkamp, A.M., Verheul, A.F., Scharringa, J., and Hoepelman, I.M. (1999). Pulmonary surfactant protein A binds to *Cryptococcus neoformans* without promoting phagocytosis. *Eur. J. Clin. Invest.* 29: 83–92.

Wesch, D., Glatzel, A., and Kabelitz, D. (2001). Differentiation of resting human peripheral blood gamma delta T cells toward Th1- or Th2-phenotype. *Cell. Immunol.* 212: 110–117.

Wormley, F.L. Jr., Steele, C., Wozniak, K., Fujihashi, K., McGhee, J.R., and Fidel, P.L., Jr. (2001). Resistance of T-cell receptor delta-chain-deficient mice to experimental *Candida albicans* vaginitis. *Infect. Immun.* 69: 7162–7164.

Yang, D., Biragyn, A., Kwak, L.W., and Oppenheim, J.J. (2002). Mammalian defensins in immunity: More than just microbicidal. *Trends Immunol.* 23: 291–296.

Zaragoza, O., Taborda, C.P., and Casadevall, A. (2003). The efficacy of complement-mediated phagocytosis of *Cryptococcus neoformans* is dependent on the location of C3 in the polysaccharide capsule and involves both direct and indirect C3-mediated interactions. *Eur. J. Immunol.* 33: 1957–1967.

Zhang, T., Kawakami, K., Qureshi, M. H., Okamura, H., Kurimoto, M., and Saito, A. (1997). Interleukin (IL)-12 and IL-18 synergistically induce the fungicidal activity of murine peritoneal exudate cells against *Cryptococcus neoformans* through production of interferon-gamma by natural killer cells. *Infect. Immun.* 65: 3594–3599.

Zhang, P., Summer, W.R., Bagby, G.J., and Nelosn, S. (2000). Innte immunity and pulmonary host defense. *Immunol. Rev.* 173: 39–51.

8

Pulmonary Cell-Mediated Immunity (CMI) to *Cryptococcus neoformans*

Dennis M. Lindell and Gary B. Huffnagle

Division of Pulmonary and Critical Care Medicine, The University of Michigan Medical School, Ann Arbor, MI.
Department of Microbiology and Immunology, University of Michigan, Ann Arbor, MI.

1. Introduction

1.1. Overview

Cryptococcus neoformans is an encapsulated yeast that primarily affects individuals with depressed T cell function. Although the incidence of cryptococcosis has declined as treatment of human immunodeficiency virus (HIV) infection with antiretroviral drugs has become more widespread, *C. neoformans* infection remains a significant cause of morbidity and mortality in acquired immune deficiency syndrome (AIDS) patients and others undergoing T cell suppressive therapies. Current antimicrobial therapy of *C. neoformans* infection is often inadequate. In patients with AIDS, amphotericin B, or a combination of amphotericin B and flucytosine are the primary drugs of choice, followed by long-term azole therapy. Resistance of *C. neoformans* to flucytosine has developed rapidly, and resistance to azoles has been reported and is likely to increase (Yamazumi et al., 2003). Consequently, alternative strategies for the management of *C. neoformans* infection are being considered, including prophylactic vaccination or passive therapy with *C. neoformans*-specific monoclonal antibodies. The successful development of these and other strategies depends upon an understanding of the mechanisms by which immunity against *C. neoformans* is generated.

Although invasive and systemic fungal infections primarily affect immunocompromised patients, there is increasing evidence that chronic fungal colonization may be a significant cause of disease, particularly in atopic individuals. Chronic fungal colonization has been linked to nasal allergies, chronic sinusitis, nasal polyps, and asthma (Ricchetti et al., 2002; Venarske and deShazo, 2002). In genetically susceptible mice, *C. neoformans* infection results in a disease, which is akin to human allergic bronchopulmonary mycosis (ABPM). Thus, experimental *C. neoformans* infection provides insight into the mechanisms by which protective and nonprotective responses to pulmonary fungal infections are generated and maintained.

1.2. The Role of T Cells/CMI in *C. neoformans* Infection

Clinically, evidence for the importance of cell-mediated immunity (CMI), and $CD4^+$ T cells in particular, for host defense against *C. neoformans* infection comes from which patients are most susceptible to cryptococcosis. Patients undergoing T cell depressive immunosuppression as treatment for hematologic malignancies (Segal et al., 2002) or following transplant surgery, as well as at those with AIDS, are dramatically more susceptible to *C. neoformans* infection. Progression to AIDS is significantly associated with a loss of T cell response to whole *C. neoformans*, and this often occurs before a drop in absolute $CD4^+$ T cell count (Hoy et al., 1988).

The importance of CMI in controlling *C. neoformans* infection has been reinforced using animal models. Congenitally athymic nude mice (*nu/nu*), severely combined immunodeficient (SCID) mice, and mice depleted of $CD4^+$ and $CD8^+$ T cells (Table 8.1) are substantially more susceptible to *C. neoformans* infection (Salkowski and Balish, 1990; Huffnagle et al., 1991a,b, 1994). T cells are required for the recruitment and activation of monocytes and macrophages, the primary effector cells for clearance of the fungus. In the absence of T cells, the pulmonary inflammatory response to *C. neoformans* is dramatically delayed and contains a large proportion of neutrophils (Table 8.1) (Huffnagle et al., 1991a,b, 1994). Adoptive transfer of T cells, but not B cells, confers protection against subsequent pulmonary challenge (Lim and Murphy, 1980; Huffnagle et al., 1991b). Thus, T cell-mediated immunity plays a critical role in the pulmonary leukocyte recruitment required to clear *C. neoformans* from the lungs.

T cells are required for: (1) recruitment of inflammatory cells, primarily monocytes, and macrophages; (2) activation of macrophages, and (3) support of antibody-mediated immunity (AMI). The type 1 cell-mediated immunity (T1) versus type 2 cell-mediated immunity (T2) nature of the lung environment dictates whether clearance or chronic infection will prevail.

2. Innate Determinants of Acquired Immunity

The innate immune response to *C. neoformans* plays a critical role in the establishment of acquired immunity. *C. neoformans* is acquired via the respiratory tract and establishes primary infection in the lungs. The resident phagocytic cells of the lungs, alveolar macrophages and dendritic cells, likely serve as antigen-presenting cells (APCs). These cells bind, internalize, process, and present fungal-derived antigens to T cells in the lung-associated lymph nodes (LALN). In addition to the roles of phagocytosis and antigen presentation, resident phagocytic cells of the innate immune system are responsible for the early production of proinflammatory mediators such as tumor necrosis factor alpha (TNF-α), IL-12, and IL-18. Phagocytes cooperate with natural killer (NK) cells, natural killer T (NKT) cells, and gamma delta T cell ($\gamma\delta$ T cell) to provide the

Table 8.1. Characteristics of T Cell-independent, T1, and T2-type Pulmonary Immune Responses to *C. neoformans*

	T cell-independent	T1	T2
Mouse strains	Athymic (nu/nu) mice, SCID, T cell depleted	CBA, Balb/C	C57/Bl6
Leukocyte recruitment	Delayed—largely neutrophils	Mono/mac, lymph	Mono/mac, lymph, eos
DTH	No	Yes	No
Early TNF, IL-12	Yes	Yes	No
IFN-γ	?	Yes	No
IL-4, IL-5, IL-10	?	No	Yes
Serum IgE	No	No	Yes
Eosinophilia/crystal deposition	No	No	Yes
Clearance	No	Yes	No
Dissemination to CNS	Universal	Uncommon	Common
Nature of infection	Progressive	Controlled	Chronic

early proinflammatory and chemotactic signals required for the establishment of CMI.

2.1. Phagocyte Recognition of *C. neoformans* via PRRs

The first step in the innate immune response to *C. neoformans* is recognition of the pathogen by phagocytes. Recognition and uptake of microbes occurs via Fc receptors, complement receptors (CR), or pattern recognition receptors (PRRs) such as mannose receptors (MR) and the toll-like receptor (TLR) family. *C. neoformans* can be taken up and presented by primary human dendritic cells, which is dependent on the presence of both MR and fragment crystallizable gamma receptor 2 (FcγR2) (Syme et al., 2002). T cell responses to *C. neoformans* mannoprotein (CnMP) are dependent upon the expression of MR by phagocytes (Mansour et al., 2002). Thus, recognition of *C. neoformans* occurs via MR, as well as possibly by other PRRs (Fig. 8.1).

2.2. Early Signal Generation: The Importance of Proinflammatory T1 Driving Cytokines

The recognition and internalization of microbes results in the production of

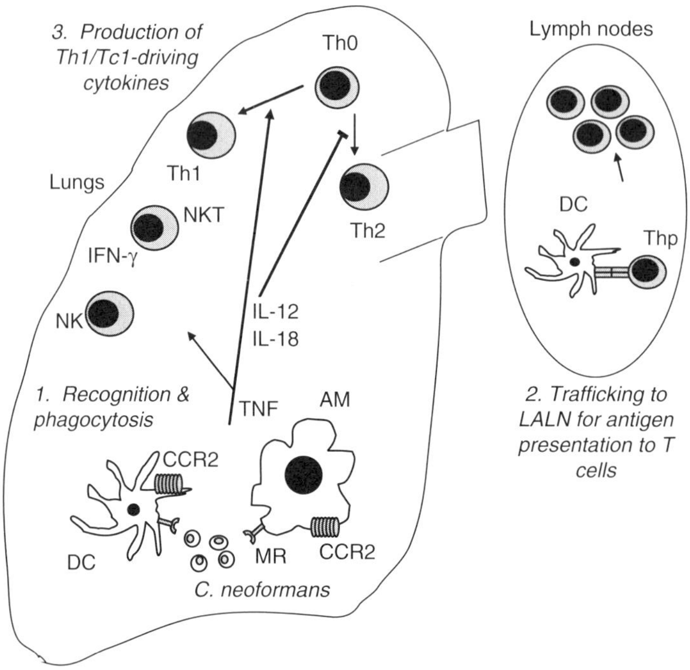

Figure 8.1. The protective innate immune response to pulmonary *C. neoformans* infection. Initial steps in the innate immune response to *C. neoformans* are the recognition and phagocytosis of the pathogen by alveolar macrophages (AM) and dendritic cells (DC), which occurs via mannose (MR) and other pattern recognition receptors (PRRs). This results in the early induction of proinflammatory mediators including TNF-α and IL-12. Subsequently, antigen-presenting cells traffic to the lung-associated lymph nodes (LALN), where they interact with antigen-specific T cells. T cells then traffic back to the lungs where their activation and polarization are affected directly and indirectly by inflammatory signals from the innate immune system such as IL-12, IL-18, and IFN-γ.

proinflammatory mediators including TNF-α, IL-12, and IL-18. The establishment of an inflammatory state induces the production of chemokines, including CCL2 monocyte chemotactic protein (MCP-1), CCL3 macrophage inflammatory protein 1 alpha (MIP1-α), and the expression of adhesion molecules on the vascular endothelium, which together coordinate the recruitment and extravasation of leukocytes.

Exposure of phagocytic cells to CnMP results in the production of proinflammatory mediators. Human monocytes cultured with CnMP produce significant amounts of IL-12 (Pitzurra et al., 2000). Activated T cells augment IL-12 production by monocytes in response to stimulation with *C. neoformans*, suggesting a positive feedback loop between monocyte/macrophages and infiltrating T cells (Retini et al., 1999).

2.2.1. TNF-α

The early induction of TNF-α is critical for the generation of T1 immunity to *C. neoformans*. TNF-α is induced in the lungs of resistant mice as early at day 2 postinfection (Herring et al., 2002). The early induction of TNF-α is critical, as a single dose of TNF-α neutralizing antibody, given at the time of pulmonary *C. neoformans* infection, prevents the development of protective CMI (Huffnagle et al., 1996). Mice given a single dose of TNF-α neutralizing antibody cannot generate *C. neoformans*-specific delayed-type hypersensitivity (DTH) responses or control growth of the fungus (Huffnagle et al., 1996). Furthermore, neutralization of TNF-α at the time of infection prevents the induction of IL-12 and interferon gamma (IFN-γ), demonstrating that TNF-α is induced proximally to, and required for, the production of IL-12 and IFN-γ. TNF-α depletion is sufficient to induce a switch from the protective T helper type 1 (Th1) response to a nonprotective T helper type 2 (Th2) phenotype (Herring et al., 2002) and increases early dissemination to the central nervous system (CNS) (Aguirre et al., 1995). One mechanism by which afferent TNF-α may act during *C. neoformans* infection is via dendritic cells. TNF-α has well-documented roles in promoting the activation, maturation, and migration of dendritic cells (Steinman, 1996). During immunization with *C. neoformans* filtrate (CneF) antigen, which generates protection against subsequent *C. neoformans* infection, neutralization of TNF-α inhibits the accumulation of Langerhans cells, myeloid, and lymphoid dendritic cells in the draining lymph nodes (Bauman et al., 2003). Thus, afferent induction of TNF-α plays a critical role in the establishment of protective Th1 immunity to *C. neoformans* possibly via the maturation and trafficking of dendritic cells (Fig. 8.1).

2.2.2. IL-12 and IL-18

Early production of IL-12 is critical to the development of Th1 immunity to *C. neoformans*. IL-12 is induced early during *C. neoformans* infection in mice (Herring et al., 2002). Similar to TNF-α neutralization, administration of anti-IL-12 neutralizing antibodies inhibits pulmonary clearance of *C. neoformans* in mice, resulting in a shift to a nonprotective Th2 immune response (Hoag et al., 1997). Additionally, mice genetically deficient in either of the heterodimeric portions of IL-12 (p35 and p40) exhibit impaired IFN-γ induction and Th2 polarization in response to *C. neoformans* infection (Decken et al., 1998). Conversely, exogenous administration of IL-12 early during pulmonary infection enhances fungal clearance and increases survival following pulmonary infection (Kawakami et al., 1996b). This occurs via the increased expression and/or production of T1 mediators, including IFN-γ, TNF-α, IL-18, as well as inducible nitric oxide synthase (iNOS).

Compared to wild-type controls, IL-18 deficient (IL-18 –/–) mice have impaired lung clearance associated with lower levels of IL-12 and IFN-γ, which is reversible upon administration of exogenous IL-18 (Kawakami et al., 2000). A number of studies have demonstrated the effectiveness of the combination of IL-12 and IL-18 at inducing IFN-γ production by T cells (Okamura et al., 1995, 1998; Micallef et al., 1996). Exogenous administration of IL-12 and IL-18 is protective against *C. neoformans* in vitro (Zhang et al., 1997) and in vivo (Kawakami et al., 1997; Qureshi et al., 1999). Thus, IL-12 and IL-18 play cooperative roles in driving Th1-mediated immunity to *C. neoformans*, both by promoting IFN-γ production (Fig. 8.1).

2.2.3. NKT Cells

A role for NKT cells on the subsequent development of Th1 responses to *C. neoformans* has been reported. The numbers of NKT cells increase in the lungs as early as day 3 postinfection. DTH responses, the differentiation of fungus-specific Th1 cells, and clearance are all impaired in variable alpha 14 positive natural killer T cell (Vα14 NKT) deficient mice, suggesting that NKT cells contribute positively to the development of T1 immunity to *C. neoformans* (Kawakami et al., 2001a). Treatment of infected mice with alpha-galactosylceramide (which stimulates NKT cells) leads to increased IFN-γ induction and enhanced clearance of mice infected intravenously with *C. neoformans* (Kawakami et al., 2001b). These results demonstrate that NKT cells may play an important supportive role in the early establishment of T1 immunity to *C. neoformans*.

2.2.4. Polymorphonuclear Neutrophil Leukocytes (PMNs)

Although neutrophils have been recognized to be a constituent of the pulmonary leukocyte infiltrate which occurs during pulmonary *C. neoformans* infection, a potential role for neutrophils in establishing CMI was only recently reported. Surprisingly, depletion of neutrophils increases the survival of mice infected intratracheally, but not intravenously with a moderately virulent strain of *C. neoformans*. Neutropenic mice have increased early lung clearance of the fungus (day 1 postinfection) and an enhancement in lung T1 and T2 cytokine profiles at week 1 postinfection (Mednick et al., 2003). Thus, neutrophils recruited to the lungs during *C. neoformans* infection play an adverse, rather than beneficial role in the development of CMI.

2.2.5. Costimulation

The role of costimulatory molecules in the induction of T cell responses has also been investigated. Human monocytes cultured with acapsular, but not encapsulated *C. neoformans* upregulate CD80 and CD86. The ability of monocytes to increase CD80 in response to encapsulated *C. neoformans* is restored by the addition of opsonic anticapsular antibody (Vecchiarelli et al., 1998). Blockade of the B7/CD28 pathway in vitro using anti-B7.1 (CD80) and anti-B7.2 (CD86) blocking antibodies results in impaired T cell proliferative responses. Thus, as would likely be expected in antigen-specific responses, blockade of the B7/CD28 pathway impairs T cell proliferative responses in vitro. The role of these molecules during infection in vivo has not been reported.

The role of cytotoxic T lymphocyte antigen-4 (CTLA-4) in *C. neoformans* infection has also been studied. CTLA-4 (CD152), which binds CD80 and CD86 on APCs, is expressed on activated T cells, and acts as a negative regulator of T cell function (Walunas et al., 1994). CTLA-4 blockade during immunization with CneF enhances DTH reactions and protection afforded by immunization with CneF (McGaha and Murphy, 2000). The induction of CTLA-4 on T cells may be an indirect mechanism of T cell suppression by *C. neoformans* as CTLA-4 is upregulated following exposure of $CD4^+$ T cells to encapsulated *C. neoformans* in the presence of accessory cells (Pietrella et al., 2001).

2.2.6. Chemokines

Chemokines are small chemoattractant molecules, which stimulate the activation and the chemotaxis of leukocytes. A variety of chemokines are produced during *C. neoformans* infection and are involved in both leukocyte trafficking and polarization of the cell-mediated immune response (Traynor and Huffnagle, 2001).

2.2.6.1. CCL2 (MCP-1)/CCR2 The chemokine receptor/ligand pair CCR2/MCP-1 plays a critical role in both afferent and efferent phases of development of CMI to *C. neoformans*. MCP-1 (CCL2) is induced in the lungs early during pulmonary *C. neoformans* infection (Traynor et al., 2000). Neutralization of MCP-1 via antibodies leads to a marked impairment in the recruitment of macrophages (95%) and $CD4^+$ T cells (76% ± 9%) at day 15 postinfection, accompanied by a decrease in cryptococcal clearance (Huffnagle et al., 1995a). $CCR2^{-/-}$ mice develop a chronic T2 response to pulmonary *C. neoformans* infection, characterized by IL-4, IL-5, eosinophilia, and tissue destruction. Neutralization of MCP-1/CCL2 during the afferent phase of the response mirrors some, but not all of the defects observed in CCR2 deficiency, suggesting that CCR2 plays a role in the development of CMI to *C. neoformans*, which is not strictly via MCP-1 (Traynor et al., 2002). In addition to the role played in polarization of CMI and lung leukocyte trafficking (discussed below), CCR2 also plays a role in trafficking of dendritic cells to the draining lymph nodes. Compared to wild-type mice, $CCR2^{-/-}$ have fewer $MHCII^+$ $CD11c^+$ cells in the lung-draining lymph nodes following pulmonary *C. neoformans* infection. Thus, CCL2 plays a critical role in chemotaxis, but CCR2 has CCL2-independent functions, which extend to innate immunity.

2.2.6.2. CCL3 (MIP1-α)/CCR5 CCR5 clearly plays a role in survival of *C. neoformans* infection and protection of the CNS against dissemination of the organism (Huffnagle et al., 1999). Pulmonary lymphocyte and leukocyte recruitment during *C. neoformans* infection, however, is not deficient in CCR5-deficient mice (Huffnagle et al., 1999). One of the ligands of CCR5, MIP1-α (CCL3) plays a role in both afferent and efferent phases of the host response to pulmonary *C. neoformans* infection. Blockade of CCL3 during the efferent phase (d7–13) of *C. neoformans* infection via neutralizing antibodies results in decreased pulmonary monocyte/macrophage and neutrophil recruitment and increased pulmonary fungal burden. This occurs, however, without a decrease in the numbers of $CD4^+$, $CD8^+$, or $B220^+$ lymphocytes, suggesting that CCL3 does not play a role in recruitment of T or B cells (Huffnagle et al., 1997). CCL3 plays a role in the afferent phase of the response, as well. Genetic CCL3 deficiency (in CCL3 knockout (KO) mice) favors the development of a nonprotective T2 response, resulting in enhanced eosinophilia and enhanced lung fungal burden (Olszewski et al., 2000, 2001).

Thus, in addition to the expected function chemokines play as chemoattractants in leukocyte trafficking to the lungs, they also serve critical roles in determining the T1 versus T2 nature of CMI to *C. neoformans*.

Taken together, these studies demonstrate that, although the innate immune response to *C. neoformans* is insufficient for clearance of the fungus, innate immune cells play critical roles in the recognition, early containment, and early signal generation required for the establishment of protective T1 cell-mediated immunity.

3. Antigen-specific (and Mitogenic) T Cell Responses

Both $CD4^+$ and $CD8^+$ T cell responses are generated in response to *C. neoformans*. This is due to the nature of the pathogen, which survives and replicates both extra- and intracellularly. T cell responses to cryptococcal mannoproteins (which are both constituents of the *C. neoformans* cell wall, as well as secreted) are associated with protection. A number of specific mannoproteins from *C. neoformans*, which induce CD4$^+$ T cell responses, have recently been characterized and cloned. These bear sequence homology to other known polysaccharide acetylase/deacetylases. Additionally, *C. neoformans* possesses mitogen activity, which can stimulate both CD4$^+$ and CD8$^+$ T cells, in a non-major histocompatibility complex (MHC) restricted manner, which may confound antigen-specific T cell responses. Other recent studies point to cross-reactivity between T cell responses to *C. neoformans* and other pathogenic fungi.

3.1. CD4$^+$ and CD8$^+$ T Cells are each Important for the Control of *C. neoformans* Infection

Experimental *C. neoformans* infection in mice generates both CD4$^+$ and CD8$^+$ T cell responses, although the pulmonary CD4$^+$ T cell response is more vigorous. In studies using human T cells, both CD4$^+$ and CD8$^+$ T cell responses are generated to *C. neoformans* (Syme et al., 1997). During pulmonary infection, CD4$^+$ T cell deficiency results in dramatically impaired fungal clearance from the lungs, increased dissemination to the CNS, and increased lethality. In the absence of CD4$^+$ T cells, mice are markedly impaired in the ability to recruit and activate monocytes and macrophages (Mody et al., 1990; Hill and Harmsen, 1991; Huffnagle et al., 1991a,b, 1994). Depletion of CD8$^+$ T cells during infection also impairs immunity, but the effect is dependent upon the virulence of the strain of *C. neoformans*. CD8$^+$ T cell depleted mice infected with a moderately virulent strain of *C. neoformans* have impaired pulmonary clear-
AQ1 ance and DTH responses (Mody et al., 1993a,b). In contrast, depletion of CD8$^+$ T cells during a highly virulent infection leads to enhanced lethality, but without altering pulmonary clearance (Mody et al., 1994). Thus, CD8$^+$ and CD4$^+$ T cells have complementary roles in the cell-mediated immune response to *C. neoformans*, and both populations mediate protection.

Animals deficient in both CD4$^+$ and CD8$^+$ T cells are even more susceptible to pulmonary *C. neoformans* infection than animals deficient in CD4$^+$ T cells alone, demonstrating that CD8$^+$ T cells mediate protection in the absence of CD4$^+$ T cells (Huffnagle et al., 1991a,b, 1994; Lindell et al., 2005b). In a number of circumstances, CD4$^+$ T cells are required for optimal CD8$^+$ T cell responses (Bennett et al., 1998; Schoenberger et al., 1998; Shedlock and Shen, 2003). Compared to CD8$^+$ T cells in CD4$^+$ T cell-sufficient mice, CD8$^+$ T cells in CD4$^+$ T cell-deficient mice expand, become activated, and traffic to the lungs (Lindell et al., 2005b). IFN-γ-producing effector CD8$^+$ T cells are present in greater numbers in *C. neoformans*-infected CD4$^+$ T cell-deficient mice relative to CD4$^+$ sufficient controls. Depletion of CD8$^+$ T cells from CD4$^+$ deficient mice or neutralization of IFN-γ in these mice results in dramatically increased pulmonary fungal load (Lindell et al., 2005b). Thus, in the absence of CD4$^+$ T cells, CD8$^+$ T cells mediate a substantial degree of protection against *C. neoformans* infection by an IFN-γ-dependent mechanism. These results suggest that CD8$^+$ T cells play a protective role against *C. neoformans* during CD4$^+$ T cell deficiency, and protection may be enhanced by augmenting the CD8$^+$ T cell response. Along these lines, successful vaccine-induced CD8$^+$ T cell-mediated immunity in CD4$^+$ T cell-deficient mice to two other pathogenic fungi (*Histoplasma capsulatum* and *Blastomyces dermatitidis*) has been demonstrated (Wuthrich et al., 2003).

3.2. The Antigen-specific T Cell Response

In culture, *C. neoformans* produces a variety of secreted products, which are shed into the culture medium. These include components of the cell wall and capsule, composed of mannoproteins (MP), glucuronoxylomannan (GXM), and galactoxylomannan (GalXM). In contrast to GXM and GalXM, which are largely regarded as having immunosuppressive effects, components of cryptococcal mannoprotein have generally been recognized as an immunopotentiating agent in the cell-mediated immune response to *C. neoformans*. Concentrated CneF antigen, which is rich in cryptococcal mannoprotein, has been used to test the ability of infected or immunized mice to mount a *C. neoformans*-specific DTH response (Murphy and Pahlavan, 1979). Immunization of mice with CneF leads to protection against subsequent *C. neoformans* challenge (Murphy et al., 1998). Additionally, peripheral T cells from patients who have recovered from *C. neoformans* infection, but not controls, exhibit proliferative responses to CneF (Hoy et al., 1989).

The role of *C. neoformans* cell-associated proteins in the protective T cell response is unclear. T cells from patients who have recovered from *C. neoformans* infection proliferate more rapidly than control T cells and produce IL-2 in response to stimulation with whole-killed *C. neoformans* (Miller and Puck, 1984). Both $CD4^+$ and $CD8^+$ T cells from mice that have resolved pulmonary *C. neoformans* infection proliferate in response to whole-killed *C. neoformans*, but immunization of mice with whole heat-killed cryptococci is nonprotective (Murphy et al., 1998).

The specific antigens within cryptococcal mannoprotein to which T cells respond have, until recently, been poorly defined. Of late, a number of immunoreactive mannoproteins have been purified and characterized. Identified by screening a library of $CD4^+$ T cell hybridomas that reacted to *C. neoformans* antigens, two mannoprotein antigens, termed MP98 and MP88, have been identified (Huang et al., 2002). MP98 bears sequence homology to polysaccharide deacetylases (Levitz et al., 2001). Immunization of mice with either the purified or recombinant protein prolongs survival in mice challenged with a virulent strain of *C. neoformans* (H99). A second immunoreactive cryptococcal protein (d25), also a putative acetylase, has been purified and cloned (Biondo et al., 2002). Immunization with d25 was found to protect mice from lethal experimental cryptococcosis in an IFN-γ-dependent fashion (Biondo et al., 2002). Recombinant d25 (rd25) induces antigen-specific T cell proliferation, as well as IL-2 and IFN-γ production by $CD4^+$ splenocytes recovered from *C. neoformans*-infected mice (Biondo et al., 2002). Thus, a number of closely related mannoproteins have been identified which serve as $CD4^+$ T cell antigens, but the specific antigens to which $CD8^+$ T cells respond remains largely unknown.

Another interesting discovery from the recent literature is that there appears to be cross-reactivity in the T cell responses to *C. neoformans* and another pathogenic fungus, *Candida albicans*. Immunization with CnMP resulted in DTH reactivity to *C. albicans* mannoprotein (CaMP) (Pietrella et al., 2002). Additionally, CaMP-induced IFN-γ production by $CD4^+$ and $CD8^+$ T cells from *C. neoformans*-infected mice. Finally, immunization with CnMP was protective against subsequent challenge with *C. albicans*. Collectively, these results suggest that mannoproteins from the two organisms have common epitopes, which stimulate T cells. These results also suggest the potential for vaccines, which protect against multiple pathogenic fungi.

3.3. The Mitogenic T Cell Response

Mitogens and superantigens are microbially derived proteins, which stimulate the proliferation of T cell in a non-MHC restricted manner. This may benefit the pathogen by the induction of a large frequency of nonspecific T cells, which interfere with the antigen-specific response by poorly understood mechanisms.

C. neoformans produces a mitogen, which can stimulate naive T cell proliferation. Normal individuals have demonstrable T cell proliferative responses to whole *C. neoformans* in vitro. The mitogenic effect is localized to proteins found in the cell wall and membrane of *C. neoformans* (Mody et al., 1996, 1999). This distinguishes the mitogenic response from the antigen-specific one, as T cells from patients who have recovered from *C. neoformans* infection who have proliferative responses to soluble CneF antigens, as well (Hoy et al., 1989). *C. neoformans* mitogen (CnM) stimulates lymphocytes from both adults and fetal cord blood to proliferate, ruling out the potential contribution of previous environmental exposure to the fungus. The mitogenic effect is similar to that of Staphylococcal enterotoxin B (SEB), a known superantigen, and requires phagocytosis and protein processing (Syme et al., 2000). The effects of CnM on human T cells have not been demonstrated in the mouse, and so the potential role of mitogenic activity on the antigen-specific response in vivo has not been determined. Nevertheless, *C. neoformans* produces a known T cell mitogen, CnM, which has the potential to interfere with antigen-specific T cell responses to *C. neoformans*.

4. Protective (T1) versus Nonprotective (T2) T Cell-Mediated Responses

Experimental cryptococcosis in mice is a clear example of the usefulness of the Th1/Th2 paradigm in infectious disease. Resistant mouse strains include CBA, Balb/C, and 129. Susceptible mice include C57/Bl6 and C3H mice. Resistance mice develop a T1 immune response characterized by the early induction of TNF-α and IL-12, production of IFN-γ, and the vigorous recruitment/activation of monocytes and macrophages (Fig. 8.3 and Table 8.1). Resistant mice clear the pulmonary infection over a period of approximately 6–8 weeks. Chronic infection is associated with a Th2-type response whose hallmarks include persistent eosinophilia, high serum immunoglobulin E (IgE) titer, and the presence of T2 cytokines IL-4, IL-5, IL-10, and IL-13 (Fig. 8.3, Table 8.1). It is noteworthy that in murine *C. neoformans* infection, C57Bl/6 mice are susceptible to chronic infection. This has limited the use of genetically engineered mice (which are predominantly on the C57Bl/6 genetic background) to study the requirements for Th1 driving immunity.

4.1. Development of the Protective T1 Response

In the afferent phase of CMI to *C. neoformans*, TNF-α, IL-12, and IFN-γ all play important roles in driving T1 responses, as discussed above. In the efferent phase of T1 responses, IFN-γ has received the most attention. IFN-γ depletion during *C. neoformans* infection leads to enhanced susceptibility and mortality (Kawakami et al., 1996a). As well as serving as early signals for the generation of T1 immunity, IFN-γ and TNF-α likely play a role as effector molecules during CMI (Fig. 8.3). Lymphocytes from immunized mice confer substantial protection against CNS dissemination when transferred to *C. neoformans*-infected SCID mice. Antibody-mediated neutralization of either TNF-α or IFN-γ leads to increased susceptibility, and neutralization of both TNF-α and IFN-γ completely abrogates protection (Aguirre et al., 1995). The role of TNF-α as en effector molecule is unclear however, because neutralization of TNF-α during the efferent phase in immunocompetent mice has little effect on the established response (Huffnagle et al., 1996).

4.2. Development of the Nonprotective T2 Response

Genetically susceptible mice (C57BL/6) also generate T cell-mediated responses to pulmonary *C. neoformans* infection. Susceptible mice generate T2 responses to *C. neoformans*, characterized by the presence of IL-4, IL-5, IL-10, IL-13, high serum IgE, eosinophilia, and chronic infection (Table 8.1 and Fig. 8.3). This disease in mice shares many hallmarks with human ABPM (Kurup and Grunig, 2002; Hernandez et al., 2004a). The results from a number of studies have demonstrated that interfering with the signals provided by T2 cytokines improves clearance of *C. neoformans* in genetically susceptible mice.

IL-4 and IL-10 have similar but distinct roles in regulating the T2 response to *C. neoformans*. Clearance of *C. neoformans* in both IL-4 KO and IL-10 KO mice is significantly greater than in wild-type C57BL/6 controls, and both IL-4 KO and IL-10 KO are protected from eosinophilia (Hernandez et al., 2005a). A decrease in T2 cytokines in the lungs occurs in both, but only IL-10 KO mice have an increase in lung TNF-α and IL-12, suggesting that IL-10 plays a role primarily in the lungs (Hernandez et al., 2005a). Conversely, IL-4 KO mice are protected from the systemic T2 response in wild-type mice and IL-10 KO mice (T2 cytokines in the LALN and high serum IgE). In IL-10 mice, a T2 response does not develop in the lungs, but does systemically. Thus, while both IL-4 and IL-10 drive polarization to a T2 phenotype, IL-10 acts locally in the lungs, whereas IL-4 acts distally in the lymph nodes. In another study, IL-4 KO mice also exhibited a shift toward T1 immunity, but had impaired footpad DTH responses (Blackstock and Murphy, 2004). These results suggest that, in addition to driving T2 responses, T2 cytokines, such as IL-4, may also play a role in potentiating T1 responses, as has been reported for other infection models (Roberts et al., 1996; Mencacci et al., 1998).

IL-5 plays a central role in mediating the T2 cell-mediated immune response. IL-5 is required for some aspects of the T2 response, including eosinophil recruitment and the deposition of eosinophilic YM1 crystals in the lungs. IL-5 production in vitro and eosinophil recruitment in vivo are blocked by depletion of $CD4^+$ (but not $CD8^+$) T cells, demonstrating that Th2 $CD4^+$ T cells are responsible for the production of IL-5 and resulting eosinophilia (Huffnagle et al., 1998).

While the absence of T2 signals decreases susceptibility to *C. neoformans* infection, exogenous addition of T2 cytokines exacerbates infection. Treatment of resistant mice with a combination of IL-4 and IL-10 increases CNS dissemination of C. *neoformans* at week 2 following pulmonary infection (Furukawa et al., 2002). Other studies have demonstrated that the pulmonary eosinophilia induced in C57/Bl6 mice can be attenuated by providing T1-driving signals, including prior *Mycobacterium bovis* Bacillus Calmette–Guerin (BCG) infection, and ligation of OX40 (Humphreys et al., 2003; Walzl et al., 2003). Thus, signals which bias the T cell response toward a Th1 phenotype may promote clearance of *C. neoformans*.

5. Effector Mechanisms of T1 and T2 Responses

There is increasing evidence from a number of experimental infection systems (including pulmonary *C. neoformans* infection) that the polarization of T cells occurs in the lungs (Baumgarth and Kelso, 1996; Howard and Zwilling, 1998; Iezzi et al., 2001; Lindell et al., 2005a). In resistant mice, $CD4^+$ T cells do not become activated or produce IFN-γ in the secondary lymphoid organs, but acquire effector function only upon reaching the lungs (Fig. 8.2) (Lindell et al., 2005a). In genetically susceptible mice, a strongly polarized T2 environment is present early in the lungs, but a mixed T1/T2 response is evident in the lymph nodes (Hernandez et al., 2005a). The acquisition of effector cytokine production occurs with a concomitant loss of proliferative capacity, as $CD4^+$ T cells from LALN and spleens of *C. neoformans*-infected mice proliferate

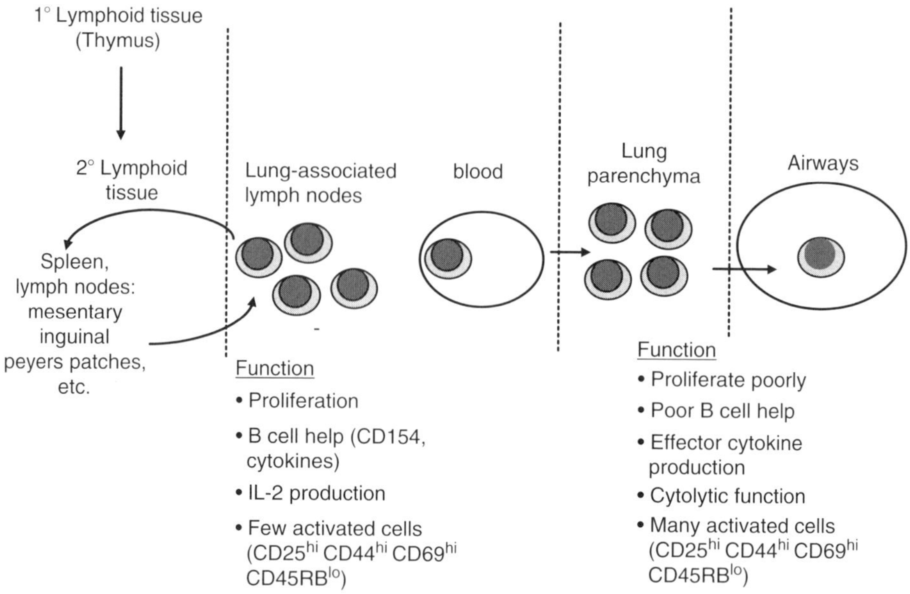

Figure 8.2. Activation and effector function by T cells during the pulmonary immune response to *C. neoformans*. T cells are in constant recirculation throughout the secondary lymphoid organs. During infection, they become trapped in the lung-associated lymph nodes. At this stage, T cells produce IL-2 and proliferate extensively, but do not express high levels of activation markers or effector cytokines. Upon trafficking to the lungs, the acquisition of effector cytokine production by T cells occurs with a concomitant loss of proliferative capacity.

extensively upon T cell antigen receptor (TCR) restimulation, whereas $CD4^+$ T cells from the effector site proliferate poorly (Fig. 8.2) (Lindell et al., 2005a). Thus, the effector mechanisms generated by T cells against pulmonary *C. neoformans* infection are dictated by the environment of the lungs.

5.1. Effector Mechanisms of the Protective T1 Response

The major effector cell in the protective T1 response to *C. neoformans* infection is the activated macrophage. IFN-γ-induced macrophage activation is a critical effector mechanism in CMI to *C. neoformans*. At the onset of cryptococcal clearance in resistant mice, iNOS mRNA expression is upregulated, as is systemic nitric oxide (NO) release (Lovchik et al., 1995). Inflammatory cells recovered from the lungs inhibited the growth of *C. neoformans* added in vitro in an NO-dependent manner (Lovchik et al., 1995). Treatment of mice with either anti-IFN-γ neutralizing antibodies or the NO synthesis inhibitor monomethyl arginine (MMA) blocks clearance of *C. neoformans*, without decreasing lung leukocyte recruitment (Lovchik et al., 1995). Other cytokines may also play a role in macrophage activation during *C. neoformans* infections. In vitro, macrophage phagocytosis and/or killing of *C. neoformans* is augmented by the exogenous addition of TNF-α and granulocyte-macrophage colony-stimulating factor (GM-CSF) (Collins and Bancroft, 1992; Chen et al., 1994; Chiller et al., 2002). Thus,

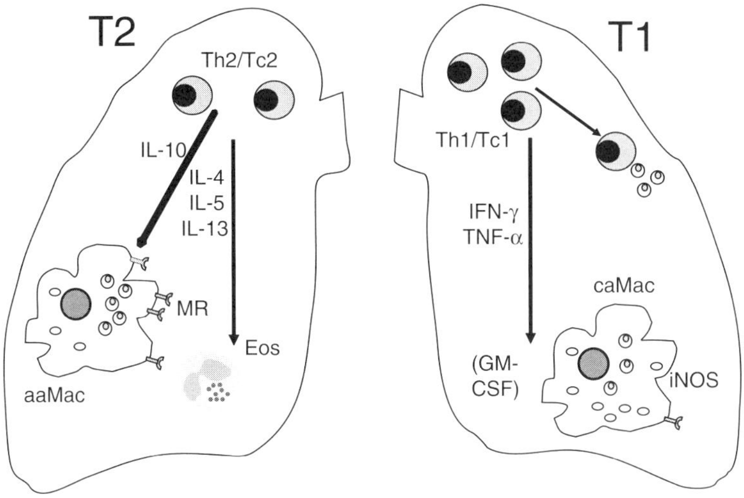

Figure 8.3. Effector cells and cytokines of the nonprotective (T2), and protective (T1) CMI to *C. neoformans* in the lungs. The nonprotective T2 response, which is characterized by the presence of IL-4, IL-5, IL-10, IL-13, high serum IgE, results in persistent eosinophilia and alternative activation of macrophages (aaMac). Alternatively activated macrophages have produced increased mannose receptor expression resulting in fungal phagocytosis, but have decreased intracellular killing and promote the development of fibrosis. In the protective T1 response, which is characterized by high levels of IFN-γ (and low levels of T2 cytokines), large numbers of classically activated macrophages (caMacs) predominate, which are able to kill *C. neoformans* in an iNOS-dependent manner. Additionally, T cells may also be directly fungicidal.

IFN-γ-mediated activation of macrophages plays a critical role in the effector phase of T1 cell-mediated response to *C. neoformans* (Fig. 8.3).

Another mechanism by which T cell may contribute to control of *C. neoformans* infection is via direct, MHC-independent anticryptococcal effects. Human lymphocytes, including IL-2 activated T cells, NK cells, and freshly isolated peripheral blood mononuclear cells (PBMCs) can inhibit the growth of *C. neoformans* (Levitz and Dupont, 1993; Levitz et al., 1994). This requires intimate association between T cells and the fungus, but without phagocytosis (Murphy et al., 1993; Levitz et al., 1994). The fungistatic activity of human lymphocytes is adversely affected by the presence of HIV (Harrison et al., 1995). More recent work characterizing direct fungicidal effects of human $CD8^+$ T cells against *C. neoformans* suggests that the effect is mediated via granulysin, and is dependent on $CD4^+$ T cells and IL-15 (Ma et al., 2002). Murine T cells from *C. neoformans*-immunized (or even naive) mice also have direct anticryptococcal effects (Muth and Murphy, 1995). These findings become more fascinating in light of the granulysin dependence of anticryptococcal activity by human $CD8^+$ T cells (Ma et al., 2002), because mice have no ortholog of granulysin. The relative contribution of $CD4^+$ versus $CD8^+$ T cells, or the $CD4^+$ dependence of $CD8^+$ mediated killing in murine T cells, have not been reported. Furthermore, whether direct anticryptococcal effects of T cells occur in vivo has not been addressed. Thus, both human and murine T cells exhibit direct antifungal activity against *C. neoformans*, but it is as yet unclear whether these occur by the same mechanisms.

5.2. Effector Mechanisms of the Nonprotective T2 Response

C. neoformans infection in C57BL/6 mice is also characterized by the presence of alternatively activated macrophages (aaMac). In contrast to classically activated macrophages (caMac), which develop during T1 conditions, alternatively activated macrophages develop in predominantly T2 conditions (Fig. 8.3). Alternatively activated macrophages produce arginase (which downregulates NO), express the chitinase-related protein YM1, have increased MR expression resulting in fungal phagocytosis, but have decreased intracellular killing and promote the development of fibrosis (Stein et al., 1992; Munder et al., 1998; Goerdt and Orfanos, 1999). While present in wild-type C57BL/6 mice later in *C. neoformans* infection, alternatively activated macrophages are significantly increased in interferon gamma homozygous deficient (IFN-γ −/−) knockout mice (Hernandez et al., 2005a).

Resistant mice generate protective T1 responses to *C. neoformans*. In contrast, susceptible mice generate cell-mediated immune responses to *C. neoformans*, but the response is T2, leading to chronic infection. The preponderance of the evidence suggests that augmenting the T1 response or neutralizing the T2 response is beneficial to the clearance of *C. neoformans*.

5.3. Cooperation between CMI and AMI

Although traditionally regarded as being independent arms of the immune system, there is increasing evidence that the efficacy of CMI and AMI depend upon cooperation between the two. While some of the mechanisms by which antibodies mediate protection (neutralization and complement fixation) can occur in the absence of cellular immunity, opsonic phagocytosis and antibody-dependent cell-mediated cytotoxicity (ADCC) require interaction with cells.

A number of studies have demonstrated the efficacy of antibodies at promoting clearance of *C. neoformans* (see Chapter 9). However, antibodies are not sufficient for clearance of the pathogen. For example, treatment of wild-type mice with a monoclonal anticapsular antibody promotes survival following intravenous *C. neoformans* infection, but protection requires $CD4^+$ T cells (Yuan et al., 1997). In other studies, protection afforded by passive antibody therapy requires nitric oxide synthase 2 (NOS2), suggesting that these antibodies mediate protection via opsonic phagocytosis or phagocyte activation (Rivera et al., 2002). Anticapsular monoclonal antibody therapy is dependent upon isotype of the antibody. Immunoglobulin G (IgG3) is nonprotective, whereas isotype switching to IgG2b and IgG1 results in protection (Yuan et al., 1998a,b). In vivo, promotion of isotype switching is presumably mediated by T cells. Thus, T cells play an important role in the efficacy of AMI to *C. neoformans*.

6. Immunomodulation of the T Cell Response by *C. neoformans*

C. neoformans produces a number of established and putative virulence factors which are described in more detail elsewhere (Buchanan and Murphy, 1998). In addition to being antiphagocytic, *C. neoformans* capsular polysaccharides have immunomodulatory properties, including the induction of IL-10, which affect the development of CMI. Different strains of *C. neoformans* vary in their capsular structure, and even a single strain can undergo phenotypic switching, which influences the magnitude and character of the host inflammatory response, as well as virulence of the fungus. Live yeast produce virulence factors, which contribute to the delay in T cell responses, as heat-killed encapsulated organisms induce more rapid responses than live organisms (Huffnagle et al., 1995a). *C. neoformans* and other pathogenic fungi produce oxylipins which can inhibit T cell proliferation and skew development of T cell responses towards nonprotective T2.

6.1. Polysaccharide Capsule

Perhaps the best-characterized virulence factor of *C. neoformans* is its capsule, which is unique among pathogenic fungi. The T cell response to encapsulated versus unencapsulated *C. neoformans* is delayed, but can be overcome by opsonization of encapsulated yeast with specific antibody (Collins and Bancroft, 1991; Syme et al., 1999).

GXM is one of the major constituents of the polysaccharide coating of *C. neoformans*, and has a number of immunomodulatory properties (Vecchiarelli, 2000). In vitro, GXM induces IL-10 production in monocytes, which dampens the proinflammatory IL-12 response normally induced by unencapsulated *C. neoformans*. IL-10 induction by GXM also serves to inhibit Th1 responses. *C. neoformans* GXM also impairs dendritic cell activation and maturation in vitro (Retini et al., 2001; Mariano Andrade et al., 2003; Vecchiarelli et al., 2003). Shed GXM may also act on APCs in vivo to dampen the proinflammatory signals generated by ingestion of the fungus. *C. neoformans* GXM may bias the Th1/Th2 balance early on. Purified capsular polysaccharide induces proliferation of $CD4^+$ T cells, which was dependent upon APCs and CD40L-mediated signaling (Almeida et al., 2001). The cytokines elaborated during this response included IL-4 and IL-10, with undetectable levels of TNF-α and IFN-γ. Thus, in addition to its numerous effects on the innate immune system, the capsular polysaccharide from *C. neoformans* may bias the immune system toward a Th2 phenotype.

GXM may also promote the apoptosis of T cells. In vitro culture of rat splenic mononuclear cells with GXM results in increased levels of T cell apoptosis (Chiapello et al., 2003). In vivo, *C. neoformans* infection also induces apoptosis in the lungs and spleens of infected rats, but whether GXM itself is responsible for this effect is unclear. Thus, GXM from *C. neoformans* may affect the development and effector phases of CMI, in addition to impairment of phagocytosis.

GXM is directly and indirectly chemotactic for leukocytes (Dong and Murphy, 1993). During infection, GXM is shed from *C. neoformans*, and the detection of serum GXM serves as a diagnostic tool for systemic *C. neoformans* infection (Hamilton et al., 1991). High concentrations of GXM in serum may affect the trafficking of T cells and other leukocytes. When administered intravenously, cryptococcal polysaccharides inhibit the influx of T cells into primary sites of infection (Dong and Murphy, 1995). One potential mechanism for this phenomenon is that GXM acts as a competitor for endogenous chemotaxins. Another mechanism is via selectins. GXM was found to cause loss of CD11a (L-selectin), which is involved in the extravasation of lymphocytes from the vasculature into the lungs (Dong et al., 1999).

Thus, cryptococcal polysaccharide may adversely affect the development of CMI to *C. neoformans* at multiple stages of the response.

6.2. Phenotypic Switching

The structure of *C. neoformans* capsule affects T cell responses in vivo. Different strains of *C. neoformans* with similar capsules differ in their T cell immunogenicity (Curtis et al., 1994; Huffnagle et al., 1995a). Additionally, even a single strain of *C. neoformans* can undergo phenotypic switching, resulting in colonies of different morphologies and capsule thicknesses. These phenotypic variants differ in the inflammatory leukocyte responses induced in mice, as well as virulence (Goldman et al., 1998). Phenotypic switching has been shown to occur in vivo during *C. neoformans* infection, which promotes a more vigorous inflammatory response and enhanced lethality (Fries et al., 2001). Phenotypic switching may contribute to the chronicity of *C. neoformans* infection by inducing overexuberant inflammatory responses.

6.3. *C. neoformans*-derived Oxylipins

C. neoformans and other pathogenic fungi produce oxylipins, which resemble mammalian prostaglandins and other eicosanoids (Noverr et al., 2002, 2003a,b). These can be produced by the fungus from arachidonic acid or synthesized de novo (Noverr et al., 2001). Prostaglandins have well-recognized immunomodulatory effects. In in vitro studies with human and murine T cells, prostaglandin E_2 (PGE_2) inhibits the production of Th1 cytokines IL-2 and IFN-γ, but not Th2 cytokines IL-4 and IL-5 (Betz and Fox, 1991; Snijdewint et al., 1993). PGE_2 also inhibits mitogen-induced T cell proliferation (Sergeeva et al., 1997). Eicosanoids are significant players in pulmonary immune responses. In an asthma model, prostaglandin D_2 (PGD_2) accelerates Th2 responses to aerosolized antigen, characterized by increased eosinophilia, lymphocytosis, and increased levels of Th2-type cytokines (Honda et al., 2003). Cumulatively, these results suggest that PGE_2 and PGD_2 promote the polarization of T cells to a T2 phenotype. The eicosanoids produced by *C. neoformans* are biologically active. In vitro, *C. neoformans*-derived prostanoid E inhibits mitogen-induced proliferation of splenocytes even better than mammalian PGE_2 (Noverr et al., 2003b). Thus, *C. neoformans*-derived oxylipins may interfere with T cell proliferation or by promoting the development of nonprotective T2 immunity.

7. Conclusion

In conclusion, during pulmonary *C. neoformans* infection, T cells serve three majors functions: (1) T cells are required for the recruitment of inflammatory cells, primarily monocytes and macrophages; (2) T cells are responsible for the activation of macrophages; (3) T cells cooperate with the antibody-mediated immune response, via promoting opsonic phagocytosis and ADCC.

The establishment of CMI depends upon the innate immune system. In addition to recognition and early containment of the fungus, innate immune cells provide critical signals, which establish a proinflammatory state, and affect the polarization of arriving T cells and macrophages. Chief among these critical early signals are TNF-α, IL-12, IL-18, and IFN-γ. In addition, a variety of chemokines, most notably CCL2/MCP-1 act both to recruit inflammatory cells and polarize the environment of the lungs.

Both $CD4^+$ and $CD8^+$ T cell responses are generated in response to *C. neoformans*. This is due to the nature of the pathogen, which survives and replicates both extra- and intracellularly. Of late, a number of cryptococcal mannoproteins have been characterized, to which protective T cell responses are generated.

During pulmonary *C. neoformans* infection, the T1 versus T2 nature of the lung environment dictates whether clearance or chronic infection will prevail. Resistant mice generate protective T1 responses to *C. neoformans*. The protective T1 response, which is characterized by the early induction of TNF-α and IL-12, and the production of large amounts of IFN-γ leads to activation of macrophages, which phagocytose and kill *C. neoformans*. In contrast, susceptible mice generate cell-mediated immune responses to *C. neoformans*, but the response is T2, leading to chronic infection. When T2 conditions dominate in the lungs, the response is characterized by the presence of T2 cytokines IL-4, IL-5, IL-10, and IL-13. Eosinophilia and the development of aaMacs are also distinguishing features of the nonprotective T2 response, and chronic infection and tissue damage result.

Chronicity of infection is also promoted by the immunomodulation of the host response by *C. neoformans*. *C. neoformans* possesses a polysaccharide capsule, and can undergo phenotypic switching. Soluble capsular polysaccharide has a number of immunosuppressive effects, and phenotypic switching may contribute to the chronicity of *C. neoformans* infection by inducing overexuberant inflammatory responses. Additionally *C. neoformans*-derived oxylipins may interfere with T cell proliferation or by promoting the development of nonprotective T2 immunity.

Thus, the nature of the immune response to *C. neoformans*, and whether clearance will take place, depends on the interplay of host and microbial factors.

List of Abbreviations

aaMac: Alternatively activated macrophage

ABPM: Allergic bronchopulmonary mycosis

ADCC: Antibody-dependent cell-mediated cytotoxicity

AIDS: Acquired immune deficiency syndrome

AMI: Antibody-mediated immunity

APC: Antigen-presenting cell

BCG: Bacillus Calmette-Guerin

caMac: Classically activated macrophage

CaMP: *Candida albicans* mannoprotein

CCL: CC chemokine ligand

CCR: CC chemokine receptor

CD: Cluster of differentiation

CMI: Cell-mediated immunity

CneF: *Cryptococcus neoformans* filtrate antigen

CnM: *Cryptococcus neoformans* mitogen

CnMP: *Cryptococcus neoformans* mannoprotein

CR: Complement receptor

CTLA-4: Cytotoxic T lymphocyte antigen-4

DTH: Delayed-type hypersensitivity

FcγR2: Fragment crystallizable gamma receptor 2

GalXM: Galactoxylomannan

GM-CSF: Granulocyte-macrophage colony-stimulating factor

GXM: Glucuronoxylomannan

HIV: human immunodeficiency virus

IFN-γ -/-: Interferon gamma homozygous deficient (knockout mouse)

IFN-γ: interferon gamma

IgE: Immunoglobulin E

IgG: Immunoglobulin G

IL: Interleukin

iNOS: Inducible nitric oxide synthase

KO: Knockout

LALN: Lung-associated lymph nodes

MCP-1: Monocyte chemotactic protein 1

MHC: Major histocompatibility complex

MIP1-α: Macrophage inflammatory protein 1 alpha

MMA: Monomethyl arginine

MP: Mannoprotein

MR: Mannose receptor

NK: Natural killer cell

NKT: Natural killer T cell

NO: Nitric oxide

NOS2: Nitric oxide synthase 2

PBMC: Peripheral blood mononuclear cell

PGD_2: Prostaglandin D_2

PGE_2: Prostaglandin E_2

PMN: Polymorphonuclear neutrophil leukocyte

PRR: Pattern recognition receptor

SCID: Severely combined immunodeficiency

SEB: Staphylococcal enterotoxin B

T1: type 1 cell-mediated immunity

T2: type 2 cell-mediated immunity

Th1: T helper type 1

Th2: T helper type 2

TLR: Toll-like receptor

TNF-α: Tumor necrosis factor alpha

Vα14 NKT: Variable alpha 14 positive natural killer T cell

γδ T cell: Gamma delta T cell

References

Aguirre, K., Havell, E.A., Gibson, G.W., and Johnson, L.L. (1995). Role of tumor necrosis factor and gamma interferon in acquired resistance to *Cryptococcus neoformans* in the central nervous system of mice. *Infect. Immun.* 63(5): 1725–1731.

Almeida, G.M., Andrade, R.M., and Bento, C.A. (2001). The capsular polysaccharides of *Cryptococcus neoformans* activate normal CD4(+) T cells in a dominant Th2 pattern. *J. Immunol.* 167(10): 5845–5851.

Arora, S., Hernandez, Y.H., Erb-Downward, J.R., McDonald, R.A., Toews, G.B., and Huffnagle, G.B. (2005a). Role of IFN-γ in regulating T2 immunity and the development of alternatively activated macrophages during *Cryptococcus neoformans* infection. *J. Immunol.* (in press).

Bauman, S.K., Huffnagle, G.B., and Murphy, J.W. (2003). Effects of tumor necrosis factor alpha on dendritic cell accumulation in lymph nodes draining the immunization site and the impact on the anticryptococcal cell-mediated immune response. *Infect. Immun.* 71(1): 68–74.

Baumgarth, N. and Kelso, A. (1996). Functionally distinct T cells in three compartments of the respiratory tract after influenza virus infection. *Eur. J. Immunol.* 26(9): 2189–2197.

Bennett, S.R., Carbone, F.R., Karamalis, F., Flavell, R.A., Miller, J.F., and Heath, W.R. (1998). Help for cytotoxic-T-cell responses is mediated by CD40 signalling. *Nature* 393(6684): 478–480.

Betz, M. and Fox, B.S. (1991). Prostaglandin E2 inhibits production of Th1 lymphokines but not of Th2 lymphokines. *J. Immunol.* 146(1): 108–113.

Biondo, C., Beninati, C., Delfino, D., Oggioni, M., Mancuso, G., Midiri, A., Bombaci, M., Tomaselli, G., and Teti, G. (2002). Identification and cloning of a cryptococcal deacetylase that produces protective immune responses. *Infect. Immun.* 70(5): 2383–2391.

Blackstock, R. and Murphy, J.W. (2004). Role of interleukin-4 in resistance to *Cryptococcus neoformans* infection. *Am. J. Respir. Cell Mol. Biol.* 30(1): 109–117.

Buchanan, K.L. and Murphy, J.W. (1998). What makes *Cryptococcus neoformans* a pathogen? *Emerg. Infect. Dis.* 4(1): 71–83.

Chen, G.H., Curtis, J.L., Mody, C.H., Christensen, P.J., Armstrong, L.R., and Toews, G.B. (1994). Effect of granulocyte-macrophage colony-stimulating factor on rat alveolar macrophage anticryptococcal activity in vitro. *J. Immunol.* 152(2): 724–734.

Chiapello, L.S., Aoki, M.P., Rubinstein, H.R., and Masih, D.T. (2003). Apoptosis induction by glucuronoxylomannan of *Cryptococcus neoformans*. *Med. Mycol.* 41(4): 347–353.

Chiller, T., Farrokhshad, K., Brummer, E., and Stevens, D.A. (2002). Effect of granulocyte colony-stimulating factor and granulocyte-macrophage colony-stimulating factor on polymorphonuclear neutrophils, monocytes or monocyte-derived macrophages combined with voriconazole against *Cryptococcus neoformans*. *Med. Mycol.* 40(1): 21–26.

Collins, H.L. and Bancroft, G.J. (1991). Encapsulation of *Cryptococcus neoformans* impairs antigen-specific T-cell responses. *Infect. Immun.* 59(11): 3883–3888.

Collins, H.L. and Bancroft, G.J. (1992). Cytokine enhancement of complement-dependent phagocytosis by macrophages: Synergy of tumor necrosis factor-alpha and granulocyte-macrophage colony-stimulating factor for phagocytosis of *Cryptococcus neoformans*. *Eur. J. Immunol.* 22(6): 1447–1454.

Curtis, J.L., Huffnagle, G.B., Chen, G.H., Warnock, M.L., Gyetko, M.R., McDonald, R.A., Scott, P.J., and Toews, G.B. (1994). Experimental murine pulmonary cryptococcosis. Differences in pulmonary inflammation and lymphocyte recruitment induced by two encapsulated strains of *Cryptococcus neoformans*. *Lab. Invest.* 71(1): 113–126.

Decken, K., Kohler, G., Palmer-Lehmann, K., Wunderlin, F., Mattner, F., Magram, J., Gately, M.K., and Alber, G. (1998). Interleukin-12 is essential for a protective Th1 response in mice infected with *Cryptococcus neoformans*. *Infect. Immun.* 66(10): 4994–5000.

Dong, Z.M. and Murphy, J.W. (1993). Mobility of human neutrophils in response to *Cryptococcus neoformans* cells, culture filtrate antigen, and individual components of the antigen. *Infect. Immun.* 61(12): 5067–5077.

Dong, Z.M. and Murphy, J.W. (1995). Intravascular cryptococcal culture filtrate (CneF) and its major component, glucuronoxylomannan, are potent inhibitors of leukocyte accumulation. *Infect. Immun.* 63(3): 770–778.

Dong, Z.M., Jackson, L., and Murphy, J.W. (1999). Mechanisms for induction of L-selectin loss from T lymphocytes by a cryptococcal polysaccharide, glucuronoxylomannan. *Infect. Immun.* 67(1): 220–229.

Fries, B.C., Taborda, C.P., Serfass, E., and Casadevall, A. (2001). Phenotypic switching of *Cryptococcus neoformans* occurs in vivo and influences the outcome of infection. *J. Clin. Invest.* 108(11): 1639–1648.

Furukawa, K., Kobayashi, M., Sasaki, H., Herndon, D.N., Pollard, R.B., and Suzuki, F. (2002). Cryptococcal encephalitis in thermally injured mice is accelerated by type 2 T-cell responses. *Crit. Care Med.* 30(7): 1419–1424.

Goerdt, S. and Orfanos, C.E. (1999). Other functions, other genes: Alternative activation of antigen-presenting cells. *Immunity* 10(2): 137–142.

Goldman, D.L., Fries, B.C., Franzot, S.P., Montella, L., and Casadevall, A. (1998). Phenotypic switching in the human pathogenic fungus *Cryptococcus neoformans* is associated with changes in virulence and pulmonary inflammatory response in rodents. *Proc. Natl. Acad. Sci. USA* 95(25): 14967–14972.

Hamilton, J.R., Noble, A., Denning, D.W., and Stevens, D.A. (1991). Performance of *Cryptococcus* antigen latex agglutination kits on serum and cerebrospinal fluid specimens of AIDS patients before and after pronase treatment. *J. Clin. Microbiol.* 29(2): 333–339.

Harrison, T.S., Kornfeld, H., and Levitz, S.M. (1995). The effect of infection with human immunodeficiency virus on the anticryptococcal activity of lymphocytes and monocytes. *J. Infect. Dis.* 172(3): 665–671.

Hernandez, Y.H., Erb-Downward, J.R., McDonald, R.A., Toews, G.B., and Huffnagle, G.B. (2005a). Distinct roles for IL-4 and IL-10 in regulating T2 immunity during allergic bronchopulmonary mycosis. *J. Immunol.* 174(2): 1027–1036.

Herring, A.C., Lee, J., McDonald, R.A., Toews, G.B., and Huffnagle, G.B. (2002). Induction of interleukin-12 and gamma interferon requires tumor necrosis factor alpha for protective T1-cell-mediated immunity to pulmonary *Cryptococcus neoformans* infection. *Infect. Immun.* 70(6): 2959–2964.

Hill, J.O. and Harmsen, A.G. (1991). Intrapulmonary growth and dissemination of an avirulent strain of *Cryptococcus neoformans* in mice depleted of CD4+ or CD8+ T cells. *J. Exp. Med.* 173(3): 755–758.

Hoag, K.A., Lipscomb, M.F., Izzo, A.A., and Street, N.E. (1997). IL-12 and IFN-gamma are required for initiating the protective Th1 response to pulmonary cryptococcosis in resistant C.B-17 mice. *Am. J. Respir. Cell Mol. Biol.* 17(6): 733–739.

Honda, K., Arima, M., Cheng, G., Taki, S., Hirata, H., Eda, F., Fukushima, F., Yamaguchi, B., Hatano, M., Tokuhisa, T., and Fukuda, T. (2003). Prostaglandin D2 reinforces Th2 type inflammatory responses of airways to low-dose antigen through bronchial expression of macrophage-derived chemokine. *J. Exp. Med.* 198(4): 533–543.

Howard, A.D. and Zwilling, B.S. (1998). Cytokine production by CD4 and CD8 T cells during the growth of *Mycobacterium tuberculosis* in mice. *Clin. Exp. Immunol.* 113(3): 443–449.

Hoy, J.F., Lewis, D.E., and Miller, G.G. (1988). Functional versus phenotypic analysis of T cells in subjects seropositive for the human immunodeficiency virus: A prospective study of in vitro responses to *Cryptococcus neoformans*. *J. Infect. Dis.* 158(5): 1071–1078.

Hoy, J.F., Murphy, J.W., and Miller, G.G. (1989). T cell response to soluble cryptococcal antigens after recovery from cryptococcal infection. *J. Infect. Dis.* 159(1): 116–119.

Huang, C., Nong, S.H., Mansour, M.K., Specht, C.A., and Levitz, S.M. (2002). Purification and characterization of a second immunoreactive mannoprotein from *Cryptococcus neoformans* that stimulates T-cell responses. *Infect. Immun.* 70(10): 5485–5493.

Huffnagle, G.B., Yates, J.L., and Lipscomb, M.F. (1991a). Immunity to a pulmonary *Cryptococcus neoformans* infection requires both CD4+ and CD8+ T cells. *J. Exp. Med.* 173(4): 793–800.

Huffnagle, G.B., Yates, J.L., and Lipscomb, M.F. (1991b). T cell-mediated immunity in the lung: A *Cryptococcus neoformans* pulmonary infection model using SCID and athymic nude mice. *Infect. Immun.* 59(4): 1423–1433.

Huffnagle, G.B., Lipscomb, M.F., Lovchik, J.A., Hoag, K.A., and Street, N.E. (1994). The role of CD4+ and CD8+ T cells in the protective inflammatory response to a pulmonary cryptococcal infection. *J. Leukoc. Biol.* 55(1): 35–42.

Huffnagle, G.B., Chen, G.H., Curtis, J.L., McDonald, R.A., Strieter, R.M., and Toews, G.B. (1995a). Down-regulation of the afferent phase of T cell-mediated pulmonary inflammation and immunity by a high melanin-producing strain of *Cryptococcus neoformans*. *J. Immunol.* 155(7): 3507–3516.

Huffnagle, G.B., Strieter, R.M., Standiford, T.J., McDonald, R.A., Burdick, M.D., Kunkel, S.L., and Toews, G.B. (1995b). The role of monocyte chemotactic protein-1 (MCP-1) in the recruitment of monocytes and CD4$^+$ T cells during a pulmonary *Cryptococcus neoformans* infection. *J. Immunol.* 155(10): 4790–4797.

Huffnagle, G.B., Toews, G.B., Burdick, M.D., Boyd, M.B., McAllister, K.S., McDonald, R.A., Kunkel, S.L., and Strieter, R.M. (1996). Afferent phase production of TNF-alpha is required for the development of protective T cell immunity to *Cryptococcus neoformans*. *J. Immunol.* 157(10): 4529–4536.

Huffnagle, G.B., Strieter, R.M., McNeil, L.K., McDonald, R.A., Burdick, M.D., Kunkel, S.L., and Toews, G.B. (1997). Macrophage inflammatory protein-1 alpha (MIP-1alpha) is required for the efferent phase of pulmonary cell-mediated immunity to a *Cryptococcus neoformans* infection. *J. Immunol.* 159(1): 318–327.

Huffnagle, G.B., Boyd, M.B., Street, N.E., and Lipscomb, M.F. (1998). IL-5 is required for eosinophil recruitment, crystal deposition, and mononuclear cell recruitment during a pulmonary *Cryptococcus neoformans* infection in genetically susceptible mice (C57BL/6). *J. Immunol.* 160(5): 2393–2400.

Huffnagle, G.B., McNeil, L.K., McDonald, R.A., Murphy, J.W., Toews, G.B., Maeda, N., and Kuziel, W.A. (1999). Cutting edge: Role of C–C chemokine receptor 5 in organ-specific and innate immunity to *Cryptococcus neoformans*. *J. Immunol.* 163(9): 4642–4646.

Humphreys, I.R., Edwards, L., Walzl, G., Rae, A.J., Dougan, G., Hill, S., and Hussell, T. (2003). OX40 Ligation on activated T cells enhances the control of *Cryptococcus neoformans* and reduces pulmonary eosinophilia. *J. Immunol.* 170(12): 6125–6132.

Iezzi, G., Scheidegger, D., and Lanzavecchia, A. (2001). Migration and function of antigen-primed nonpolarized T lymphocytes in vivo. *J. Exp. Med.* 193(8): 987–993.

Kawakami, K., Tohyama, M., Teruya, K., Kudeken, N., Xie, Q., and Saito, A. (1996a). Contribution of interferon-gamma in protecting mice during pulmonary and disseminated infection with *Cryptococcus neoformans*. *FEMS Immunol. Med. Microbiol.* 13(2): 123–130.

Kawakami, K., Tohyama, M., Xie, Q., and Saito, A. (1996b). IL-12 protects mice against pulmonary and disseminated infection caused by *Cryptococcus neoformans*. *Clin. Exp. Immunol.* 104(2): 208–214.

Kawakami, K., Qureshi, M.H., Zhang, T., Okamura, H., Kurimoto, M., and Saito, A. (1997). IL-18 protects mice against pulmonary and disseminated infection with *Cryptococcus neoformans* by inducing IFN-gamma production. *J. Immunol.* 159(11): 5528–5534.

Kawakami, K., Koguchi, Y., Qureshi, M.H., Kinjo, Y., Yara, S., Miyazato, A., Kurimoto, M., Takeda, K., Akira, S., and Saito, A. (2000). Reduced host resistance and Th1 response to *Cryptococcus neoformans* in interleukin-18 deficient mice. *FEMS Microbiol. Lett.* 186(1): 121–126.

Kawakami, K., Kinjo, Y., Uezu, K., Yara, S., Miyagi, K., Koguchi, Y., Nakayama, T., Taniguchi, M., and Saito, A. (2001a). Monocyte chemoattractant protein-1-dependent increase of V alpha 14 NKT cells in lungs and their roles in Th1 response and host defense in cryptococcal infection. *J. Immunol.* 167(11): 6525–6532.

Kawakami, K., Kinjo, Y., Yara, S., Koguchi, Y., Uezu, K., Nakayama, T., Taniguchi, M., and Saito, A. (2001b). Activation of Vα14$^+$ natural killer T cells by α-galactosylceramide results in development of Th1 response and local host resistance in mice infected with *Cryptococcus neoformans*. *Infect. Immun.* 69(1): 213–220.

Kurup, V.P. and Grunig, G. (2002). Animal models of allergic bronchopulmonary aspergillosis. *Mycopathologia* 153(4): 165–177.

Levitz, S.M. and Dupont, M.P. (1993). Phenotypic and functional characterization of human lymphocytes activated by interleukin-2 to directly inhibit growth of *Cryptococcus neoformans* in vitro. *J. Clin. Invest.* 91(4): 1490–1498.

Levitz, S.M., Dupont, M.P., and Smail, E.H. (1994). Direct activity of human T lymphocytes and natural killer cells against *Cryptococcus neoformans*. *Infect. Immun.* 62(1): 194–202.

Levitz, S.M., Nong, S., Mansour, M.K., Huang, C., and Specht, C.A. (2001). Molecular characterization of a mannoprotein with homology to chitin deacetylases that stimulates T cell responses to *Cryptococcus neoformans*. *Proc. Natl. Acad. Sci. USA* 98(18): 10422–10427.

Lim, T.S. and Murphy, J.W. (1980). Transfer of immunity to cryptococcosis by T-enriched splenic lymphocytes from *Cryptococcus neoformans*-sensitized mice. *Infect. Immun.* 30(1): 5–11.

Lindell, D.M., G.B. Toews, R.A. McDonald and G.B. Huffnagle (2005a). Distinct Compartmentalization of CD4+ T Cell Effector function versus Proliferative Capacity During Pulmonary Cryptococcosis. Submitted for publication.

Lindell, D.M., G.B. Toews, R.A. McDonald and G.B. Huffnagle (2005b). Generation of Antifungal Effector CD8+ T cells in the Absence of CD4+ T cells During Cryptococcus neoformans Infection. Submitted for publication.

Lovchik, J.A., Lyons, C.R., and Lipscomb, M.F. (1995). A role for gamma interferon-induced nitric oxide in pulmonary clearance of *Cryptococcus neoformans*. *Am. J. Respir. Cell Mol. Biol.* 13(1): 116–124.

Ma, L.L., Spurrell, J.C., Wang, J.F., Neely, G.G., Epelman, S., Krensky, A.M., and Mody, C.H. (2002). CD8 T cell-mediated killing of *Cryptococcus neoformans* requires granulysin and is dependent on CD4 T cells and IL-15. *J. Immunol.* 169(10): 5787–5795.

Mansour, M.K., Schlesinger, L.S., and Levitz, S.M. (2002). Optimal T cell responses to *Cryptococcus neoformans* mannoprotein are dependent on recognition of conjugated carbohydrates by mannose receptors. *J. Immunol.* 168(6): 2872–2879.

Mariano Andrade, R., Monteiro Almeida, G., Alexandre DosReis, G., and Alves Melo Bento, C. (2003). Glucuronoxylomannan of *Cryptococcus neoformans* exacerbates in vitro yeast cell growth by interleukin 10-dependent inhibition of CD4+ T lymphocyte responses. *Cell. Immunol.* 222(2): 116–125.

McGaha, T. and Murphy, J.W. (2000). CTLA-4 down-regulates the protective anticryptococcal cell-mediated immune response. *Infect. Immun.* 68(8): 4624–4630.

Mednick, A.J., Feldmesser, M., Rivera, J., and Casadevall, A. (2003). Neutropenia alters lung cytokine production in mice and reduces their susceptibility to pulmonary cryptococcosis. *Eur. J. Immunol.* 33(6): 1744–1753.

Mencacci, A., Del Sero, G., Cenci, E., d'Ostiani, C.F., Bacci, A., Montagnoli, C., Kopf, M., and Romani, L. (1998). Endogenous interleukin 4 is required for development of protective CD4+ T helper type 1 cell responses to *Candida albicans*. *J. Exp. Med.* 187(3): 307–317.

Micallef, M.J., Ohtsuki, T., Kohno, K., Tanabe, F., Ushio, S., Namba, M., Tanimoto, T., Torigoe, K., Fujii, M., Ikeda, M., Fukuda, S., and Kurimoto, M. (1996). Interferon-gamma-inducing factor enhances T helper 1 cytokine production by stimulated human T cells: Synergism with interleukin-12 for interferon-gamma production. *Eur. J. Immunol.* 26(7): 1647–1651.

Miller, G.P. and Puck, J. (1984). In vitro human lymphocyte responses to *Cryptococcus neoformans*. Evidence for primary and secondary responses in normals and infected subjects. *J. Immunol.* 133(1): 166–172.

Mody, C.H., Lipscomb, M.F., Street, N.E., and Toews, G.B. (1990). Depletion of CD4+ (L3T4+) lymphocytes in vivo impairs murine host defense to *Cryptococcus neoformans*. *J. Immunol.* 144(4): 1472–1477.

Mody, C.H., Chen, G.H., Jackson, C., Curtis, J.L., and Toews, G.B. (1993a). Depletion of murine CD8+ T cells in vivo decreases pulmonary clearance of a moderately virulent strain of *Cryptococcus neoformans*. *J. Lab. Clin. Med.* 121(6): 765–773.

Mody, C.H., Paine, R. III, Jackson, C.J., and Toews, G.B. (1993b). CD8 cells mediate delayed hypersensitivity following intrapulmonary infection with *Cryptococcus neoformans*. *Chest* 103(2 Suppl.): 118S.

Mody, C.H., Chen, G.H., Jackson, C., Curtis, J.L., and Toews, G.B. (1994). In vivo depletion of murine CD8 positive T cells impairs survival during infection with a highly virulent strain of *Cryptococcus neoformans*. *Mycopathologia* 125(1): 7–17.

Mody, C.H., Sims, K.L., Wood, C.J., Syme, R.M., Spurrell, J.C., and Sexton, M.M. (1996). Proteins in the cell wall and membrane of *Cryptococcus neoformans* stimulate lymphocytes from both adults and fetal cord blood to proliferate. *Infect. Immun.* 64(11): 4811–4819.

Mody, C.H., Wood, C.J., Syme, R.M., and Spurrell, J.C. (1999). The cell wall and membrane of *Cryptococcus neoformans* possess a mitogen for human T lymphocytes. *Infect. Immun.* 67(2): 936–941.

Munder, M., Eichmann, K., and Modolell, M. (1998). Alternative metabolic states in murine macrophages reflected by the nitric oxide synthase/arginase balance: Competitive regulation by CD4+ T cells correlates with Th1/Th2 phenotype. *J. Immunol.* 160(11): 5347–5354.

Murphy, J.W. and Pahlavan, N. (1979). Cryptococcal culture filtrate antigen for detection of delayed-type hypersensitivity in cryptococcosis. *Infect. Immun.* 25(1): 284–292.

Murphy, J.W., Hidore, M.R., and Wong, S.C. (1993). Direct interactions of human lymphocytes with the yeast-like organism, *Cryptococcus neoformans*. *J. Clin. Invest.* 91(4): 1553–1566.

Murphy, J.W., Schafer, F., Casadevall, A., and Adesina, A. (1998). Antigen-induced protective and nonprotective cell-mediated immune components against *Cryptococcus neoformans*. *Infect. Immun.* 66(6): 2632–2639.

Muth, S.M. and Murphy, J.W. (1995). Direct anticryptococcal activity of lymphocytes from *Cryptococcus neoformans*-immunized mice. *Infect. Immun.* 63(5): 1637–1644.

Noverr, M.C., Phare, S.M., Toews, G.B., Coffey, M.J., and Huffnagle, G.B. (2001). Pathogenic yeasts *Cryptococcus neoformans* and *Candida albicans* produce immunomodulatory prostaglandins. *Infect. Immun.* 69(5): 2957–2963.

Noverr, M.C., Toews, G.B., and Huffnagle, G.B. (2002). Production of prostaglandins and leukotrienes by pathogenic fungi. *Infect. Immun.* 70(1): 400–402.

Noverr, M.C., Cox, G.M., Perfect, J.R., and Huffnagle, G.B. (2003a). Role of PLB1 in pulmonary inflammation and cryptococcal eicosanoid production. *Infect. Immun.* 71(3): 1538–1547.

Noverr, M.C., Erb-Downward, J.R., and Huffnagle, G.B. (2003b). Production of eicosanoids and other oxylipins by pathogenic eukaryotic microbes. *Clin. Microbiol. Rev.* 16(3): 517–533.

Okamura, H., Tsutsi, H., Komatsu, T., Yutsudo, M., Hakura, A., Tanimoto, T., Torigoe, K., Okura, T., Nukada, Y., Hattori, K., and et al. (1995). Cloning of a new cytokine that induces IFN-gamma production by T cells. *Nature* 378(6552): 88–91.

Okamura, H., Tsutsui, H., Kashiwamura, S., Yoshimoto, T., and Nakanishi, K. (1998). Interleukin-18: A novel cytokine that augments both innate and acquired immunity. *Adv. Immunol.* 70: 281–312.

Olszewski, M.A., Huffnagle, G.B., McDonald, R.A., Lindell, D.M., Moore, B.B., Cook, D.N., and Toews, G.B. (2000). The role of macrophage inflammatory protein-1 alpha/CCL3 in regulation of T cell-mediated immunity to *Cryptococcus neoformans* infection. *J. Immunol.* 165(11): 6429–6436.

Olszewski, M.A., Huffnagle, G.B., Traynor, T.R., McDonald, R.A., Cook, D.N., and Toews, G.B. (2001). Regulatory effects of macrophage inflammatory protein 1α/CCL3 on the development of immunity to *Cryptococcus neoformans* depend on expression of early inflammatory cytokines. *Infect. Immun.* 69(10): 6256–6263.

Pietrella, D., Perito, S., Bistoni, F., and Vecchiarelli, A. (2001). Cytotoxic T lymphocyte antigen costimulation influences T-cell activation in response to *Cryptococcus neoformans*. *Infect. Immun.* 69(3): 1508–1514.

Pietrella, D., Mazzolla, R., Lupo, P., Pitzurra, L., Gomez, M.J., Cherniak, R., and Vecchiarelli, A. (2002). Mannoprotein from *Cryptococcus neoformans* promotes T-helper type 1 anticandidal responses in mice. *Infect. Immun.* 70(12): 6621–6627.

Pitzurra, L., Cherniak, R., Giammarioli, M., Perito, S., Bistoni, F., and Vecchiarelli, A. (2000). Early induction of interleukin-12 by human monocytes exposed to *Cryptococcus neoformans* mannoproteins. *Infect. Immun.* 68(2): 558–563.

Qureshi, M.H., Zhang, T., Koguchi, Y., Nakashima, K., Okamura, H., Kurimoto, M., and Kawakami, K. (1999). Combined effects of IL-12 and IL-18 on the clinical course and local cytokine production in murine pulmonary infection with *Cryptococcus neoformans*. *Eur. J. Immunol.* 29(2): 643–649.

Retini, C., Casadevall, A., Pietrella, D., Monari, C., Palazzetti, B., and Vecchiarelli, A. (1999). Specific activated T cells regulate IL-12 production by human monocytes stimulated with *Cryptococcus neoformans*. *J. Immunol.* 162(3): 1618–1623.

Retini, C., Kozel, T.R., Pietrella, D., Monari, C., Bistoni, F., and Vecchiarelli, A. (2001). Interdependency of interleukin-10 and interleukin-12 in regulation of T-cell differentiation and effector function of monocytes in response to stimulation with *Cryptococcus neoformans*. *Infect. Immun.* 69(10): 6064–6073.

Ricchetti, A., Landis, B.N., Maffioli, A., Giger, R., Zeng, C., and Lacroix, J.S. (2002). Effect of anti-fungal nasal lavage with amphotericin B on nasal polyposis. *J. Laryngol. Otol.* 116(4): 261–263.

Rivera, J., Mukherjee, J., Weiss, L.M., and Casadevall, A. (2002). Antibody efficacy in murine pulmonary *Cryptococcus neoformans* infection: A role for nitric oxide. *J. Immunol.* 168(7): 3419–3427.

Roberts, C.W., Ferguson, D.J., Jebbari, H., Satoskar, A., Bluethmann, H., and Alexander, J. (1996). Different roles for interleukin-4 during the course of *Toxoplasma gondii* infection. *Infect. Immun.* 64(3): 897–904.

Salkowski, C.A. and Balish, E. (1990). Pathogenesis of *Cryptococcus neoformans* in congenitally immunodeficient beige athymic mice. *Infect. Immun.* 58(10): 3300–3306.

Schoenberger, S.P., Toes, R.E., van der Voort, E.I., Offringa, R., and Melief, C.J. (1998). T-cell help for cytotoxic T lymphocytes is mediated by CD40–CD40L interactions. *Nature* 393(6684): 480–483.

Segal, B.H., Bow, E.J., and Menichetti, F. (2002). Fungal infections in nontransplant patients with hematologic malignancies. *Infect. Dis. Clin. North Am.* 16(4): 935–964, vii.

Sergeeva, M.G., Gonchar, M.V., Mevkh, A.T., and Varfolomeyev, S.D. (1997). Prostaglandin E2 biphasic control of lymphocyte proliferation: Inhibition by picomolar concentrations. *FEBS Lett.* 418(3): 235–238.

Shedlock, D.J. and Shen, A. (2003). Requirement for CD4 T cell help in generating functional CD8 T cell memory. *Science* 300(5617): 337–339.

Snijdewint, F.G., Kalinski, P., Wierenga, E.A., Bos, J.D., and Kapsenberg, M.L. (1993). Prostaglandin E2 differentially modulates cytokine secretion profiles of human T helper lymphocytes. *J. Immunol.* 150(12): 5321–5329.

Stein, M., Keshav, S., Harris, N., and Gordon, S. (1992). Interleukin 4 potently enhances murine macrophage mannose receptor activity: A marker of alternative immunologic macrophage activation. *J. Exp. Med.* 176(1): 287–292.

Steinman, R.M. (1996). Dendritic cells and immune-based therapies. *Exp. Hematol.* 24(8): 859–862.

Syme, R.M., Wood, C.J., Wong, H., and Mody, C.H. (1997). Both $CD4^+$ and $CD8^+$ human lymphocytes are activated and proliferate in response to *Cryptococcus neoformans*. *Immunology* 92(2): 194–200.

Syme, R.M., Bruno, T.F., Kozel, T.R., and Mody, C.H. (1999). The capsule of *Cryptococcus neoformans* reduces T-lymphocyte proliferation by reducing phagocytosis, which can be restored with anticapsular antibody. *Infect. Immun.* 67(9): 4620–4627.

Syme, R.M., Spurrell, J.C., Ma, L.L., Green, F.H., and Mody, C.H. (2000). Phagocytosis and protein processing are required for presentation of *Cryptococcus neoformans* mitogen to T lymphocytes. *Infect. Immun.* 68(11): 6147–6153.

Syme, R.M., Spurrell, J.C.L., Amankwah, E.K., Green, F.H.Y., and Mody, C.H. (2002). Primary dendritic cells phagocytose *Cryptococcus neoformans* via mannose receptors and Fcγ receptor II for presentation to T lymphocytes. *Infect. Immun.* 70(11): 5972–5981.

Traynor, T.R. and Huffnagle, G.B. (2001). Role of chemokines in fungal infections. *Med. Mycol.* 39(1): 41–50.

Traynor, T.R., Kuziel, W.A., Toews, G.B., and Huffnagle, G.B. (2000). CCR2 expression determines T1 versus T2 polarization during pulmonary *Cryptococcus neoformans* infection. *J. Immunol.* 164(4): 2021–2027.

Traynor, T.R., Herring, A.C., Dorf, M.E., Kuziel, W.A., Toews, G.B., and Huffnagle, G.B. (2002). Differential roles of CC chemokine ligand 2/monocyte chemotactic protein-1 and CCR2 in the development of T1 immunity. *J. Immunol.* 168(9): 4659–4666.

Vecchiarelli, A. (2000). Immunoregulation by capsular components of *Cryptococcus neoformans*. *Med. Mycol.* 38(6): 407–417.

Vecchiarelli, A., Monari, C., Retini, C., Pietrella, D., Palazzetti, B., Pitzurra, L., and Casadevall, A. (1998). *Cryptococcus neoformans* differently regulates B7-1 (CD80) and B7-2 (CD86) expression on human monocytes. *Eur. J. Immunol.* 28(1): 114–121.

Vecchiarelli, A., Pietrella, D., Lupo, P., Bistoni, F., McFadden, D.C., and Casadevall, A. (2003). The polysaccharide capsule of *Cryptococcus neoformans* interferes with human dendritic cell maturation and activation. *J. Leukoc. Biol.* 74(3): 370–378.

Venarske, D.L. and deShazo, R.D. (2002). Sinobronchial allergic mycosis: The SAM syndrome. *Chest* 121(5): 1670–1676.

Walunas, T.L., Lenschow, D.J., Bakker, C.Y., Linsley, P.S., Freeman, G.J., Green, J.M., Thompson, C.B., and Bluestone, J.A. (1994). CTLA-4 can function as a negative regulator of T cell activation. *Immunity* 1(5): 405–413.

Walzl, G., Humphreys, I.R., Marshall, B.G., Edwards, L., Openshaw, P.J.M., Shaw, R.J., and Hussell, T. (2003). Prior exposure to live *Mycobacterium bovis* BCG decreases *Cryptococcus neoformans*-induced lung eosinophilia in a gamma interferon-dependent manner. *Infect. Immun.* 71(6): 3384–3391.

Wuthrich, M., Filutowicz, H.I., Warner, T., Deepe, G.S. Jr., and Klein, B.S. (2003). Vaccine immunity to pathogenic fungi overcomes the requirement for CD4 help in exogenous antigen presentation to $CD8^+$ T cells: Implications for vaccine development in immune-deficient hosts. *J. Exp. Med.* 197(11): 1405–1416.

Yamazumi, T., Pfaller, M.A., Messer, S.A., Houston, A.K., Boyken, L., Hollis, R.J., Furuta, I., and Jones, R.N. (2003). Characterization of heteroresistance to fluconazole among clinical isolates of *Cryptococcus neoformans*. *J. Clin. Microbiol.* 41(1): 267–272.

Yuan, R.R., Casadevall, A., Oh, J., and Scharff, M.D. (1997). T cells cooperate with passive antibody to modify *Cryptococcus neoformans* infection in mice. *Proc. Natl. Acad. Sci. USA* 94(6): 2483–2488.

Yuan, R., Clynes, R., Oh, J., Ravetch, J.V., and Scharff, M.D. (1998a). Antibody-mediated modulation of *Cryptococcus neoformans* infection is dependent on distinct Fc receptor functions and IgG subclasses. *J. Exp. Med.* 187(4): 641–648.

Yuan, R.R., Spira, G., Oh, J., Paizi, M., Casadevall, A., and Scharff, M.D. (1998b). Isotype switching increases efficacy of antibody protection against *Cryptococcus neoformans* infection in mice. *Infect. Immun.* 66(3): 1057–1062.

Zhang, T., Kawakami, K., Qureshi, M.H., Okamura, H., Kurimoto, M., and Saito, A. (1997). Interleukin-12 (IL-12) and IL-18 synergistically induce the fungicidal activity of murine peritoneal exudate cells against *Cryptococcus neoformans* through production of gamma interferon by natural killer cells. *Infect. Immun.* 65(9): 3594–3599.

9

Antibody-Mediated Immunity to Fungi in the Lungs

Marta Feldmesser and Arturo Casadevall

Division of Infectious Diseases, Department of Medicine, Albert Einstein College of Medicine, Bronx, New York.
Department of Microbiology and Immunology, Albert Einstein College of Medicine, Bronx, New York.
Division of Infectious Diseases, Department of Obstetrics & Gynecology and Women's Health, Albert Einstein College of Medicine, Bronx, New York.

1. Introduction

With the notable exception of *Candida* spp., infection with most fungal pathogens is acquired by inhalation and the lung is the most common site of primary infection. A common theme in fungal pathogenesis is that a significant proportion of primary infections are either subclinical or cause minimal symptoms and that primary pulmonary infection may regress spontaneously, particularly in immunocompetent hosts. Recognition that cell-mediated immune responses are crucial for host defense has deflected interest away from study of the role of antibody (Ab) in immune responses to invasive disease. The premise that cell-mediated responses are critical for host defense is supported by the association of disease with conditions where T cell immunity is impaired and granulomatous inflammation is linked with containment of disease in the lung. However, impaired cell-mediated responses also are accompanied by defects in humoral immunity and the relative contribution of each harm to host defense is unknown.

Insight into the role of Ab responses in host immunity to fungal infections has been provided by several patterns of investigation, including direct measurement of Ab or Ab-producing cells in this location. However, much of the Ab present in the lung is derived from systemic responses. Recently, fungal immunology research has focused primarily on determining the factors that allow the development of protective T_H1-associated responses. Toward that end, Ab responses are sometimes measured as part of characterization of the cytokine milieu following pulmonary infection. Study of animals with defects in Ab production due to targeted gene disruption has been applied to the investigation of the role of Ab. Substantial insight about Ab function has been provided by the effect of specific passive Ab on fungal disease in the lung. Here, we review what is known about Ab immunity to several pathogens in the lung.

2. Overview of Antibody Responses in the Lung

2.1. Naturally Occurring and Specific Ab

Ab present in the absence of specific antigenic challenge may differ from that produced in response to infection. The constitutively produced "natural" Ab pool is important for innate immunity. Natural Abs are mostly IgM and can bind to pathogens or antigens to which the host has never been exposed (Boes, 2000). After infection, specific Ab is produced that may function later in the course of subacute or chronic infection or as part of memory responses. Specific Ab responses are characterized by higher frequencies of IgG and higher affinity Abs to particular antigens. Thus, Ab from specific responses may function differently in response to infection than that present at the onset of infection. Two distinct lineages of B cells are responsible for Ab production in the lung that may differ in their relative contributions to innate compared to specific immune responses. In contrast to conventional bone marrow-derived B cells (B2 B cells) that are responsible for most Ab produced in response to antigenic challenge, B1 B cells maintain themselves by self-renewal for the life of the animal (Ishida et al., 1992). This population is rarely found in primary or secondary lymphoid tissue and, though predominantly studied in the peritoneum, is enriched in the pleural compartment (Marcos et al., 1989; Ishida et al., 1992). These cells produce a restricted repertoire of low-affinity Abs that are highly cross-reactive with self-determinants, do not mature by somatic mutation, and generate most of the IgM found in serum (Baumgarth et al., 1999). B1 B cells preferentially recognize T lymphocyte-independent antigens, such as polysaccharides and phospholipids (Kantor and Herzenberg, 1993).

2.2. Compartments in the Lung

2.2.1. *Upper Airways*

The lung may be viewed as divided into two compartments: larger airways, including bronchi, and the distal airways. Such distinction is relevant for consideration of Ab-mediated immunity, as regional responses differ in terms of the origin of Ab present, stimuli for local Ab production, and type of Ab produced (Kunkel and Butcher, 2003). The larger airways are part of the common mucosal immune system that includes not only other parts of the respiratory tract (trachea, nares, and pharynx), but also other mucosal compartments, including the gastrointestinal tract and the vagina. In these locations, a substantial proportion of Ab production occurs locally and Ab responses are highly influenced by cytokine production not only by classical immune cells, but also by the respiratory epithelium. Unlike the organized lymphoid systems found in other mucosal compartments (mucosal-associated lymphoid tissue (MALT)), in bronchus-associated lymphoid tissue (BALT), a typical compartment is not seen in many species, including humans, and, in most studies, no germinal centers are found (Pabst and Gehrke, 1990). Further, the M (microfold) cells that are responsible for antigen sampling in the intestinal lumen have not been identified in normal respiratory mucosa (Pilette et al., 2001). Thus, it has been proposed that additional cell types are responsible for stimulating local Ab production in the normal host (Salvi and Holgate, 1999).

The predominant Ab found in the upper airway is IgA. IgA may exist in dimeric or monomeric forms. Monomeric serum IgA is produced mainly in the bone marrow, while in the respiratory tract, locally produced IgA is predominantly dimeric (Salvi and Holgate, 1999). In addition to those made by host immune cells of hematopoietic origin, bronchial epithelial cells provide cytokines that are important for IgA production, including IL-10, transforming growth factor (TGF)-β, IL-5, and IL-6 (Cromwell et al., 1992; Magnan et al., 1994; Bonfield et al., 1995; Salvi et al., 1999). IgA produced by Ab-secreting cells in the lung interstitium or derived from the systemic circulation is transported from these sites to luminal surfaces by transcytosis. IgA is bound by the polymeric Ig receptor (pIgR) found on basolateral surfaces of bronchial epithelial cells and on endothelial cells. Following endocytosis, pIgR bound to IgA may be transported to the apical membrane, where proteolytic cleavage results in release of secretory (S) IgA, consisting of polymeric IgA attached to secretory component (SC), the residua of the pIgR (Pilette et al., 2001).

In the airway lumen, the major function attributed to IgA is "immune exclusion"—by binding to microbes or their antigens, these components are prevented from adhering to host tissue and their clearance is facilitated (Reynolds, 1987; Salvi and Holgate, 1999). The polymeric nature of SIgA enhances its capacity for agglutination. Traditionally, IgA has been viewed as an isotype that removes microbes or microbial components while not triggering proinflammatory responses, such as complement activation or Ab-dependent cellular cytotoxicity (ADCC). More recently, IgA has been shown to be capable of inducing proinflammatory effects through complement activation or Fc receptor (FcR) binding (Kerr, 1990; Arulanandam et al., 2001; Pilette et al., 2001).

IgG, which is monomeric, is present in the tracheobronchial tree, though in amounts far below those of IgA. Further, far fewer Ab-secreting cells in the bronchial mucosa produce IgG than IgA (Soutar, 1976). IgG can enter the upper airway by passive diffusion or transudation from serum or following production by plasma cells in the bronchial mucosa (Soutar, 1976; Lamm, 1997; Brandtzaeg et al., 1997). The functions of IgG are discussed below.

IgM is detected in bronchoalveolar lavage fluid only in very low concentrations, a feature that is attributed to the large size of the pentameric form of the Ab, resulting in less transudation from plasma (Burnett, 1986; Reynolds, 1987). Nonetheless, IgM is found in BAL fluid in concentrations higher than can be explained by simple diffusion from the blood (Burnett, 1986). IgM-producing cells are found in the bronchial mucosa and, like IgA, pentameric IgM can be transcytosed via the poly-IgR and released in conjunction with SC. IgM is the isotype that activates complement most efficiently and, because of its polymeric structure, IgM can agglutinate antigens strongly (Burnett, 1986). Thus, like IgA, IgM in the airways can function in immune exclusion. IgE is present in both serum and bronchoalveolar lavage fluids at low concentrations (Burnett, 1986). This isotype, which may be produced by B cells in the bronchial mucosa, is an important mediator of hypersensitivity responses to inhaled antigens, the subject of another chapter that will not be considered further here.

2.2.2. Distal Airways

In contrast, the lower lung compartment, including the alveolar space, is not considered part of the common mucosal immune system (Zuercher et al., 2002). Rather, Ab responses in the distal lung are believed to reflect systemic responses. In fluid obtained by lavage of the distal airways of normal human lung, immunoglobulin accounts for approximately 14% of the total protein content, yet cells of B lymphocyte lineage represent less than 1% of all cells recovered from BAL (Merrill et al., 1985; Reynolds, 1988; Hance et al., 1988). IgA predominates in fluid obtained by distal airway lavage, accounting for about half of the total immunoglobulin. IgA-producing cells are found in the lamina propria of bronchioles but are absent from terminal bronchioles and alveolar epithelium (Soutar, 1976). The proportion of IgG in this compartment is increased compared to the upper airways.

IgG in the distal airway is derived largely from plasma (Reynolds, 1988). Proteins significantly larger than 150 kDa are excluded from passage into the alveolar space, but IgG can pass freely by transudation (Reynolds, 1987). Alveolar macrophages may downregulate local Ab production (Kaltreider et al., 1986; Blumenthal et al., 2001). Human alveolar macrophages can preferentially inhibit IgG and IgM production by B cells in response to stimulation with T cell-independent antigens, while having little effect on IgA synthesis (Wilkes et al., 1993). Of the human IgG subclasses, IgG1 is most abundant in serum, followed by IgG2, IgG3, and then IgG4. IgG4 is present at higher Ig-to-albumin ratios in BAL fluid than in serum (Reynolds, 1987). Local production of IgG4 and possibly IgG3 is thought to be higher than that of IgG1 or IgG2 (Merrill et al., 1985). Antigenic challenge may alter the location of Ab production within the lung. In the terminal airway of normal human lung, Ab-producing cells are localized to the interstitium and little synthesis occurs on the alveolar epithelial layer (Hance et al., 1988). Following antigenic challenge, Ab-producing cells are found in the alveolar space. These cells are derived from the blood but can mature in the lung (Bice et al., 1987). Specific Ab responses in this compartment result from the development of Ab-secreting cells in regional lymph nodes with subsequent homing of these cells back to the airway based upon selective expression of adhesion molecules (Kaltreider et al., 1987; Kunkel and Butcher, 2003).

The mechanism of action of IgG largely is mediated by binding to FcRs. Activation receptors for IgG are present on most immune effector cells, including monocytes, macrophages, neutrophils, dendritic cells, NK cells, eosinophils, and platelets, but are not found on T cells (Fanger et al., 1996; Ravetch and Bolland, 2001). In addition, FcγRs have been identified on cells of the human alveolar epithelial type II cell line A549, suggesting the potential for receptor-mediated interaction with Ab (Salik et al., 1999). Inhibitory FcRs are present on macrophages, neutrophils, B cells, and mast cells, but not T cells or NK cells (Ravetch and Bolland, 2001). Activation through FcγRs results in phagocytosis, degranulation, ADCC, transcription of cytokine genes, and release of inflammatory mediators (Ravetch and Bolland, 2001). In the airspace, IgG functions as an opsonin, triggering phagocytosis of microorganisms by macrophages, neutrophils, and dendritic cells. While 25% of human alveolar macrophages can bind IgG3 and 10% bind IgG4, no significant binding of IgG1 or IgG2 is observed, suggesting that IgG3 and IgG4 may be the most important subclasses for opsonization of microbial pathogens (Burnett, 1986). Complement activation by the classical pathway resulting in the generation of complement breakdown products generates additional opsonic fragments, including C3b, and fragments with chemotactic properties, such as C5a. Human IgG1, IgG2, and IgG3 can activate complement via classical pathway, while IgG4 does not (Burnett, 1986).

3. Ab-Mediated Immunity: Specific Pathogens

3.1. *Aspergillus fumigatus*

Aspergillus fumigatus causes disease through allergy induction or tissue destruction resulting from fungal growth. Apart from hypersensitivity responses, pulmonary diseases due to *A. fumigatus* include aspergillomas, fungal masses that grow in preexisting cavities, and invasive aspergillosis, which occurs most commonly in severely immunocompromised hosts. Conidia (spores) are the infectious particles and are typically 2 to 3 μm in size, enabling them to reach the distal airway (Latge, 1999).

Abs to *A. fumigatus* antigens are found in the serum of normal hosts, appearing in late infancy and increasing with age (Bardana et al., 1972; Bardana, 1974). Presumably, these responses occur because of exposure to *A. fumigatus*, but the possibility that they represent responses to cross-reactive antigens cannot be excluded. IgG, IgA, and IgM to *A. fumigatus* antigens are found in bronchial secretions of 58%, 83%, and 5%, respectively, of patients without aspergillosis (Schonheyder et al., 1983). In contrast, all of those tested had serum IgG, while fewer had IgA. Monomeric IgA was detected more frequently than sIgA in bronchial secretions, suggesting that this Ab reached the lung from the systemic circulation. However, the presence of SC also suggested that local Ab synthesis occurs. It has been proposed that the response occurring in the absence of disease prevents the development of hypersensitivity reactions to *A. fumigatus* antigens.

Initial efforts to characterize Ab responses to pulmonary aspergillosis beyond the context of hypersensitivity reactions focused on study of patients with aspergilloma. Multiple studies have documented the development of serum IgG responses to *A. fumigatus* antigens, while IgM and IgA responses have been variably documented (Bardana et al., 1972; Bardana, 1974; Schonheyder et al., 1982; Kostiala et al., 1984; Huizinga et al., 1985; Reen, 1988; Kurup et al., 1988; Reijula et al., 1991). In a study of Ab responses in patients with aspergilloma, only IgG1 binding to *A. fumigatus* culture filtrate antigens was elevated compared to isotypes found in control sera (Kurup et al., 1990). In contrast, the traditional view has been that the degree of immunocompromise in patients with invasive aspergillosis prevents the development of systemic Ab responses and Ab titers fall as disease becomes more severe (Young and Bennett,

1971; Matthews et al., 1985; Weig et al., 2001).

The effect of Ab on pathogenesis or host responses to pulmonary aspergillosis is unclear. The presence of serum IgA to a high molecular weight fraction correlated inversely with the ability to culture *A. fumigatus* from the respiratory tract of patients with cystic fibrosis, suggesting that sIgA could protect against airway colonization (Schonheyder et al., 1985). In the case of aspergilloma, the presence of Abs with specificities not found in the absence of disease was suggested to limit fungal invasion (Bardana et al., 1972; Kobayashi et al., 1993). However, direct demonstration of a role for Ab is lacking. In vitro, rabbit alveolar macrophages more effectively kill *A. fumigatus* conidia in the presence of immune serum than normal serum, though phagocytosis is not altered (Kurup, 1984). Abs capable of mediating ADCC have been demonstrated in sera of patients with aspergilloma (Kurup et al., 1985). Study of aspergillosis in chicks found that appearance of serum Ab reactive with hyphal fragments correlated with resistance to pulmonary infection and that development of serum precipitins coincided with hyphal clearance from the lung (Taylor and Burroughs, 1973). However, mice with targeted disruption of the IgM constant region (μMT mice), in whom B cell development is arrested at the pre-B cell stage and who do not have surface IgM (Kitamura et al., 1991), had lower lung fungal burden following intranasal (i.n.) infection, compared to wild-type controls (Montagnoli et al., 2003). When cyclophosphamide was given to induce neutropenia, prolonged survival and lower fungal burden were demonstrated in infected μMT mice. These findings could be interpreted as suggesting that neither Ab nor B cells are required for resistance to invasive pulmonary aspergillosis. However, in these mice, compensatory changes in other potentially important cell populations have been demonstrated in response to infection with other pathogens (van der Heyde et al., 1996). Thus, only limited conclusion can be drawn from these experiments. In addition, passive transfer of normal mouse serum to nonneutropenic μMT mice resulted in further control of fungal burden compared to those that did not receive serum (Montagnoli et al., 2003), maintaining the possibility that naturally occurring Ab is beneficial to the host.

In summary, the literature regarding Ab responses to pulmonary infection with *A. fumigatus* contains studies in which a variety of crude antigen preparations were used that were not standardized for content, strain, or form of the organism. Evaluation of systemic responses in patients with aspergilloma revealed that systemic IgG is made in response to pulmonary disease. More recently, the use of purified or recombinant Ags has provided reagents to characterize Ab responses. However, our understanding of Ab responses in the lung remains rudimentary, as does our understanding of the contribution of Ab to immunity or pathogenesis of pulmonary *A. fumigatus* infections.

3.2. *Blastomyces dermatitidis*

Following inhalation of *Blastomyces dermatitidis* conidia, germination and phase transition to the yeast form occur in the lung. Primary infection results in pneumonia that most commonly resolves spontaneously, though bronchial ulceration can lead to endobronchial spread, resulting in fulminant infection (Sarosi and Davies, 1979). Chronic disease can ensue that may be associated with dissemination to any organ, though the lung frequently remains involved.

Serological testing for *B. dermatitidis* historically was less sensitive or specific than with other dimorphic fungal pathogens. Based upon studies using an enzyme immunoassay (EIA) to A antigen, a yeast filtrate antigen preparation containing numerous proteins and glycoproteins, acute pulmonary blastomycosis is believed to cause short-lived systemic Ab responses in patients with self-limited disease or who are effectively treated. No correlation was found between serological results and symptomatic or severe acute infections (Kaufman et al., 1973; Klein et al., 1987). In chronic infection, higher titers correlate with the presence of disseminated disease (Klein et al., 1986; Turner et al., 1986).

In a murine model of *B. dermatitidis* infection, plasma cells were present in perivascular spaces adjacent to inflammatory foci 1 to 3 weeks following intratracheal (i.t.) infection. At this time, peribronchial lymph nodes became fully developed with germinal centers and medullary accumulations that contained plasma cells (Williams et al., 1994). These findings support the view that both local Ab synthesis and regional lymph node stimulation contribute to Ab responses to pulmonary *B. dermatitidis* infection. In this model, serum Ab to A antigen was not detected by EIA until 35 days after infection, suggesting either that this test was insensitive or that Ab was being produced to antigens other than those contained in A antigen preparations.

As with *A. fumigatus*, B cell-deficient μMT mice are more resistant than wild-type littermate controls to lethal i.n. infection with *B. dermatitidis*, with significantly prolonged survival and lower lung fungal burdens 20 days after infection (Wuthrich and Klein, 2000). Though these results have been proposed to indicate that the favoring of a T_H1-like phenotype may enhance resistance, as recognized by the investigators, T_H phenotypes have not been measured directly in this system (Wuthrich and Klein, 2000). Thus, though a possible interpretation of these experiments is that Ab induced by infection is deleterious, alternative possibilities cannot be excluded.

3.3. *Coccidioides immitis*

In approximately 60% of immunocompetent hosts, primary *Coccidioides immitis* infection in the lung is asymptomatic or mild enough so that affected individuals do not seek medical care (Pappagianis, 2001). Common features of primary pneumonia include the presence of unilateral infiltrates, hilar adenopathy, and pleural effusions. Complete resolution usually occurs, though a few die from acute pneumonia and ~0.5% of infected immunocompetent individuals develop disseminated disease (Stevens, 1995). Higher Ab titers correlate with more severe disease, such that those with localized disease in the lung and draining lymph nodes rarely have complement fixation (CF) titers, which detect IgG binding to a chitinase (Johnson and Pappagianis, 1992), above 1:16, though higher titers occasionally have been seen in patients with prominent tracheobronchial or mediastinal lymphadenopathy (Pappagianis and Zimmer, 1990). Chronic cavitary disease has been associated with persistent serum tube precipitin (TP) Abs, whose formation results from a reaction of IgM with several *C. immitis* macromolecules and a 21kDa serine proteinase (Smith et al., 1950; Cole et al., 1991).

For *C. immitis*, very little is known about the local Ab response in the lung. Pulmonary Ab isotype concentrations have not been measured and pathogenesis of pulmonary infection in the selective absence of Ab has not been studied. Smith et al. (1950) reported testing of simultaneous pleural fluid and serum samples from 13 patients with coccidioidal hydropneumothorax. These investigators found that CF titers are the same in pleural fluid as in serum in a few paired samples, while titers are higher in serum in the remainder. This finding is in concert with the view that systemic synthesis may be more important than local synthesis as a source for Ab in pleural fluid.

The role of Ab in host defense or pathogenesis is unknown with respect to pulmonary coccidioidomycosis. The finding that higher Ab titers correlate with more severe and disseminated disease has been cited as evidence to support a harmful role (Cox and Arnold, 1979). In vitro, alveolar macrophages from rhesus macaques phagocytose *C. immitis* endospores and spherules without the need for exogenous opsonin. Phagolysosomal fusion is impaired in comparison to that observed following phagocytosis of *Candida albicans*, this macrophage population is unable to kill the organism and intracellular replication ensues. Immune serum from an infected macaque containing CF Abs, but not TP Abs, did not enhance phagocytosis, phagolysosomal fusion, or fungal killing (Beaman and Holmberg, 1980). This finding suggests that Ab occurring in response to infection does not directly enhance macrophage effector function in the lung, but a range of variables have not been explored, including the roles of Ab specificity, isotype, and quantity.

3.4. *Cryptococcus neoformans*

In the overwhelming majority of normal humans, initial infection with *Cryptococcus neoformans* presumably can be eradicated by the immune response or may become latent, with the organisms contained in a granuloma within a subpleural nodule. Disseminated infection may follow initial infection in certain individuals or may follow reactivation of latent disease in circumstances of acquired immunodeficiency (Garcia-Hermoso et al., 1999). Serologic studies indicate that the prevalence of Abs reactive with *C. neoformans* protein and polysaccharide antigens among individuals with and without a history of cryptocococcosis is high (Abadi and Pirofski, 1999; Fleuridor et al., 1999; Goldman et al., 2001). A study of over 100 children in New York City that assayed serum Ab for *C. neoformans* protein antigens found that >70% of children older than 5 years of age were seropositive and concluded that initial cryptococcal infection occurred in early childhood (Goldman et al., 2001).

The role of the natural Ab response in defense against *C. neoformans* infection in the lung is uncertain, but there is some evidence from rat, mouse, and human studies suggesting that the type of Ab response elicited correlates with the outcome of infection. In rat pulmonary infection, granuloma formation coincides with the appearance of serum Ab opsonins, suggesting a temporal association between a humoral response and control of infection (Goldman et al., 1994). Furthermore, the establishment of persistent infection is associated with downregulation of both cellular and humoral immune responses to *C. neoformans* (Goldman et al., 2000). Pulmonary *C. neoformans* infection in mice elicits Abs to both the capsular polysaccharide and protein antigens. Among protein antigens, heat shock protein 70 is a major target of the humoral response (Kakeya et al., 1997). In BALB/c mice, pulmonary infection elicits serum Abs that produce immunofluorescence patterns associated with nonprotective Abs (Zaragoza and Casadevall, 2004). Although both IgM and IgG were produced in response to infection, staining of yeast cells in alveolar spaces revealed only IgG, suggesting that only this isotype crossed into the alveolar space.

In summary, the biological relevance of the Ab response to *C. neoformans* pulmonary infection is uncertain. In rats and humans, circumstantial evidence supports an association between this response and resistance to infection. Interestingly, both species are relatively resistant to cryptococcosis. In contrast, for mice, there is currently no evidence that the natural Ab response contributes to defense against pulmonary cryptococcosis and this species is considered highly susceptible. In fact, a comparison of C.B.-17 (resistant) and BALB/c (susceptible) mice suggested that a genetic difference at the immunoglobulin heavy chain locus was responsible for the genetic difference in susceptibility (Lovchik et al., 1999).

3.5. *Histoplasma capsulatum*

Histoplasma capsulatum is an endemic fungus found in the Ohio–Mississippi river valley and certain parts of the Caribbean and South America. A different variety of the fungus is found in Africa that is known as *Histoplasma duboisii*. Human *H. capsulatum* infection is associated with strong Ab responses to fungal antigens, including ribosomes and histoplasmin (Raman et al., 1990). Isotype analysis reveals that all types of histoplasmosis are associated with elevated levels of IgG and IgA and depressed levels of IgM (Caldwell et al., 1983). A significant proportion of the Abs elicited by *H. capsulatum* infection are cross-reactive with other fungi such as *B. dermatitidis*, *C. neoformans*, and *C. albicans* (Raman et al., 1990), contributing to the difficulties with using serology for diagnosis and in associating Ab responses with outcomes to infection.

At this time there is no evidence to support the view that natural Ab responses to *H. capsulatum* contribute to host defense. B cell-deficient μMT mice are not more susceptible to experimental pulmonary histoplasmosis than wild-type mice (Allendorfer et al., 1999). However, as discussed in Section 4.2 below, the absence of evidence should not be construed as absence of Ab efficacy against *H. capsulatum*.

3.6. *Paracoccidioides brasiliensis*

Primary pulmonary infection with *Paracoccidioides brasiliensis* results in the development of two forms of disease—the acute (juvenile) form that is associated with extensive lymphoreticular involvement and the more common chronic (adult) form, which may be uni- or multicentric. While the lung may be involved in both forms, unicentric disease may not be accompanied by detectable infection in the lung (Brummer et al., 1993). Both human disease and animal models are characterized by the presence of high titers of specific Abs to *P. brasiliensis* antigens in the serum and disease progression correlates with Ab titer, which reflects the extent of dissemination (Greer and McMurray, 1981; Defaveri et al., 1982; Biagioni et al., 1984; Tani et al., 1987; Castaneda et al., 1988).

Comparison of mice with isolated pulmonary paracoccidioidomycosis to those with disseminated disease provides a window into the effect of systemic Ab responses on pulmonary disease. Study of pulmonary infection in resistant A/Sn mice and susceptible B10.6 mice, whose differing susceptibility to *P. brasiliensis* maps to the pbr locus, showed that A/Sn mice have higher lung fungal burdens than do B10.6 mice but similar patterns of pulmonary pathology, despite the finding that the former do not develop disseminated disease. Comparable increases in the numbers of Ig^+ cells in the lungs by 4 weeks after infection are found in these strains (Cano et al., 2000). Both mouse strains produce Ab of all IgG subclasses, though A/Sn mice have higher serum titers of IgG2a and IgG3 than do B10.A mice, while the latter produce IgG1 and IgG2b earlier than they produce IgG2a and IgG3 (Cano et al., 1995). These findings are consistent with patterns of cytokine measurement in lung homogenates from infected mice, which show that, in both resistant and susceptible mice, a mixed T_H1–T_H2 cytokine response is detected in the lung, though higher concentrations of IFN-γ, IL-4, IL-5, and IL-10, but not IL-2, are found in the lungs of susceptible mice (Cano et al., 1998). These results raised the possibility that IgG2a and IgG3, isotypes produced in the context of T_H1-associated responses, played a role in preventing dissemination. However, anti-IFN-γ treatment abrogated resistance to dissemination in A/Sn mice while increasing total specific Ig, IgG1, Ig2a, and IgG2b concentrations in this strain, without altering IgG3, suggesting that Ab was not mediating this control. Conversely, administration of IL-12, an important regulator of T_H1-associated cytokine production, on days 0 through 5 after i.t. infection to B10.A mice did not alter lung fungal burden but reduced dissemination (Arruda et al., 2002). Lung inflammation was enhanced from 1 to 8 weeks after infection and, while 1 week after infection, lung IFN-γ concentration was increased, at the latter time, lung concentrations of both T_H1- and T_H2-associated cytokines and serum IgG1 and IgG3 titers were lower than in control mice. These findings suggest that a more T_H1-like environment results in containment within the lung but argue against a causal role for Ab in these effects (Carvalhaes et al., 1986).

In summary, systemic Ab responses correlate with the cytokine milieu found in the lung and manipulation has produced alterations in relative proportions of Ab isotypes that would be predicted based upon our current understanding of the role of cytokines in isotype switching. At present, we know little of Ab function in pathogenesis or protection in the specific environment of the lung during paracoccidioidomycosis.

4. Effect of Exogenous Antibody Administration on Pulmonary Fungal Infection

The ability of systemic Ab to influence the course of pulmonary infection is amply illustrated by experiments where administration of exogenous Ab to a nonimmune host changes the outcome of infection to the benefit of the host. In the preantibiotic era, horse immune sera was demonstrated to be highly effective for therapy of human *Streptococcus pneumoniae* pneumonia when administered shortly after the onset of symptoms (Casadevall and Scharff, 1994). Today, Ab therapy is used for the prophylaxis and therapy of respiratory syncytial virus pulmonary infections (Groothuis et al., 1993). Among the medically important fungi, the ability of exogenous Ab to influence experimental murine pulmonary infection has been studied for *C. neoformans*, *H. capsulatum*, *P. brasiliensis*, *B. dermatitidis*, and *A. fumigatus*.

4.1. *C. neoformans*

Systemic administration of an IgG1 to *C. neoformans* capsular glucuronoxylomannan prior to experimental pulmonary infection significantly prolonged survival for Ab-treated A/J and C57BL/6 mice without a reduction in pulmonary fungal burden in the first 4 weeks of infection (Feldmesser and Casadevall, 1997; Feldmesser et al., 1998). Approximately 80% of Ab-treated A/J mice survived pulmonary infection and a third of these mice cleared the infection from their lungs (Fig. 9.1). Ab-treated and control mice manifested differences in the appearance of the inflammatory response, with Ab-treated mice having more localized disease. For C57BL/6 mice, Ab administration was associated with significant reduction in the number of granules per eosinophil, indicating increased degranulation and/or a change in eosinophil physiology (Feldmesser et al., 1998).

In vitro, specific Ab is a potent opsonin for *C. neoformans* and addition of capsule-binding IgG to suspensions of macrophages and yeast cells resulted in transient reduction of fungal colony-forming units (CFUs), consistent with enhanced killing of yeast cells by macrophages (Mukherjee et al., 1995, 1996). However, the observation that passive Ab was protective without significant reductions in lung CFU early in infection made the hypothesis that Ab functioned primarily as an opsonin less attractive. In fact, the observation that *C. neoformans* is rapidly phagocytosed by lung alveolar macrophages irrespective of Ab administration argued against a mechanism of Ab-mediated protection based on enhanced opsonization of yeast cells (Feldmesser et al., 2000). This result, combined with differences in inflammation, suggested that Ab was mediating protective effects in the lung

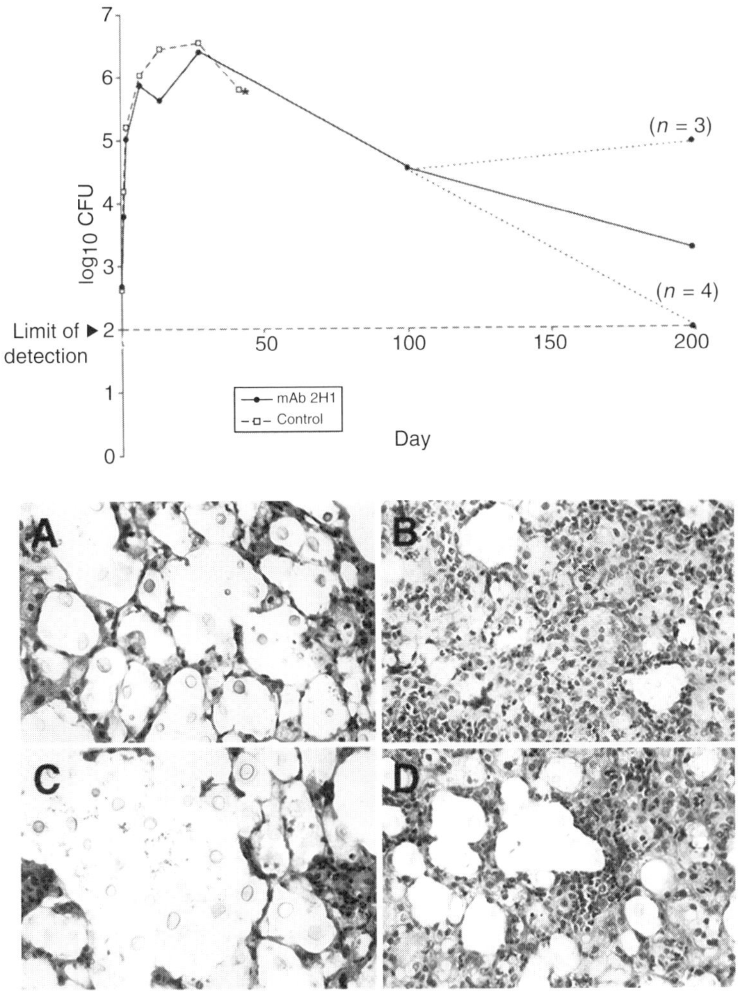

Figure 9.1. Top: The relationship between lung CFU and time in control and mAb 2H1-treated mice following i.t. infection with 10^4 *C. neoformans* yeast. MAb 2H1 (1 mg/mouse) was given intraperitoneally 24 h prior to infection. Values represent means. Broken lines from day 100 to day 199 represent the curves when day 199 mice were separated into those with detectable lung CFU (upper line) and those for whom CFU were not detectable (lower line). Asterisk (*) indicates point after which CFU data could not be obtained from control animals because they began to die rapidly. For control mice, n = 10, 9, 8, 10, 12, 13, and 4 at 2, 24, 48 h, 7, 14, 28, and 42 days, respectively. For mAb 2H1-treated mice, n = 10, 10, 10, 11, 10, 27, 4, and 7 at 2, 24, 48 h, 7, 14, 28, 100, and 199 days, respectively. Because the curves are derived from multiple experiments, statistical analysis was not included. Bottom: A and C, day 28 lungs of two control mice show a predominance of extracellular *C. neoformans*. Organisms were able to grow freely in the alveolar space outside of inflammatory foci. B and D, day 28 lungs of two mAb 2H1-treated mice show granulomatous inflammation and predominantly intracellular *C. neoformans* (arrows). In mAb 2H1-treated mice, organisms were usually contained within foci of inflammation; H&E stain, X250. Reproduced with permission from *J. Immunol.* 1997; 158: 790–799. Copyright 1997. The American Association of Immunologists, Inc.

of *C. neoformans*-infected mice by altering the inflammatory response in a manner that reduced host damage.

The hypothesis that Ab was protective through immunomodulatory effects was tested by comparing cytokine and leukocyte responses in the lung of A/J mice infected with *C. neoformans* in the presence and absence of exogenously administered IgG1. Despite the histological differences associated with the inflammatory response to *C. neoformans* in the presence and absence of exogenous IgG1 mAb, fluorescence-activated cell sorter analysis of lung homogenates revealed no significant differences in the number of leukocytes in mAb-treated and control mice (Feldmesser et al., 2002). However, cytokine and cellular marker analysis of lung homogenates revealed quantitative differences between mAb-treated and control mice that, alone or in combination, may have been responsible for the beneficial effect of Ab. Specifically, mAb-treated mice had more granulocytes at day 14 and higher macrophage CD86 surface expression on day 28. At day 7, analysis of lung homogenates revealed that mAb-treated mice had higher amounts of IL-10, a trend toward lower amounts of IFN-γ and a smaller increase in IL-4. Since control of *C. neoformans* infection in the lung requires granuloma formation, which implies at T_H1-polarized response, the observation of higher levels of IL-10 and a trend towards lower levels of IFN-γ would appear paradoxical. However, the observation that control mice die and mAb-treated mice survive despite comparable lung CFUs suggest that mortality in control mice is probably mediated by factors other than microbial burden and implies the possibility of immune-mediated damage. In this scenario, the higher levels of IL-10 and lower levels of IFN-γ may serve to downregulate the intensity of the inflammatory response and reduce lung damage. According to this view, the histological differences between mAb-treated and control mice could reflect better organization of the inflammatory cell infiltrate in mAb-treated mice as a consequence of downregulation of the immune response by higher amounts of IL-10 and lower amounts of IFN-γ. The increased numbers of granulocytes at day 14 could provide additional effector cells against *C. neoformans* and the higher expression of CD86 in macrophages may reflect enhanced functional capacity.

Analysis of inflammatory responses in inducible NO synthase (NOS2)-sufficient and -deficient C57BL/6 mice provides additional support for the theme that exogenous Ab mediates protection by modulating the cellular immune response (Rivera et al., 2002). $NOS2^{-/-}$ mice were more susceptible to *C. neoformans* infection than wild-type controls despite lower lung CFUs. Exogenous IgG1 mAb was protective against pulmonary infection in C57BL/6 mice but had no effect in $NOS2^{-/-}$ mice. Histological examination indicated a florid inflammatory response in $NOS2^{-/-}$ mice, consistent with the view that the increased susceptibility was a function of host inflammatory damage as a consequence of immune regulatory defects in the absence of NOS. The intense inflammatory response in $NOS2^{-/-}$ mice was paralleled by significantly higher lung levels of IFN-γ, MCP-1, and MIP-1α than observed in parental mice with *C. neoformans* infection. In this system, the only measurable cytokine differences in parental C57BL/6 mice were modest increases in both IL-4 and IFN-γ concentrations in IgG1 mAb-treated mice. However, in $NOS2^{-/-}$ mice, exogenous IgG1 mAb administration was associated with major reductions in IFN-γ, MCP-1, and MIP-1α concentrations, although the decrease was not sufficient to reduce the level of these cytokines to those measured in parental mice. The inefficacy of exogenous IgG1 mAb in $NOS2^{-/-}$ mice illustrates the inability of Ab to mediate protection in the absence of a major regulator of the immune response. Furthermore, the differences in cytokine and inflammatory response measured in the presence and absence of exogenous IgG1 mAb illustrate a dependence on genetic background for the type of effects mediated by specific Ab.

The mechanism of exogenous Ab-mediated protection against *C. neoformans* in the lung can be considered in the context of the "damage–response" framework of microbial pathogenesis, which posits that the relevant outcome of the host–microbe interaction is the amount of damage incurred by the host and that damage can originate from the microbe, the host, or both (Casadevall and Pirofski, 2003). According to this synthesis, the amount of damage as a function of immune response is a parabolic relationship where most host damage occurs in situations of weak or strong immune responses (Fig. 9.2A). Since there is ample evidence that cell-mediated immunity makes a critical contribution to host defense for *C. neoformans*, one can place the intensity of the cell-mediated response in the *x*-axis (Fig. 9.2B). Hence, Ab-mediated protection can be envisioned as reducing inflammatory damage. Although this scheme is almost certainly a simplification of a very complex process, it provides a construct for understanding how Ab-associated increases in T_H2-related cytokines and/or reductions in T_H1-related cytokines are implicated in Ab-mediated protection of a process that is dependent on competent cell-mediated responses.

In summary, IgG1 mAb to *C. neoformans* polysaccharide is protective against cryptococcal infection in mice by a mechanism that involves modulation of the immune response through changes in both T_H1- and T_H2-associated cytokines. IgG1 mAb administration produced different effects on the cytokine profile of A/J and C57BL/6 mice infected with *C. neoformans*, suggesting that Ab-mediated protection may be achieved through different combinations of changes to the cytokine response to infection. An emerging theme in these studies is the view that exogenous Ab protects mice by reducing immune-mediated damage to the lung. Reduced damage can promote or result in a more effective inflammatory response, which effectively controls the infection and reduces mortality (Casadevall and Pirofski, 2003).

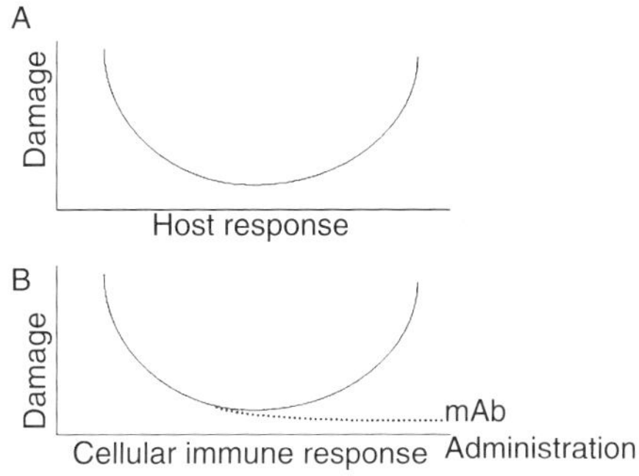

Figure 9.2. (A) The damage-response framework proposes that host damage is a function of the host response with damage occurring primarily in hosts that mount weak or strong responses. In this synthesis, administration of Ab to hosts capable of mounting strong immune responses translates into protective efficacy by reducing the amount of host-mediated damage. *C. neoformans* has been proposed to be a Class II pathogen in humans (Casadevall and Pirofski, 1999) but behaves as a Class III pathogen in mice, since both immunocompetent and immunocompromised mice are susceptible to experimental infection. (B) Ab administration to mice alters the Class III curve to resemble that of Class II, whereby normal mice are less susceptible. However, passive Ab is not effective in mice with defective cell-mediated immunity and, consequently, the left part of the curve is not affected by exogenous Ab.

4.2. *H. capsulatum*

An IgM mAb to a surface histone-like protein of *H. capsulatum* prolonged survival in lethally infected mice when the Ab was incubated with conidia prior to infection (Nosanchuk et al., 2003). Systemic administration of the

IgM mAb prior to infection had only a modest effect on survival, presumably because of poor penetration of IgM into the alveolar space. Ab-mediated protection against *H. capsulatum* was associated with comparable CFUs and reduced inflammation relative to control mice. mAb-treated mice had higher levels of IL-4 and IL-6 at day 2 of infection and increased levels of IFN-γ at day 7. These results echo the findings with Ab-mediated protection against *C. neoformans*, with the important caveats that those studies used IgG1 instead of IgM and that the observed cytokine changes are different. Although that study established that Ab can modify the course of infection to the benefit of the host, these data do not necessarily imply that similar Abs are elicited in the course of infection. In fact, analysis of the mouse Ab response revealed no serum Abs to this histone-like protein in the course of natural infection, suggesting that this protein is a cryptic antigen in infection. Hence, one explanation for difficulty in establishing an important role for Ab in host defense to *H. capsulatum* is that the response to infection does not include the generation of certain protective Abs.

4.3. *P. brasiliensis*

Concomitant administration of two IgG1 mAbs to the 70 kDa glycoprotein antigen of *P. brasiliensis* resulted in beneficial outcome in an i.t. model of *P. brasiliensis* (de Mattos Grosso et al., 2003). This antigen is predominantly located intracellularly but also can be detected in culture supernatant and in the urine of patients with the acute form of paracoccidioidomycosis (Salina et al., 1998; de Mattos Grosso et al., 2003). Gp70 can inhibit phagocytosis of particles via both mannose receptors and FcRs on peritoneal macrophages, reduces NO production by nonactivated peritoneal macrophages and decreases H_2O_2 production by resting or activated peritoneal macrophages. Administration of the mAbs significantly reduced CFU in the lungs of mice 45 days after infection with *P. brasiliensis*, compared to controls. Sole administration of one of the mAbs, which binds a protein epitope, had no effect, while a trend toward reduction in lung fungal burden followed single administration of the other, whose gp70 binding capacity is inhibited by carbohydrate. While lungs of control mice contained inflammatory cellular infiltrates and well-organized granulomas with large numbers of predominantly intracellular yeast, in mice that received both mAbs, the parenchyma was preserved and neither granuloma nor yeast cells were observed (de Mattos Grosso et al., 2003). Effects on survival have not been reported. In contrast, beneficial outcome was not seen following passive administration of IgG2a mAbs to the laminin-binding immunodominant gp43 antigen of *P. brasiliensis* (de Mattos Grosso et al., 2003).

4.4. *B. dermatitidis*

In contrast to the experience with *C. neoformans*, *H. capsulatum*, and *P. brasiliensis*, administration of IgG1 mAbs to the BAD-1 antigen (formerly known as WI-1) prior to i.n. infection did not result in improved outcome (Wuthrich and Klein, 2000). In some experiments there was the suggestion that mAb administration enhanced infection, as indicated by a worse outcome. In vitro, these mAbs were opsonic but did not enhance fungicidal activity of murine macrophages-like cells against *B. dermatitidis*.

4.5. *A. fumigatus*

For *A. fumigatus*, polyclonal serum obtained from mice immunized with fungal elastase (alkaline protease) inhibited in vitro enzymatic activity and passive transfer of immune serum-protected immunocompetent mice from death in response to a very high conidial inoculum, but did not prolong survival in immunocompromised mice (Frosco et al., 1994). Administration of elastase-binding IgG1 mAbs to corticosteroid-immunosuppressed mice did not prolong survival or alter lung histopathology following i.n. infection, whether administered singly or in combinations capable of inhibiting 100% of enzymatic activity in vitro (Frosco et al., 1992, 1994). The inability of passive transfer to confer host benefit may be related to properties of the mAbs. In addition, the lack of effect observed in this model may be related to the target antigen, as *A. fumigatus* isolates with disruption of this gene do not display reduced virulence in low-dose pulmonary infection models (Tang et al., 1993), a feature that could be related to redundancy of function among *A. fumigatus* proteases.

In contrast, an anti-idiotypic mAb (IgM) of *Pichia anomala* killer toxin that binds to a receptor involved in β-glucan cell wall synthesis prevents infection with *A. fumigatus* in murine models of T lymphocyte-depleted bone marrow transplantation and neutropenia (Cenci et al., 2002). Pulmonary pathology and lung fungal burden were markedly reduced in mice that received mAb in comparison to control mice. The efficacy of this mAb, which has broad specificity against bacteria, fungi, and parasites (Polonelli et al., 1997; Conti et al., 2000; Savoia et al., 2002) and primarily affects hyphal growth, provides support for the view that mAbs may be useful for prevention of *A. fumigatus* infections in immunocompromised hosts.

5. Conclusion

In summary, for the fungal pathogens that establish primary infection in the lung, most existing evidence suggests that Ab responses elicited in individuals with disease do not contribute to host defense. While for the dimorphic fungi, systemic Ab responses correlate with severity of disease, in invasive aspergillosis, spread of infection correlates with decreasing Ab titers. However, direct study of both the Ab response in the pulmonary compartment and the role of Ab-mediated immunity during infection, particularly in the context of T_H1-associated responses, has been limited. In contrast, mounting evidence supports that passive administration of specific mAbs can confer host benefit, at least in part by limiting host damage. Such mAbs may be different from those elicited as part of the Ab response to infection.

References

Abadi, J. and Pirofski, L. (1999). Antibodies reactive with the cryptococcal capsular polysaccharide glucuronoxylomannan are present in sera from children with and without human immunodeficiency virus infection. *J. Infect. Dis.* 180: 915–919.

Allendorfer, R., Brunner, G.D., and Deepe, G.S. Jr. (1999). Complex requirements for nascent and memory immunity in pulmonary histoplasmosis. *J. Immunol.* 162: 7389–7396.

Arruda, C., Franco, M.F., Kashino, S.S., Nascimento, F.R., Fazioli, R.A., Vaz, C.A., Russo, M., and Calich, V.L. (2002). Interleukin-12 protects mice against disseminated infection caused by *Paracoccidioides brasiliensis* but enhances pulmonary inflammation. *Clin. Immunol.* 103: 185–195.

Arulanandam, B.P., Raeder, R.H., Nedrud, J.G., Bucher, D.J., Le, J., and Metzger, D.W. (2001). IgA immunodeficiency leads to inadequate Th cell priming and increased susceptibility to influenza virus infection. *J. Immunol.* 166: 226–231.

Bardana, E.J. Jr. (1974). Measurement of humoral antibodies to aspergilli. *Ann. NY Acad. Sci.* 221: 64–75.

Bardana, E.J. Jr., McClatchy, J.K., Farr, R.S., and Minden, P. (1972). The primary interaction of antibody to components of aspergilli. II. Antibodies in sera from normal persons and from patients with aspergillosis. *J. Allergy Clin. Immunol.* 50: 222–234.

Baumgarth, N., Herman, O.C., Jager, G.C., Brown, L., Herzenberg, L.A., and Herzenberg, L.A. (1999). Innate and acquired humoral immunities to influenza virus are mediated by distinct arms of the immune system. *Proc. Natl. Acad. Sci. USA* 96: 2250–2255.

Beaman, L. and Holmberg, C.A. (1980). In vitro response of alveolar macrophages to infection with *Coccidioides immitis*. *Infect. Immun.* 28: 594–600.

Biagioni, L., Souza, M.J., Chamma, L.G., Mendes, R.P., Marques, S.A., Mota, N.G., and Franco, M. (1984). Serology of paracoccidioidomycosis. II. Correlation between class-specific antibodies and clinical forms of the disease. *Trans. R. Soc. Trop. Med. Hyg.* 78: 617–621.

Bice, D.E., Gray, R.H., Evans, M.J., and Muggenburg, B.A. (1987). Identification of plasma cells in lung alveoli and interstitial tissues after localized lung immunization. *J. Leukoc. Biol.* 41: 1–7.

Blumenthal, R.L., Campbell, D.E., Hwang, P., DeKruyff, R.H., Frankel, L.R., and Umetsu, D.T. (2001). Human alveolar macrophages induce functional inactivation in antigen-specific CD4 T cells. *J. Allergy Clin. Immunol.* 107: 258–264.

Boes, M. (2000). Role of natural and immune IgM antibodies in immune responses. *Mol. Immunol.* 37: 1141–1149.

Bonfield, T.L., Konstan, M.W., Burfeind, P., Panuska, J.R., Hilliard, J.B., and Berger, M. (1995). Normal bronchial epithelial cells constitutively produce the anti-inflammatory cytokine interleukin-10, which is downregulated in cystic fibrosis. *Am. J. Respir. Cell Mol. Biol.* 13: 257–261.

Brandtzaeg, P., Jahnsen, F.L., Farstad, I.N., and Haraldsen, G. (1997). Mucosal immunology of the upper airways: An overview. *Ann. N Y Acad. Sci.* 830: 1–18.

Brummer, E., Castaneda, E., and Restrepo, A. (1993). Paracoccidioidomycosis: An update. *Clin. Microbiol. Rev.* 6: 89–117.

Burnett, D. (1986). Immunoglobulins in the lung. *Thorax* 41: 337–344.

Caldwell, C.W., Sprouse, R.F., and Everett, E.D. (1983). Antigen-specific immunoglobulins in patients with acute pulmonary, chronic pulmonary, or disseminated histoplasmosis. *Diagn. Microbiol. Infect. Dis.* 1: 49–57.

Cano, L.E., Singer-Vermes, L.M., Vaz, C.A., Russo, M., and Calich, V.L. (1995). Pulmonary paracoccidioidomycosis in resistant and susceptible mice: Relationship among progression of infection, bronchoalveolar cell activation, cellular immune response, and specific isotype patterns. *Infect. Immun.* 63: 1777–1783.

Cano, L.E., Kashino, S.S., Arruda, C., Andre, D., Xidieh, C.F., Singer-Vermes, L.M., Vaz, C.A., Burger, E., and Calich, V.L. (1998). Protective role of gamma interferon in experimental pulmonary paracoccidioidomycosis. *Infect. Immun.* 66: 800–806.

Cano, L.E., Singer-Vermes, L.M., Costa, T.A., Mengel, J.O., Xidieh, C.F., Arruda, C., Andre, D.C., Vaz, C.A., Burger, E., and Calich, V.L. (2000). Depletion of CD8(+) T cells in vivo impairs host defense of mice resistant and susceptible to pulmonary paracoccidioidomycosis. *Infect. Immun.* 68: 352–359.

Carvalhaes, M.S., da Silva, W.D., Birman, E.G., Sant'Anna, O.A., Abrahamsohn, P., and Kipnis, T.L. (1986). Experimental paracoccidioidomycosis in high and low antibody-producer mice. I. Evolution of the disease, its correlation with the humoral immune response and the patterns of tissue lesions. *Ann. Inst. Pasteur Immunol.* 137C: 127–141.

Casadevall, A. and Pirofski, L.A. (1999). Host–pathogen interactions: Redefining the basic concepts of virulence and pathogenicity. *Infect. Immun.* 67: 3703–3713.

Casadevall, A. and Pirofski, L.A. (2003). Antibody-mediated regulation of cellular immunity and the inflammatory response. *Trends Immunol.* 24: 474–478.

Casadevall, A. and Scharff, M.D. (1994). Serum therapy revisited: Animal models of infection and development of passive antibody therapy. *Antimicrob. Agents Chemother.* 38: 1695–1702.

Castaneda, E., Brummer, E., Pappagianis, D., and Stevens, D.A. (1988). Impairment of cellular but not humoral immune responses in chronic pulmonary and disseminated paracoccidioidomycosis in mice. *Infect. Immun.* 56: 1771–1777.

Cenci, E., Mencacci, A., Spreca, A., Montagnoli, C., Bacci, A., Perruccio, K., Velardi, A., Magliani, W., Conti, S., Polonelli, L., and Romani, L. (2002). Protection of killer antiidiotypic antibodies against early Invasive aspergillosis in a murine model of allogeneic T-cell-depleted bone marrow transplantation. *Infect. Immun.* 70: 2375–2382.

Cole, G.T., Kruse, D., and Seshan, K.R. (1991). Antigen complex of *Coccidioides immitis* which elicits a precipitin antibody response in patients. *Infect. Immun.* 59: 2434–2446.

Conti, S., Magliani, W., Arseni, S., Dieci, E., Frazzi, R., Salati, A., Varaldo, P.E., and Polonelli, L. (2000). In vitro activity of monoclonal and recombinant yeast killer toxin-like antibodies against antibiotic-resistant Gram-positive cocci. *Mol. Med.* 6: 613–619.

Cox, R.A. and Arnold, D.R. (1979). Immunoglobulin E in coccidioidomycosis. *J. Immunol.* 123: 194–200.

Cromwell, O., Hamid, Q., Corrigan, C.J., Barkans, J., Meng, Q., Collins, P.D., and Kay, A.B. (1992). Expression and generation of interleukin-8, IL-6 and granulocyte-macrophage colony-stimulating factor by bronchial epithelial cells and enhancement by IL-1 beta and tumour necrosis factor-alpha. *Immunology* 77: 330–337.

de Mattos Grosso, D., de Almeida, S.R., Mariano, M., and Lopes, J.D. (2003). Characterization of gp70 and anti-gp70 monoclonal antibodies in *Paracoccidioides brasiliensis* pathogenesis. *Infect. Immun.* 71: 6534–6542.

Defaveri, J., Rezkallah-Iwasso, M.T., and de Franco, M.F. (1982). Experimental pulmonary paracoccidioidomycosis in mice: Morphology and correlation of lesions with humoral and cellular immune response. *Mycopathologia* 77: 3–11.

Fanger, N.A., Wardwell, K., Shen, L., Tedder, T.F., and Guyre, P.M. (1996). Type I (CD64) and type II (CD32) Fc gamma receptor-mediated phagocytosis by human blood dendritic cells. *J. Immunol.* 157: 541–548.

Feldmesser, M. and Casadevall, A. (1997). Effect of serum IgG1 to *Cryptococcus neoformans* glucuronoxylomannan on murine pulmonary infection. *J. Immunol.* 158: 790–799.

Feldmesser, M., Kress, Y., and Casadevall, A. (1998). Effect of antibody to capsular polysaccharide on eosinophilic pneumonia in murine infection with *Cryptococcus neoformans*. *J. Infect. Dis.* 177: 1639–1646.

Feldmesser, M., Kress, Y., Novikoff, P., and Casadevall, A. (2000). *Cryptococcus neoformans* is a facultative intracellular pathogen in murine pulmonary infection. *Infect. Immun.* 68: 4225–4237.

Feldmesser, M., Mednick, A., and Casadevall, A. (2002). Antibody-mediated protection in murine *Cryptococcus neoformans* infection is associated with pleotrophic effects on cytokine and leukocyte responses. *Infect. Immun.* 70: 1571–1580.

Fleuridor, R., Lyles, R.H., and Pirofski, L. (1999). Quantitative and qualitative differences in the serum antibody profiles of human immunodeficiency virus-infected persons with and without *Cryptococcus neoformans* meningitis [In Process Citation]. *J. Infect. Dis.* 180: 1526–1535.

Frosco, M., Fahed, C., Chase, T. Jr., and Macmillan, J.D. (1992). Inhibition of *Aspergillus fumigatus* elastase with monoclonal antibodies produced by using denatured elastase as an immunogen. *Infect. Immun.* 60: 735–741.

Frosco, M.B., Chase, T. Jr., and Macmillan, J.D. (1994). The effect of elastase-specific monoclonal and polyclonal antibodies on the virulence of *Aspergillus fumigatus* in immunocompromised mice. *Mycopathologia* 125: 65–76.

Garcia-Hermoso, D., Janbon, G., and Dromer, F. (1999). Epidemiological evidence for dormant *Cryptococcus neoformans* infection. *J. Clin. Microbiol.* 37: 3204–3209.

Goldman, D., Lee, S.C., and Casadevall, A. (1994). Pathogenesis of pulmonary *Cryptococcus neoformans* infection in the rat. *Infect. Immun.* 62: 4755–4761.

Goldman, D.L., Lee, S.C., Mednick, A.J., Montella, L., and Casadevall, A. (2000). Persistent *Cryptococcus neoformans* pulmonary infection in the rat is associated with intracellular parasitism, decreased inducible nitric oxide synthase expression, and altered antibody responsiveness to cryptococcal polysaccharide. *Infect. Immun.* 68: 832–838.

Goldman, D.L., Khine, H., Abadi, J., Lindenberg, D.J., Pirofski, L., Niang, R., and Casadevall, A. (2001). Serologic evidence for *Cryptococcus neoformans* infection in early childhood. *Pediatrics* 107: E66.

Greer, D.L. and McMurray, D.N. (1981). Pathogenesis and immune response to *Paracoccidioides brasiliensis* in the fructivorous bat, *Artibeus lituratus*. *Sabouraudia* 19: 165–178.

Groothuis, J.R., Simoes, E.A., Levin, M.J., Hall, C.B., Long, C.E., Rodriguez, W.J., Arrobio, J., Meissner, H.C., Fulton, D.R., and Welliver, R.C. (1993). Prophylactic administration of respiratory syncytial virus immune globulin to high-risk infants and young children. The respiratory syncytial virus immune globulin study group. *N. Engl. J. Med.* 329: 1524–1530.

Hance, A.J., Saltini, C., and Crystal, R.G. (1988). Does de novo immunoglobulin synthesis occur on the epithelial surface of the human lower respiratory tract? *Am. Rev. Respir. Dis.* 137: 17–24.

Huizinga, M., Stevens, E., and Berrens, L. (1985). Detection of class-specific antibodies against *Aspergillus fumigatus* antigens in various pulmonary diseases. *Ann. Inst. Pasteur Immunol.* 136C: 343–352.

Ishida, H., Hastings, R., Kearney, J., and Howard, M. (1992). Continuous anti-interleukin 10 antibody administration depletes mice of Ly-1 B cells but not conventional B cells. *J. Exp. Med.* 175: 1213–1220.

Johnson, S.M. and Pappagianis, D. (1992). The coccidioidal complement fixation and immunodiffusion-complement fixation antigen is a chitinase. *Infect. Immun.* 60: 2588–2592.

Kakeya, H., Udono, H., Ikuno, N., Yamamoto, Y., Mitsutake, K., Miyazaki, T., Tomono, K., Koga, H., Tashiro, T., Nakayama, E., and Kohno, S. (1997). A 77-kilodalton protein of *Cryptococcus neoformans*, a member of the heat shock protein 70 family, is a major antigen detected in the sera of mice with pulmonary cryptococcosis. *Infect. Immun.* 65: 1653–1658.

Kaltreider, H.B., Caldwell, J.L., and Byrd, P.K. (1986). The capacity of normal murine alveolar macrophages to function as antigen-presenting cells for the initiation of primary antibody-forming cell responses to sheep erythrocytes in vitro. *Am. Rev. Respir. Dis.* 133: 1097–1104.

Kaltreider, H.B., Curtis, J.L., and Arraj, S.M. (1987). The mechanism of appearance of specific antibody-forming cells in lungs of inbred mice after immunization with sheep erythrocytes intratracheally. II. Dose-dependence and kinetics of appearance of antibody-forming cells in hilar lymph nodes and lungs of unprimed and primed mice. *Am. Rev. Respir. Dis.* 135: 87–92.

Kantor, A.B. and Herzenberg, L.A. (1993). Origin of murine B cell lineages. *Annu. Rev. Immunol.* 11: 501–538.

Kaufman, L., McLaughlin, D.W., Clark, M.J., and Blumer, S. (1973). Specific immunodiffusion test for blastomycosis. *Appl. Microbiol.* 26: 244–247.

Kerr, M.A. (1990). The structure and function of human IgA. *Biochem.* J. 271: 285–296.

Kitamura, D., Roes, J., Kuhn, R., and Rajewsky, K. (1991). A B cell-deficient mouse by targeted disruption of the membrane exon of the immunoglobulin mu chain gene. *Nature* 350: 423–426.

Klein, B.S., Kuritsky, J.N., Chappell, W.A., Kaufman, L., Green, J., Davies, S.F., Williams, J.E., and Sarosi, G.A. (1986). Comparison of the enzyme immunoassay, immunodiffusion, and complement fixation tests in detecting antibody in human serum to the A antigen of *Blastomyces dermatitidis*. *Am. Rev. Respir. Dis.* 133: 144–148.

Klein, B.S., Vergeront, J.M., Kaufman, L., Bradsher, R.W., Kumar, U.N., Mathai, G., Varkey, B., and Davis, J.P. (1987). Serological tests for blastomycosis: Assessments during a large point-source outbreak in Wisconsin. *J. Infect. Dis.* 155: 262–268.

Kobayashi, H., Debeaupuis, J.P., Bouchara, J.P., and Latgé, J.P. (1993). An 88-kilodalton antigen secreted by *Aspergillus fumigatus*. *Infect. Immun.* 61: 4767–4771.

Kostiala, A.I., Stenius-Aarniala, B., and Alanko, K. (1984). Analysis of antibodies to *Aspergillus fumigatus* antigens by class-specific enzyme-linked immunosorbent assay in patients with pulmonary aspergillosis. *Diagn. Microbiol. Infect. Dis.* 2: 37–49.

Kunkel, E.J. and Butcher, E.C. (2003). Plasma-cell homing. *Nat. Rev. Immunol.* 3: 822–829.

Kurup, V.P. (1984). Interaction of *Aspergillus fumigatus* spores and pulmonary alveolar macrophages of rabbits. *Immunobiology* 166: 53–61.

Kurup, V.P., Nair, M.P., Schwartz, S.A., and Fink, J.N. (1985). Serum antibodies and their role in antibody-dependent cell-mediated cytotoxicity in aspergillosis. *Immunobiology* 169: 362–371.

Kurup, V.P., Ramasamy, M., Greenberger, P.A., and Fink, J.N. (1988). Isolation and characterization of a relevant *Aspergillus fumigatus* antigen with IgG- and IgE-binding activity. *Int. Arch. Allergy Appl. Immunol.* 86: 176–182.

Kurup, V.P., Resnick, A., Kalbfleish, J., and Fink, J.N. (1990). Antibody isotype responses in *Aspergillus*-induced diseases. *J. Lab. Clin. Med.* 115: 298–303.

Lamm, M.E. (1997). Interaction of antigens and antibodies at mucosal surfaces. *Annu. Rev. Microbiol.* 51: 311–340.

Latgé, J.P. (1999). *Aspergillus fumigatus* and aspergillosis. *Clin. Microbiol. Rev.* 12: 310–350.

Lovchik, J.A., Wilder, J.A., Huffnagle, G.B., Riblet, R., Lyons, C.R., and Lipscomb, M.F. (1999). Ig heavy chain complex-linked genes influence the immune response in a murine cryptococcal infection. *J. Immunol.* 163: 3907–3913.

Magnan, A., Frachon, I., Rain, B., Peuchmaur, M., Monti, G., Lenot, B., Fattal, M., Simonneau, G., Galanaud, P., and Emilie, D. (1994). Transforming growth factor beta in normal human lung: Preferential location in bronchial epithelial cells. *Thorax* 49: 789–792.

Marcos, M.A., Huetz, F., Pereira, P., Andreu, J.L., Martinez, A., and Coutinho, A. (1989). Further evidence for coelomic-associated B lymphocytes. *Eur. J. Immunol.* 19: 2031–2035.

Matthews, R., Burnie, J.P., Fox, A., and Tabaqchali, S. (1985). Immunoblot analysis of serological responses in invasive aspergillosis. *J. Clin. Pathol.* 38: 1300–1303.

Merrill, W.W., Naegel, G.P., Olchowski, J.J., and Reynolds, H.Y. (1985). Immunoglobulin G subclass proteins in serum and lavage fluid of normal subjects. Quantitation and comparison with immunoglobulins A and E. *Am. Rev. Respir. Dis.* 131: 584–587.

Montagnoli, C., Bozza, S., Bacci, A., Gaziano, R., Mosci, P., Morschhauser, J., Pitzurra, L., Kopf, M., Cutler, J., and Romani, L. (2003). A role for antibodies in the generation of memory antifungal immunity. *Eur. J. Immunol.* 33: 1193–1204.

Mukherjee, S., Lee, S.C., and Casadevall, A. (1995). Antibodies to *Cryptococcus neoformans* glucuronoxylomannan enhance antifungal activity of murine macrophages. *Infect. Immun.* 63: 573–579.

Mukherjee, S., Feldmesser, M., and Casadevall, A. (1996). J774 murine macrophage-like cell interactions with *Cryptococcus neoformans* in the presence and absence of opsonins. *J. Infect. Dis.* 173: 1222–1231.

Nosanchuk, J.D., Steenbergen, J.N., Shi, L., Deepe, G.S. Jr., and Casadevall, A. (2003). Antibodies to a cell surface histone-like protein protect against *Histoplasma capsulatum*. *J. Clin. Invest.* 112: 1164–1175.

Pabst, R. and Gehrke, I. (1990). Is the bronchus-associated lymphoid tissue (BALT) an integral structure of the lung in normal mammals, including humans? *Am. J. Respir. Cell Mol. Biol.* 3: 131–135.

Pappagianis, D. (2001). Serologic studies in coccidioidomycosis. *Semin. Respir. Infect.* 16: 242–250.

Pappagianis, D. and Zimmer, B.L. (1990). Serology of coccidioidomycosis. *Clin. Microbiol. Rev.* 3: 247–268.

Pilette, C., Ouadrhiri, Y., Godding, V., Vaerman, J.P., and Sibille, Y. (2001). Lung mucosal immunity: Immunoglobulin-A revisited. *Eur. Respir. J.* 18: 571–588.

Polonelli, L., Seguy, N., Conti, S., Gerloni, M., Bertolotti, D., Cantelli, C., Magliani, W., and Cailliez, J.C. (1997). Monoclonal yeast killer toxin-like candidacidal anti-idiotypic antibodies. *Clin. Diagn. Lab. Immunol.* 4: 142–146.

Raman, C., Khardori, N., Von Behren, L.A., Wheat, L.J., and Tewari, R.P. (1990). Evaluation of an ELISA for the detection of anti-Histoplasma ribosomal and antihistoplasmin antibodies in histoplasmosis. *J. Clin. Lab. Anal.* 4: 199–207.

Ravetch, J.V. and Bolland, S. (2001). IgG Fc receptors. *Annu. Rev. Immunol.* 19: 275–290.

Reen, D.J. (1988). Assessment of immunoblotting in the investigation of specific immune responses during infection. *Biochem. Soc. Trans.* 16: 132–134.

Reijula, K.E., Kurup, V.P., and Fink, J.N. (1991). Ultrastructural demonstration of specific IgG and IgE antibodies binding to *Aspergillus fumigatus* from patients with aspergillosis. *J. Allergy Clin. Immunol.* 87: 683–688.

Reynolds, H.Y. (1987). Identification and role of immunoglobulins in respiratory secretions. *Eur. J. Respir. Dis. Suppl.* 153: 103–116.

Reynolds, H.Y. (1988). Immunoglobulin G and its function in the human respiratory tract. *Mayo Clin. Proc.* 63: 161–174.

Rivera, J., Mukherjee, J., Weiss, L.M., and Casadevall, A. (2002). Antibody efficacy in murine pulmonary *Cryptococcus neoformans* infection: A role for nitric oxide. *J. Immunol.* 168: 3419–3427.

Salik, E., Tyorkin, M., Mohan, S., George, I., Becker, K., Oei, E., Kalb, T., and Sperber, K. (1999). Antigen trafficking and accessory cell function in respiratory epithelial cells. *Am. J. Respir. Cell Mol. Biol.* 21: 365–379.

Salina, M.A., Shikanai-Yasuda, M.A., Mendes, R.P., Barraviera, B., and Mendes Giannini, M.J. (1998). Detection of circulating *Paracoccidioides brasiliensis* antigen in urine of paracoccidioidomycosis patients before and during treatment. *J. Clin. Microbiol.* 36: 1723–1728.

Salvi, S. and Holgate, S.T. (1999). Could the airway epithelium play an important role in mucosal immunoglobulin A production? *Clin. Exp. Allergy* 29: 1597–1605.

Salvi, S., Semper, A., Blomberg, A., Holloway, J., Jaffar, Z., Papi, A., Teran, L., Polosa, R., Kelly, F., Sandstrom, T., Holgate, S., and Frew, A. (1999). Interleukin-5 production by human airway epithelial cells. *Am. J. Respir. Cell Mol. Biol.* 20: 984–991.

Sarosi, G.A. and Davies, S.F. (1979). Blastomycosis. *Am. Rev. Respir. Dis.* 120: 911–938.

Savoia, D., Avanzini, C., Conti, S., Magliani, V., Frazzi, R., and Polonelli, L. (2002). In vitro leishmanicidal activity of a monoclonal antibody mimicking a yeast killer toxin. *J. Eukaryot. Microbiol.* 49: 319–323.

Schonheyder, H., Andersen, P., and Stenderup, A. (1982). Serum antibodies to *Aspergillus fumigatus* in patients with pulmonary aspergillosis detected by immunofluorescence. *Acta Pathol. Microbiol. Immunol. Scand. [B]* 90: 273–279.

Schonheyder, H., Andersen, P., and Pedersen, A.T. (1983). Antibodies against *Aspergillus fumigatus* in bronchial secretions from patients without aspergillosis. *Acta Pathol. Microbiol. Immunol. Scand. [B]* 91: 187–191.

Schonheyder, H., Jensen, T., Hoiby, N., Andersen, P., and Koch, C. (1985). Frequency of *Aspergillus fumigatus* isolates and antibodies to aspergillus antigens in cystic fibrosis. *Acta Pathol. Microbiol. Immunol. Scand. [B]* 93: 105–112.

Smith, C.E., Saito, M.T., Beard, R.R., Kepp, R.M., Clark, R.W., and Eddie, B.U. (1950). Serological tests in the diagnosis and prognosis of coccidioidomycosis. *Am. J. Hyg.* 52: 1–21.

Soutar, C.A. (1976). Distribution of plasma cells and other cells containing immunoglobulin in the respiratory tract of normal man and class of immunoglobulin contained therein. *Thorax* 31: 158–166.

Stevens, D.A. (1995). Coccidioidomycosis. *N. Engl. J. Med.* 332: 1077–1082.

Tang, C.M., Cohen, J., Krausz, T., Van Noorden, S., and Holden, D.W. (1993). The alkaline protease of *Aspergillus fumigatus* is not a virulence determinant in two murine models of invasive pulmonary aspergillosis. *Infect. Immun.* 61: 1650–1656.

Tani, E.M., Franco, M., Peracoli, M.T., and Montenegro, M.R. (1987). Experimental pulmonary paracoccidioidomycosis in the Syrian hamster: Morphology and correlation of lesions with the immune response. *J. Med. Vet. Mycol.* 25: 291–300.

Taylor, J.J. and Burroughs, E.J. (1973). Experimental avian aspergillosis. *Mycopathol. Mycol. Appl.* 51: 131–141.

Turner, S., Kaufman, L., and Jalbert, M. (1986). Diagnostic assessment of an enzyme-linked immunosorbent assay for human and canine blastomycosis. *J. Clin. Microbiol.* 23: 294–297.

van der Heyde, H.C., Elloso, M.M., Chang, W.L., Pepper, B.J., Batchelder, J., and Weidanz, W.P. (1996). Expansion of the gammadelta T cell subset in vivo during bloodstage malaria in B cell-deficient mice. *J. Leukoc. Biol.* 60: 221–229.

Weig, M., Frosch, M., Tintelnot, K., Haas, A., Gross, U., Linsmeier, B., and Heesemann, J. (2001). Use of recombinant mitogillin for improved serodiagnosis of *Aspergillus fumigatus*-associated diseases. *J. Clin. Microbiol.* 39: 1721–1730.

Wilkes, D.S., Yarbrough, W.C. Jr., and Weissler, J.C. (1993). Human alveolar macrophages inhibit immunoglobulin production in response to direct B cell mitogen. *Am. J. Respir. Cell Mol. Biol.* 9: 141–147.

Williams, J.E., Moser, S.A., Turner, S.H., and Standard, P.G. (1994). Development of pulmonary infection in mice inoculated with *Blastomyces dermatitidis* conidia. *Am. J. Respir. Crit. Care Med.* 149: 500–509.

Wuthrich, M. and Klein, B.S. (2000). Investigation of anti-WI-1 adhesin antibody-mediated protection in experimental pulmonary blastomycosis. *J. Infect. Dis.* 181: 1720–1728.

Young, R.C. and Bennett, J.E. (1971). Invasive aspergillosis. Absence of detectable antibody response. *Am. Rev. Respir. Dis.* 104: 710–716.

Zaragoza, O. and Casadevall, A. (2004). Antibodies produced in response to *Cryptococcus neoformans* pulmonary infection in mice have characteristics of non-protective antibodies. *Infect. Immun.* 72: 4271–4274.

Zuercher, A.W., Jiang, H.Q., Thurnheer, M.C., Cuff, C.F., and Cebra, J.J. (2002). Distinct mechanisms for cross-protection of the upper versus lower respiratory tract through intestinal priming. *J. Immunol.* 169: 3920–3925.

10

Pulmonary Paracoccidioidomycosis

Vera Lúcia Garcia Calich and Maria Heloísa Souza Lima Blotta

Department of Immunology, Institute of Biomedical Sciences, University of São Paulo (USP) Faculty of Medical Sciences, Department of Clinical Pathology, State University of Campinas (UNICAMP), São Paulo, Brazil.

1. Introduction

1.1. The Human Disease

Paracoccidioidomycosis (PCM), first described by Lutz in 1908 (Lutz, 1908), is caused by the thermally dimorphic fungus *Paracoccidioides brasiliensis*. This endemic infection is the most prevalent deep mycosis in Latin America (reviewed by Franco, 1987; Franco et al., 1989; Brummer et al., 1993). The frequency of pulmonary lesions suggests that inhalation of airborne propagules is the main route of infection (Restrepo, 1988). Most exposed subjects develop an asymptomatic pulmonary infection (PCM-infection) although some individuals present clinical manifestations. The disease presents a wide spectrum of clinical and pathological manifestations, ranging from benign and localized to severe and disseminated forms (Fava Netto et al., 1969; Mendes and Raphael, 1971; Franco et al., 1989). According to the current classification (Franco, 1987), paracoccidioidomycosis infection (PI) is defined as an asymptomatic infection caused by *P. brasiliensis* in healthy individuals who live in endemic areas and are positive to the paracoccidioidin skin test. The adult or chronic progressive form of the disease (AF) predominantly affects adult males, with a high frequency of pulmonary, skin, adrenal, and visceral involvement. About 90% of the patients with the adult form present pulmonary involvement (Brummer et al., 1993). The symptoms are nonspecific and include cough, expectoration, shortness of breath, weight loss, fever, and anorexia.

In clear contrast to the adult type, the acute or juvenile type (JF) equally affects young patients of both sexes. The JF is characterized by systemic lymph node involvement, hepatosplenomegaly, and bone marrow dysfunction, resembling a lymphoproliferative disease. Patients with AF usually exhibit low levels of specific antibodies and adequate cellular immune responses, while those with the JF typically show high levels of specific antibodies, polyclonal activation of B cells, antigenemia, and impaired cellular immune responses (Fig. 10.1) (Franco, 1987; Restrepo, 1988; Brummer et al., 1993; Montenegro and Franco, 1994; Camargo and Franco, 2000).

It is well known that early lung infection is difficult to be clinically recognized and the animal models of pulmonary infection have facilitated characterizing the cells, cytokines, and regulatory mechanisms that play a fundamental role in the development of protective immune responses. This chapter will present the main immunological aspects, which regulate host–*P. brasiliensis* interactions with a special emphasis on lung involvement, both in the human pathology and in animal models. Aspects of fungal structure, morphology, dimorphism physiology, genetics, and immunodiagnosis were recently reviewed elsewhere (Camargo and Franco, 2000; Restrepo et al., 2001; Borges-Welmsley et al., 2002; San-Blas et al., 2002).

1.2. The Isogenic Murine Model of Resistance/Susceptibility

Our laboratory established a genetically controlled murine model of PCM, which allowed us to investigate several parameters of host–parasite interactions. Eleven different inbred mouse strains infected intraperitoneally (i.p.) with five million yeast cells from *P. brasiliensis* showed four distinct patterns of susceptibility: susceptible (B10.A, B10D2/oSn, B10D2/nSn), intermediate (BALB/c, C57Bl/10, CBA, C3H/FeJ), resistant (C3H/HeJ), and highly resistant (A/Sn, A/J, DBA/2). Our results clearly showed that those differences are not controlled by the H-2 locus or by the presence of the C5 component of the complement system (Calich et al., 1985). Furthermore, congenic mouse strains differing only at the C5 locus (B10D2/old and B10D2/new) develop similar pattern of disease (Burger et al., 1985).

As prototypes of the polarized behavior, B10.A and A/Sn (or A/J) mice were studied regarding their innate and adaptative immune responses after *P. brasiliensis*

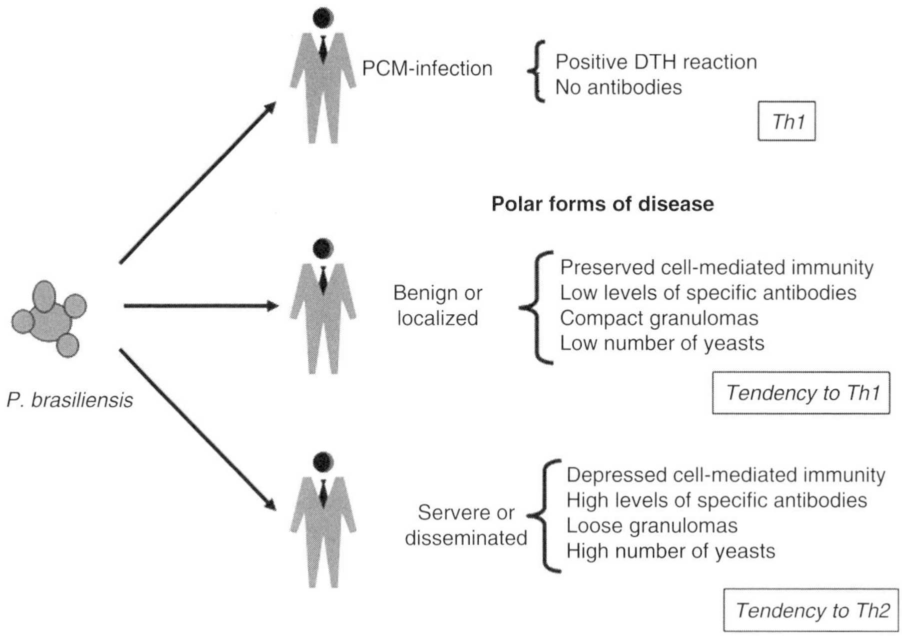

Figure 10.1. Main features of polar clinical forms of human paracoccidioidomycosis (PCM).

infection. Most of those results were recently reviewed (Calich et al., 1994, 1998; Calich and Kashino, 1998) and clearly show the diverging immune responses mounted by susceptible and resistant animals. One important characteristic of our model is the similarity with the human disease, B10.A mice mimicking the progressive, severe forms of the disease and A/Sn mice showing a pattern of immune response similar to the regressive or localized forms of the infection. As in the human disease, our experimental model demonstrated that resistance is associated with immune responses that favor cellular immunity and activation of phagocytes, whereas susceptibility is associated with impairment of cellular immune responses and preferential activation of B cells. This general pattern of immunological reactivity, also observed in other chronic infectious diseases, led us to postulate that resistance in experimental PCM is associated with a preferential Th1 activation, whereas susceptibility is associated with a predominant Th2 pattern (Fig. 10.2) (Calich et al., 1994; Murphy et al., 1994; Calich and Kashino, 1998). As will be discussed in this chapter, the resistance mechanisms to *P. brasiliensis* are very complex processes and the Th1/Th2 dichotomy can only partially explain the immunoregulatory mechanisms associated with the progressive and regressive forms of PCM.

After an intratracheal (i.t.) infection, the susceptibility and resistance patterns observed in the i.p. model were maintained as reflected both by the higher mortality rates of the B10.A mice when compared to the A/Sn ones, and by the pattern of fungal dissemination developed (Cano et al., 1995). Susceptible mice were not able to restrain the infection to the lungs, allowing dissemination to the liver and spleen after 2 months of infection and thus developing a chronic disseminated form

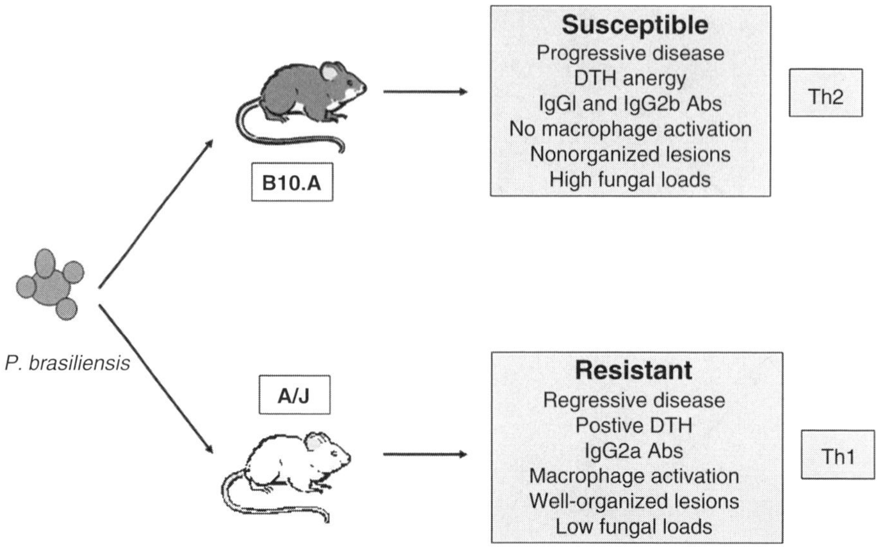

Figure 10.2. The resistance/susceptibility murine model of paracoccidioidomycosis.

of the disease; in the resistant mice, on the other hand, no dissemination was observed, characterizing a pulmonary-restricted chronic disease.

In this chapter, the results of the isogenic pulmonary model will be presented in counterpoint to the equivalent knowledge existent in the human disease or in other experimental models using similar approaches.

2. Innate Immune Response

There is an increasing body of evidence on the importance of innate immunity mechanisms not only in the control of early pathogen growth but also in determining the type of adaptative immune response subsequently developed by infected hosts. Several mechanisms of innate immunity, like the activation of complement proteins, natural killer (NK) cells, phagocytic cells, production of inflammatory cytokines and chemokines have been shown to play an important role in the early response to *P. brasiliensis* infection.

2.1. Genetic Control of Susceptibility

Clinical studies suggested that susceptibility to *P. brasiliensis* is dependent on several factors, including the host's genetic background and hormonal function (reviewed by Brummer et al., 1993; Borges-Welmsley et al., 2002; San-Blas et al., 2002). A fungal receptor for estrogen was characterized and appears to block the conversion of conidia or mycelium to the infecting yeast form (Loose et al., 1983). This finding may explain the unusual susceptibility of male individuals of endemic areas. Early clinical studies have also demonstrated that PCM is more frequent among certain ethnic groups such as Japanese individuals and among members of some families living in endemic regions (Lacaz, 1956; Fava Netto et al., 1965). In addition, an association between PCM and known genetic markers such as HLA-A9, HLA-B13, and HLA-B40 was also described (Restrepo et al., 1983; Lacerda et al., 1988; Goldani et al., 1991).

Genetic studies performed by our group with the mouse strains presenting polar behavior after i.p. infection with *P. brasiliensis* have shown the existence of an autosomal dominant gene (*Pbr* gene), which appears to be similar to the *Nramp* gene (Forbes and Gross, 2001) that control resistance to infection (Calich et al., 1987).

2.2. Early Lung Inflammation

Animal models of pulmonary infection have allowed the characterization of cells, humoral factors, and regulatory mechanisms that play an essential role in the early inflammation, which will influence the adaptative immunity that develops further.

Comparing the early influx of inflammatory cells to the lungs of susceptible and resistant mice, Cano (1995) demonstrated an equivalent mononuclear cell influx but a more prominent migration of neutrophil and eosinophil PMN cells into the lung of susceptible mice. Furthermore, only in susceptible mice this early (24 h after infection) PMN inflammatory influx affects disease outcome and the acquired immunity further established (Pina, 2002).

As described in other infectious diseases, in murine PCM chemokines appear to play a major role in regulating the migration of specific leukocytes subsets in both the acute and chronic inflammatory processes. A recent study showed an association between high levels of RANTES, MCP-1, IP-10, and Mig and mononuclear cell recruitment to the lungs of *P. brasiliensis*-infected C57BL/6 mice (Souto et al., 2003).

2.3. Macrophages and Nitric Oxide

The infection by *P. brasiliensis* occurs by inhalation of airborne propagules of the mycelial phase of the fungus, which reach the lungs, eventually evade the host defenses, and disseminate via the bloodstream and/or lymphatics to virtually all parts of the body (reviewed by Restrepo, 1988; Franco et al., 1989; Brummer et al., 1993). Alveolar macrophages (AM) are believed to be important in the initial containment of the microorganisms through nonspecific or innate immune mechanisms. AM or dendritic cells also phagocytose particles and microbial organisms and carry them via lymphatics to regional hilar lymph nodes, where specific immune responses are believed to be generated. Thus, AM may be involved in the innate and acquired immune responses to *P. brasiliensis* both as accessory cells and as target of cytotoxic T lymphocytes in the regional lymph nodes.

P. brasiliensis proliferates *ex vivo* in a variety of mouse macrophages, including resident peritoneal, alveolar, and peripheral blood derived monocytes until the cells are lysed and killed by as yet unknown mechanism. However, the immunological activation of these cells efficiently inhibits fungal growth (Brummer, 1994; Brummer et al., 1988). When alveolar macrophages were analyzed after pulmonary infection, absence of hydrogen peroxide production was observed with cells obtained from susceptible mice whereas macrophages from resistant mice produced increasing levels of this metabolite in the course of disease (Cano et al., 1995). These different activities parallel the delayed-type hypersensitivity (DTH) anergy and the evident DTH reactivity developed by susceptible and resistant mice, respectively.

Despite several studies showing the nitric oxide (NO)-dependent fungal killing of IFN-γ activated macrophages (Cano et al., 1994; Gonzalez, et al., 2000), a dual role for NO was also described since NO production is important for fungal killing but is also associated with immunosuppression (Bocca et al., 1988; Nascimento et al., 2002).

Prostaglandins (Soares et al., 2001) and gp43 (Popi et al., 2002), the immunodominant antigen from *P. brasiliensis* (Travassos et al., 1995), were shown to inhibit macrophage function and were postulated to be involved in the evasion mechanism of fungal cells, facilitating their homing in the host tissues of infected hosts. In addition, gp43 has been shown to bind laminin, fibronectin, and collagen, and is considered an important adhesin that allows *P. brasiliensis* interaction with extracellular matrix components (Vicentini et al., 1994; Mendes-Giannini et al., 2000). Laminin-coated yeasts appear to enhance fungal pathogenicity in a model of testicle infection of hamster (Vicentini et al., 1994), but this was not the case in the pulmonary model of murine infection where laminin treatment decreased the pathogenicity of yeast cells to susceptible mice (André et al., 2004).

Other studies also employing B10.A and A/J mice showed that gp43 is preferentially presented by dendritic cells, resulting in Th1 immunity in resistant mice whereas B cells are the main antigen-presenting cells (APCs) which direct a strong activation of Th2 lymphocytes in susceptible mice (Almeida et al., 1998; Ferreira et al., 2003).

We have performed recent studies on the effect of *P. brasiliensis* infection of normal alveolar macrophages recovered from lungs of A/J and B10.A mice and results appear to demonstrate an opposite behavior of these cells. Normal alveolar macrophages of B10.A mice, in vitro infected with *P. brasiliensis* yeasts, can be activated by small doses of exogenously added IFN-γ, secrete high levels of IL-12, nitric oxide, and display a very efficient fungal killing activity. In contrast, macrophages from A/J mice were poorly activated by low doses of IFN-γ, secrete low amounts of IL-12, NO, and present a poor fungicidal ability concomitant with the production of high levels of IL-10. Thus, alveolar macrophages of susceptible mice seem to be more efficient than those of resistant mice and interaction of *P. brasiliensis* with these cells probably occurs through different macrophage receptors. This different behavior appears to explain the apparently discrepant result we observed when the pulmonary model of infection was described: at the beginning of infection higher number of viable yeast cells were recovered from lungs of resistant mice as compared with susceptible ones (Cano et al., 1995). Furthermore, IFN-γ, the most efficient macrophage activator was found in higher levels in the lung homogenates of susceptible mice (Cano et al., 1998). Thus, the innate immunity appears to be much more efficient in the susceptible mice than in resistant animals. This hyperactivity is concomitant with production of high levels of NO that, besides its effect restraining fungal growth, can interfere with acquired immune responses, leading to a subsequent immunosuppression of T cell-mediated immunity (Pina and Calich, unpublished data; Nascimento et al., 2002).

2.4. Polymorphonuclear Leukocytes

Several investigations demonstrated that murine PMN leukocytes are able to kill *P. brasiliensis* yeasts through the oxidative metabolism (reviewed by McEwen et al., 1987; Brummer, 1994). In a air pouch model of infection and compared with PMN leukocytes from susceptible mice, cells from A/J mice presented superior fungicidal ability associated with their enhanced oxidative burst (Meloni Bruneri et al., 1996). The antifungal activity of murine and human PMN leukocytes can be enhanced by IFN-γ, granulocyte-macrophage colony-stimulating factor (GM-CSF), or IL-1β but not by TNF-α or IL-8 (Kurita et al., 2000).

The early in vivo depletion of PMN cells resulted in a more severe and disseminated disease of susceptible but not in resistant mice. Interestingly, the more severe disease of B10.A mice was concomitant with increased production of proinflammatory cytokines (IFN-γ and IL-12). So, the genetic pattern of hosts influences the effect of this important cell of natural immunity in controlling murine PCM. We also investigated the role of PMN leucocytes in the acquired phase of immune response developed by susceptible mice subcutaneously (s.c.) vaccinated with viable *P. brasiliensis* yeast cells and 15 days later challenged by the i.t. route. Both groups developed immunoprotection and no significant differences were found between vaccinated and vaccinated-PMN-depleted mice showing that in secondary PCM, even in hosts of susceptible genetic background, PMN cells do not play a protective role (Pina, 2002).

We have extended our studies on the effect of PMN cells depletion on the natural immunity mounted by athymic and euthymic BALB/c mice infected i.t. with *P. brasiliensis*. Equivalent to that observed with resistant A/J mice, in vivo depletion of these cells did not modify the pulmonary disease and mortality data of these mouse strains. The pulmonary cytokines, however, were significantly altered by PMN cell depletion (Valente-Ferreira and Calich, unpublished results). In conclusion, the role of PMN cells in pulmonary PCM is clearly dependent on the genetic pattern of hosts and more prominent in the innate phase of immunity. These cells, however, can actively participate in the control of fungal growth inside granulomatous lesions due to their ability to produce reactive oxygen intermediates and to secrete cytokines and chemokines.

2.5. NK Cells

Several studies have described the important role of NK cells controlling intracellular infections and aberrant cells. In some pathologies however, this cell has a more ambiguous role probably due to different degrees of maturation, diverse physiologic behavior in different biological compartments, preferential use of activating or deactivating receptors and, probably, the existence of different NK cell subpopulations (reviewed by Colucci et al., 2003). There is not much information about the role of NK cell in *P. brasiliensis* infection, but the few available investigations in this area suggest that the function of this lymphocyte subpopulation is complex and varies according to the type of host or site these cells were obtained. In the peripheral blood of human PCM patients NK cells were found in elevated number but they displayed low cytotoxic activity (Peraçoli et al., 1991). In vitro studies showed a direct inhibitory effect of murine NK cells on *P. brasiliensis* growth (Jimenez and Murphy, 1984) and in a hamster model of infection, NK cell was shown to be activated in the first weeks of infection followed by an impairment of its activity associated with depressed cell-mediated immunity (Peraçoli et al., 1995).

Our findings of illness exacerbation in euthymic and athymic BALB/c mice after in vivo depletion of IL-12 or IFN-γ suggested that NK cells, another important mediator of innate immunity, would have a protective role in pulmonary PCM. Preliminary results showed that in vivo depletion of NK cells by anti-Asialo GM1 polyclonal antibody results in a more severe disease of both mouse strains. The depletion effect was more pronounced in the NK-depleted athymic than euthymic mice. NK cell depletion led to increased antibody production by the former strain but did not modify the humoral immunity of euthymic animals. Hence, NK cells seem to have a protective effect in pulmonary PCM and its effect appears to be more prominent in T-cell deficient than in T-cell sufficient mice. Further experiments, however, suggested a more complex function of NK cell in the pulmonary PCM. In vivo depletion of NK cells in *scid* BALB/c mice, deficient in both T and B cells, caused a less disseminated infection to liver and spleen indicating that the presence of B and T cells can modify the behavior of NK lymphocytes (Valente-Ferreira and Calich, unpublished observations). In addition, the important role of additional mechanisms of innate immunity in pulmonary PCM was further emphasized by the prolonged survival time of NK-cell-depleted and untreated *scid* mice which survived several weeks after infection. In another mouse strain (C57BL/6), NK cell depletion by the anti-NK PK136 mAb also induced lower fungal loads in the liver and spleen (Valente-Ferreira and Calich, unpublished observations), once more indicating that NK cells can exert a protective or a disease-promoting effect in pulmonary PCM, depending on the genetic background and immunological status of the host.

2.6. Cytokines

2.6.1. IFN-γ

P. brasiliensis growth in *nude* or *scid* mice remains relatively constant for the first weeks followed by a loss of control of infection that ultimately results in the death of the animal (Burger et al., 1996a,b; Valente-Ferreira et al., unpublished results). Initial survival and control of fungal loads appear to be dependent upon production of pulmonary cytokines, mainly IFN-γ (Cano et al., 1998).

In resistant and susceptible mouse strains to *P. brasiliensis* infection neutralization of endogenous IFN-γ induced exacerbation of the pulmonary infection, earlier fungal dissemination to the liver and spleen, impairment of the specific cellular immune response, and increased humoral immunity. In addition, neutralization of IFN-γ changes the focal granulomatous lesions found in the lungs of B10.A and A/Sn mice into coalescent granulomas, which destroy the pulmonary architecture (Cano et al., 1998). We also investigated the role of IFN-γ in the innate immunity of athymic and euthymic BALB/c mice comparing the effect of its depletion with that conferred by depletion of IL-12, PMN, or NK cells. Again, IFN-γ was shown to be the most important protective mediator in pulmonary PCM and its neutralization by monoclonal antibodies at the first days of infection results in a more severe disease. However, diminished survival time was detected only in the athymic strain demonstrating a more prominent role of this mediator in mice deficient of T cell immunity (Valente-Ferreira and Calich, unpublished observations). These results suggest that, irrespective of the mouse strain, IFN-γ plays a protective role and this cytokine is the major mediator of resistance against *P. brasiliensis* infection in mice.

IFN-γ knockout (KO) and TNF-α receptor p55 KO C57Bl/6 mice were shown to develop a more severe disease associated with the presence of incipient granulomas in IFN-γ KO mice and nonorganized granulomas in p55 KO mice (Souto et al., 2000). In accordance with other investigations using C57Bl/6 mice (Bocca et al., 1998; Nascimento et al., 2002), resistance to *P. brasiliensis* was concluded to be mediated by endogenous TNF-α and IFN-γ, which regulate granuloma formation, induce NO production but also induce a marked T cell unresponsiveness. Further investigation using IFN-γ KO mice showed that this cytokine is a major regulator of chemokine synthesis and subsequent mobilization of inflammatory cells into the lungs of C57BL/6-infected mice (Souto et al., 2003).

Although the cell type responsible for the production of IFN-γ during the early phase of immune response remains to be identified, cells of the innate immune system such as NK cells appear to be an important source in other fungal infections. Type 1 $CD4^+$ and $CD8^+$ T cells further expanded appear to be the other important source of IFN-γ.

In human disease IFN-γ production was associated with resistance (Oliveira et al., 2002) and clinical remission (Karhawi et al., 2000; Benard et al., 2001). Individuals with PCM infection, with no signs or symptoms of disease, present higher percentage of $CD8^+$/IFN-γ^+, $CD4^+$/TNF-α^+, and $CD4^+$/IL-2^+ T cells as compared to AF and FJ patients, confirming Th1 response and supporting the resistance phenotype exhibited by this group (Mamoni et al., unpublished observations).

2.6.2. IL-12

IL-12 is a critical cytokine, which stimulates IFN-γ production and proliferation of activated T cells and NK cells. In experimental pulmonary PCM, early treatment with recombinant IL-12 leads to a less disseminated disease but induced an augmented pulmonary mononuclear cell inflammation and an early increase in pulmonary IFN-γ. The less disseminated infection was concomitant with decreased cytokine and specific antibody production. These results show that IL-12 administration induces a less severe infection but the high inflammatory response detected in the lungs precludes its possible use as a new therapeutic tool for severe PCM (Arruda et al., 2002).

To further elucidate the role of IL-12 in murine PCM, IL-12 KO C57BL/6 mice and their wild-type (WT) controls were infected i.t. with *P. brasiliensis* (Deepe et al., 2000). IL-12 deficient mice presented increased number of *P. brasiliensis* yeasts in the lungs accompanied by a highly increased dissemination to liver and spleen (respectively 10,000- and 1,000-fold higher in KO than WT mice). The higher colony-forming units (CFU) counts detected in IL-12 KO mice paralleled the precocious mortality of these animals. The most severe disease developed by IL-12 KO mice was accompanied by increased production of specific antibodies and loose granulomas, which replace almost all the pulmonary structure. Metastatic lesions, containing high number of yeast cells, were observed in almost all examined organs (heart, thymus, kidney, intestines, etc) of IL-12 KO mice (Deepe et al., 2000).

Three different schedules of IL-12 depletion by mAb induced a more severe disease in resistant and susceptible mice but the effects were more evident in the susceptible strain. Usually, the increased fungal loads in the lungs of IL-12 depleted mice were concomitant with higher levels of antibodies and cytokines (TNF-α, IFN-γ, GM-CSF, IL-3, IL-4, IL-5, and IL-10). In IL-12 depleted mice, the pulmonary granulomatous reaction changed to nonorganized lesions containing considerable numbers of eosinophils and pulmonary fibrosis whose intensity depended on the protocol and mice strain employed. In conclusion, depletion of endogenous IL-12 caused a more severe PCM but its effects on the immune response to *P. brasiliensis* varied depending on the resistance pattern of hosts and protocol of treatment employed (Deepe et al., 2000; Calich and Molinari-Madlum, unpublished observations).

Using athymic and euthymic BALB/c mice we could also verify that systemic or local depletion of IL-12 aggravated pulmonary PCM once more indicating that this cytokine, besides IFN-γ, is one important mediator of innate defense against *P. brasiliensis* (Valente-Ferreira and Calich, unpublished observations).

AM from patients with PCM are able to produce more IL-12 than PBMC, indicating a local immune response to the fungus in the lungs (Fornazim et al., 2003).

2.6.3. IL-4

In most fungal infections IL-4, the most significant Th2 cytokine, is an important determinant of susceptibility or resistance of hosts. IL-4 depletion by mAb enhances the protective immunity to fungi in experimental models of infection (Romani et al., 1992; Magee and Cox, 1995). IL-4 can activate or deactivate phagocytes inhibiting or enhancing the killing functions of these cells (Hart et al., 1989; Stein et al., 1992). Furthermore, besides its well-known Th2 inducing activity, IL-4 can promote the differentiation of Th1 cells due to its IL-12 promoting activity on dendritic cells (Mencacci et al., 1998).

To assess the role of IL-4 in the innate and adaptative immune response to *P. brasiliensis*, the pulmonary infection was studied in IL-4-deficient mice (IL-$4^{-/-}$) of the C57BL/6 background and their wild-type counterparts. Alveolar macrophages from infected IL-$4^{-/-}$ mice, activated or not by exogenous IFN-γ, controlled in vitro fungal growth more efficiently than macrophages from WT mice and this activity paralleled their enhanced ability to produce nitric oxide. At the acquired phase of immunity lower pulmonary and hepatic fungal loads in IL-4$^{-/-}$ mice were associated with increased production of IFN-γ but a clear shift to a Th1 pattern was not characterized since IL-4$^{-/-}$ mice did not alter DTH anergy or IL-2 levels. In IL-4$^{-/-}$ mice, well-organized granulomas restraining fungal cells replaced the more extensive lesions containing high number of fungi and inflammatory leukocytes developed by IL-4-sufficient mice. These results clearly showed that genetically determined deficiency of IL-4 can exert a protective role in pulmonary PCM (Pina et al., 2004). To further assess the role of IL-4, pulmonary PCM was studied in IL-4-depleted susceptible (B10.A) and intermediate (C57Bl/6) mice. Unexpectedly, in IL-4-depleted B10.A mice enhanced pulmonary infection was seen but the levels of pulmonary cytokines and specific antibodies have not changed. In contrast, IL-4 neutralization of C57BL/6 mice resulted in a less severe pulmonary disease associated with impaired synthesis of Th2 cytokines in the lungs and liver. Lung pathology was equivalent in IL-4-depleted and untreated B10.A mice. In IL-4-depleted C57BL/6 mice, however, smaller and well-organized granulomas replaced the more extensive lesions developed by untreated controls. These results clearly showed that IL-4 can play a protective or a disease-promoting effect in pulmonary PCM depending on the genetic background of the host (Arruda et al., 2004).

In humans, an indirect participation of IL-4 in the JF of the disease was confirmed by the preferential induction of IgE and IgG4 isotypes (Baida et al., 1999; Biselli et al., 2001; Mamoni et al., 2001, 2002). In addition, production of IL-4 and IL-5 was described in patients with active PCM (Mello et al., 2002) and in patients with the JF of the disease (Oliveira et al., 2002). However, in several patients with the chronic form of PCM increased levels of IL-4 was not found, indicating that other immune mechanisms may also account for the severity of the disease (Benard et al., 2001; Campanelli et al., 2003). Even in the i.p. model of infection, susceptibility was not clearly linked to IL-4 production since antigen-stimulated lymph node cells produce IL-10 but not IL-4 during the initial 8 weeks of infection (Kashino et al., 2000). This finding appears to indicate that IL-10 secreting cells (regulatory T cells?) are important regulators of murine PCM and several mechanisms may account for genetic susceptibility to *P. brasiliensis* infection.

2.6.4. IL-10

IL-10 production is well preserved in human PCM, regardless of the clinical form (Karhawi et al., 2000; Benard et al., 2001; Fornari et al., 2001; Oliveira et al., 2002). Moreover, a negative correlation between production of IL-12 and IL-10 was also demonstrated. In vitro treatment of mononuclear blood cells with anti-IL-10 monoclonal antibodies added of rIL-12 not only reverted lymphoproliferative anergy but also induced the synthesis of elevated levels of IFN-γ (Romano et al., 2002). In the i.p. model of murine PCM, IL-10 was also the most prominent and early Th2 cytokine observed after antigen stimulation of lymph node cells from susceptible mice (Calich and Kashino, 1998; Kashino et al., 2000), whereas resistant mice present a delayed secretion of this cytokine. Interestingly, in kinetic studies it was shown that antigen-stimulated lymph node cells from resistant mice produce IL-10 later than the susceptible strain. In accordance, in PI individuals an early and high IFN-γ and IL-2 mRNA expression in PBMC is followed by late and low IL-10 mRNA expression (Mamoni et al., unpublished results). These data both in animals and human suggest that the delayed IL-10 production may have a role in allowing the establishment of a potent Th1 response, sufficient to avoid the development of the disease. In addition, the production of IL-10 in a late phase may have a beneficial effect by damping the production of type 1 cytokines and restraining their inflammatory effects on host tissues.

In another experimental PCM study, it was observed that when T cells from resistant mice were stimulated in vitro with B lymphocytes as APC from susceptible animals, very high levels of IL-10 were observed and vice versa (Almeida et al., 1998). These results emphasize the importance of different T cell subsets in PCM infection and the reciprocal regulation between the innate and adaptive immune systems in the development of optimal antifungal immunity.

The influence of IL-10 was further investigated in the pulmonary model of PCM using C57BL/6 IL-10 KO mice and their WT counterparts. At week 8 of infection, decreased (more than 1000-folds) fungal burdens were detected in the lungs and almost no fungal cells were detected in the livers and spleens. This picture was more prominent at week 16 after infection where IL-10 deficient mice present almost no yeasts in the lungs but wild-type mice showed around 6.0 $\log_{10}$ CFUs. This much less severe disease was accompanied by low levels of IgG antibodies but almost no differences in the amounts of cytokines in affected organs. So, differently from other experimental situations where decreased fungal loads induced diminished cytokine secretion, *P. brasiliensis* infection in IL-10 KO mice courses with high levels of cytokines. This finding is consistent with the inhibitory activity of IL-10 on cytokine secretion. The typical pulmonary lesion of wild-type C57BL/6 mice is well organized, surrounded by lymphocytes, and contains a very large number of yeast cells in active growth, detected by evident multiple budding yeast cells. In IL-10 KO mice, no granulomas and no yeast cells were detected in the lungs but a small inflammatory reaction still persisted. Even in Grocott-stained preparations no fungal cells could be observed.

2.6.5. Cytokines: Main Conclusions

IFN-γ is the most important protective cytokine to susceptible, intermediate, and resistant mice. TNF-α and IL-12 are also very important protective cytokines. IL-4 has a dual role (protective or disease-promoting) in pulmonary PCM depending on the genetic pattern of the host. Despite the less severe disease induced by administration of rIL-12, the strong inflammatory reaction in the lungs demonstrated the harmful effect of this cytokine. IL-10 appears to be the most important macrophage-deactivating cytokine in pulmonary PCM and its genetic absence appears to result in the aseptic cure of infected mice. Altogether, studies with cytokine-deficient mice showed that the Th1/Th2 paradigm can clearly be applied to explain fungal growth (or dissemination) in liver and spleen: IL-4 and IL-10 are disease-promoting cytokines while IL-12 and IFN-γ are protective ones. However, the control of fungal growth in the lungs is more complex and both Th1 (e.g., IL-12) and Th2 cytokines (e.g., IL-4) can have antagonistic effects. IL-10 is a disease-promoting cytokine and appears to have a more prominent role in the control of pulmonary PCM than IL-4 (Fig. 10.3).

3. Adaptive Immunity

Epidemiological studies have estimated that in endemic areas more than 10 million individuals could be infected with *P. brasiliensis* (Restrepo et al., 2001). Most of them, however, do not develop the disease demonstrating the protective effect of the adaptative immune response. T cell-mediated immunity has been recognized as the main protective mechanism through its ability to secrete cytokines, to activate phagocytes for fungal killing, to exert a putative cytotoxic effect on infected cells, to

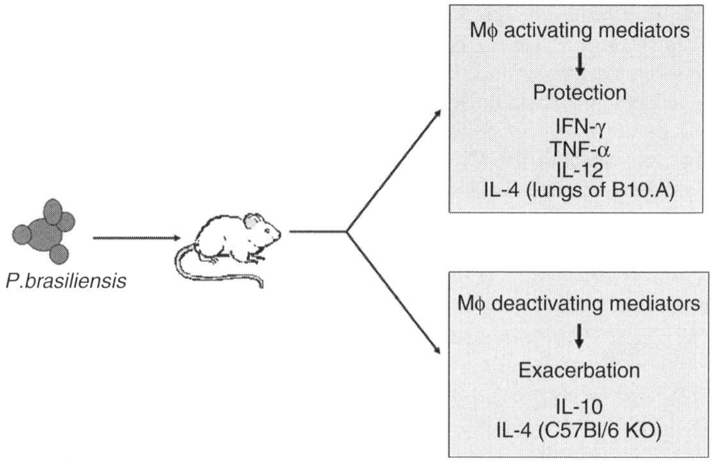

Figure 10.3. Cytokines in the pulmonary murine model of paracoccidioidomycosis. Studies were performed in vivo using cytokine-depleted or genetically cytokine-deficient mice.

control antibody production, and to regulate granuloma formation, an effective tissue response that limits fungal evasion.

3.1. Granulomatous Lesions

The organization of granulomatous lesions in *P. brasiliensis* infection is independent of the acquired immunity of patients, but the control of these lesions depends on the immunological status of the patients (Burger et al., 1996a; Xidieh et al., 1999). The tissular host response to *P. brasiliensis* is a typical epithelioid granulomatous inflammation with variable numbers of yeast cells and areas of suppuration. The epithelial tubercles can present central areas of necrosis, presence of variable numbers of giant cells, aggregates of PMN leukocytes in close association with fungal cells, a lymphomononuclear halo and fibrosis. B lymphocytes and plasma cells, usually secreting IgG antibodies, are also present in different numbers and stages of maturation (Montenegro and Franco, 1994; Camargo and Franco, 2000). Pioneer studies have demonstrated the correlation of organized granulomas and the presence of cellular immunity. Several experimental models confirmed such an association and a correlation between the number of giant cells, presence of a peripheral halo of lymphocytes, and cell-mediated immunity to *P. brasiliensis* antigens has been demonstrated with Pb18-infected Swiss mice (Coelho et al., 1994; Calich et al., 1998; Soares et al., 2000).

The multiple nonorganized lesions of susceptible mice present a little encapsulation mainly composed of type II collagen fibers whereas resistant mice develop residual or well-organized granulomas largely constituted by type I collagen and high expression of decorin, which appears to be a marker of the fibrogenic process (Xidieh et al., 1997; Nishikaku and Burger, 2003).

In vivo neutralization of cytokines or experiments using cytokine gene-deleted mice clearly showed that endogenous IFN-γ, TNF-α, and IL-12 are involved in the organization of the granulomatous lesions in the lungs and its absence leads to loose, nonorganized inflammatory reactions (Cano et al., 1998; Deepe et al., 2000; Souto et al., 2000). In contrast, absence or IL-4 neutralization induces the presence of smaller, well-organized granulomas circumscribed by a small halo of mononuclear leukocytes (Arruda et al., 2004; Pina et al., 2004).

Neworal et al. (2003) analyzed lymph nodes of patients with the JF of PCM and found a high expression of anti-inflammatory cytokines (IL-10 and TGF-β). Similarly in another study it was demonstrated that loose lesions of patients with severe disease present a high frequency of IL-5 and IL-10 positive cells. On the contrary, the well-organized lesions usually associated with the benign form of the infection present many cells positive for IL-2 and IFN-γ (Pagliari and Soto, 2003).

3.2. Bronchoalveolar Lavage Fluid

Analysis of bronchoalveolar lavage fluid (BALF) has been an important tool to follow the pulmonary infection caused by *P. brasiliensis*. The cellular and molecular composition of this material can bring information not only on the local inflammation but also on the adaptative immune response associated with progressive and regressive character of infection. Few studies available in experimental and human PCM report an increased number of different cell types such as neutrophils, lymphocytes, $CD4^+$, or $CD8^+$ T cells or even multinucleated giant cells in the BALF of infected individuals (Boscardin et al., 1985; Tapia et al., 1991; Cano, 1995; Vilani-Moreno et al., 1998; Calvi et al., 2003; Fornazim et al., 2003). A fact to be taken into consideration is that the majority of the patients involved in the studies were smokers and the correlation between smoking and increased number of alveolar macrophages and neutrophils is well known (Goldstein et al., 1990). However, the increase in lymphocytes is not a common finding in smokers, suggesting they are a result of the fungal infection itself.

Recent investigations in patients have compared the activity of AM with monocytes obtained from peripheral blood of same PCM patient. In both investigations predominance of macrophages associated with the presence of neutrophils and/or lymphocytes was described in BALF (Calvi et al., 2003; Fornazim et al., 2003). Compared with peripheral blood monocytes, cultured AM spontaneously secreted higher amounts of IL-6, TNF-α, and MIP-1α and presented a higher expression of adhesion and costimulatory molecules (HLA-class II antigen, ICAM-1, and B7-2) (Fornazim et al., 2003). The expression of HLA class II, ICAM-1, and B7-2 in alveolar macrophages seems to indicate a preserved and active macrophage function in patients with PCM. Another interesting finding was the increased number of $CD8^+$ T cells in PCM BALF. MIP-1α was shown to promote chemotaxis of lymphocytes selectively recruiting $CD8^+$ T cells (Serody et al., 2000). As better discussed below, a protective role for $CD8^+$ T cells was observed in experimental PCM since its depletion induces a more severe and disseminated disease in both resistant and susceptible mice (Cano et al., 2000).

Recent study performed by Calvi et al. (2003) showed an equivalent fungicidal ability and hydrogen peroxide production when alveolar macrophages and blood monocytes from PCM patients were compared. In contrast, Bretaña et al. (1995) described a low percentage of alveolar macrophages expressing MHC class II antigen in BALF of patients with PCM as compared with other pulmonary diseases and this fact was understood as a defect in activation of macrophages with consequences in the processing and defense functions against *P. brasiliensis*.

Studies in the pulmonary model of infection clearly demonstrated that the degree of alveolar macrophage activation depends on the severity of the disease and host's immune response. Thus, in the course of the infection, resistant mice presented increased macrophage activation concomitant with positive DTH reactions whereas absence of macrophage activation and anergy of DTH reactions were found in susceptible mice

(Cano et al., 1995). In addition, the presence of multinucleated giant cells was more evident in resistant mice at the acquired phase of immunity (Cano, 1995). Interestingly, IL-4 and IFN-γ have been reported to induce giant cell formation (McInnes and Rennick, 1988; Most et al., 1991) and the trapping of *Cryptococcus neoformans* to the site of infection was shown to be associated with the presence of $CD4^+$ T cells which cause the formation of multinucleated giant cells (Hill, 1992). Both IL-4 and IFN-γ were found in lung homogenates of resistant and susceptible mice (Cano et al., 1998), but $CD4^+$ T cells were found to play an important role only in the immunity of resistant mice (Calich, 2003).

3.3. Humoral Immunity as a Marker of T Cell Immunity

Although in some fungal infections specific antibodies may have a protective role (reviewed by Casadevall et al., 2002) in human, and experimental PCM antibody production is a marker of disease severity. Thus, patients with the acute or chronic disseminated forms of disease have high titers of antibodies, polyclonal activation of B cells, and circulating immune complexes (reviewed by Camargo and Cano, 1994; Camargo and Franco, 2000). Additionally, significant titers of antibodies can persist after successful treatment of the disease suggesting that they have no protective role. Some experimental models reproduced these findings of human disease but the isogenic murine model of PCM first elucidated the role of T cells and cytokines in determining the isotype and amount of antibody produced.

Studying murine PCM in athymic BALB/c mice and their euthymic counterparts it was verified that most of the *P. brasiliensis* components are T-dependent antigens although some of them, including gp43, can directly activate B cells without the help of $CD4^+$ T cells (Burger et al., 1996b). Immunoblotting studies also showed that both resistant and susceptible mice can produce antibodies to major *P. brasiliensis* components but susceptible mice are able to react with minor antigens not recognized by the resistant animals (Vaz et al., 1998). In the pulmonary model of infection, the more severe disease of susceptible mice was associated with increased production of IgG1 and IgG2b (Cano et al., 1995), which are respectively regulated by IL-4 and TGF-α (McIntire et al., 1993; Snapper et al., 1997). Conversely, the regressive pulmonary disease of resistant mice was associated with predominant secretion of IgG2a (Cano et al., 1995), a recognized IFN-γ-regulated isotype (Snapper and Paul, 1987).

The production of polyclonal IgE was associated with impairment of T cell-mediated immunity in patients with PCM (Arango and Yarzabal, 1982). JF patients present high titers of IgE (Biselli et al., 2001; Mamoni et al., 2001, 2002) and IgG4 anti-gp43 (Baida et al., 1999; Mamoni et al., 2002), the immunodominant and specific molecule of *P. brasiliensis*. Elevated levels of IgG4 and IgE were also observed in patients with the multifocal adult form of the disease. From the clinical point of view, these are patients with disseminated disease with lymph node involvement. This group is illustrative of the heterogeneity of the AF of PCM, ranging from isolated lesions in the respiratory tract to widely disseminated forms.

A strong positive correlation between specific IgE levels and IgG4, IgA, and eosinophilia was described for patients with the JF of PCM (Mamoni et al., 2002). The authors observed significantly higher numbers and percentages of peripheral eosinophils in JF compared to AF patients. The degree of eosinophilia was positively correlated with IgE levels and both parameters decreased with treatment. These results are in accordance with those of Benard et al. (1996), who showed an inverse correlation between eosinophil levels and T cell function, evaluated by the in vitro proliferative response to *P. brasiliensis* antigens. They also agree with the observation of high levels of IL-5 and peripheral blood eosinophilia detected in susceptible mice (Kashino et al., 2000). A recent paper suggested that eosinophils, through toxic granule proteins, could participate in the pathophysiology of PCM (Wagner et al., 1998).

In experimental PCM a preferential secretion of specific IgA was associated with progressive disease in susceptible mice (Kashino et al., 2000). However, the data concerning IgA antibodies production in the two forms of human PCM is scarce and controversial (Bueno et al., 1997; Baida et al., 1999). Higher IgA-specific antibodies amounts were detected in the JF rather than in the AF of PCM in addition to increased levels of TGF-β (Mamoni et al., 2002). TGF-β is a cytokine responsible for IgA switch (McIntire et al., 1993), in addition to a variety of other immunologic effects such as inhibition of the proliferative response of T cells and impairment of macrophages activation (Clark and Coker, 1998). TGF-β was also detected in lymph nodes from patients with the JF of PCM, probably promoting a local anti-inflammatory response (Neworal et al., 2003).

3.4. Cellular Immunity

It has long been appreciated that T cells are essential for containing fungal infections (Huffnagle and Deepe, 2003; Koguchi and Kawakami, 2002; Romani, 2004) and it has been postulated that $CD4^+$ T cells are the principal lymphocytes involved in the protective immune response to *P. brasiliensis*. Several investigations have reported the association between anergy in DTH reactions and low lymphoproliferative responses with the severe forms of PCM (Benard et al., 1995; 1997). In relation to lymphocyte subpopulations, decreased percentage of T cells associated with normal or elevated number of B lymphocytes was described in human patients. In addition, a significant fall in the CD4/CD8 ratio was found in the peripheral blood of patients with both the acute and chronic forms of the disease. The increased number of $CD8^+$ T lymphocytes was associated with enhanced suppressive activity of Con-A activated lymphocytes (reviewed by Musatti et al., 1994). The mechanisms involved in the imbalance of lymphocyte subsets remain unclear.

3.4.1. Cytokines and Immunoregulation

More recently it has been shown in experimental and human PCM that fungal antigens induce the production of Th1 or Th2 cytokines according to the severity of the disease (Calich and Kashino, 1998; Cano et al., 1998; Benard et al., 2001; Oliveira et al., 2002). This fact indicates that fungal antigens are mainly processed in the endosomal MHC class II pathway and are subsequently presented to $CD4^+$, class II-restricted T cells. However, the low frequency of PCM in patients with HIV infection (Goldani and Sugar, 1995) seems not to support this pathway as the principal mode of antigen presentation to T cells. Furthermore, recent findings in the pulmonary model of infection using CD4-depleted, CD8-depleted, CD4 KO, and CD8 KO mice, described below, appear to indicate the important function of $CD8^+$ T lymphocytes in the control of fungal growth in pulmonary PCM.

Peripheral blood lymphocytes from patients with both the AF and JF of PCM proliferate poorly and produce low or undetectable levels of the Th1 cytokines IFN-γ and IL-2 in response to gp43, as compared to healthy *P. brasiliensis* sensitized individuals (Benard et al., 2001). IL-4 and IL-5 were detected in patients with active PCM (Mello et al., 2002) and in JF patients (Oliveira et al., 2002), suggesting the preferential activation of Th2 cells. Another Th2 feature well characterized in PCM is the blood eosinophilia observed in some JF patients and susceptible mice (Benard et al., 1996; Kashino et al., 2000; Mamoni et al., 2002). The lymphoproliferative response and IFN-γ production can be restored by concomitant treatment of peripheral blood leukocytes with recombinant IL-12 and anti-IL-10, showing a synergistic action of these reagents (Romano et al., 2002). Altogether these data have been used to explain the immunosuppression of PCM patients.

Recent investigations have described different mechanisms underlying T cell dysfunction in human PCM. Campanelli et al. (2003) detected an overexpression of anexin V^+ and FasL in T cells of patients with PCM, suggesting the activation of cell death mechanisms during the disease. These data confirmed previous findings of gp43-induced apoptosis of cells from PCM patients (Cacere et al., 2002). In addition to anexin V^+ and FasL, an overexpression of CTLA-4, a critical costimulatory molecule that downregulates T cell activation, was also observed in antigen-stimulated T cells from PCM patients. In conclusion, besides cytokines imbalances, other inhibitory mechanisms can actively participate in the T cell unresponsiveness of PCM patients.

3.4.2. T Cell Subsets

The evidences on the role of T cell subsets in human and experimental PCM are scarce and mainly indirect. Almost no investigations discriminate the role played by $CD4^+$ and $CD8^+$ T cells in the immunopathogenesis and immunoregulation of human and experimental disease. This fact led us to study the contribution of $CD4^+$ and $CD8^+$ T lymphocyte subsets to protective immune responses against *P. brasiliensis* infection (Calich, 2003). Experiments were performed using susceptible (B10.A) and resistant (A/J) mice as well as CD4 KO and CD8 KO mice in a C57BL/6 background. Previous in vivo studies using our murine model of pulmonary PCM demonstrated that $CD8^+$ T lymphocytes played a protective function in the immune response mounted by susceptible and resistant mice to *P. brasiliensis* infection. Moreover, only in susceptible mice a regulatory $CD8^+$ T cell subset was present and was able to suppress DTH reactions (Cano et al., 2000). Further studies on pulmonary cytokines demonstrated that depletion of $CD8^+$ T cells of resistant mice led to decreased levels of IL-2 concomitant with augmented levels of IL-4 indicating a predominant type 1 behavior of these cells. In susceptible mice, however, the increment in the IL-10 and IFN-γ levels induced by anti-CD8 mAb treatment indicated the presence of both type 1 and type 2 $CD8^+$ T cells (Chiarella, 2003).

In contrast with other infectious pathologies, depletion of $CD4^+$ T cells of B10.A and A/J mice by mAb did not increase the severity of the disease induced by a low virulent *P. brasiliensis* isolate (Cano, 1995). With a virulent isolate a different effect was seen in resistant and susceptible mice. Thus, in vivo depletion of $CD4^+$ T cells did not affect the severe disease developed by the susceptible strain whereas in resistant mice a consecutive action of protective (Th1) and disease-promoting (Th2) $CD4^+$ T cells was characterized. In both mouse strains antibody production was mainly $CD4^+$ T cell-dependent. Yet, positive DTH reactions of resistant mice were mediated by T $CD4^+$ lymphocytes and the DTH anergy of B10.A mice was governed by $CD8^+$ T cells (T-suppressor cells?). These findings appear to have special relevance since the contribution of $CD4^+$ and $CD8^+$ T cells to *P. brasiliensis* immunity was determined concurrently for comparison (Calich, 2003).

Preliminary studies with CD4-KO and CD8-KO mice confirmed the important role of both $CD8^+$ and $CD4^+$ lymphocytes in the immunoprotection of pulmonary PCM. Genetic deficiency of $CD8^+$ or $CD4^+$ T cells results in a more severe disease only at late phases of infection confirming the important protective function of natural immunity in pulmonary PCM. In the C57BL/6 mice the protective effect of $CD8^+$ cells was superior to that conferred by $CD4^+$ T cells (Arruda and Calich, unpublished observations; Calich, 2003). These clear results indicate that the importance of $CD8^+$ T cells is underestimated in PCM but also suggest that $CD8^+$ T cell immunity against *P. brasiliensis* needs conventional $CD4^+$ T cells to maintain protective immunity.

The results obtained with mice deleted or deficient of $CD4^+$ or $CD8^+$ T cells appear to suggest the following picture regarding the participation of T cell subsets in the immunopathogenesis of murine PCM. Resistant and susceptible strains develop protective type 1 $CD8^+$ T lymphocytes but only susceptible mice present concomitant activation of type 2 or CD8-suppressor cells. Resistant and susceptible mice develop Th2 $CD4^+$ T cells, which regulate antibody production although only resistant mice mount an early protective Th1 immune response. In this scenario, the only protective cell in susceptible hosts is the $CD8^+$ subpopulation that was unable to overcome the negative effect of Th2 cells, CD8-suppressor lymphocytes, and excessive production of nitric oxide. In resistant mice, the protective $CD8^+$ T cell subset is supported by a Th1 $CD4^+$ subset, which regulate Th2 cells resulting in a balanced and protective immune response (Fig. 10.4).

3.4.3. Immunoprotection

Both susceptible and resistant mice inoculated with *P. brasiliensis* by the s.c. route develop a self-healing infection. B10.A mice, however, mount a more evident DTH response that can be elicited with a fungal infecting dose 100-fold lower than that required to prime A/J mice. This interesting finding demonstrates that susceptible mice have a high T cell reactivity, which could be further explored by vaccinating procedures.

The role of cytokines and lymphocyte subsets in secondary PCM was investigated in our laboratory. The protective immunity against a pulmonary challenge conferred by a previous subcutaneous inoculation of fungal cells was assessed using B10.A and A/J mice. Immunoprotection was achieved only in B10.A mice and was associated with low fungal loads, reversal of DTH anergy, and a more intense pulmonary inflammatory response

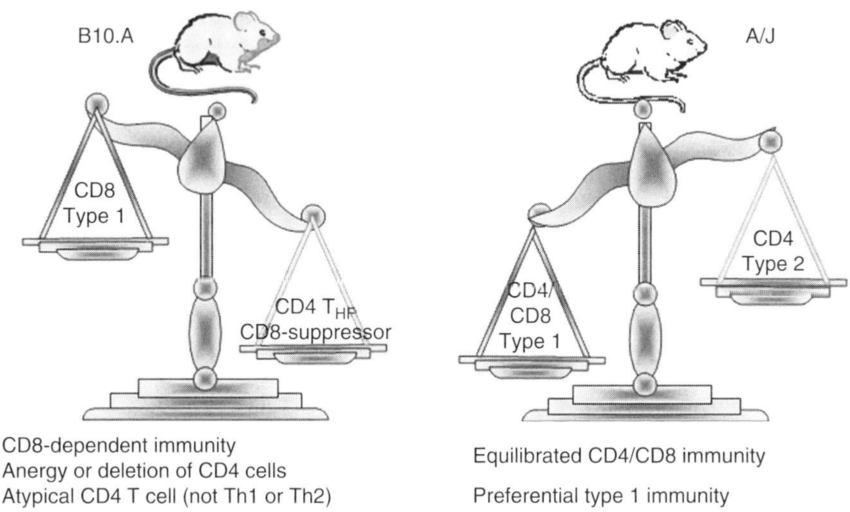

Figure 10.4. Role of T cell subsets in the murine model of paracoccidioidomycosis. Susceptible (B10.A) mice appear to mount a concomitant type-1 and type-2 $CD8^+$ T cell immunity that does not compensate the anergy or deletion of protective Th1 $CD4^+$ T cells. A preferential type-1 immunity composed by $CD4^+$ and $CD8^+$ T lymphocytes associated with Th2 cells appears to determine the regressive pattern of infection of resistant (A/J) mice.

that probably restrained the local growth and spread of the fungus. This vaccinating procedure conferred a sterilizing immunity to B10.A mice, since late in the infection no fungal cells could be isolated from pretreated mice whereas all nonvaccinated animals died of an overwhelming infection (Arruda, 1999). The immunoprotection was long-lasting and could also be induced by a nonvirulent fungal isolate. The in vivo depletion of $CD4^+$ and $CD8^+$ T cells as well as of endogenous IFN-γ and IL-12 led to impaired immunoprotection suggesting that this phenomenon is multimediated and requires the function of both T cell subpopulations and the activity of proinflammatory cytokines. As the previous s.c. infection did not alter the disease outcome of resistant A/J mice, we could demonstrate that the genetic background of hosts determines the success or failure of a vaccinating procedure and, interestingly, the susceptible background is more reactive to fungal components and prone to develop protective immunity than the resistant one.

BALB/c mice, which have an intermediate pattern of susceptibility to *P. brasiliensis* infection, can develop a protective Th1 immune response to gp43 immunization and after a DNA-based vaccination using the gp43 gene. Furthermore, the immunodominant T-cell epitope in gp43 has been mapped to a 15-residue sequence and immunization with the corresponding polypeptide induces partial immunoprotection against a virulent fungal isolate (Taborda et al., 1998; Pinto et al., 2000).

In conclusion, $CD8^+$ T lymphocytes are very important protective cells in primary and secondary PCM. These lymphocytes can also act as regulatory cells of cellular immunity in susceptible hosts. Protective Th1 $CD4^+$ T lymphocytes were only detected in resistant mice and susceptibility of B10.A mice was not abolished by depletion of $CD4^+$ T cells or IL-4. This behavior indicates that susceptibility of B10.A mice is not mainly controlled by $CD4^+$ T cells (Th2 subset) and other regulatory mechanisms such as excessive production of nitric oxide (Nascimento et al., 2002) and anergy or deletion of T lymphocytes can play a role in the defective immunity developed by susceptible hosts. In the C57BL/6 background, however, a clear Th1/Th2 mechanism of immunoregulation could be demonstrated (Arruda et al., 2004; Pina et al., 2004) although even in this strain NO production plays a very important effect in controlling T cell responsiveness (Bocca et al., 1988; Nascimento et al., 2002).

4. Concluding Remarks: A Hypothesis on the Mechanisms of Resistance and Susceptibility to *P. brasiliensis*

In human disease the Th1/Th2 dichotomy of $CD4^+$ T cells immune response appears to partially explain the behavior of PCM patients and healthy infected individuals. So, the most evident Th1 immunity is observed when lymphocytes from healthy infected subjects or cured patients are in vitro activated by gp43 and a clear production of IL-2 and IFN-γ is concomitant with a vigorous lymphoproliferative response. The JF or acute form of the disease appears to be the Th2 pole of reactivity, in which IL-4, IL-5, and IL-10 are produced and associated with low T cell proliferation, which however can be reverted by in vitro treatment with rIL-12 and anti-IL-10 antibodies. The severe form of the chronic disease also appears to present a Th2 pattern of reactivity. Several individuals of the chronic form of PCM, however, do not display polarized Th1/Th2 immune responses and their hyporesponsiveness appear not to be linked to imbalanced cytokine synthesis and may be due to other immunoregulatory mechanisms such as T cell anergy or deletion by apoptosis. The roles played by T cell subsets, however, remain unclear.

The concomitant analysis on the functional activity of macrophages and T cell subsets in the mechanisms of resistance and susceptibility to *P. brasiliensis* infection encouraged us to propose a general model on the immunopathogenesis of pulmonary PCM. Alveolar macrophages of susceptible mice are very reactive to *P. brasiliensis* components and proinflammatory mediators are secreted by cells involved in the innate immunity of lungs. The high production of IL-12 stimulate NK cells to secrete elevated amounts of IFN-γ that induces the secretion of high levels of nitric oxide by macrophages which develop a very efficient fungicidal ability. Anti-inflammatory cytokines such as IL-10 and/or TGF-β are secreted in low levels. Also, such behavior is similar to the previously described M1 or reductive macrophages (Mills et al., 2000; Murata et al., 2002) and results in a very effective innate immunity and precocious control of fungal growth. This behavior is adequate to the activation of Th1 $CD4^+$ cells. The excessive and continuous production of NO, however, inhibits the initial development of $CD4^+$ T cell immunity by active induction of T cell anergy or deletion. The elevated expression of costimulatory molecules (MHC class I, CD40, B7, for example) by macrophages can directly activate $CD8^+$ T cells without the help of $CD4^+$ T lymphocytes (Albert et al., 1998; Ridge et al., 1998). The high production of antibodies could be ascribed to a nonclassical Th cell subset recently described, the T Helper–Follicular subpopulation (T_{HF}). This population localizes preferentially to lymph node germinal centers, does not secrete typical Th2 cytokines but is very efficient in helping B cell antibody production (Breitfeld et al., 2000). This pattern of immunity could explain the very efficient mechanism of natural immunity resulting, however, in poor T cell-mediated immunity (Fig. 10.5). It could also explain the

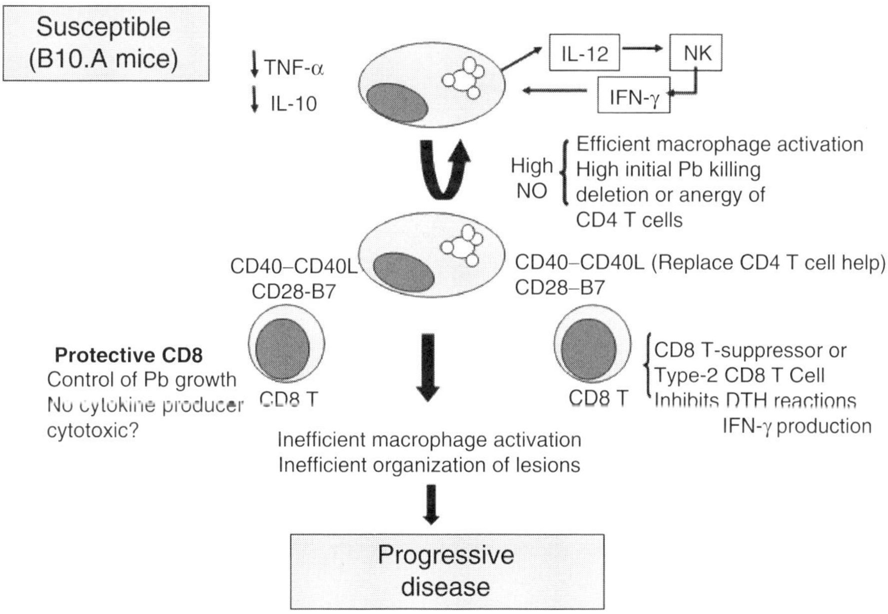

Figure 10.5. Hypothesis on the innate and acquired immunological mechanisms leading to resistance to *P. brasiliensis* infection. At the innate phase of immunity, macrophages from resistant mice secrete low amounts of IL-12 associated with high levels of IL-10, resulting in impaired nitric oxide (NO) secretion and inefficient fungal clearance. However, the slow but prevalent type-1 acquired immunity mediated by both $CD4^+$ and $CD8^+$ T cells is able to induce efficient macrophage activation and regressive disease.

DTH anergy, the nonorganized lesions, the high levels of antibodies, and the progressive disease developed by susceptible mice and JF patients.

Alveolar macrophages from resistant mice respond to *P. brasiliensis* infection by secreting low amounts of IL-12, but high levels of IL-10 and TNF-α. This behavior results in poor NK cell activation, IFN-γ production, NO secretion, and inefficient fungal killing at initial times of infection. This activity is similar to that previously described for M2 or oxidative macrophages (Mills et al., 2000; Murata et al., 2002) and characterizes the low efficient natural immunity of resistant mice. The production of cytokines and NO in low levels does not impair T cell immunity. So, resistant animals slowly develop *P. brasiliensis* specific $CD4^+$ and $CD8^+$ T lymphocytes, which control fungal growth and organize lesion morphology (Fig. 10.6).

The present hypothesis does not exclude the previously proposed Th1/Th2 model of *P. brasiliensis* control. It tries, however, to put together many results of innate and acquired immunity observed in the murine pulmonary model of infection, which eventually may contribute to enhance our knowledge on the immunopathogenesis of human PCM.

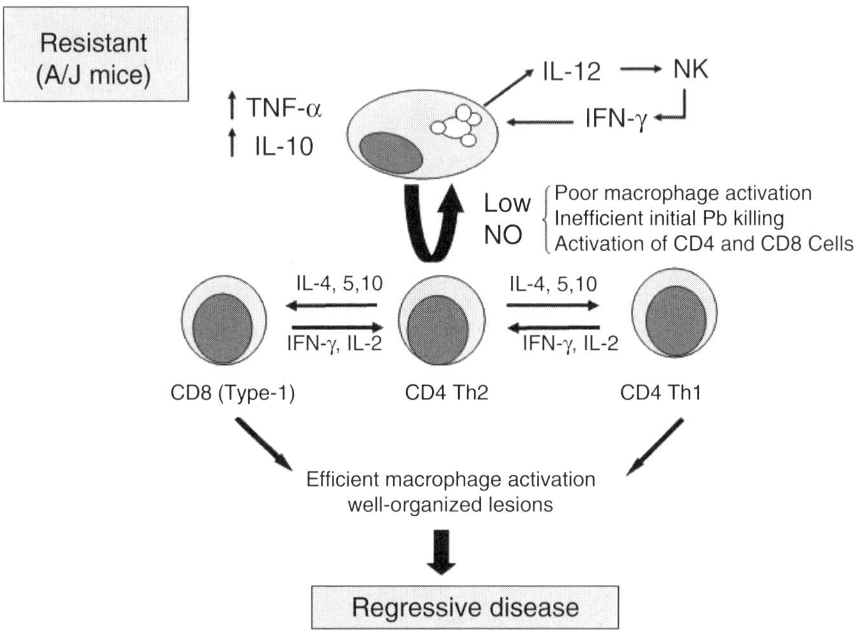

Figure 10.6. Hypothesis on the innate and acquired immunological mechanisms leading to susceptibility to *P. brasiliensis* infection. At the initial stage of infection, macrophages from susceptible mice secrete high amounts of IL-12 and nitric oxide (NO), resulting in efficient fungal clearance. However, excessive NO secretion induces anergy or deletion of $CD4^+$ T cells. The expression of high levels of costimulatory molecules by antigen-presenting cells induces a preferential activation of $CD8^+$ T cells that is not sufficient to efficiently activate macrophages and to control disease progression.

References

Albert, M., Sauter, B., and Bhardwaj, N. (1998). Dendritic cells acquire antigen from apoptotic cells and induce class I-restricted CTLs. *Nature* 392: 86–89.

Almeida, S.R., Moraes, J.Z., Camargo, Z.P., Geztesi, J.L., Mariano, M., and Lopes, J.D. (1998). Pattern of immune response to gp43 from *P. brasiliensis* in susceptible and resistant mice is influenced by antigen-presenting cells. *Clin. Immunol.* 190: 68–76.

André, D.C., Lopes, J.D., Franco, M.F., Vaz, C.A.C., and Calich, V.L.G. (2004). Binding of laminin to *Paracoccidioides brasiliensis* induces a less severe pulmonary paracoccidioidomycosis caused by virulent and low-virulent isolates. *Microbes Infect.* 6: 549–559.

Arango, M. and Yarzabal, L. (1982). T-cell dysfunction and hyperimmunoglobulinemia E in paracoccidioidomycosis. *Mycopathologia* 79: 115–119.

Arruda, C. (1999). Paracoccidioidomicose pulmonar experimental: Imunoproteção induzida pela inoculação subcutânea prévia do fungo, PhD Thesis, Instituto de Ciências Biomédicas, Universidade de São Paulo, São Paulo.

Arruda, C., Franco, M.F., Kashino, S.S., Nascimento, F.R.F., Fazioli, R.A., Vaz, C.A.C., Russo, M., and Calich, V.L.G. (2002). IL-12 protects mice against disseminated infection caused by *Paracoccidioides brasiliensis* but enhances pulmonary inflammation. *Clin. Immunol.* 103: 185–195.

Arruda, C., Valente-Ferreira, R.C., Pina, A., Kashino, S.S., Fazioli, R.A., Vaz, C.A.C., Franco, M.F., and Calich, V.L.G. (2004). Dual role of IL-4 in pulmonary paracoccidioidomycosis: Endogenous IL-4 can induce protection or exacerbation of disease depending on the host genetic pattern. *Infect. Immun.* 72: 3932–3940.

Baida, H.B., Biselli, P.J.C., Juvenale, M., Del Negro, G., Mendes-Giannini, M.J.S., Duarte, A.J.S., and Benard, G. (1999). Differential antibody isotype expression to the major *Paracoccidioides brasiliensis* antigen in juvenile and adult form paracoccidioidomycosis. *Microbes Infect.* 1: 273–278.

Benard, G., Durandy, A., Assis, C.M., Hong, M., Orii, A.N.M., Sato, N.M., Mendes-Giannini, M.J.S., Lacaz, C.S., and Duarte, A.J.S. (1995). Responses of T and B lymphocytes to a *Paracoccidioides brasiliensis* cell wall extract in healthy sensitized and nonsensitized subjects. *Am. J. Trop. Med. Hyg.* 53: 189–194.

Benard, G., Hong, M.A., Del Negro, G.M.B., Batista, L., Shikanai-Yasuda, M.A., and Duarte, A.J. (1996). Antigen-specific immunosuppression in paracoccidioidomycosis. *Am. J. Trop. Med. Hyg.* 50: 7–12.

Benard, G., Mendes-Giannini, M.J.S., Juvenale, M., Miranda, E.T., and Duarte A.J. (1997). Immunosuppression in paracoccidioidomycosis: T cell hyporesponsiveness to two *Paracoccidioides brasiliensis* glycoproteins that elicit strong humoral immune response. *J. Infect. Dis.* 175: 1263–1267.

Benard, G., Romano, C.C., Cacere, C.R., Juvenale, M., Mendes-Giannini, M.J.S., and Duarte, A.J. (2001). Imbalance of IL-2, IFN-gamma and IL-10 secretion in the immunosuppression associated with human paracoccidioidomycosis. *Cytokine* 13: 248–252.

Biselli, P.J., Juvenale, M., Mendes-Giannini, M.J.S., Duarte, A.J., and Benard, G. (2001). IgE antibody response to the main antigenic component of *Paracoccidioides brasiliensis* in patients with paracoccidioidomycosis. *Med. Mycol.* 39: 475–478.

Bocca, A.L., Hayashi, E.E, Pinheiro, A.G., Furianetto, A.B., Campanelli, A.P., Cunha, F.Q., and Figueiredo, F. (1988). Treatment of *Paracoccidioides brasiliensis* infected mice with a nitric oxide inhibitor prevents the failure of cell-mediated immune responses. *J. Immunol.* 162: 3056–3063.

Borges-Welmsley, M.I., Chen, D., Shu, X., and Welmsley, A.R. (2002). The pathobiology of *Paracoccidioides brasiliensis*. *Trends Microbiol.* 10: 80–87.

Boscardin, R.N., Brandão, H., and Balla, A. (1985). Bronchoalveolar lavage findings in pulmonary paracoccidioidomycosis. *J. Med. Vet. Mycol.* 23: 143–146.

Breitfeld, D., Ohl, L., Kremmer, E., Ellwart, J., Sallusto, F., Lipp, M., and Forster, R. (2000). Follicular B helper T cells express CXC chemokine receptor, localize to B-cell follicles, and support immunoglobulin production. *J. Exp. Med.* 111: 1545–1522.

Bretaña, A., Goihman-Yahr, M., Tapia, F.J., Istúriz, G., Viloria, N., Carrasquero, M., Saavedra, N., Albornoz, M.C., Pereira, J., Román, A., and Gómez, M.H. (1995). Comparative ultrastructure and immunolabeling of MHC-II antigens of alveolar macrophages obtained from patients with paracoccidioidomycosis and other lung diseases. *J. Leukoc. Biol.* 57: 101–109.

Brummer, E. (1994). Interaction of *Paracoccidioides brasiliensis* with host defense cells. In M. Franco, C.S. Lacaz, A. Restrepo, and G. Del Negro (eds), *Paracoccidioidomycosis*. CRC Press, Boca Raton, Florida, pp. 213–224.

Brummer, E., Hanson, L.H., and Stevens, D.A. (1988). Gamma-interferon activation of macrophages for killing of *Paracoccidioides brasiliensis*: Evidence for non-oxidative mechanisms. *Int. J. Immunopharmacol.* 10: 945–952.

Brummer, E., Castañeda, E., and Restrepo, A. (1993). Paracoccidioidomycosis: An update. *Clin. Microbiol. Rev.* 6: 89–117.

Bueno, J.P., Mendes-Giannini, M.J.S., Del Negro, G.M.B., Assis, C.M., Takiguti, C.A., and Shikanai-Yasuda, M.A. (1997). IgG, IgM, IgA antibody response for the diagnosis and follow-up of paracoccidioidomycosis: Comparison of counterimmunoelectrophoresis and complement fixation. *J. Med. Vet. Mycol.* 35: 213–217.

Burger, E., Singer-Vermes, L.M., and Calich, V.L.G. (1985). Role of C5 in experimental murine paracoccidioidomycosis. *J. Infect. Dis.* 152: 425.

Burger, E., Miyaji, M., Sano, A., Calich, V.L.G., Nishimura, K., and Lenzi, H.L. (1996a). Histopathology of paracoccidioidomycotic infection in athymic and euthymic mice: A sequential study. *Am. J. Trop. Med. Hyg.* 55: 235–242.

Burger, E., Vaz, C.A.C., Sano, A., Calich, V.L.G., Singer-Vermes, L.M., Xidieh, C.F., Kashino, S.S., Nishimura, K., and Miyaji, M. (1996b). *Paracoccidioides brasiliensis* infection in nude mice: Studies with isolates differing in virulence and definition of their T-cell-dependent and T-cell independent components. *Am. J. Trop. Med. Hyg.* 55: 391–398.

Cacere, C.R., Romano, C.C., Mendes-Giannini, M.J.S., Duarte, A.J., and Benard, G. (2002). The role of apoptosis in the antigen-specific T cell hyporesponsiveness of paracoccidioidomycosis patients. *Clin. Immunol.* 105: 215–222.

Calich, V.L.G. (2003). Control of pulmonary paracoccidioidomycosis by T cell subsets. In *Proceedings of the 15th Congress of the International Society for Human and Animal Mycology*, San Antonio, Texas, pp. 281–282.

Calich, V.L.G. and Kashino, S.S. (1998). Cytokines produced by susceptible and resistant mice in the course of *Paracoccidioides brasiliensis* infection. *Braz. J. Med. Exper. Biol.* 31: 615–623.

Calich, V.L.G., Singer-Vermes, L.M., and Burger, E. (1985). Susceptibility and resistance of inbred mice to *Paracoccidioides brasiliensis*. *Br. J. Exp. Pathol.* 66: 585–594.

Calich, V.L.G., Burger, E., Kashino, S.S., Fazioli, R.A., and Singer-Vermes, L.M. (1987). Resistance to *Paracoccidioides brasiliensis* in mice is controlled by a single dominant autosomal gene. *Infect. Immun.* 55: 1919–1923.

Calich, V.L.G., Singer-Vermes, L.M., Russo, M., Vaz, C.A.C., and Burger, E. (1994). Immunogenetics in paracoccidioidomycosis. In M. Franco, C.S. Lacaz, A. Restrepo-Moreno, and G. Del Negro (eds), *Paracoccidioidomycosis*. CRC Press, Boca Raton, Florida, pp. 151–173.

Calich, V.L.G., Vaz, C.A.C., and Burger, E. (1998). Immunity to *Paracoccidioides brasiliensis* infection. *Res. Immunol.* 149: 407–416.

Calvi, S.A., Soares, A.M.V.C., Peraçoli, M.T.S., Franco, M., Ruiz, R.L. Jr., Marcondes-Machado, J., Fecchio, D., Mattos, M.C.I., and Mendes, R.P. (2003). Study of bronchoalveolar lavage fluid in paracoccidioidomycosis: Cytopathology and alveolar macrophage function in response to gamma interferon; comparison with blood leukocytes. *Microbes Infect.* 5: 1373–1379.

Camargo, Z.P. and Cano, L.E. (1994). Humoral Immunity. In M. Franco, C.S. Lacaz, A. Restrepo, and G. Del Negro (eds), *Paracoccidioidomycosis*. CRC Press, Boca Raton, Florida, pp. 187–197.

Camargo, Z.P. and Franco, M.F. (2000). Current knowledge on pathogenesis and immunodiagnosis of paracoccidioidomycosis. *Rev. Iberoam. Micol.* 17: 41–48.

Campanelli, A.P., Martins, G.A., Souto, J.T., Pereira, M.S., Livonesi, M.C., Martinez, R., and Silva, J.S. (2003). Fas–Fas ligand (CD95–CD95L) and cytotoxic T lymphocyte antigen-4 engagement mediate T cell unresponsiveness in patients with paracoccidioidomycosis. *J. Infect. Dis.* 187: 1496–1505.

Cano, L.E. (1995). Paracoccidioidomicose pulmonar experimental. Caracterização do modelo de infecção intratraqueal em camundongos resistentes e susceptíveis; participação do IFN-γ células T $CD4^+$ e $CD8^+$ na resistência ao fungo, PhD Thesis, Instituto de Ciências Biomédicas, Universidade de São Paulo, São Paulo.

Cano, L.E., Gómez, B., Brummer, E., Restrepo, A., and Stevens, D.A. (1994). Inhibitory effect of deferoxamine or macrophage activation on transformation of *Paracoccidioides brasiliensis* conidia by ingested macrophages: Reversal by holotransferrin. *Infect. Immun.* 62: 1494–1496.

Cano, L.E., Singer-Vermes, L.M., Vaz, C.A.C., Russo, M., and Calich V.L.G. (1995). Pulmonary paracoccidioidomycosis in resistant and susceptible mice: Relationship among progression of infection, bronchoalveolar cell activation, cellular immune response and specific isotype patterns. *Infect. Immun.* 63: 1777–1783.

Cano, L.E., Kashino, S.S., Arruda, C., André, D., Xidieh, C.F., Singer-Vermes, L.M., Vaz, C.A.C., Burger, E., and Calich, V.L.G. (1998). Protective role of interferon-gamma in experimental pulmonary paracoccidioidomycosis. *Infect. Immun.* 66: 800–806.

Cano, L.E., Singer-Vermes, L.M., Mengel, J.A., Xidieh, C.F., Arruda, C., André, D.C., Vaz, C.A.C., Burger, E., and Calich, V.L.G. (2000). Depletion of CD8 T cells *in vivo* impairs host defense of resistant and susceptible mice to pulmonary paracoccidioidomycosis. *Infect. Immun.* 68: 352–359.

Casadevall, A., Feldmesser, M., and Pirofski, L.A. (2002). Induced humoral immunity and vaccination against major human fungal pathogens. *Curr. Opin. Microbiol.* 5: 386–391.

Chiarella, A.P. (2003). Caracterização da função das células TCD4$^+$ e T CD8$^+$ na paracoccidioidomicose pulmonar de camundongos isogênicos. Características imunopatológicas da paracoccidioidomicose experimental, MSc Dissertation, Instituto de Ciências Biomédicas, Universidade de São Paulo, São Paulo.

Clark, D.A. and Coker, R. (1998). Transforming growth factor-beta (TGF-β) *Int. J. Biochem. Cell Biol.* 30: 293–298.

Coelho, K.I.R., Defaveri, J., Rezkalllah-Iwasso, M.T., and Peraçoli, T.S. (1994). In M. Franco, C.S. Lacaz, A. Restrepo, and G.D. Negro (eds), *Paracoccidioidomycosis*. CRC Press, Boca Raton, FL, pp. 87–102.

Colucci, F., Caligiuri, M.A., and Di Santo, J.P. (2003). What does it take to make a natural killer? *Nature Rev.* 3: 413–425.

Deepe, G.S., Romani, L., Calich, V.L.G., Huffnagle, G., Arruda, C., Molinari-Madlum, E.E.I.W., and Perfect, J.R. (2000). Knockout mice as experimental models of virulence. *Med. Mycol.* 38: 87–98.

Fava Netto, C., Castro, R.M., Gonçalves, A.P., and Dillon, N.L. (1965). Ocorrência familiar de blastomicose sul-americana. A propósito de 14 casos. *Rev. Inst. Med. Trop. São Paulo* 11: 177–184.

Fava Netto, C., Vegas, V.S., Sciannaméa, I.M., and Guarnieri, E.D.B. (1969). Antígeno polisacarídico *do Paracoccidioides brasiliensis*. Estudo do tempo de cultivo do *P. brasiliensis* necessário ao preparo do antígeno. *Rev. Inst. Med. Trop. São Paulo* 11: 177–181.

Ferreira, K.S., Lopes, J.D., and Almeida, S.R. (2003). Regulation of T helper differentiation in vivo by gp43 from *Paracoccidioides brasiliensis* provided by different antigen-presenting cells. *Scand. J. Immunol.* 58: 290–297.

Forbes, J.R. and Gross, P. (2001). Divalent-metal transport by NRAMP proteins at the interface of host–pathogen interactions. *Trends Microbiol.* 9: 397–403.

Fornari, M.C., Bava, A.J., Guereño, M.T., Berardi, V.E., Silaf, R., Negroni, R., and Diez, R.A. (2001). High serum interleukin-10 and tumor necrosis factor alpha levels in chronic paracoccidioidomycosis. *Clin. Diag. Lab. Immunol.* 8: 1036–1038.

Fornazim, M.C., Balthazar, A., Quagliato, R. Jr., Mamoni, R.L., Garcia, C., and Blotta, M.H.S.L. (2003). Evaluation of bronchoalveolar cells in pulmonary paracoccidioidomycosis. *Eur. Resp. J.* 22: 895–899.

Franco, M. (1987). Host–parasite relationships in paracoccidioidomycosis. *J. Med. Vet. Mycol.* 25: 5–18.

Franco, M.F., Mendes, R.P., Moscardi-Bachi, M., Reskallah-Iwasso, M.T., and Montenegro, M.R. (1989). Paracoccidioidomycosis. *Baillières Clin. Trop. Méd. Comum.* 4: 185–220.

Goldani, L.Z. and Sugar, A.M. (1995). Paracoccidioidomycosis and AIDS: An overview. *Clin. Infect. Dis.* 21: 1275–1281.

Goldani, L.Z., Monteiro, C.M.C., Donadi, D.A., Martinez, R., and Voltarelli, J.C. (1991). HLA in Brazilian patients with paracoccidioidomycosis. *Mycopathologia* 114: 89–96.

Goldstein, R.A., Rohatgi, P.K., Bergofsky, E.H., Block, E.R., Daniele, R.P., Dantzker, D.R., Davis, G.S., Hunninghake, G.W., King, T.E. Jr., Metzger, W.J., Rankin, J.A., Reynolds, H.Y., and Turino, G.M. (1990). Clinical role of bronchoalveolar lavage in adults with pulmonary diseases. *Am. Rev. Respir. Dis.* 142: 481–486.

Gonzalez, A., de Gregori, W., Velez, D., Restrepo, A., and Cano, L.E. (2000). Nitric oxide participation in the fungicidal mechanism of interferon-gamma activated murine macrophages against *Paracoccidioides brasiliensis*. *Infect. Immun.* 68: 2546–2552.

Hart, P.H., Vitti, G.F., Burgess, D.R., Whitty, G.A., Piccoli, D.S., and Hamilton, J.A. (1989). Potential anti-inflammatory effects of interleukin-4: Suppression of human monocyte tumor necrosis factor. *Proc. Natl. Acad. Sci. USA* 86: 3803–3807.

Hill, J.O. (1992). CD4+ T cells cause multinucleated giant cell to form around *Cryptococcus neoformans* and confine the yeast within the primary site of infection in the respiratory tract. *J. Exp. Med.* 175: 1685–1695.

Huffnagle, G.B. and Deepe, G.S. (2003). Innate and adaptive determinants of host susceptibility to medically important fungi. *Curr. Opin. Microbiol.* 6: 344–350.

Jimenez, B.E. and Murphy, J.W. (1984). In vitro effects of natural killer cells against *Paracoccidioides brasiliensis*. *Infect. Immun.* 46: 552–558.

Karhawi, A.S.K., Colombo, A.L., and Salomão, R. (2000). Production of IFN-γ is impaired in patients with paracoccidioidomycosis during active disease and is restored after clinical remission. *Med. Mycol.* 38: 225–229.

Kashino, S.S., Fazioli, R.A., Cafalli-Favati, C., Meloni-Bruneri, L.H., Vaz, C.A.C., Burger, E., and Calich, V.L.G. (2000). Resistance to *Paracoccidiodes brasiliensis* infection is linked to a preferential Th1 immune response whereas susceptibility is associated with absence of IFN-γ production. *J. Interferon Cytokine Res.* 20: 89–97.

Koguchi, Y. and Kawakami, K. (2002). Cryptococcal infection and Th1–Th2 cytokine balance. *Int. Rev. Immunol.* 21: 423–438.

Kurita, N., Oarada, M., Miyaji, M., and Ito, E. (2000). Effect of cytokines on antifungal activity of human polymorphonuclear leukocytes against yeast cells of *Paracoccidioides brasiliensis*. *Med. Mycol.* 38: 177–182.

Lacaz, C.S. (1956) South American blastomycosis. *Am. Fac. Med. Univ. São Paulo* 29: 7–18.

Lacerda, G.B., Arce-Gomes, B., and Telles-Filho, F.Q. (1988). Increased frequency of HLA-B40 in patients with paracoccidioidomycosis. *J. Med. Vet. Mycol.* 26: 253–259.

Loose, D.S., Stover, E.P., Restrepo, A., Stevens, D.A., and Feldman, D. (1983). Estradiol binds to a receptor-like cytosol binding protein and initiates a biological response in *Paracoccidioides brasiliensis*. *Proc. Natl. Acad. Sci. USA* 80: 7659–7663.

Lutz, A. (1908). Uma micose pseudo-coccídica localizada na boca e observada no Brasil: Contribuição ao conhecimento das hipho-blastomicoses Americana. *Brasil Med.* 22: 121–124.

Magee, D.M. and Cox, R.A. (1995). Roles of interferon and interleukin-4 in genetically determined resistance to *Coccidioides immitis*. *Infect. Immun.* 63: 3514–3519.

Mamoni, R.L., Rossi, C.L., Camargo, Z.P., and Blotta, M.H.S.L. (2001). Capture enzyme-linked immunosorbent assay to detect specific immunoglobulin E in sera of patients with paracoccidioidomycosis. *Am. J. Trop. Med. Hyg.* 65: 237–241.

Mamoni, R.L., Nouer, R.A.M.S., Oliveira, S.A., Musatti, C.C., Rossi, C.L., Camargo, Z.P., and Blotta, M.H.S.L. (2002). Enhanced production of specific IgG4, IgE, IgA and TGF-β in sera from patients with the juvenile form of paracoccidioidomycosis. *Med. Mycol.* 40: 1–7.

McEwen, J.G., Brummer, E., Stevens, D.A., and Restrepo, A. (1987). Effect of murine polymorphonuclear leukocytes on the yeast form of *Paracoccidioides brasiliensis*. *Am. J. Trop. Med. Hyg.* 36: 603–608.

McInnes, A. and Rennick, D.M. (1988). Interleukin-4 induces cultured monocytes/macrophages to form giant multinucleated cells. *J. Exp. Med.* 167: 598–611.

McIntire, T.M., Klinman, D.R., Rothman, P., Lugo, M., Dash, J.R., Mond, J.J., and Snapper, C.M. (1993). Transforming growth factor β1 selectively stimulates immunoglobulin G2b by lipopolysaccharide-activated murine B cells. *J. Exp. Med.* 177: 1031–1037.

Mello, L.M., Silva-Vergara, M.L., and Rodrigues, V. Jr. (2002). Patients with active infection with *Paracoccidioides brasiliensis* present a Th2 immune response characterized by high interleukin-4 and interleukin-5 production. *Human Immunol.* 63: 149–154.

Meloni-Bruneri, L.H., Campa, A., Abdalla, D.S.P., Calich, V.L.G., and Burger, E. (1996). Neutrophils from air-pouches of resistant mice to *Paracoccidioides brasiliensis* infection are more activated and efficient in killing the fungi than those of susceptible ones. *J. Leukoc. Biol.* 59: 526–533.

Mencacci, A., Del Sero, G., Cenci, E., D'Ostiani, C.F., Bacci, A., Montagnoli, C., Kopf, M., and

Romani, L. (1998). Endogenous interleukin-4 is required for development of protective CD4+ T helper type-1 cell responses to *Candida albicans*. *J. Exp. Med.* 187: 307–317.

Mendes, E. and Raphael, A. (1971). Impaired delayed hypersensitivity in patients with South American blastomycosis. *J. Allergy* 47: 17–22.

Mendes-Giannini, M.J.S., Taylor, M.L., Bouchara, J.B., Burger, E., Calich, V.L.G., Escalante, E.D., Hanna, S.A., Lenzi, H.L., Machado, M.P., Myiaji, M., Monteiro da Silva, J.L., Mota, E.M., Restrepo, A., Restrepo, S., Tronchin, G., Vicenzi, L.R., Xidieh, C.F., and Zenteno, E. (2000). Pathogenesis II. Fungal responses to host responses: Interaction of host cells with fungi. *Med. Mycol.* 38: 113–123.

Mills, C.D., Kinkaid, K., Alt, J.M., Heilman, M.J., and Annete, M.H. (2000). M1/M2 macrophages paradigm. *J. Immunol.* 164: 6166–6173.

Montenegro, M.R. and Franco, M. (1994). Pathology. In M. Franco, C.S. Lacaz, A. Restrepo-Moreno, and G.D. Negro (eds), *Paracoccidioidomycosis*. CRC Press, Boca Raton, FL, pp. 131–147.

Most, J., Neumayer, H.P., and Dierich, N.M.P. (1991). Cytokine-induced generation of multinucleated giant cells "in vitro" requires interferon-gamma and expression of LFA-1. *Eur. J. Immunol.* 20: 1661–1667.

Murata, Y., Shimamura, T., and Hamuro, J. (2002). The polarization of T(h)1/T(h)2 balance is dependent on the intracellular thiol redox status of macrophages due to the distinctive cytokine production. *Int. Immunol.* 14: 201–212.

Murphy, J.W., Wu-hsieh, A., Singer-Vermes, L.M., Ferrante, A., Moser, S., Russo, M., Vaz, C.A.C., Burger, E., Calich, V.L.G., Kowanko, I.C., Rathjen, D.A., Martin, A.J., Buci, R.C., and Chen, Q. (1994). Cytokines in the host response to mycotic agents. *J. Med. Vet. Mycol.* 32: 203–210.

Musatti, C.C., Peraçoli, M.T.S., Soares, A.M.V.C., and Reskallah-Iwasso, M.T. (1994). Cell-mediated immunity in patients with paracoccidioidomycosis. In M. Franco, C.S. Lacaz, A. Restrepo, and G. Del Negro, (eds), *Paracoccidioidomycosis*. CRC Press, Boca Raton, FL, pp. 175–186.

Nascimento, F.R., Calich, V.L.G., Rodriguez, D., and Russo. M. (2002). Dual role for nitric oxide in paracoccidioidomycosis: Essential for resistance, but overproduction associated with susceptibility. *J. Immunol.* 168: 4593–4600.

Neworal, E.P.M., Altemani, A., Mamoni, R.L., Noronha, I.L., and Blotta, M.H.S.L. (2003). Immunocytochemical localization of cytokines and inducible nitric oxide synthase (iNOS) in oral mucosa and lymph nodes of patients with paracoccidioidomycosis. *Cytokine* 21: 1–8.

Nishikaku, A.S. and Burger, E. (2003). Immunohistochemical demonstration of TGF-β and decorin in paracoccidioidal granulomas. *Braz. J. Med. Biol. Res.* 36: 10723–10728.

Oliveira, S.J., Mamoni, R.L., Musatti, C.C., Papaiordanou, P.M., and Blotta, M.H. (2002). Cytokines and lymphocyte proliferation in juvenile and adult forms of paracoccidioidomycosis: Comparison with infected and non-infected controls. *Microbes Infect.* 4: 139–144.

Pagliari, C. and Sotto, M.N. (2003). Dendritic cells and pattern of cytokines in paracoccidioidomycosis skin lesions. *Am. J. Dermatopathol.* 25: 107–112.

Peraçoli, M.T., Soares, A.M., Mendes, R.P., Marques, S.A., Pereira, P.C., and Reskallah-Iwasso, M.T. (1991). Studies of natural killer cells in patients with paracoccidioidomycosis. *J. Med. Vet. Mycol.* 29: 373–380.

Peraçoli, M.T., Fortes, M.R., Da Silva, M.F., and Montenegro, M.R. (1995). Natural killer cell activity in experimental paracoccidioidomycosis of the Syrian hamster. *Rev. Inst. Med. Trop. São Paulo* 37: 129–136.

Pina, A. (2002). Efeito da depleção de leucócitos PMN em camundongos resistentes e susceptíveis à paracoccidioidomicose pulmonar, MSc Dissertation, Instituto de Ciências Biomédicas, Universidade de São Paulo, São Paulo.

Pina, A., Valente-Ferreira, R.C., Vaz, C.A.C., Molinari-Madlum, E.E.I.W., Keller, A.C., and Calich, V.L.G. (2004). Absence of IL-4 determines a less severe pulmonary paracoccidioidomycosis associated with impaired Th2 response. *Infect. Immun.* 72: 2369–2378.

Pinto, A.R. (2000). DNA-based vaccination against murine paracoccidioidomycosis using *gp43* gene from *Paracoccidioides brasiliensis*. *Vaccine* 18: 3030–3058.

Popi, A.F., Lopes, J.D., and Mariano, M. (2002). GP43 from *Paracoccidioides brasiliensis* inhibits macrophage functions. An evasion mechanism of the fungus. *Cell. Immunol.* 218: 87–94.

Restrepo, A. (1988). Immune responses to *Paracoccidioides brasiliensis* in human and animal hosts. In M.R. McGinnis (ed.), *Current*

Topics in Medical Mycology, Vol. 2. Springer, New York, pp. 235–239.
Restrepo, F.M., Restrepo, M., and Restrepo, A. (1983). Blood groups and HLA antigens in paracoccidioidomycosis. *Sabouraudia* 21: 35–42.
Restrepo, A., McEwen, J.G., and Castaneda, E. (2001). The habitat of *Paracoccidioides brasiliensis*: How far from solving the riddle? *Med. Mycol.* 39: 233–241.
Ridge, J.P., Di Rosos, F., and Maztinger, P. (1998). A conditioned dendritic cell can be a temporal bridge between a CD4$^+$ T helper cell and a T-killer cell. *Nature* 393: 474–478.
Romani, L. (2004). Immunity to fungal infections. *Nat. Rev.* 4: 1–13.
Romani, L., Mencacci, A., Grohmann, U., Mocci, S., Mosci, P., Puccetti, P., and Bistoni, F. (1992). Neutralizing antibody to interleukin-4 induces systemic protection and T helper 1-associated immunity in murine candidiasis. *J. Exp. Med.* 176: 19–25.
Romano, C.C., Mendes-Giannini, M.J.S., Duarte, A.J.S., and Benard, G. (2002). IL-12 and neutralization of endogenous IL-10 revert the in vitro antigen-specific cellular immunosuppression of paracoccidioidomycosis patients. *Cytokine* 18: 149–157.
San-Blas, G., Niño-Vega, G., and Iturriaga, T. (2002). *Paracoccidioides brasiliensis* and paracoccidioid0mycosis: Molecular approaches to morphogenesis, diagnosis, epidemiology, taxonomy and genetics. *Med. Mycol.* 40: 225–242.
Serody, J.S., Burkett, S.E., and Panoskaltsis-Mortari, A. (2000). T lymphocyte production of macrophage inflammatory protein-1α is critical to the recruitment of CD8$^+$ T cells to the liver, lung and spleen during graft-versus-host disease. *Blood* 96: 2973–2980.
Snapper, C.M. and Paul, W.E. (1987). Interferon-γ and B stimulatory factor-I reciprocally regulate Ig isotype production. *Science* 236: 944–947.
Snapper, C.M., Marcu, K.B., and Zelazowsky, P. (1997). Immunoglobulin class switch: Beyond accessibility. *Immunity* 6: 217–223.
Soares, A.M.V.C., Peraçoli, M.T.S., and Santos, R.R. (2000). Correlation among immune response, morphogenesis of granulomatous reaction and spleen lymphoid structure in murine experimental paracoccidioidomycosis. *Med. Mycol.* 38: 371–377.
Soares, A.M., Calvi, S.A., Peraçoli, M.T., Fernandez, A.C., Dias, L.A., and Dos Anjos, A.R. (2001). Modulatory effect of prostaglandins on human monocytes activation for killing of high- and low-virulence strains of *Paracoccidioides brasiliensis*. *Immunology* 102: 480–485.
Souto, J.F., Figueiredo, F., Furlanetto, A., Pfeffer, K., Rossi, M.A., and Silva, J.S. (2000). Interferon-γ and tumor necrosis factor-α determines resistance to *Paracoccidioides brasiliensis* infection. *Am. J. Pathol.* 156: 1811–1820.
Souto, J.T., Aliberti, J.C., Campanelli, A.P., Livonesi, M., Maffei, C.M.L., Ferreira, B.R., Travassos, L.R., Martinez, R., Rossi, M.A., and Silva, J.S. (2003). Chemokine production and leukocyte recruitment to the lungs of *Paracoccidioides brasili*ensis-infected mice is modulated by interferon-γ. *Am. J. Pathol.* 163: 583–590.
Stein, M., Keslav, S., Harris, N., and Gordon, S. (1992). Interleukin-4 potently enhances murine macrophage mannose receptor activity: A marker of alternative immunologic macrophage activation. *J. Exp. Med.* 176: 287–292.
Taborda, C.P., Juliano, M.A., Puccia, R., Franco, M., and Travassos, L.R. (1998). Mapping the T cell epitope in the major gp43 glycoprotein of *Paracoccidioides brasiliensis* which induces a Th1 immune response protective against infection in BALB/c mice. *Infect. Immun.* 66: 786–793.
Tapia, F.J., Goihman-Yahr, M., Cácere, A., and Dittmar, G. (1991). Leukocyte immunophenotypes in bronchoalveolar lavage fluid and blood of paracoccidioidomycosis, sarcoidisis and silicosis. *Histol. Histopathol.* 6: 395–402.
Travassos, L.R., Puccia, R., Cisalpino, P., Taborda, C.P., Rodrigues, M., Silveira, J.S., and Almeida, I.G. (1995). Biochemistry and molecular biology of the main antigen of *Paracoccidioides brasiliensis*. *Arch. Med. Res.* 26: 297–304.
Vaz, C.A.C., Singer-Vermes, L.M., and Calich, V.L.G. (1998). Comparative studies on the antibody repertoire produced by susceptible and resistant mice to virulent and nonvirulent *Paracoccidioides brasiliensis* isolates. *Am. J. Trop. Med. Hyg.* 59: 971–977.
Vicentini, A.P., Gesztesi, J.L., Franco, M.F., De Souza, W., Moraes, J.Z., Travassos, L.R., and Lopes, J.D. (1994). Binding of *Paracoccidioides brasiliensis* to laminin through surface glycoprotein gp43 leads to enhancement of fungal pathogenesis. *Infect. Immun.* 62: 1465–1469.
Vilani-Moreno, F., Fecchio, D., Mattos, M.C.I., Moscardi-Bacchi, M., Defaveri, J., and Franco,

M. (1998). Study of pulmonary experimental paracoccidioidomycosis by analysis of bronchoalveolar lavage cells: Resistant vs. susceptible mice. *Mycopathologia* 141: 79–91.

Wagner, J.M., Franco, M., Kephart, G.M., and Gleich, G.J. (1998). Localization of eosinophil granule major basic protein in paracoccidioidomycosis lesions. *Am. J. Trop. Med. Hyg.* 59: 66–72.

Xidieh, C.F., Lenzi, H.L., Calich, V.L.G., and Burger, E. (1999). Influence of the genetic background on the pattern of lesions developed by resistant and susceptible mice infected with *Paracoccidioides brasiliensis. Med. Microbiol. Immunol.* 188: 42–49.

11

The Innate and Acquired Pulmonary Immune Response to *Aspergillus fumigatus*

Jane M. Schuh[1] and Cory M. Hogaboam[2]

1. An Introduction to *Aspergillus*

1.1. *Aspergillus* in the Environment

Aspergillus is a filamentous, saprophytic fungal genus whose essential role in nature is the aerobic decomposition of organic material (Pitt, 1994). *Aspergillus* is a truly ubiquitous fungus. In addition to being found in soil and plant debris, it is found year-round in homes, schools, workplaces, libraries, and in such improbable places as the sand of the Sahara desert (Buckingham and Hansell, 2003). With a diameter of only 2–3 μm, an *Aspergillus*

[1] Department of Veterinary and Microbiology Sciences, North Dakota State University, Fargo, ND, USA.
[2] Department of Pathology, University of Michigan School of Medicine, Medical Science I, Room 5214, 1301 Catherine Road, Ann Arbor, MI 48109-0602, USA.

spore, or conidium, is quite small. Thousands of conidia are shed into the air from the asexual fruiting bodies of the fungi, called conidiophores (Latge, 2001).

While the vast majority of more than 185 species of *Aspergillus* pose no threat to humans, at least 19 species are known opportunistic pathogens (Stevens et al., 2000). Foremost among the pathogenic varieties is *Aspergillus fumigatus*. *A. fumigatus* is unique among the *Aspergillus* species in that it can grow at temperatures from 20°C to 50°C and survive at temperatures above 55°C. Concentrations of *A. fumigatus* in either indoor or outdoor air range from 1 to 100 conidia/m^3, permitting the average person to inhale several hundred conidia per day (Latge, 2001). Mature conidia are dark green, with a hydrophobic outer cell wall that aids in the spore's ability to stay airborne as well as in its adhesion to lung surfaces. *A. fumigatus* has no specific nutritional requirements; it needs only moisture and a carbon source to grow (Latge, 2001). The fungus grows quickly. At ideal growth conditions, *A. fumigatus* can produce mature conidia in a matter of days.

1.2. *Aspergillus* as an Opportunistic Pathogen of Man

Typically, *A. fumigatus* is considered to be a rather weak opportunistic pathogen, mainly responsible for allergic reactions in sensitized individuals. Fungal sinusitis, fungal asthma, and alveolitis are allergic responses elicited by *A. fumigatus* that are typically mild and require minimal therapeutic intervention. Allergic bronchopulmonary aspergillosis (ABPA) is primarily an allergic disease in which the fungus is retained in, but contained to, the bronchioles (Bosken et al., 1988). It may present clinically at any point in a spectrum of disease ranging from very mild fungal asthma to very aggressive disease that can progress to invasive aspergillosis (IA). Pulmonary aspergilloma and IA are *Aspergillus*-induced infections involving mycelial colonization of the lung itself. In at-risk populations, these fungal infections, particularly IA, are very serious and frequently fatal. There is considerable overlap between the various forms of *Aspergillus*-induced disease. ABPA may progress to aspergilloma or IA. Aspergilloma patients may develop allergic disease consistent with ABPA, or they may progress to IA. Although other species of *Aspergillus* can initiate disease, *A. fumigatus* is the dominant pathogenic species and is responsible for 90% of human mycoses (Kurup and Kumar, 1991). The growing population of severely immunocompromised patients—those with diseases that directly impact immune cells or those who are undergoing immunosuppressive medical treatment—are particularly vulnerable to *Aspergillus* infection, morbidity, and mortality.

2. The Innate Pulmonary Response to *A. fumigatus*

2.1. The Lung

At the interface between the body and the environment, the human lung must counter numerous chemical, biological, and mechanical assaults while maintaining the gas exchange that is critical to life. To prevent pulmonary infection while maintaining the operation of the lung, a robust innate immune response is imperative. A number of factors come together to compose the antigen-nonspecific defense of the innate immune response. Innate immunity in the lung allows the host an immediate reaction that is capable of eliminating unwanted microbes before they can colonize the respiratory tract. It is made up of anatomical barriers and commensal organisms that limit access to pulmonary tissue, humoral products to recruit leukocytes and aid in phagocytosis, and cellular surveillance to directly phagocytose and kill invading pathogens.

2.2. The Barriers of the Lung: Mechanical and Humoral Mediators

There are a number of mechanisms that limit microbial colonization in the human respiratory tract. For example, human body temperature performs an important role in innate immunity. It is sufficiently high to discourage most microbes from colonizing the host. In addition, many types of infection trigger a fever, which limits the growth or replication of the prospective pathogen by further increasing the host's temperature. *A. fumigatus* grows well in a wide temperature range and optimally at 37°C, the human body temperature. The thermotolerant nature of this fungus may be the single most important factor in its success as an opportunistic pathogen of humans.

Size and hydrophobicity permit *A. fumigatus* conidia to remain airborne for extended periods of time, allowing the fungus to contact the human respiratory tract. Unimpeded, conidia are sufficiently small to reach even the tiny alveoli of the lung; however, skin and mucous membranes provide physical barriers and platforms that allow cilia and mucus to trap and remove the spores from the upper airway. In addition, there are a number of host-protective humoral products that are normally present in the lung and that augment the cellular immune response to a pathogen. For example, surfactant proteins A and D enhance both phagocytosis and killing ability of macrophages and neutrophils, and binding of fungal surface proteins by C3 and C5 activate the complement system (Kozel et al., 1989; Madan et al., 1997a). Interestingly, a number of humoral products that are used against *A. fumigatus* in host defense have been commandeered by the fungus for use as adherence molecules. The conidia can attach to hydrophobic binding pockets found in the superstructure of a number of host products. Not only are structural molecules such as collagen, fibrinogen, and laminin used by the fungus for adhesion to pulmonary matrix, but it can also use host defense molecules such as complement and surfactant proteins (Annaix et al., 1992; Sturtevant and Latge, 1992; Bouchara et al., 1997; Madan et al., 1997a,b; Tronchin et al., 1997).

Fungi have ensured their ecological niche in the environment by developing strategies to promote colony success. Unfortunately, the same products that make *A. fumigatus* an excellent agent of decomposition in a compost heap make it a formidable pathogen in a compromised host. *A. fumigatus* produces a number of toxins that aid in fungal colonization by damaging pulmonary epithelial cells, slowing ciliary action, and killing local immune cells (Latge, 2001). These toxins may be physiologically active in the minute amounts that are present in the conidial cell wall, but even more so in a very large inoculum of conidia or an established colony, would produce more of these toxins and proteases that would result in increased injury. In addition, fungal species are notorious for generating abiotic products that are injurious to bacteria, killing their primary competitors and significantly promoting fungal dissemination in their natural habitat. In order to effectively colonize the human respiratory tract, *A. fumigatus* must successfully compete for space and nutrients against the microorganisms that already inhabit that space. Bacterial antagonism by commensal microbes impedes fungal maturation that would lead to the increased production of toxic products. This explains, in part, the increased risk of serious fungal disease associated with immunosuppressive therapies that not only limit the effectiveness of the immune cells but may also disrupt the normal flora of the host.

2.3. The Cellular Mediators of Innate Immunity in the Lung

In a healthy, nonatopic host, the relatively few invading organisms that avoid the barriers of the innate immune response are eliminated by innate cellular responses (Fig. 11.1). Resident alveolar macrophages are the main phagocytic cells triggered innately in the lung. They phagocytose inhaled conidia, killing the spores before they can germinate to the potentially invasive hyphal form (Waldorf, 1989). Lectin interactions are believed to trigger phagocytosis of conidia by alveolar macrophages, but the specifics of this interaction are still being studied (Ezekowitz, 2003). The majority (~90%) of *A. fumigatus* conidia are phagocytosed within 2 h of in vitro inoculation (Philippe et al., 2003). In the in vitro setting, phagocytosis of conidia does not require humoral opsonins. However, the accessibility of immunoglobulins and complement in vivo are likely to have significant impact on phagocytosis (Kozel et al., 1989). The recognition of pathogenic, nonpathogenic, and even dead conidia does not appear to be different, as phagocytosis occurs at comparable rates in all of these situations (Jahn et al., 1998). Ostensibly, the phagocytosed conidia are not differentiated from general particulate debris until they start to swell within the macrophage at which time conidial killing is commenced. The alveolar macrophage has at least a few methods to kill the potentially pathogenic intruder. The phagocytosed conidium moves through the normal phagocytic compartments

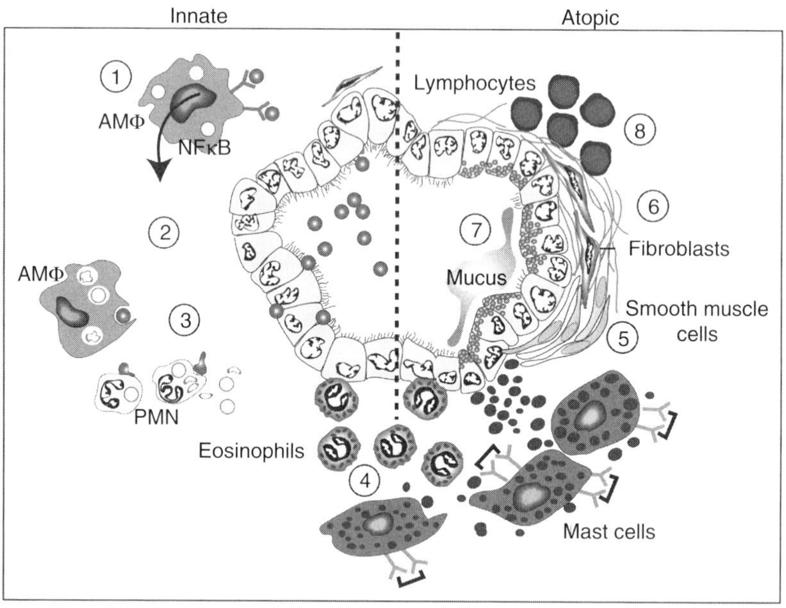

Figure 11.1. *Aspergillus fumigatus*: the innate and atopic response in an immunocompetent host. *Innate response* (1) alveolar macrophages phagocytose conidia through nonspecific means. Pathogen-associated pattern molecules bind to TLR2 and TLR4 on the macrophage's surface and signal through the NFκB pathway. (2) Activated epithelial signaling joins that of the alveolar macrophage to recruit and activate inflammatory cells. (3) Recruited macrophages and neutrophils phagocytose and kill conidia and germinating hyphae, respectively. *Atopic response* (4) in the sensitized host, eosinophils are recruited to the airways and *Aspergillus*-specific IgE binds to mast cells via the Fc receptor. Cross-linking of the IgE by *Aspergillus* antigens causes degranulation, directly affecting airway reactivity. (5) Smooth muscle cell hyperplasia, (6) peribronchial fibrosis, and (7) goblet cell hyperplasia are consequences of the remodeling of the atopic airway that is driven by (8) Th2-associated lymphocytes, which produce IL-13, IL-4, and IL-5.

and enters an acidified phagolysosome where killing can occur (Ibrahim-Granet et al., 2003). Alveolar macrophages use nonoxidative killing mechanisms, such as defensins, to eliminate growing conidia (Morgenstern et al., 1997), but reactive oxygen intermediates may also play an important role, as has been shown in vitro, in killing germinating conidia (Philippe et al., 2003). It has recently been demonstrated that while corticosteroid treatment does not reduce the phagocytic properties of alveolar macrophages, it dramatically impacts the production of reactive oxidant intermediates, suggesting that fungal infection as a consequence of high-dose steroid treatment may be due to the inability to produce these important mediators (Philippe et al., 2003). Mature conidia of *A. fumigatus* are characteristically dark green with conspicuous cell wall ornamentation, called rodlets. Mutated strains that do not produce the pigment, and subsequently do not produce the outer cell wall ornamentation, are promptly phagocytosed and killed much more readily than wild-type spores. The selective advantage of the coat components is probably related to their ability to scavenge reactive oxygen intermediates and to evade binding by immune response molecules (Jahn et al., 2000).

The innate immune system does not recognize every possible antigen; rather, it recognizes a few (~1000) highly conserved structures that are present on a multitude of microorganisms. These structures are collectively known as pathogen-associated molecular patterns (PAMPs). The pattern recognition molecules of resident alveolar macrophages recognize PAMPs on the fungal cell wall. One class of pattern recognition molecule, the toll-like receptors (TLRs), is largely responsible for the recognition of fungal PAMPs by alveolar macrophages. TLRs are mediators that play roles in both the innate response and the activation of the adaptive immune response. All ten of the known TLRs consist of a leucine-rich extracellular domain and a conserved intracellular Toll/IL-1 receptor (TIR) signaling domain (Kopp and Medzhitov, 1999). Upon binding of the PAMP, the intracellular peptide interacts with other TIRs and recruits adaptor proteins to the complex. This in turn dictates the activation of the signaling cascade to follow. TLR2 and TLR4 have been identified as the primary pattern recognition molecules responsible for the detection of *A. fumigatus* (Meier et al., 2003). TLR2 is responsible for the recognition of both conidia and hyphae, while TLR4 is believed to be restricted to the detection of conidia (Mambula et al., 2002; Meier et al., 2003). The inflammatory response is essential for the elimination or isolation of microbes in affected tissue as well as facilitating repair of injured tissues. NFκB is an important nuclear transcription factor and is vital for the initiation and amplification of inflammatory responses in a number of different signaling pathways. In vitro studies with manipulated macrophage cell lines and *ex vivo* experiments with elicited peritoneal macrophages support a role for TLR2, TLR4, the coreceptor CD14, and adaptor signaling proteins such as MyD88 in the signaling pathways that lead to NFκB translocation in response to *A. fumigatus* (Mambula et al., 2002; Meier et al., 2003). It is obvious, however, that these results should lead to further studies using alveolar macrophages to clarify differences in various macrophage lines and types. Tumor necrosis factor alpha (TNF-α), proinflammatory cytokines, and chemokines that are products of NFκB activation recruit and activate neutrophils and more monocytes/macrophages to the area of inflammation and augment phagocytic activity by innate immune cells already present in the lung (Mambula et al., 2002).

Hyphae and germinating conidia that are too large to be phagocytosed by macrophages are eliminated by recruited neutrophils (Waldorf, 1989). In contrast to the macrophage, which phagocytoses conidia, the neutrophil kills germinating hyphae by releasing cytoplasmic granules and reactive oxygen intermediates (Diamond and

Clark, 1982; Levitz and Diamond, 1985; Levitz and Farrell, 1990). Both reactive oxidant-producing enzymes, such as myeloperoxidase (MPO) and NADPH-oxidase, and granules containing nonoxidative molecules such as defensins are utilized for killing (Diamond and Clark, 1982; Aratani et al., 2002). Individuals with chronic granulomatous disease, neutropenia as a result of chemotherapy, or other conditions that limit the recruitment or effectiveness of the neutrophil population are at particular risk of IA (Cohen et al., 1981; Levitz and Diamond, 1985). Experimentally, neutropenia induced by cyclophosphamide treatment yields a mouse that develops invasive fungal disease within days of encountering the fungus. In a healthy host, the neutrophil-mediated response is rapid and results in efficient killing. Fifty percent of the contacted hyphae are killed within 2 h (Roilides et al., 1993, 1998). Platelets are also important mediators necessary to eliminate hyphae. They facilitate hyphal killing by attaching to the germinating hyphae as they begin to infiltrate the vasculature (Christin et al., 1998).

3. The Adaptive Immune Response to *A. fumigatus*

3.1. The T Cell Response to *A. fumigatus*: Protective Immunity and T Cell Skewing

Although frequently considered separate distinct entities, the acquired immune response is a continuation of the innate response. Innate immunity educates the adaptive response to take the most appropriate measures that will remove an offending organism or, barring its removal, to protect the host. In addition, innate immunity still functions in a fungal infection even if there is an acquired response directed against the fungus. The difference comes when the initial response to the fungus is unsuccessful to remove the infection before the adaptive immune response takes over and then mediates the chronicity of the response. In the case of *A. fumigatus*, innate immune responses and an initial Th1-type response, characterized by interferon gamma (IFN-γ) and interleukin (IL)-12 production with a robust cellular response, is superceded by a Th2-associated response that is responsible for much of the immunopathology that is seen in the chronic allergic disease, which is the most typical form of *Aspergillus*-induced disease seen in the general population (Hogaboam et al., 2000; Blease et al., 2002).

While the fungus produces a number of potentially damaging proteases and toxins, mutants deficient in any one of these products frequently remain pathogenic in an immunocompromised host (Hogan et al., 1996). The disease pattern elicited by *A. fumigatus* infection; therefore, is primarily dependent upon the reaction of the host's immune system, not the virulence of the pathogen itself. As such, there is a spectrum of disease in which symptoms may range from subclinical to grossly incapacitating while technically residing under the same clinical diagnosis. For example, ABPA may present as fungal-induced asthma, but it may progress to invasive disease. Aspergilloma patients may be asymptomatic or critically ill. Cases of IA rarely have a mild-case scenario: this disease is uniformly serious and frequently fatal.

3.2. ABPA and Allergic Responses in the Lung

ABPA (Fig. 11.2) is an allergic disease that is primarily seen in asthmatics. While ABPA is believed to be underdiagnosed, estimates of ABPA among asthmatics are as high as 25% (Wark and Gibson, 2001) and 35% in cystic fibrosis patients (Knutsen and Slavin, 1991). This disease is characterized by grossly elevated *Aspergillus*-specific immunoglobulins (IgE, IgG, and IgA) as well as bronchopulmonary and serum eosinophilia (Greenberger, 1997). An

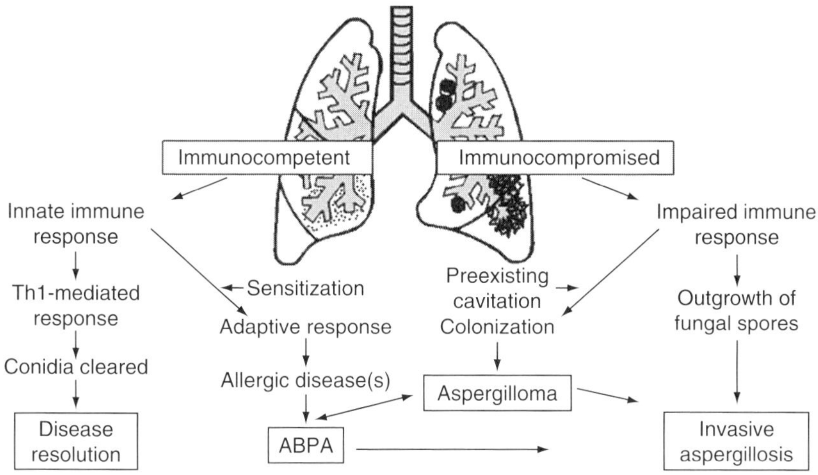

Figure 11.2. The generation of *Aspergillus*-induced disease. In the immunocompetent lung, the innate immune response kills and clears the conidia with full resolution. The atopic, adaptive response in a sensitized host allows for the generation of allergic diseases including ABPA. In the immunocompromised host, the impaired general immunity allows colonization of preexisting cavities (aspergilloma) or saprophytic growth of the fungus (invasive aspergillosis). Either ABPA or aspergilloma may provoke the other disease and may also lead to more serious invasive disease.

immediate hypersensitivity reaction, mediated by both humoral and cellular responses is evident in asthmatics that encounter a concentrated conidial inoculum (Schatz and Hamburger, 1979). The ensuing immune reaction results in chronic mucus hypersecretion with bronchial plugging, bronchiectasis, bronchospasm, and bronchial edema. Many of these sequela are mimicked in experimental murine models using *A. fumigatus* as an inducing agent (Hogaboam et al., 2000). ABPA is confined to the bronchioles, which differentiates it from infective *Aspergillus* diseases; however, proteinases produced by *Aspergillus* in chronic ABPA can, over time, damage the bronchial epithelium and may lead to an invasive disease course (Saraceno et al., 1997).

3.3. Aspergilloma and Colonization of the Airway

Mycetoma is a term used to describe a free-floating fungus ball within a preexisting lung cavity. Mycetomas are usually caused by *Aspergillus* (called aspergillomas), but may also be associated with other types of fungi (Buckingham and Hansell, 2003). Aspergilloma is primarily a colonization of spaces in the upper lobes of the lung (Fig. 11.2). The conidia germinate and grow in existing necrotized cavities left by previous disease processes such as tuberculosis or sarcoidosis. Aspergillomas occur in 10–15% of all patients with cavitating lung disease (Addrizzo-Harris et al., 1997). Typically, the cavity is fibrotic with a necrotizing inner layer and a rich blood supply, giving it a propensity to bleed (Logan and Muller, 1996; Regnard et al., 2000). Hemoptysis is most frequently internal and minor but may be massive and even fatal (Judson and Stevens, 2001). The combination of the growing *Aspergillus* hyphae, proteinaceous matrix, mucus, and cellular debris make up the body of the aspergilloma (Latge, 1999). As with other *Aspergillus*-induced diseases, aspergilloma traverses a wide range of symptomology. The treatment course depends upon the amount of dysfunction that the patient experiences.

Aspergillomas are difficult to treat with traditional antifungal therapy due to the lack of blood supply within the cavity itself. As a result, they may require computed tomography (CT)- or fluoroscopy-guided intracavitary treatment. In advanced cases, surgical resection of the lung is the most successful therapeutic course, allowing that the underlying pulmonary disease and the patient's general health permit invasive surgery (Jewkes et al., 1983; Chatzimichalis et al., 1998; Regnard et al., 2000).

3.4. IA and Destruction of the Airway and Pulmonary Vasculature

Fungi are unique among the common household allergens in that they are live entities capable of infection under certain conditions. This is not to say that dead conidia cannot act as allergens; indeed they do. But the ability of *A. fumigatus* to grow in the conditions of the lung presents a more complex medical scenario than a typical allergen. While serious fungal disease is rarely seen in the general population, because of the increasing population of severely immunosuppressed patients (either due to disease or treatment), *A. fumigatus* is an emerging pathogen that is a chief cause of mortality in transplant patients, AIDS sufferers, and neutropenic patients (Cohen et al., 1981; Gerson et al., 1984). In IA, the conidia overcome whatever marginal immune response the lung can mount and survive to germinate and produce an invasive mycelial mat that can severely damage the airway and/or vasculature (Fig. 11.2). IA may have a particularly rapid disease progression with as little as 1–2 weeks from onset to death (Latge, 1999). IA can be categorized into two main types based upon the primary structure that is attacked. Airway IA involves the attack of the bronchial tree with subsequent destruction of the lung tissue, and angioinvasive aspergillosis involves the attack of the pulmonary artery branches with dissemination of the fungus to the brain and other vital organs. In practice, angioinvasive and airway invasive forms may coincide in one patient due to the proximity of the bronchioles and the vasculature. Fulminant disease is due to dissemination through the vasculature, although dissemination is not necessary for mortality. IA can affect any organ of the body, but especially the lungs, heart, brain, and kidneys. Late in the course of the disease, the nervous system, skin, and other organs may become affected.

4. Concluding Remarks

Epidemiological studies, clinical research, and anecdotal evidence illustrate a mounting risk for the development of fungus-related diseases throughout the world. The reason for an increased incidence of fungal allergic disease is not well understood, but is probably linked to the general increase in allergic asthma and allergy in developed countries. *Aspergillus* is an emerging pathogen in the increasing population of individuals who are immunocompromised to an extent that they can no longer mount an effective response against the opportunistic pathogen. Much of the pulmonary pathology seen in *Aspergillus*-associated diseases is, in fact, a result of the poor integrity of the lung, allowing the colonization by the fungus or the inadequate response of an immune system debilitated either by treatment or disease. Our insufficient knowledge of human fungal allergy and infection highlights the need for animal models that more closely represent the clinical condition. There have been recent advances in early detection of IA and potential therapeutic targets that specifically intervene at the junction between host protection and immunopathology (Blease et al., 2001; Blease and Raymon, 2003; Pinel et al., 2003; Schuh et al., 2003; Challier et al., 2004; Kwak et al., 2004). The increased understanding of the nature of pulmonary fungal aspergillosis immunology will in turn fuel research for more specific and appropriate ways to combat the potentially devastating diseases that this fungus instigates.

Acknowledgments

We thank Robin Kunkel for her graphic illustration of innate and atopic responses to *A. fumigatus* (Fig. 11.1).

References

Addrizzo-Harris, D.J., Harkin, T.J., McGuinness, G., Naidich, D.P., and Rom, W.N. (1997). Pulmonary aspergilloma and AIDS. A comparison of HIV-infected and HIV-negative individuals. *Chest* 111(3): 612–618.

Annaix, V., Bouchara, J.P., Larcher, G., Chabasse, D., and Tronchin, G. (1992). Specific binding of human fibrinogen fragment D to *Aspergillus fumigatus* conidia. *Infect. Immun.* 60(5): 1747–1755.

Aratani, Y., Kura, F., Watanabe, H., Akagawa, H., Takano, Y., Suzuki, K., Dinauer, M.C., Maeda, N., and Koyama, H. (2002). Relative contributions of myeloperoxidase and NADPH-oxidase to the early host defense against pulmonary infections with *Candida albicans* and *Aspergillus fumigatus*. *Med. Mycol.* 40(6): 557–563.

Blease, K. and Raymon, H.K. (2003). Small molecule inhibitors of cell signaling: Novel future therapeutics for asthma and chronic obstructive pulmonary diseases. *Curr. Opin. Investig. Drugs* 4(5): 544–551.

Blease, K., Jakubzick, C., Schuh, J.M., Joshi, B.H., Puri, R.K., and Hogaboam, C.M. (2001). IL-13 fusion cytotoxin ameliorates chronic fungal-induced allergic airway disease in mice. *J. Immunol.* 167(11): 6583–6592.

Blease, K., Schuh, J.M., Jakubzick, C., Lukacs, N.W., Kunkel, S.L., Joshi, B.H., Puri, R.K., Kaplan, M.H., and Hogaboam, C.M. (2002). Stat6-deficient mice develop airway hyperresponsiveness and peribronchial fibrosis during chronic fungal asthma. *Am. J. Pathol.* 160(2): 481–490.

Bosken, C.H., Myers, J.L., Greenberger, P.A., and Katzenstein, A.L. (1988). Pathologic features of allergic bronchopulmonary aspergillosis. *Am. J. Surg. Pathol.* 12(3): 216–222.

Bouchara, J.P., Sanchez, M., Chevailler, A., Marot-Leblond, A., Lissitzky, J.C., Tronchin, G., and Chabasse, D. (1997). Sialic acid-dependent recognition of laminin and fibrinogen by *Aspergillus fumigatus* conidia. *Infect. Immun.* 65(7): 2717–2724.

Buckingham, S.J. and Hansell, D.M. (2003). Aspergillus in the lung: Diverse and coincident forms. *Eur. Radiol.* 13(8): 1786–1800.

Challier, S., Boyer, S., Abachin, E., and Berche, P. (2004). Development of a serum-based Taqman real-time PCR assay for diagnosis of invasive aspergillosis. *J. Clin. Microbiol.* 42(2): 844–846.

Chatzimichalis, A., Massard, G., Kessler, R., Barsotti, P., Claudon, B., Ojard-Chillet, J., and Wihlm, J.M. (1998). Bronchopulmonary aspergilloma: A reappraisal. *Ann. Thorac. Surg.* 65(4): 927–929.

Christin, L., Wysong, D.R., Meshulam, T., Hastey, R., Simons, E.R., and Diamond, R.D. (1998). Human platelets damage *Aspergillus fumigatus* hyphae and may supplement killing by neutrophils. *Infect. Immun.* 66(3): 1181–1189.

Cohen, M.S., Isturiz, R.E., Malech, H.L., Root, R.K., Wilfert, C.M., Gutman, L., and Buckley, R.H. (1981). Fungal infection in chronic granulomatous disease. The importance of the phagocyte in defense against fungi. *Am. J. Med.* 71(1): 59–66.

Diamond, R.D. and Clark, R.A. (1982). Damage to *Aspergillus fumigatus* and *Rhizopus oryzae* hyphae by oxidative and nonoxidative microbicidal products of human neutrophils in vitro. *Infect. Immun.* 38(2): 487–495.

Ezekowitz, R.A. (2003). Role of the mannose-binding lectin in innate immunity. *J. Infect. Dis.* 187(Suppl. 2): S335–S339.

Gerson, S.L., Talbot, G.H., Hurwitz, S., Strom, B.L., Lusk, E.J., and Cassileth, P.A. (1984). Prolonged granulocytopenia: The major risk factor for invasive pulmonary aspergillosis in patients with acute leukemia. *Ann. Intern. Med.* 100(3): 345–351.

Greenberger, P.A. (1997). Immunologic aspects of lung diseases and cystic fibrosis. *JAMA* 278(22): 1924–1930.

Hogaboam, C.M., Blease, K., Mehrad, B., Steinhauser, M.L., Standiford, T.J., Kunkel, S.L., and Lukacs, N.W. (2000). Chronic airway hyperreactivity, goblet cell hyperplasia, and peribronchial fibrosis during allergic airway disease induced by *Aspergillus fumigatus*. *Am. J. Pathol.* 156: 723–732.

Hogan, L.H., Klein, B.S., and Levitz, S.M. (1996). Virulence factors of medically important fungi. *Clin. Microbiol. Rev.* 9(4): 469–488.

Ibrahim-Granet, O., Philippe, B., Boleti, H., Boisvieux-Ulrich, E., Grenet, D., Stern, M., and Latge, J.P. (2003). Phagocytosis and intracellular fate of *Aspergillus fumigatus* conidia in alveolar macrophages. *Infect. Immun.* 71(2): 891–903.

Jahn, B., Rampp, A., Dick, C., Jahn, A., Palmer, M., and Bhakdi, S. (1998). Accumulation of amphotericin B in human macrophages enhances activity against *Aspergillus fumigatus* conidia: Quantification of conidial kill at the single-cell level. *Antimicrob. Agents Chemother.* 42(10): 2569–2575.

Jahn, B., Boukhallouk, F., Lotz, J., Langfelder, K., Wanner, G., and Brakhage, A.A. (2000). Interaction of human phagocytes with pigmentless *Aspergillus conidia. Infect. Immun.* 68(6): 3736–3739.

Jewkes, J., Kay, P.H., Paneth, M., and Citron, K.M. (1983). Pulmonary aspergilloma: Analysis of prognosis in relation to haemoptysis and survey of treatment. *Thorax* 38(8): 572–578.

Judson, M.A. and Stevens, D.A. (2001). The treatment of pulmonary aspergilloma. *Curr. Opin. Investig. Drugs* 2(10): 1375–1377.

Knutsen, A.P. and Slavin, R.G. (1991). Allergic bronchopulmonary aspergillosis in patients with cystic fibrosis. *Clin. Rev. Allergy* 9(1–2): 103–118.

Kopp, E.B. and Medzhitov, R. (1999). The toll-receptor family and control of innate immunity. *Curr. Opin. Immunol.* 11(1): 13–18.

Kozel, T.R., Wilson, M.A., Farrell, T.P., and Levitz, S.M. (1989). Activation of C3 and binding to *Aspergillus fumigatus* conidia and hyphae. *Infect. Immun.* 57(11): 3412–3417.

Kurup, V.P. and Kumar, A. (1991). Immunodiagnosis of aspergillosis. *Clin. Microbiol. Rev.* 4(4): 439–456.

Kwak, E.J., Husain, S., Obman, A., Meinke, L., Stout, J., Kusne, S., Wagener, M.M., and Singh, N. (2004). Efficacy of galactomannan antigen in the Platelia *Aspergillus* enzyme immunoassay for diagnosis of invasive aspergillosis in liver transplant recipients. *J. Clin. Microbiol.* 42(1): 435–438.

Latge, J.P. (1999). *Aspergillus fumigatus* and aspergillosis. *Clin. Microbiol. Rev.* 12(2): 310–350.

Latge, J.P. (2001). The pathobiology of *Aspergillus fumigatus. Trends Microbiol.* 9(8): 382–389.

Levitz, S.M. and Diamond, R.D. (1985). Mechanisms of resistance of *Aspergillus fumigatus* conidia to killing by neutrophils in vitro. *J. Infect. Dis.* 152(1): 33–42.

Levitz, S.M. and Farrell, T.P. (1990). Human neutrophil degranulation stimulated by *Aspergillus fumigatus. J. Leukoc. Biol.* 47(2): 170–175.

Logan, P.M. and Muller, N.L. (1996). High-resolution computed tomography and pathologic findings in pulmonary aspergillosis: A pictorial essay. *Can. Assoc. Radiol. J.* 47(6): 444–452.

Madan, T., Eggleton, P., Kishore, U., Strong, P., Aggrawal, S.S., Sarma, P.U., and Reid, K.B. (1997a). Binding of pulmonary surfactant proteins A and D to *Aspergillus fumigatus* conidia enhances phagocytosis and killing by human neutrophils and alveolar macrophages. *Infect. Immun.* 65(8): 3171–3179.

Madan, T., Kishore, U., Shah, A., Eggleton, P., Strong, P., Wang, J.Y., Aggrawal, S.S., Sarma, P.U., and Reid, K.B. (1997b). Lung surfactant proteins A and D can inhibit specific IgE binding to the allergens of *Aspergillus fumigatus* and block allergen-induced histamine release from human basophils. *Clin. Exp. Immunol.* 110(2): 241–249.

Mambula, S.S., Sau, K., Henneke, P., Golenbock, D.T., and Levitz, S.M. (2002). Toll-like receptor (TLR) signaling in response to *Aspergillus fumigatus. J. Biol. Chem.* 277(42): 39320–39326.

Meier, A., Kirschning, C.J., Nikolaus, T., Wagner, H., Heesemann, J., and Ebel, F. (2003). Toll-like receptor (TLR) 2 and TLR4 are essential for *Aspergillus*-induced activation of murine macrophages. *Cell. Microbiol.* 5(8): 561–570.

Morgenstern, D.E., Gifford, M.A., Li, L.L., Doerschuk, C.M., and Dinauer, M.C. (1997). Absence of respiratory burst in X-linked chronic granulomatous disease mice leads to abnormalities in both host defense and inflammatory response to *Aspergillus fumigatus. J. Exp. Med.* 185(2): 207–218.

Philippe, B., Ibrahim-Granet, O., Prevost, M.C., Gougerot-Pocidalo, M.A., Sanchez Perez, M., Van der Meeren, A., and Latge, J.P. (2003). Killing of *Aspergillus fumigatus* by alveolar macrophages is mediated by reactive oxidant intermediates. *Infect. Immun.* 71(6): 3034–3042.

Pinel, C., Fricker-Hidalgo, H., Lebeau, B., Garban, F., Hamidfar, R., Ambroise-Thomas, P., and Grillot, R. (2003). Detection of circulating *Aspergillus fumigatus* galactomannan: Value and limits of the Platelia test for diagnosing invasive aspergillosis. *J. Clin. Microbiol.* 41(5): 2184–2186.

Pitt, J.I. (1994). The current role of *Aspergillus* and *Penicillium* in human and animal health. *J. Med. Vet. Mycol.* 32(Suppl. 1): 17–32.

Regnard, J.F., Icard, P., Nicolosi, M., Spagiarri, L., Magdeleinat, P., Jauffret, B., and Levasseur,

P. (2000). Aspergilloma: A series of 89 surgical cases. *Ann. Thorac. Surg.* 69(3): 898–903.

Roilides, E., Uhlig, K., Venzon, D., Pizzo, P.A., and Walsh, T.J. (1993). Enhancement of oxidative response and damage caused by human neutrophils to *Aspergillus fumigatus* hyphae by granulocyte colony-stimulating factor and gamma interferon. *Infect. Immun.* 61(4): 1185–1193.

Roilides, E., Dimitriadou-Georgiadou, A., Sein, T., Kadiltsoglou, I., and Walsh, T.J. (1998). Tumor necrosis factor alpha enhances antifungal activities of polymorphonuclear and mononuclear phagocytes against *Aspergillus fumigatus*. *Infect. Immun.* 66(12): 5999–6003.

Saraceno, J.L., Phelps, D.T., Ferro, T.J., Futerfas, R., and Schwartz, D.B. (1997). Chronic necrotizing pulmonary aspergillosis: Approach to management. *Chest* 112(2): 541–548.

Schatz, M. and Hamburger, R.N. (1979). Allergic bronchopulmonary aspergillosis. *Conn. Med.* 43(8): 486.

Schuh, J.M., Blease, K., Bruhl, H., Mack, M., and Hogaboam, C.M. (2003). Intrapulmonary targeting of RANTES/CCL5-responsive cells prevents chronic fungal asthma. *Eur. J. Immunol.* 33(11): 3080–3090.

Stevens, D.A., Kan, V.L., Judson, M.A., Morrison, V.A., Dummer, S., Denning, D.W., Bennett, J.E., Walsh, T.J., Patterson, T.F., and Pankey, G.A. (2000). Practice guidelines for diseases caused by *Aspergillus*. Infectious Diseases Society of America. *Clin. Infect. Dis.* 30(4): 696–709.

Sturtevant, J. and Latge, J.P. (1992). Participation of complement in the phagocytosis of the conidia of *Aspergillus fumigatus* by human polymorphonuclear cells. *J. Infect. Dis.* 166(3): 580–586.

Tronchin, G., Esnault, K., Renier, G., Filmon, R., Chabasse, D., and Bouchara, J.P. (1997). Expression and identification of a laminin-binding protein in *Aspergillus fumigatus* conidia. *Infect. Immun.* 65(1): 9–15.

Waldorf, A.R. (1989). Pulmonary defense mechanisms against opportunistic fungal pathogens. *Immunol. Ser.* 47: 243–271.

Wark, P.A. and Gibson, P.G. (2001). Allergic bronchopulmonary aspergillosis: New concepts of pathogenesis and treatment. *Respirology* 6(1): 1–7.

12

Fungal Hypersensitivity in the Lungs

Viswanath P. Kurup[1] and Alan P. Knutsen[2]

[1] Department of Pediatrics, Allergy, Immunology Division, Medical College of Wisconsin and Research Service, Veterans Affairs Medical Center, Milwaukee, WI.
[2] Pediatrics Research Institute, St Louis University Health Sciences, St Louis, MO.

1. Introduction

Hypersensitivity lung diseases are caused by a number of allergens from diverse sources and origins, of which, fungi constitute a major group. Allergen has been defined as the substance that is involved in atopy where induction of specific immunoglobulin E (IgE) antibody results from the exposure and sensitization to allergens. Although fungi are associated with a number of allergic and nonallergic diseases in humans, respiratory allergy constitutes a major group (Kurup and Fink, 1993; Kurup et al., 2002; Kurup, 2003; 2004). Majority of the fungi associated with allergy in humans are caused by freely distributed saprophytic fungi and constitute only a very small percentage of the sum total of all known fungi (Kurup, 2003).

The allergic conditions most frequently recognized are allergic rhinitis, conjunctivitis, and bronchial asthma (Katzenstein et al., 1983; Kurup, 1989; Kurup and Fink, 1993). In the pathogenesis of atopic diseases, the immune responses result from the interaction of the host immune system and the allergens. There are a number of modulating environmental factors that have also been identified or suggested in the pathogenesis of allergy. Exposure to allergens and sensitization can result from inhalation, contact, ingestion, or by injection. The major clinical manifestations induced by allergens include sneezing, nasal discharge, coughing, wheezing, and shortness of breath with evidence of reversible airway obstruction, urticaria, angioedema, and anaphylaxis (Kurup, 2004).

Allergy to fungi results from exposure and sensitization to outdoor and indoor molds and affects a substantial number of patients (Kozak et al., 1979; Burge, 1985; Vijay et al., 1998). Fungi present in both indoor and outdoor air are generally considered as important cause of mold-induced allergy. The concentrations of the fungi in the outdoor environment vary depending on the climate, vegetation, and many other factors, while the concentration of indoor fungi depends on moisture content, ventilation, presence and absence of carpets, pets, and houseplants (Gravesen, 1999).

Fungi are eukaryotic, nonchlorophyllus organism that exist in nature predominantly as saprophytic organisms (Hawksworth et al., 1994). A fewer number of fungi cause plant and animal diseases, while several fungi produce economically useful metabolites including antibiotics, vitamins, enzymes, and flavors. In spite of the fewer fungi that are associated with the production of toxins and other potent deleterious agents, the impact of such fungi in health and disease are significant. The inhalation of fungal spores or mycelial fragments of the fungi contaminating both indoor and outdoor environments cause allergy in susceptible individuals. The prevalence of fungal allergy is estimated to be about 6% in the general population, while it constitutes 20% to 30% of allergy in atopic individuals (Wuethrich, 1989; Vijay et al., 1998).

Fungal allergy also follows the same induction pathway as do other allergies caused by pollen, house dust, etc. These diseases result from exposure to spores, respirable hyphal fragments, or metabolites of fungi. The spores of fungi and fragments of vegetative hyphae are usually very small and most of them can penetrate the smaller airways of the lung and mediate allergic reactions. The allergens of fungi are heterogeneous and are partly shared by a number of fungi as indicated by their cross-reactivity (Kurup et al., 2000b; Kurup and Fink, 2002). Knowledge of the antigens, their biochemical and immunological characteristics, and their structure and function are important in understanding the pathogenesis of the disease, laboratory diagnosis, and even in patient care (Kurup, 2003).

Although fungi cause a number of allergic diseases, the majority of them are restricted to respiratory tract. They include allergic asthma, allergic bronchopulmonary mycoses, and hypersensitivity pneumonitis. Other related allergic diseases caused by fungi are allergic rhinitis and sinusitis. In this chapter, we will concentrate on allergic conditions of the lungs resulting from the first three diseases.

2. Allergic Asthma

Asthma is a complex clinical syndrome characterized by airway obstruction and cellular inflammation. Allergic asthma is caused by the sensitization to allergens belonging to a number of different sources including fungi (Kurup, 2003; 2004). There are two types of responses in asthma, the acute asthmatic response that occur within minutes after the exposure to the allergens, and the late-phase reaction occurring 3–4 h after exposure to the allergens. The immediate response results from the release of mediators, such as histamine, tryptase, leukotrienes, and vasoactive mediators, which induce airway mucosal edema, smooth muscle contractions, and mucus release (Busse et al., 2003). The cross-linking resulting from allergen binding to IgE on the surface of basophils/mast cells causes mediator release. The mediators cause smooth muscle hyperresponsiveness and results in anaphylaxis, leading to asphyxia and death if not attended in time. The late-phase reaction results in cytokines, such as interleukin-4 (IL-4), IL-5, and IL-13 and chemokines like RANTES, eotaxin, membrane cofactor protein (MCP)-1, MCP-2, MCP-3, and MIP-1α released by lymphocytes and accessory cells. These factors and Th2 T cells coordinate a cellular influx of activated eosinophils, neutrophils, and T-lymphocytes to the late asthmatic response. These activated inflammatory cells further release more mediators, which results in aggravation of late asthmatic reaction that leads to increased airway obstruction and chronic asthma. Allergic asthma is characterized by airway epithelial cell disruption, mucus hypersecretion, subepithelial collagen deposition, and interstitial inflammation. The mechanisms governing the preferential recruitment and activation of these participating cells have been a primary focus directed at discovering therapeutic strategies. Although a large number of fungi have been reported as capable of causing allergic asthma the most predominant ones are those belonging to the genera *Alternaria*, *Aspergillus*, *Cladosporium*, and *Penicillium* (Kurup et al., 2002). Animal models of asthma using some of these antigens have contributed to our understanding of the immunopathogenesis of allergic asthma (Kurup and Grunig, 2001).

2.1. Immunopathogenesis in Allergic Asthma

Asthma is characterized clinically by the presence of reversible airflow obstruction, cough, and increased bronchial smooth muscle hyperresponsiveness. Asthmatic subjects on inhalation of specific allergen experience both early (5–20 min; EAR) and late (2–4 h; LAR) broncho constriction lasting for 1 h and 2 to 12 h, respectively (Krishna et al., 2001). The acute asthmatic response is initiated by the release of short-lived mediators from mast cells and other airway cells. These mediators include histamine, tryptase, prostaglandins, and leukotrienes, which induce airway mucosal edema, smooth muscle contraction, and mucus release. In the LAR, there is a large influx of neutrophils into the bronchial mucosa. The neutrophils discharge their granular secretion to the airways playing a major role in the early part of the LAR. Twenty-four hours after allergen challenge, there is significant eosinophilia (Busse et al., 2003). This was further confirmed by the presence of enhanced levels of IL-5 in the bronchoalveolar fluid. Thus, the early-phase reaction seems to be modulated by IgE while the late-phase is due to activated T cells and eosinophils and their mediators.

Although it is fairly well understood that $CD4^+$ Th2 effector T cells play an important role in the pathogenesis of allergy and asthma, it is not understood as to how the Th2 response is initially induced. Similarly, it is not known how the role and effect of other lymphoid and nonlymphoid cell types facilitate or downregulate Th2-mediated lung inflammation. The immune responses detected in this condition are the result of interplay of both innate and acquired immunities. The immunopathogenesis of asthma is more or less similar to allergic bronchopulmonary aspergillosis (ABPA) except in severity.

2.2. Cytokines in Allergic Asthma

The Th2 subtype of T cells produce IL-4, IL-5, IL-9, and IL-13, but not interferon gamma (IFN-γ) and IL-2 (Kurup and Grunig, 2001; Krishna et al., 2001). The Th1 subtype of T cells produce IL-2, IFN-γ, and tumor necrosis factor beta (TNF-β). IL-4 and IL-13 are instrumental in isotype switching of B cells, while IFN-γ inhibits B cell activation and IgE synthesis. Frequently, the severity of asthma and bronchial hyperreactivity have been directly correlated with the presence of activated T cells and eosinophils that secrete IL-5 (Kurup and Grunig, 2001). These cytokines are induced by a number of cells including T cells, eosinophils, mast cells, and some of the epithelial and endothelial cells.

Several cytokines are expressed by the bronchial epithelium include IL-1β, IL-5, IL-6, and granulocyte-macrophage colony-stimulating factor (GM-CSF). IL-5 and GM-CSF play a major role in the survival, recruitment, and activation of eosinophils. Other cytokines produced by epithelial cells are IL-11 and TNF-α. These cytokines can activate B cells and monocytes and induce synthesis of other important cytokines and chemokines such as IL-6, IL-8, and RANTES. They can also upregulate adhesion molecules intercellular adhesion molecule 1 (ICAM-1), -2, VCAM-1, and E-selectins and actively participate in the trafficking of various effector and accessory cells (Busse et al., 2003).

2.3. Chemokines and Receptors in Allergic Asthma

For the direct migration and activation of various effector cells, chemokines are produced by a number of different cells. Chemokines, a group of small molecular weight factors, fall into four different subtypes based on their structure (Hogaboam et al., 2003). They participate in various functions including antigen processing, receptor-induced recruitment of dendritic cells, thymocytes, and other cells of the lymphoid organs (Rothenberg, 2000). This migration is effected by MIP-3β and the constitutively expressed CCR6 receptor. T-lymphocytes express CCR1, CCR2, CCR- 7, and CXCR4. However, there is differential expression of CCR3, CCR4, CCR8, and CXCR4 on Th2 cells and CCR5, CXCR3, and CXCR6 on Th1 cells. Eosinophils express CCR3 and CXCR4. B cells express CXCR4 and CXCR5, and stromal cells surrounding B-lymphocytes express SDF-1, while MIP-3β is expressed by dendritic cells in T cell area. Thus, chemokines produced by dendritic cells, B-lymphocytes, and endothelial cells play an important role in the selective recruitment of activated CD4+ Th2 lymphocytes and eosinophils in allergic inflammatory responses and CD4+ Th1 cells, monocytes and neutrophils in Th1 cell-mediated inflammatory responses. This results in enhanced proliferation of B cells, leading to differentiation of plasma cells and synthesis of IL-4-mediated IgE production, where CD40/CD154 (CD40L) interaction is essential (Busse et al., 2003).

Recent studies suggest that CC-chemokines like RANTES, MCP-1, MCP-3, and eotaxins also play a major role in recruiting inflammatory cells (Rothenberg, 2000). It has been shown that eotaxin-expressing cells increase dramatically in the site of inflammation and has been correlated with methacholine challenge. The results indicate that CC-chemokine exerted epithelial and endothelial damage through the induction CCR3 receptor contribute to infiltration of eosinophils to the local tissues. In this connection RANTES is more effective than eotaxin and is constitutively produced in the tissues. MCP-1, although less effective for eosinophils, activate basophils and induce secretion of leukotriene C (LTC) and histamine (Rothenberg, 2000). Histochemical studies indicate that MCP-1 recruit macrophages and activate basophils thus playing a major role in the inflammatory pathogenesis of bronchial asthma (Bischoff et al., 1992; Sousa et al., 1994). Among the CXC chemokines, IL-8 plays a major role as a chemoattractant for neutrophils and T-lymphocytes (Davis et al., 1995). IL-8 has been detectable in both the protein level in the BAL and in the mRNA level in the epithelial cells of the bronchi and other airways of asthmatic patients, but not in the normal controls.

2.4. Airway Remodeling in Allergic Asthma

Although asthmatic patients show marked airway hyperreactivity the exact mechanism and the underlying factors are not well understood. Airway remodeling resulting from the destruction of the airway integrity is considered as a potent cause. It has been suggested that the various factors and mediators mentioned before have an adverse effect on the smooth muscle and fibroblasts; of particular interest are metalloproteinases, transforming growth factor beta (TGF-β), epithelial growth factor (EGF), and platelet-derived growth factor (PDGF) (Kauffman, 2003). In addition, proteases present in the antigens also have been shown to play a major role in the destruction of tight junctions of the airway epithelium (Tomee et al., 1997).

To examine airway remodeling, investigators have studied the relationship of the epithelial mesenchymal trophic unit (EMTU) and allergic inflammation. The EMTU is comprised of bronchial epithelium, basement membrane, myofibroblasts, and smooth muscle cells. Remodeling of the EMTU is normally present in the bronchial morphogenesis of the airway during development of airways (Zhang et al., 1999; Richter et al., 2001). Relative levels of EGF and TGF-β act in opposing fashion in normal lung development to promote, EGF>TGF-β, or to inhibit, TGF-β>EGF, in the growth and elongation of the airway. It has been proposed that injury to the bronchial epithelium due to inflammation that occurs in asthma, reactivates the EMTU resulting in remodeling of the airways (Davies et al., 2003). Evidence has emerged that myofibroblasts in the lamina reticulosis play a central role in the EMTU. Exposure of the epithelium to allergen causes myofibroblasts to migrate toward the smooth muscle. Members of the TGF-β family are the most potent mediators of fibroblast–myofibroblast transformation, indeed TGF-β stimulates fibroblast deposition of collagens I and III. The extracellular matrix (ECM) is comprised of collagen, fibronectin, vitronectin, and lamina, which are important to maintain the contractile phenotype of the smooth muscle.

In addition to TGF-β, IL-11 and IL-17 have been associated with airway remodeling. IL-11 promotes the accumulation of myofibroblasts and myocytes and is secreted by bronchial fibroblasts and epithelial cells. Its level has been observed to correlate with severity of asthma. IL-17 stimulates bronchial fibroblasts to synthesize higher levels of IL-6 and IL-11, both profibrotic cytokines. Smooth muscle hyperplasia and hypertrophy are thought to be the result of smooth muscle cell stimulation by the growth factors including PDGF, endothelin-1, and EGF produced by epithelial cells and macrophages in inflamed airways (Davies et al., 2003).

2.5. Allergens Associated with Allergic Asthma

A number of fungi have been implicated in allergy and considered capable of inducing asthma are listed in Table 12.1 (Vijay et al., 1998). In most instances, sensitization with more than one fungus has been reported. Because of the cross-reactivity and sharing of antigenic epitopes it is not easy to ascertain the role of individual allergens in the allergic process. Both indoor and outdoor fungal allergens have been reported as causing allergic asthma (Kurup et al., 2002). Antigens extracted from the molds usually show immediate skin test reactivity in these

Table 12.1. Fungi Associated Frequently with Allergic Asthma

Phycomycetes	**Basidiomycetes (cont.)**	**Deuteromycetes (cont.)**
Phytophthora	*Lentinus*	*Fusarium*
Plasmophora	*Pleurotus*	*Gliocladium*
Mucor	*Polyporus*	*Helminthosporium*
Rhizopus	*Psilocybe*	*Monilia*
Ascomycetes	*Puccinia*	*Neurospora*
Chaetomium	*Tilletia*	*Nigrospora*
Claviceps	*Urocystis*	*Paecilomyces*
Daldinia	*Ustilago*	*Penicillium*
Didymella	**Deuteromycetes (fungi imperfecti)**	*Phoma*
Eurotium	*Acremonium*	*Pyrenochaeta*
Microsphaera	*Alternaria*	*Scopulariopsis*
Yeasts	*Aspergillus*	*Sporotrichum*
Candida	*Aureobasidium*	*Stachybotrys*
Rhodotorula	*Botrytis*	*Stemphylium*
Saccharomyces	*Cephalosporium*	*Torula*
Basidiomycetes	*Chrysosporium*	*Trichoderma*
Agaricus	*Cladosporium*	*Trichophyton*
Calvatia	*Coniosporium*	*Ulocladium*
Cantharellus	*Curvularia*	*Wallemia*
Cyathus	*Cylindrocarpon*	
Ganoderma	*Drechslera*	
Geastrum	*Epicoccum*	

patients. Although a large number of allergens from these fungi have been characterized, limited numbers only are available in pure form.

3. Allergic Bronchopulmonary Mycoses

Allergic bronchopulmonary mycoses (ABPM) is a disabling lung disease seen frequently in atopic individuals. ABPM is characterized by clinical, immunologic, radiologic, and pathologic findings that range from mild asthma to end-stage fibrotic disease (Greenberger, 1988, 2003). Although several fungi, such as *Curvularia*, *Geotrichum*, *Dreschlera*, and *Candida* sp., have been reported as causing ABPM, the most predominant organism associated with the condition is *Aspergillus fumigatus* (Greenberger, 1988; Kurup and Apter, 1998). Hence, we will concentrate our discussion on ABPA. The pathogenesis of ABPM follows the same course as classic asthma with unique cellular immune responses and pathophysiology stemming from the responses of T cells (Kurup et al., 1998b). The activation of specific T-helper cells leads to the cytokine cascade with IgE production and recruitment of eosinophils and mast cells. ABPA appears as a secondary complication in patients with allergic asthma and cystic fibrosis and is characterized by fleeting pulmonary infiltration, immediate skin test reactivity to *Aspergillus* antigen, elevated serum total IgE, peripheral blood eosinophilia, and precipitating antibodies to *A. fumigatus* antigens in the serum (Greenberger, 2003). Specific IgE, IgG, and IgA antibodies to *A. fumigatus* have been shown to be present in substantial amounts in the sera of patients with ABPA compared to skin test positive asthmatics (Greenberger, 1988; Kurup, 2000). In ABPA patients, soluble IL-2 receptor (sCD25) concentration has been shown to be markedly increased compared to normals and non-ABPA asthmatics (Brown et al., 1995).

3.1. Immunology of Allergic Bronchopulmonary Aspergillosis

The immune response in ABPA is very complex and diverse types of immunological responses can be demonstrable in ABPA. Immediate cutaneous reactivity to *Aspergillus* antigens mediated by IgE through mast cell degranulation and release of classical mediators including histamine is universal in all ABPA patients. A good number of ABPA patients also demonstrate late reaction (Arthus reaction) to *Aspergillus* allergens resulting from immune complex activation of alternate complement activation pathway. The specific IgG and *Aspergillus* antigen complex trigger the release of cystenyl leukotrienes C-4, which in turn promotes mucus production, bronchial constriction, hyperemia, and edema. However, the lack of vasculitis or deposition of complement and immunoglobulin in the vessel walls suggests ABPA as a nonimmune complex-mediated disease, even though there are strong antibody responses in all ABPA patients and the presence of circulating immune complexes in some ABPA patients. Lung biopsy specimens from patients with ABPA show *Aspergillus*-specific IgE in the germinal centers, whereas IgG antibodies could be detected in the lung parenchyma. Antibody directed cell-mediated cytotoxicity has also been reported in some patients (Kurup et al., 1985). Similarly in a few ABPA patients cell-mediated immunity (CMI) evidenced by delayed skin test response and enhanced antigen-induced T cell stimulation have been demonstrated (Knutsen et al., 1998).

3.2. Cell-Mediated Immunity

The most striking characteristics of ABPA are the enhanced IgE expression, Th2 cytokine profile, and recruitment and activation of eosinophils (Kurup and Apter,

1998). Peripheral blood lymphocytes (PBMC) demonstrate *A. fumigatus* allergen-induced proliferation, while B cells spontaneously produce IgE in in vitro cultures due to in vivo activation (Knutsen et al., 1998). Upon stimulation, $CD4^+$ Th2 cells from ABPA patients secrete cytokines, IL-4, IL-5, IL-10, and IL-13, of which IL-4 and IL-13 enhances the expression of IgE, while IL-5 enhances eosinophil recruitment and activation. IFN-γ, a Th1 cytokine participates in the tissue inflammation when produced and is important in switching of IgG subclasses. Th1 cytokines support a Th1 response and suppress the Th2 response particularly IgE production and eosinophil recruitment. Activated basophils also secrete Th2 cytokines and stimulate further activation of Th2 pathway, resulting in enhanced IgE and eosinophil production (Kurup et al., 1998b).

Analysis of cells from bronchial biopsies from ABPA patients revealed a mixture of cell types including macrophages, eosinophils, and lymphocytes. Eosinophils predominate both the bronchoalveolar lavage fluid (BALF) and lung tissues. The eosinophils on activation release their mediators such as major basic proteins (MBP), eosinophil peroxidase (EPO), and eosinophilic cationic protein (ECP). These products cause inflammation in the lung and continue to sustain the ongoing immunological and inflammatory responses. Hence, the Th2 cytokine IL-5 is very important in the activation of eosinophils and is important in the development of ABPA (Knutsen et al., 1998; Kurup et al., 1998b). However, in murine models of ABPA, eosinophils do not appear to be critical in mediating tissue damage or causing airway hyperreactivity (Kurup et al., 1997). IL-5 gene knockout mice or those treated with anti-IL-5 antibodies still develop the full spectrum of ABPA (Corry et al., 1998; Ford et al., 2001). In the lung biopsies, in addition to eosinophils other cell types such as T cells, B cells, and natural killer (NK) cells have also been reported.

3.3. Humoral Immunity

Patients with ABPA develop greater amounts of IgE, IgG, and IgA than patients with atopic asthma who do not have ABPA (Brummund et al., 1987; Greenberger, 2003). The specific IgE antibody to *A. fumigatus* represents only a fraction of the total elevated IgE antibody levels; however, there is evidence of *A. fumigatus*-specific IgE production in bronchial lymphoid tissues of ABPA patients. Lung biopsies from ABPA patients showed the presence of specific IgE-bearing B cells in the lymphoid follicles. The protein antigen of *A. fumigatus* reacts frequently with serum IgG_1 and IgG_2 antibodies in patients with ABPA (Brummund et al., 1987). The polysaccharides and glycoprotein antigens demonstrate significant response to IgG in aspergilloma, but with less reactivity than with ABPA sera.

3.4. Cytokines and Receptors in ABPA

Several cytokines are produced by activated T cells, which include IL-4, IL-5, IL-6, IL-9, IL-10, and IL13. IL-4 and IL-13 are instrumental in IgE switching of B cells (Knutsen et al., 1998; Kurup et al., 1998b). Although IL-4 is essential for IgE isotype switching, this cytokine alone is not sufficient for IgE transcription and expression. In order for IgE secretion to occur, a second signal mediated by the cognate T and B cell interactions via CD40–C40L is essential (Zhang et al., 1991). CD40 is a member of the TNFR superfamily, is a 50-kDa integral membrane glycoprotein that was identified originally on B lymphocytes. Along with cell–cell and –cytokine interaction costimulatory molecule interactions, such as CD28 and CD80/86 and CD27 and CD70 are essential for sustaining the expression of IgE (Kobate et al., 1995; Mathur et al., 1999). It has been demonstrated that CD23 and soluble

CD23 also augment B cell IgE synthesis. The high levels of IL-5 production by activated T lymphocytes explains eosinophilia demonstrated in ABPA. Several chemokines also actively interact with the immune system and modulate the pathogenic responses. Of particular interest are MIP-1α, MCP, RANTES, and eotaxin that are actively involved in the activation of eosinophils (Hogaboam et al., 2003).

The $CD4^+$ Th2 cytokine, IL-4 plays a central role in the allergic inflammatory responses observed in ABPA (Brown et al., 1995; Kurup et al., 1997, 1998b) (Fig. 12.1). IL-4 upregulates cellular activity through the binding to the IL-4Rα receptor (Nelms et al., 1999; Bacharier and Geha, 2000). There are two IL-4 receptors (IL-4R), type 1 and type 2. IL-4R type 1 is a heterodimer comprised of the IL-4Rα chain and Cγ chain and is present on immune cells, such as T cells, B cells, eosinophils, mast cells, and dendritic cells; whereas IL-4R type 2 is comprised of IL-4Rα and IL-13Rα and is present on immune cells, bronchial epithelium, and vascular endothelium. IL-4 stimulates both type 1 and type 2 IL-4 receptors, whereas IL-13 stimulates only type 2 IL-4 receptor. From the distribution of IL-4 type 1 and 2 receptors, it is evident that IL-4

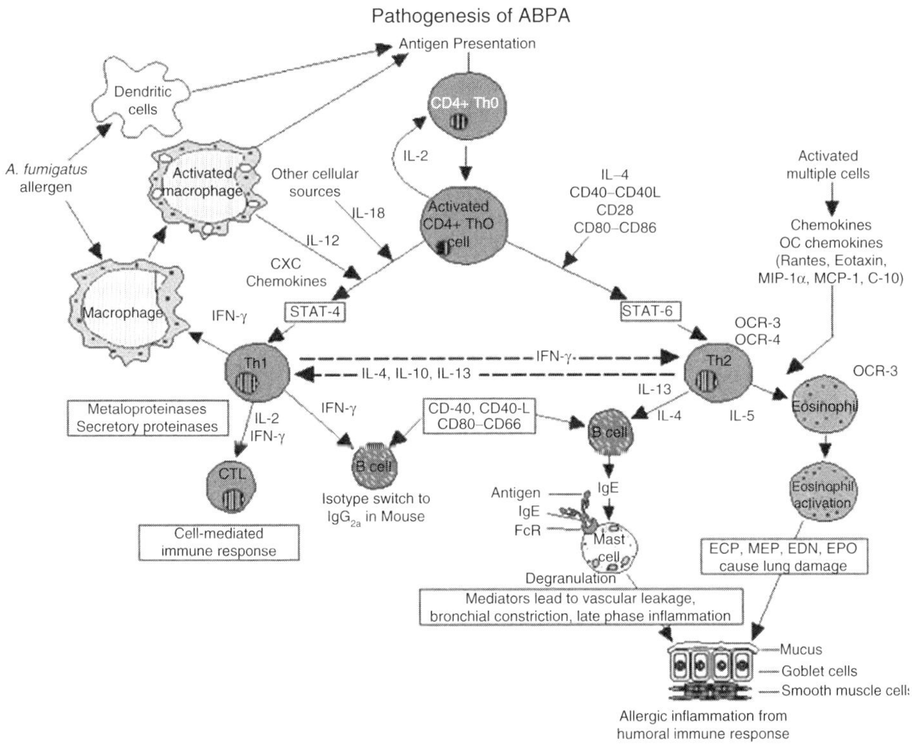

Figure 12.1. Schematic illustration of the current understanding of the pathogenesis of ABPA.

and IL-13 play key roles in the allergic inflammatory responses in allergic fungal bronchopulmonary diseases, including isotype switch of B cells to IgE synthesis.

3.5. Chemokines and Chemokine Receptors

Emerging experimental data, particularly from animal model studies of allergic aspergillosis, indicates a major role for chemokines and their receptors. Acute airway disease in mice due to *A. fumigatus* demonstrates the importance of RANTES, C10, eotaxin, and eotaxin-2 in the recruitment of eosinophils in the lungs. In the chronic model of *Aspergillus*-induced allergy, inflammation in the lung, enhanced eosinophilia, elevated levels of IgE, reversible airway obstruction, goblet cell hyperplasia, and peribronchial fibrosis (Hogaboam et al., 2000). The contribution of chemokine receptors such as CCR1, CCR2, CCR5, and CXCR2 have been studied in relation to the development of chronic fungal allergy (Hogaboam et al., 2003). The contribution of individual receptors have been studied using targeted knockout mice. The chemokine receptor CCR1 through its interactions with macrophage inflammatory protein-1 alpha (MIP-1α/CCL3) contributes to remodeling responses such as goblet cell hyperplasia and peribronchial fibrosis during chronic asthma without any impact on innate immune response and airway hyperresponsiveness. CCR2 and its ligand monocytic chemoattractant protein-1 (MCP-1/CCL2) are critical in the clearance of fungal spores. However, after the clearance of fungal spores, MCP-1/CCL2 and CCR2 are major contributors in the airway remodeling and airway hyperreactivity. CCR5 modulates movement of eosinophils and T cells into the lungs and appear to inhibit innate response by alveolar macrophages towards *A. fumigatus*. These results from animal model studies indicate the involvement of a complex and specific role for chemokines and their receptors in allergic aspergillosis (Fig. 12.1).

3.6. T and B cell Epitopes

T cell lines generated against Asp f 1 from ABPA patients were $CD4^+$ $CD25^+$ T cells (Knutsen et al., 1994). These cell lines showed a cytokine profile of IL-4^+ and IFN-γ and the lymphoproliferation was inhibited by anti-IL-4 and not by anti-IL-2, indicating an autocrine response. Recent studies demonstrating single nucleotide polymorphisms of the IL-4 receptor and increased sensitivity to IL-4 stimulation is probably responsible for this earlier observation. T cell clones having a Th2 type were also generated against Asp f 1 from allergic asthmatics. However, Th1 type of T cells could be generated with tetanus antigen from these patients. This indicates that Th2 response in ABPA is specific to *Aspergillus* antigens and not the result of a generalized Th2 skewing.

The T cell clones generated from ABPA patients against Asp f 2 showed more of a Th2 type of response (Rathore et al., 2001). These clones were stimulated with Asp f 2 deletion mutants and synthetic overlapping peptides to define the T cell epitopes. Two of the synthetic peptides aa54–68 and aa60–74 were able to induce significant proliferation of two T cell clones. Both clones represent $CD4^+$ Th2 type, but differed in their ability to secrete cytokines, IL-4, and IL-5.

Synthetic peptides from Asp f 1 and f 2 were studied for their binding to IgE from patients. A number of linear epitopes have been identified (Kurup et al., 1996; Banerjee et al., 1999). The peptides of Asp f 1 synthesized based on the predicted T cell epitope demonstrated different responses by spleen cells of mice exposed to antigens of *Aspergillus*. A "C" terminal peptide of Asp f 1 induced a Th1 response, while another peptide aa53–68 induced a Th2 response. Thus the Th2 skewing in experimental animals is antigen dependent as in the case of human ABPA (Kurup et al., 1998a).

3.7. HLA-Restriction in ABPA

Studies have been directed to understand the unique T cell antigen receptor (TCR) recognition (T cell epitopes), TCR-Vβ restriction, and HLA-class II restriction in promoting enhanced Th2 responses in ABPA (Chauhan et al., 1996, 1997, 2000). Analysis of T cell epitope mapping has revealed that there were three immunodominant regions of the Asp f 1 protein in ABPA patients that is recognized by TCR (Knutsen, 2003). These findings were similar to that demonstrated with other experimental models of allergy. T cell clones generated against house dust mite allergens from nonatopic individuals proliferated in response to allergen stimulation but did not support IgE synthesis, whereas the T cell clone from atopic patients did (Tsitoura et al., 1996). Furthermore, TCR epitope mapping studies revealed limited number of epitopes reacting with TCR, TCR-Vβ restriction or usage, and HLA-class II restriction. Four major Vβ chains, Vβ 3, 6, 13, and 14, react to Asp f 1. This will allow for the evaluation whether mutations of the epitope might alter the T cell cytokine and/or lymphoproliferative responses for potential immunotherapy of ABPA. Recently, Chauhan et al. (2000) identified that there is HLA-DR2 and DR5 restriction in patients with ABPA. Furthermore, they also demonstrated restricted genotypes within HLA-DR2 and DR5. In particular, HLA-DRB1*1501 and 1503 were reported to provide high relative risk. On the other hand, 40% to 44% of non-ABPA atopic *Aspergillus*-sensitive individuals have the HLA-DR2 and/or DR5 type. Further studies indicated that the presence of HLA-DQ2 (especially DQB1*0201) provided protection from the development of ABPA. Thus, certain genotypes of HLA-DR2 and DR5 may be necessary but not sufficient to cause ABPA.

3.8. Airway Remodeling

Mucosal defense of airways of healthy individuals is a highly efficient barrier in eliminating antigens and microorganisms. Exposure to *A. fumigatus* allergens as spores, fragments of hyphae, or limited growth of the organism in the bronchus results in the release of various antigenic components. These include peroxidases, proteases, ribotoxins, catalases, and many other immunogenic or toxic components (Kauffman and Tomee, 1998). These secretory products have a direct effect on the pulmonary epithelium and subsequent inflammatory process. The integrity of the pulmonary epithelium is disrupted by these products of *A. fumigatus* resulting in the shedding of epithelial layers and exposure to the bronchoalveolar lymphoid tissue (BALT). The BALT initiates and maintains an immune system response to *Aspergillus* with subsequent trafficking to the peripheral lymphoid system (Tomee et al., 1997). The physical barrier prevents penetration of large molecules and particles. Particles are frequently removed by the ciliary movement of the epithelial cells, phagocytic cells, and mucus secreting cells, particularly goblet cells. The airway epithelial tight junctions retain the integrity of the airway epithelium and actively prevent the transport of molecules between the epithelial cells and across the epithelium. The secretory cells present in the epithelium and their products such as mucin, defensive proteins, and enzymes together constitute a protective environment in the airway (Tomee et al., 1997; Kauffman and Tomee, 1998).

The allergic inflammatory response in ABPA appears to be more intense than in asthmatic and may result in severe changes in the airway structure or remodeling. Spores of *A. fumigatus* trapped in the airway release proinflammatory cytokines and growth factors that mediate both inflammatory responses and airway remodeling (Kauffman, 2003). It has been shown that *A. fumigatus* release proteolytic enzymes with elastolytic and collagenolytic activities and play a major role in the airway injury and destruction. The damaging effect on the epithelial layer is also caused by proinflammatory chemokines and cytokines, IL-6, IL-8, and MCP-1 produced by epithelial cells of the airways. Factors released by the eosinophils in response to *A. fumigatus* such as MBP, ECP, EPO, etc. also play a role in epithelial damage. Thus, the airway remodeling results from proteases of *A. fumigatus*, proinflammatory cytokines, and factors produced by eosinophils and other cells (Tomee et al., 1997; Hogaboam et al., 2000; Kauffman, 2003).

Damage to the bronchial epithelium and Th2 cytokines together cause disturbances of the EMTU. Both IL-4 and IL-13 cause epithelial activation and fibroblast activation. The IL-4/IL-13 receptors on bronchial epithelium is comprised of IL-4Rα/IL-13Rα heterodimer. In in vitro cultures of bronchial epithelial cells, IL-4, and IL-13 increased expression of STAT-6, GM-CSF, and IL-8. Kauffman and associates (Tomee et al., 1997; Kauffman and Tomee, 1998; Kauffman, 2003) have shown that proteases of *A. fumigatus* and *Alternaria* disrupt normal bronchial epithelium and result in IL-6 and TNF-α secretion. IL-4/IL-13 also enhanced fibroblast eotaxin secretion, which might explain the accumulation of eosinophils beneath the lamina reticularis. In ABPA, where there is increased sensitivity to IL-4 stimulation probably due to IL-4R polymorphisms, the bronchial epithelium and EMTU probably respond to *Aspergillus* antigens and IL-4/IL-13 stimulations that result in increased fibrosis and accounting for the increased risk of bronchiectasis and fibrosis.

Airway remodeling is characterized by changes involving epithelial cell hyperplasia and metaplasia, collagen deposition, thickening of the lamina reticularis, smooth muscle hyperplasia, and proliferation of airways and blood vessels (Chakir et al., 2003; Davies et al., 2003). Airway hyperreactivity (AHR) by morphometric analysis may be due to adventitial thickening of the airways to a large extent. Investigators have proposed that airway inflammation, which is central to asthma, may not explain fully the AHR and airway remodeling. In support of this, anti-IL-5 mAb effectively reduces bronchial epithelium of eosinophils by 50%, but does not improve AHR (Menzies-Gow et al., 2003).

3.9. Animal Models of ABPA

Animal models of *Aspergillus*-induced allergy demonstrated high levels of total IgE, *Aspergillus*-specific IgG_1, peripheral and lung eosinophilia, pulmonary inflammation, and airway hyperreactivity (Kurup et al., 1992; Kurup and Grunig, 2001). Elevated levels of antigen-induced IL-4, IL-5, and IL-13 have been demonstrated in the spleen cell cultures of sensitized animals. The induction of a Th2-type response was evidenced by the enhanced IL-4, IL-5, and IL-13 production and the inhibition of the same with IFN-γ (Kurup et al., 1997). Subsequent studies using various knockout mice provided a more clear picture of the immunopathogenesis (Fig. 12.1). The pathogenesis in the model was found to be the result of T cells as the IgE knockout, IL-4 knockout, and IL-5 knockout mice still developed the disease in spite of the lack of IgE and eosinophil responses (Kurup et al., 1997, 1999; Mehlhop et al., 1997). However, animals depleted of T cells failed to show any disease activity. When such animals were reconstituted with T cells from previously sensitized mice-induced airway inflammation and hyperreactivity (Corry et al., 1998). Another Th2 cytokine, IL-13, has been found to induce airway inflammatory responses (characterized by eosinophils and T cells), airway hyperreactivity, and airway remodeling (Blease et al., 2001a,b; Hogaboam et al., 2003). However, by neutralizing IL-13 with polyclonal antibodies or eliminating IL-13 responsive cells using chimeric IL-13 and *Pseudomonas* endotoxin A failed to prevent *Aspergillus* conidia clearance from sensitized mice (Blease et al., 2001a,b).

Exposure to *Aspergillus* antigens not only induce a predominant Th2 response, but also demonstrate a Th1 cytokine networking in the lungs representing IL-12 and IL-18 (Hogaboam et al., 2000; Blease et al., 2001c). Neutralization of IL-18 resulted in marked increase in the growth and persistence of *A. fumigatus* in the lungs of challenged mice (Blease et al., 2001c). However, it was noted that endogenous IL-10 is necessary for regulating the innate immune response and for developing allergic syndrome. Mice depleted of IL-10 gene demonstrated enhanced Th1 (IFN-γ) and Th2 (IL-4 and IL-5) type cytokines compared to wild-type mice exposed to *Aspergillus* antigen (Grunig et al., 1997). These results from animal model studies suggest that immunomodulatory cytokines such as IL-10, IL-12, and IL-18 have a marked effect on the experimental murine allergic aspergillosis (Grunig et al., 1997; Hogaboam et al., 2000; Blease et al., 2001c). Indeed, *A. fumigatus* antigen Asp f 2, f 3, and f 4 stimulate human PBMC to secrete IL-10. Although not fully understood, the chemokines and their receptors also play a major role in the pathogenesis of ABPA (Fig. 12.1).

3.10. Allergens Associated with ABPM

Although several fungi like *Aspergillus*, *Penicillium*, *Fusarium*, *Curvularia*, etc. are implicated in ABPM, by far the most predominant organism recognized is *A. fumigatus* (Table 12.2). In recent years, considerable progress has been made in purifying relevant allergens from *A. fumigatus*. These allergens have been used in studying antibody response and cell-mediated immunity (Kurup, 2003; 2004; Kurup et al., 2000a). Some of these allergens have been used in animal model studies to understand their role in the immunopathogenesis.

Table 12.2. Fungi Associated with Allergic Bronchopulmonary Mycoses

Aspergillus fumigatus
Aspergillus niger
Curvularia
Candida albicans
Dreschlera
Fusarium sp.
Geotrichum
Helminthosporium

4. Hypersensitivity Pneumonitis

Hypersensitivity pneumonitis (HP), also called extrinsic allergic alveolitis, is an allergic lung disease caused by a number of antigens including several fungi and actinomycetes (Patel et al., 2001; Kurup and Fink, 2002; Fink and Zacharisen, 2003). HP caused by inhalant allergens can progress to disabling and even to end-stage fatal lung disease. The common fungi associated with hypersensitivity pneumonitis are numerous, but *Aspergillus* and *Penicillium* are the most predominant with a number of scattered reports implicating many other fungi (Table 12.3). The exposure to airborne antigens occurs in various occupations, hobbies, and environmental contamination in air-handling equipments. Serum-precipitating antibodies to the offending inhaled antigen is usually elevated. However, the immunopathogenesis is believed to be the result of cell-mediated immunity, particularly through the interactions of $CD8^+$ cytotoxic lymphocytes and macrophages (Fig. 12.2 and Table 12.4).

Table 12.3. Fungi Associated with Hypersensitivity Pneumonitis

Aspergillus
Curvularia
Aureobasidium
Penicillium
Chaetomium
Trichosporon
Cephalosporium
Cryptococcus

Pulmonary function tests show restrictive defects and diffusion abnormalities with hypoxemia, especially after exercise or enhanced activity. Radiographic changes vary according to the stage of the disease and are best evaluated by high-resolution computed tomography (CT) scan. In most instances, a history of exposure to the antigen and presence of IgG antibodies to the antigen provide a suggestive diagnosis of HP. However, in more obscure cases, bronchoalveolar lavage, lung biopsy, and history of environmental exposure are indicated for conclusive diagnosis (Bourke et al., 2001; Patel et al., 2001; Fink and Zacharisen, 2003).

4.1. Acute Hypersensitivity Pneumonitis

Macrophages after ingesting antigen particles or antigen–antibody complexes become

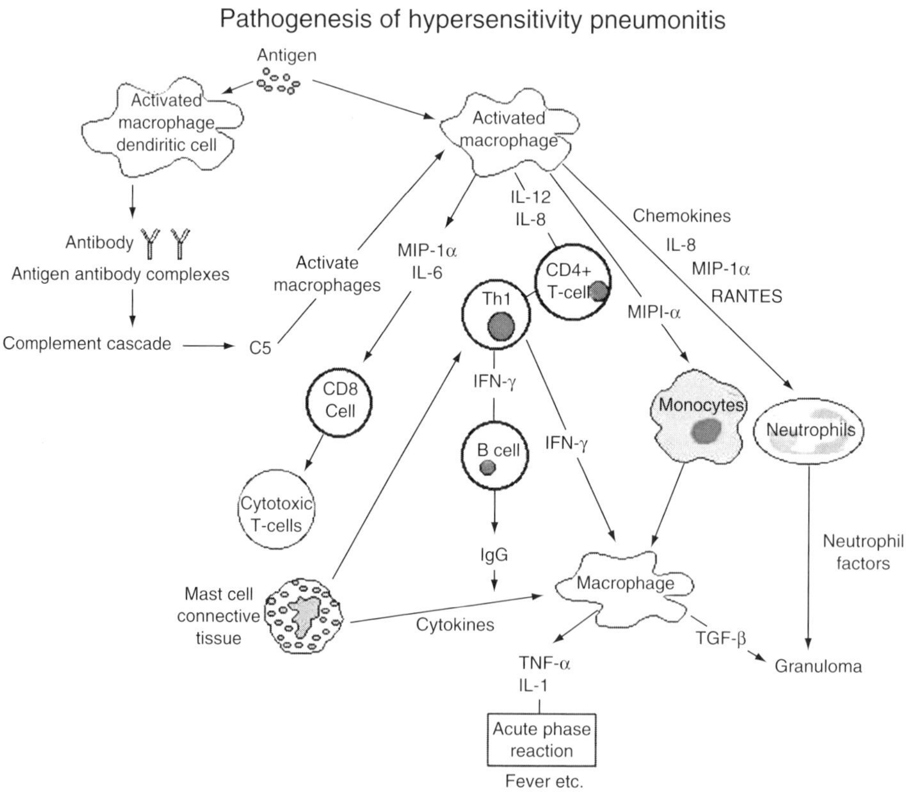

Figure 12.2. Schematic presentation of the current understanding of the pathogenesis of hypersensitivity pneumonitis.

Table 12.4. Summary of Immunopathogenesis of Hypersensitivity Pneumonitis and ABPA

Parameter	Hypersensitivity pneumonitis	ABPA[a]
BALF cells	Lymphocytes, monocytes	Eosinophils, lymphocytes, monocytes
BALF T cells	$CD8^+ > CD4^+$ $CD3^+TCR\gamma\delta^+$	$CD4^+$:$CD8^+$ ratio 2:1
BALF NK cells	Present	$CD23^+CD56^+$
B cell follicles	Present	IgE^+
T helper cells	Th1	Th2
T activation markers	$CD25^+CD4^+$ DR^+CD8^+	$CD25^+$ sCD25
Cytokine synthesis	IFN-γ, TNF-α, IL-1, IL-10, IL-12 IL-16	IL-4, IL-5, IL-10, TGF-β IFN-γ
Chemokines	IL-8, MCP-1, MCP-1α	Eotaxin, RANTES, MCP-1, MIP-1α
T cytotoxic cells	$CD8^+$ increased in BALF	
T suppressor function	Normal	
B cells	Normal	CD23 CD86 expression
Immunoglobulins	Normal	IgE
Antibody to antigen	IgG, IgA	IgE, IgG, IgA
Immune complexes	Present	Reported
Monocytes	CD80 and CD86	CD86/CD23 expression on monocyte-derived dendritic cells
Adhesion molecules	ICAM	VCAM, ICAM
HLA restriction	HLA-DRB1*1305 HLA-DQB1*0402	HLA-DR2 (DR15, DR16) DRB1*1501, 1502, 1503, 1601 and HLA-DR5 DRB1*1101, 1103, 1104, 1202 HLA-DQ2 (DQB1*0201)
TCR-Vβ restriction	Unknown	Vβ3, β6, β13, β14
Polymorphisms	TNF-α promoter region	IL-4Rα polymorphisms: I50 V, various cytoplasmic
Mast cell degranulation	Absent	Present
Basophil hyperactivity	Absent	Present

[a]Between ABPA and allergic asthma, the difference was only quantitative.

activated and secrete chemokines and cytokines. Chemokine IL-8, induced during activation of macrophage, attract neutrophils to the site. Compared to IgE-mediated responses in asthma and ABPA, where eosinophils form a major cell type, in HP it is mostly neutrophils. Other chemokines produced are MIP-1α and RANTES. Although MIP-1α is a major chemotactic factor of activation for monocyte/macrophages and lymphocytes, it is also involved in the differentiation of $CD4^+$ Th0 cells to Th1 cells (Fink and Zacharisen, 2003).

IFN-γ is essential for inflammation and granuloma formation in HP (Gudmundsson and Hunninghake, 1997). In a mouse model it has been shown that $CD4^+$ Th1 cells produce IFN-γ, which activates macrophages and develop granuloma. However, IL-10 was shown to counteract this response (Gudmundsson et al., 1998). Cytokines produced by the activation of macrophages include TNF-α and IL-1 and may be the cause of fever and acute phase response in HP (Yamasaki et al., 1999). Macrophages from mice sensitized to *Saccharopolyspora faeni*, secrete IL-12, which contribute to the differentiation of Th0 cells to Th1 T cells (Schuyler et al., 2002). BALF from patients frequently show enhanced presence of IL-12 receptor. IL-6 produced by macrophage promotes the terminal differentiation of B cells to antibody-secreting plasma cells and in the maturation of $CD8^+$ cytotoxic T cells. The role of costimulatory molecules in the immunopathogenesis of murine HP has also been studied (Isreal-Assayag et al., 1999). Activated macrophages show increased expression of CD80/86, while activated T cells show expression of CD28 on T cells. By blocking the CD28–CD80/86 interaction, the inflammation can be reduced considerably in the mouse model of HP.

Following exposure to antigen, the $CD4^+$ Th1 cells appear in the BAL fluid, but will diminish their numbers and show a gradual increase in $CD8^+$ cells. This is in contrast to sarcoidosis where $CD4^+$ cells show predominance over other cells. However, in IgE-mediated allergy, a predominant Th2 response over Th1 response was the norm (Table 12.4).

4.2. Subacute Hypersensitivity Pneumonitis

Prolonged exposure to the antigens results in granuloma formation in the lungs. The macrophages in response to various chemotactic factors are activated and recruited to the lungs. These macrophages in response to MIP-1α become transformed into epithelial cells and multinucleated giant cells (Suga et al., 1997). Plasma cells develop in large numbers in the interstitial and lymphoid follicles and is a result of the cognizant interactions between the $CD4^+$ $CD154^+$ T lymphocytes with CD40 bearing B lymphocytes (Fig. 12.2). This results in the local production of antibody in the lungs.

4.3. Chronic Hypersensitivity Pneumonitis

The activated macrophages produce TGF-β, a potent stimulator of fibrosis and angiogenesis (Yamasaki et al., 1999; Semenzato et al., 2000; Chouchakova et al., 2001). BAL fluids in experimental HP in mouse model and in patients showed procollagen, FAS ligand, CD40 ligand, fibronectin, and enhanced number of mast cells. All these factors contribute to enhanced inflammation and progression to fibrosis. Although a substantial number of mast cells have been identified in the lavage of the lungs, no histamine-mediated inflammation was detected and it is assumed that these mast cells may be responsible for the cytokines needed for sustaining and progression of the granuloma formation and for promoting fibrosis.

4.4. Histopathology

The histopathologic findings of HP vary with the stage of the disease. In acute and subacute stages, the inflammatory response noted in the histopathology of lung biopsies mirrors the findings of BAL studies (Patel et al., 2001; Fink and Zacharisen, 2003). Little only is known of the histology of acute HP, but an acute bronchiolitis with neutrophilic infiltrate in the alveoli and respiratory bronchioles has been described. In the subacute stage, a nonspecific interstitial pneumonia is identified. Alveolar and interstitial inflammation is composed of predominantly lymphocytes, macrophages, and plasma cells. Macrophages with foamy cytoplasm surrounded by large numbers of mononuclear cells are unique to HP. Noncaseating granulomata in the peribronchial interstitium and an organizing pneumonia and interstitial fibrosis are also present in the subacute stage and chronic stages. Immunophenotyping studies reveal a predominance of $CD8^+$ T cells and NK cells. B cell follicular formation may be seen in interstitial spaces. Immunofluorescence studies have detected antigen in the alveolar spaces and in the interstitium. Immunoglobulin and complement have only been rarely demonstrated. Lymphoid interstitial pneumonia and HP are the most common features in infectious pneumonia in children, and these two are pathologically identical to their adult counterparts.

Chronic HP has a more distinctive appearance when all components of the characteristic triad are present: bronchiolocentric cellular interstitial pneumonia, poorly formed noncaseating granulomata, and bronchiolitis obliterans. Of these, the most consistent histologic manifestation is the peribronchial interstitial inflammation composed mostly of lymphocytes with some macrophages and plasma cells. Eosinophils are typically absent or scant. Granulomas are present in approximately 65% of patients. The intraluminal fibrosis is also present in two thirds of HP. As the disease progresses, a nonspecific interstitial fibrosis resembling interstitial pneumonia or end-stage pulmonary fibrosis with lymphoid aggregates may be present. A resulting honeycombing or cystic change occurs due to the peripheral destruction of alveoli. Since similar histologic findings are seen in collagen vascular diseases, drug hypersensitivity reactions, and infection, the diagnosis of HP cannot be made by histology alone. It requires clinical, serologic, roentgenographic, and BAL correlation.

4.5. Cell-Mediated Immunity

Cell-mediated immune reactivity within the bronchoalveolar lymphoid tissue (BALT) appears to be the key site of response to these various small-inhaled antigens in patients with HP and in experimental murine models (Gudmundsson and Hunninghake, 1997; Yamasaki et al., 1999; Semenzato et al., 2000; Chouchakova et al., 2001). T cells obtained from peripheral blood and bronchoalveolar lavage (BAL) demonstrate lymphoproliferative responses to eliciting antigen, which differentiates symptomatic patients from asymptomatic exposed individuals. There are both $CD4^+$ and $CD8^+$ T cells found in BAL and lung tissue with a preponderance of $CD8^+$ T cells. The $CD8^+$ T cells are probably T cytotoxic cells, as T-suppressor function is decreased. Furthermore, there are increased numbers of $CD3^+TCR\gamma\delta^+$ T cells, which usually have T-cytotoxic activity. NK cells similarly are increased in both BAL and lung tissue. Thus, in active disease there are increased numbers of pulmonary macrophages, cytotoxic T cells and NK cells, the effector cells of cellular cytotoxicity.

$CD4^+$ T cells in HP secrete IFN-γ, IL-2, IL-16, and TNF-α, typical of a Th1 cytokine pattern. Monocyte cytokine synthesis is also increased with secretion of IL-8, IL-12, TNF-α, IL-6, and some IL-1. Thus, monocyte and T cell cytokines favor a Th1 cell-mediated immune response (Fig. 12.2). Recently, polymorphism of the TNF-α promoter gene has been identified, which would result in increase of TNF-α synthesis. In addition, there is some evidence for decreased IL-10 synthesis, which might promote a Th1 response. Investigators have also identified endotoxins in some protein antigen preparations, suggesting their role in eliciting an inflammatory response directly. Lipopolysaccharides are potent stimulators of macrophages, principally through toll-like receptors (TLR). This results in increased monocyte cytokine synthesis of IL-8, IL-12, and TNF-α, which would promote a cell-mediated inflammatory response.

Chemokines. Chemokines, such as increased IL-8, MIP-1α, and MCP-1 have been identified in HP and would favor a monocyte, neutrophil, and Th1 T cell inflammatory response. Likewise, increased expression of adhesion molecules such as L-, E-, and P-selectins, ICAM, and CD11/CD18 interactions would also favor a Th1 cell-mediated inflammatory infiltration (Semenzato et al., 2000; Fink and Zacharisen, 2003).

HLA-DR restriction. Previous studies suggested that HLA restriction with HLA-Bw40 may play a role (Diaz de la Vega et al., 1980); however, this association has not been confirmed. HLA-class II restriction has been identified in pigeon breeder's disease where an increased frequency of HLA-DRB1*1305 and decreased frequency of HLA-DQB1*0402 have been reported (Fink and Zacharisen, 2003).

4.6. Humoral Immunity

The presence of IgG complement-fixing antibody is the serologic hallmark of HP; IgA and IgM antibodies have also been detected. However, immune complex deposition has only rarely been reported. Complement activation and release of C5a, a strong chemotactic factor for neutrophils, contributes to the neutrophil infiltration seen in early exposure to the antigens (<48 h). Increased expression of FcγRIII receptors on macrophages has been reported, suggesting a role of macrophage involvement (Chouchakova et al., 2001). IgG antibodies may also play a role through antibody-dependent cell-mediated cell cytotoxicity (ADCC) by K cells.

4.7. Immunopathogenesis of HP

HP is not a uniform disease entity, but represents a complex dynamic clinical syndrome that manifests as different patterns during the course of time. In addition, the list of etiologic agents is long and new sources of antigens are frequently identified. Environmental factors play a major role in the pathogenesis of HP (Bourke et al., 2001). Our current understanding of the immunopathogenesis of HP is presented in Fig. 12.2.

Both cell-mediated and antibody-mediated immune responses play a major role in the pathogenesis of HP. Although most of our current knowledge on immunopathogenesis is derived from information originating from animal models, these findings have been confirmed by studies using lung lavages from patients. Most exposed individuals develop high levels of IgG antibody to the antigens. However, antibody alone is not sufficient to cause disease and requires the presence of $CD8^+$ cytotoxic lymphocytes. It has been shown that the immunopathology of HP is CD8-macrophage-mediated, but is also controlled by the Th1/Th2 balance as the disease is severe when shifted to a Th1 response and less severe when a Th2 response predominates (Gudmundsson et al., 1998; Schuyler et al., 2002). The factors responsible for the development of the more complex immune reactions in human beings are poorly defined. Although the immunopathogenesis of acute, subacute, and chronic phases of HP overlap, the alveolitis process leading to granuloma formation and ultimate fibrosis will be considered separately to obtain a better perspective. A number of glycoproteins have been detected in BAL fluid collected during acute-phase hypersensitivity reactions. These include elevated levels of vitronectin, fibronectin, and the fibroblast-derived collagen metabolite procollagen-III peptide. These molecules participate in airway remodeling and fibrosis.

4.8. Antigen Associated with HP

A large number of antigens have been implicated in HP (Patel et al., 2001; Kurup and Fink, 2002; Fink and Zacharisen, 2003). Microbial antigens, particularly fungi and actinomycetes, constitute a major proportion of all antigens (Table 12.3). The exposure to these antigens occurs in various occupations and results from both indoor and outdoor contamination with the antigens. The prevalence of the etiologic agents varies from country to country and depends on climatic and other factors. Farmer's lung, a disease predominantly seen among farmers, is caused by thermophilic actinomycetes and *Aspergillus* sp., while *Trichosporon cutaneum* and *Cryptococcus* species have been implicated in summer-type HP prevalent in southern part of Japan. Ventilation system induced HP is caused by thermophilic actinomycetes and several fungi. Humidifier and damp atmosphere induced HP are caused by *Aureobasidium*, *Chaetomium*, *Cephalosporium*, *Curvularia*, *Penicillium*, and *Rhodotorula*. There are a number of isolated reports of HP resulting numerous fungi and actinomycetes have appeared in the literature in the recent years.

5. Immunotherapy in Fungal Hypersensitivity

Specific immunotherapy and vaccination are the probable means for controlling the type I allergy. All the earlier studies concentrated mainly on the crude allergens as immunotherapeutic agents. As a result of a more clearer understanding of the pathogenesis of the disease, attempts have been directed to reverse the Th2 type of response to a Th0 or Th1 response. Several major directions have been taken in immunotherapy of IgE-mediated allergy, including peptide immunotherapy, immunotherapy using immunostimulatory sequences (ISS-ODN), and naked DNA vaccination (Kurup, 2003; 2004).

Allergen-specific therapy may aim for prophylaxis of atopy, induction of tolerance, or modification of ongoing immune responses (Hoyne et al., 1994; Svirshchevskaya et al., 2001). Although attempts have been made with different allergens to induce T cell nonresponsiveness in patients by selectively administering major T cell epitopes, no such studies have been carried out with any of the fungal allergens. We studied Asp f 2, a major *A. fumigatus* allergen and constructed a number of deletion and point mutants (Tang et al., 2000). Some of these mutated proteins, while showing T cell proliferation with patients' cells, failed to bind to IgE in the sera of patients and mice immunized with the allergen. These candidate allergens for immunotherapy need further evaluation (Hoyne et al., 1994; Banerjee et al., 2001).

While studying synthetic peptides representing sequences of Asp f 1, we identified two peptides, Peptide #5 and Peptide #10 showing cytokine specificity. Peptide #5 NGYDGNGKLIKGRTPI elicited a Th2 type of cytokine response and Peptide #10 KVFCGIVAHQRGN a Th1 type of cytokine response in immunized mice (Kurup et al., 1996). Intravenous immunization of mice with two other epitopes of Asp f 1 prevented them from elaborating the immune response on subsequent challenge with *A. fumigatus* antigens (Svirshchevskaya et al., 2001). The potential role for these synthetic peptides as immunotherapeutic agent in allergic aspergillosis needs further evaluation.

A number of studies have appeared emphasizing the usefulness of immunostimulatory CpG oligonucleotides (CpG-ODN) in vaccination against IgE-mediated allergy

(Banerjee et al., 2001). Immunization with DNA-based vaccines, such as plasmid DNA of major *A. fumigatus* antigens or allergen and ISS-ODN coadministered, result in reversing the Th2 response to a predominantly Th1 response. There was a marked shift to a Th1 type of response as evidenced by the threefold increase in specific serum IgG2a in ISS-ODN-treated BALB/c mice compared to mice treated with antigen alone. Blood eosinophil counts of ISS-treated group were significantly less compared to that of antigen-immunized group. Pulmonary histology revealed less eosinophilic infiltration in the perivascular and peribronchial regions of CpG-ODN-treated mice. Periodic acid Schiff (PAS) staining of lung sections also indicate enhanced mucus glycoconjugate production in mice without CpG compared to CpG-injected animals. These results suggest that the immune deviation induced by CpG motifs may alter the Th2 type allergic responses in *A. fumigatus*-sensitized mice and hence, may be a possible candidate for immunotherapy in allergic aspergillosis.

Immunotherapy for HP is neither available nor any attempt has been made in investigating the role in experimental models. The large number of antigens implicated in this immunologically complex disease may be a major factor and concern in the success of immunomodulatory therapies.

Acknowledgments

This study was supported by U.S. Veterans Administration Medical Research and Cystic Fibrosis Foundation. The editorial assistance of Donna Schrubbe is gratefully acknowledged.

References

Bacharier, L.B. and Geha, R.S. (2000). Molecular mechanisms of IgE regulation. *J. Allergy Clin. Immunol.* 105: S547–S558.

Banerjee, B., Greenberger, P.A., Fink, J.N., and Kurup, V.P. (1999). Conformational and linear B-cell epitopes of Asp f 2, a major allergen of *Aspergillus fumigatus*, bind differently to immunoglobulin E antibody in the sera of allergic bronchopulmonary aspergillosis patients. *Infect. Immun.* 67: 2284–2291.

Banerjee, B., Xia, J.Q., Rickaby, D.A., Henderson, J.D., Kelly, K.J., Fink, J.N., and Kurup, V.P. (2001). Modulation of airway inflammatory CpG oligodeoxynucleotide in a murine model of aspergillosis (abstract). *J. Allergy Clin. Immunol.* 107: S216.

Bischoff, S.C., Krieger, M., Brunner, T., and Dahinden, C.A. (1992). Monocyte chemoattractant proteins-1 is a potent activator of basophils. *J. Exp. Med.* 175: 1271–1275.

Blease, K., Jakubzick, C., Westwick, J., Lucas, N., Kunkel, S.L., and Hogaboam, C.M. (2001a). Therapeutic effect of IL-13 immunoneutralization during chronic experimental fungal asthma. *J. Immunol.* 166: 5219–5224.

Blease, K., Jakubzick, C., Schuh, J.M., Joshi, B.H., Puri, R.K., and Hogaboam, C.M. (2001b). IL-13 fusion cytotoxin ameliorates chronic fungal induced allergic airway disease in mice. *J. Immunol.* 167: 6583–6592.

Blease, K., Kunkel, S.L., and Hogaboam, C.M. (2001c). IL-18 modulates chronic fungal asthma in a murine model: Putative involvement of T cell-like receptor-2. *Inflamm. Res.* 50: 552–560.

Bourke, S.J., Dalphin, J.C., Boyd, G., McSharry, C., Baldwin, C.I., and Calvert, J.E. (2001). Hypersensitivity pneumonitis: Current concepts. *Eur. Respir. J.* 32: 81s–92s.

Brown, J.E., Greenberger, P.A., and Yarnold, P.R. (1995). Soluble serum interleukin-2 receptors in patients with asthma and allergic bronchopulmonary aspergillosis. *Ann. Allergy Asthma Immunol.* 74: 484–488.

Brummund, W., Resnick, A., Fink, J.N., and Kurup, V.P. (1987). *Aspergillus fumigatus*-specific antibodies in allergic bronchopulmonary aspergillosis and aspergilloma: Evidence for a polyclonal antibody response. *J. Clin. Microbiol.* 25: 5–9.

Burge, H.A. (1985). Fungus allergens. *Clin. Rev. Allergy* 3: 319–329.

Busse, W.W., O'Bryne, P.M., and Holgate, S.T. (2003). Asthma pathogenesis. In N.F. Adkinson Jr., J.W. Yunginger, W.W. Busse, B.S. Bochner, S.T. Holgate, and F.E.R. Simons (eds),

Middleton's Allergy Principles and Practice, Vol. 6. Mosby, Philadelphia, pp. 1175–1207.

Chakir, J., Shannon, J., Molet, S., Fukakusa, M., Elias, J., Laviolette, M., Boulet, L.P., and Hamid, Q. (2003). Airway remodeling-associated mediators in moderate to severe asthma: Effect of steroids on TGF-β, IL-11, IL-17 and type I and type III collagen expression. *J. Allergy Clin. Immunol.* 111: 1293–1298.

Chauhan, B.A., Knutsen, A.P., Hutcheson, P.S., Slavin, R.G., and Bellone, C.J. (1996). T cell subsets, epitope mapping, and HLA-restriction in patients with allergic bronchopulmonary aspergillosis. *J. Clin. Invest.* 97: 2324–2331.

Chauhan, B., Santiago, L., Kirschmann, D.A., Hauptfield, V., Knutsen, A.P., Hutcheson, P.S., Woulfe, S.L., Slavin, R.G., Schwartz, H.J., and Bellone, C.J. (1997). The association of HLA-DR alleles and T-cell activation with allergic bronchopulmonary aspergillosis. *J. Immunol.* 159: 4072–4076.

Chauhan, B., Santiago, L., Hutcheson, P.S., Schwartz, H.J., Spitznagel, E., Castro, M., Slavin, R.G., and Bellone, C.J. (2000). Evidence for the involvement of two different MHC class II regions in susceptibility or protection in allergic bronchopulmonary aspergillosis. *J. Allergy Clin. Immunol.* 106: 723–729.

Chouchakova, N., Skokowa, J., Baumann, U., Tschernig, T., Philippens, K.M., Nieswandt, B., Schmidt, R.E., and Gessner, J.E. (2001). Fc gamma RIII-mediated production of TNF-alpha induces immune complex alveolitis independently of CXC chemokines generation. *J. Immunol.* 166: 5193–5200.

Corry, D.B., Grunig, G., Hadeiba, H., Kurup, V.P., Warnock, M.L., Sheppard, D., Rennick, D.M., and Locksley, R.M. (1998). Requirements for allergen-induced airway hyperreactivity in T and B cell-deficient mice. *Mol. Med.* 4: 344–355.

Davies, D.E., Wicks, J., Powell, R.M., Puddicome, S.M., and Holgate, S.T. (2003). Airway remodeling in asthma: New insights. *J. Allergy Clin. Immunol.* 111: 215–225.

Davis, R.J., Wang, J.H., Trigg, C.J., and Devalia, J.L. (1995). Expression of GM-CSF, IL-8 and RANTES in the bronchial epithelium of mild asthmatics is down-regulated by inhaled beclomethasone dipropionate. *Int. Arch. Allergy Immunol.* 107: 428–429.

Diaz de la Vega, V., Bialostosky, D., Lupi, E., Castro, G., Barrios, R., and Reyes, P.A. (1980). Familial pigeon breeder's disease. Possible association with HLA-Bw40 antigen. *Rev. Invest. Clin.* 32: 401–407.

Fink, J.N. and Zacharisen, M.C. (2003). Hypersensitivity pneumonitis. In N.F. Adkinson Jr., J.W. Yunginger, W.W. Busse, B.S. Bochner, S.T. Holgate, and F.E.R. Simons (eds). Mosby, St. Louis, pp. 1373–1390.

Ford, J.G., Rennick, D., Donaldson, D.D., Venkayya, R., McArthur, C., Hansell, E., Kurup, V.P., Warnock, M., and Grunig, G. (2001). IL-13 and IFN-γ: Interactions in lung inflammation. *J. Immunol.* 167: 1769–1777.

Gravesen, S. (1999). Microfungal contamination of damp buildings: Biological aspects. In E. Johanning (ed.), *Bioaerosols, Fungi, and Mycotoxins*. Eastern New York Occupational and Environmental Health Center, New York, pp. 505–511.

Greenberger, P.A. (1988). Allergic bronchopulmonary aspergillosis. *Clin. Chest Med.* 1: 599–608.

Greenberger, P.A. (2003). Allergic bronchopulmonary aspergillosis. In N.F. Adkinson Jr., J.W. Yunginger, W.W. Busse, B.S. Bochner, S.T. Holgate, and F.E.R. Simons (eds), *Middleton's Allergy Principles and Practice*, Vol. 6. Mosby, Philadelphia, pp. 1353–1371.

Grunig, G., Corry, D.B., Leach, M.W., Seymour, B.W.P., Kurup, V.P., and Rennick, D.M. (1997). Interleukin-10 is a natural suppressor of cytokine production and inflammation in a murine model of allergic bronchopulmonary aspergillosis. *J. Exp. Med.* 185: 1089–1099.

Gudmundsson, G. and Hunninghake, G.W. (1997). Interferon-gamma is necessary for the expression of hypersensitivity pneumonitis. *J. Clin. Invest.* 99: 2386–2390.

Gudmundsson, G., Bosch, A., Davidson, B.L., Berg, D.J., and Hunninghake, G.W. (1998). Interleukin-10 modulates the severity of hypersensitivity pneumonitis in mice. *Am. J. Respir. Cell Mol. Biol.* 19: 812–818.

Hawksworth, D.L., Sutton, B.C., and Ainsworth, G.C. (1994). *Ainsworth & Bisby's Dictionary of the Fungi*. International Mycological Institute, University Press, Cambridge.

Hogaboam, C.M., Blease, K., Mehrad, B., Steinhauser, M.L., Standiford, T.J., Kunkel, S.L., and Lukacs, N.W. (2000). Chronic airway hyperreactivity, goblet cell hyperplasia, and peribronchial fibrosis during allergic airway disease induced by *Aspergillus fumigatus*. *Am. J. Pathol.* 156: 723–732.

Hogaboam, C.M., Blease, K., and Schuh, J.M. (2003). Cytokines and chemokines in allergic bronchopulmonary aspergillosis and experimental *Aspergillus*-induced allergic airway or asthmatic disease. *Front. Biosci.* 8: e147–156.

Hoyne, C.F., Callow, M.G., Kuo, M.C., and Thomas, W.R. (1994). Inhibition of T-cell responses by feeding peptides containing major and cryptic epitopes: Studies with Der p 1 allergen. *Immunology* 83: 190–195.

Isreal-Assayag, E., Fournier, M., and Cormier, Y. (1999). Blockade of T cell costimulation by CTLA4-Ig inhibits lung inflammation in murine hypersensitivity pneumonitis. *J. Immunol.* 163: 6794–6799.

Katzenstein, A.A., Sale, S.R., and Greenberger, P.A. (1983). Allergic *Aspergillus* sinusitis: A newly recognized form of sinusitis. *J. Allergy Clin. Immunol.* 72: 89–98.

Kauffman, H. ·(2003). Immunopathogenesis of allergic bronchopulmonary aspergillosis and airway remodeling. *Front. Biosci.* 8: e190–196.

Kauffman, H.F. and Tomee, J.F.C. (1998). Inflammatory cells and airway defense against *Aspergillus fumigatus*. In V.P. Kurup and A.J. Apter (eds) *Immunology and Allergy Clinics of North America*, Vol. 18. W.B. Saunders, Philadelphia, pp. 619–640.

Knutsen, A.P. (2003). Immunopathogenesis of allergic bronchopulmonary aspergillosis. *Front. Biosci.* 8: d589–602.

Knutsen, A.P., Mueller, K.R., Levine, A.D., Chauhan, B., Hutcheson, P., and Slavin, R.G. (1994). Characterization of Asp f 1 $CD4^+$ T cell lines in allergic bronchopulmonary aspergillosis. *J. Allergy Clin. Immunol.* 94: 215–221.

Knutsen, A.P., Chauhan, B., and Slavin, R.G. (1998). Cell-mediated immunity in allergic bronchopulmonary aspergillosis. *Immunol. Allergy Clin. North Am.* 18: 575–599.

Kobate, T., Jacquot, S., Kozlowski, S., Agematsu, K., Schlossman, S.F., and Morimoto, C. (1995). CD27–CD70 interaction regulate B-cell activation by T-cells. *Proc. Natl. Acad. Sci. USA* 92: 11249–11253.

Kozak, P.P. Jr., Gallup, J., Cummins, L.H., and Gilmman, S.A. (1979). Factors of importance in determining the prevalence of indoor molds. *Ann. Allergy* 43: 88–94.

Krishna, M.T., Salvi, S.S., and Holgate, S.T. (2001). Pathogenesis of asthma. In R.R. Rich, T.A. Fleisher, W.T. Shearer, B.L. Kotzin, and H.W. Schroeder Jr. (eds), *Clinical Immunology Principles and Practice*. Mosby, New York, pp. 49.1–49.12.

Kurup, V.P. (1989). Hypersensitivity pneumonitis due to sensitization with thermophilic actinomycetes. *Immunol. Allergy Clin. North Am.* 9: 285–306.

Kurup, V.P. (2000). Immunopathogenesis of fungal induced asthma and allergy. *Proceedings of International Symposium on Recent Advances in Molecular Biology, Allergy and Immunology*, pp. 81–94.

Kurup, V.P. (2003). Fungal allergens. *Curr. Allergy Asthma Rep.* 3: 416–423.

Kurup, V.P. (2004). Fungal Allergy. In D.K. Arora (ed.), *Fungal Biotechnology*, 2nd edition. Marcel Dekker, New York, pp. 515–525.

Kurup, V.P. and Apter, A.J. (eds) (1998). *Immunology and Allergy Clinics of North America*, Vol. 18. W.B. Saunders, Philadelphia.

Kurup, V.P. and Fink, J.N. (1993). Fungal allergy. In J.W. Murphy,, H. Friedman, and M. Bendinelli (eds), *Fungal Infections and Immune Responses*. Plenum Press, New York, pp. 393–404.

Kurup, V.P. and Fink, J.N. (2002). Immunological tests for evaluation of hypersensitivity pneumonitis and allergic bronchopulmonary aspergillosis. In N.R. Rose, R.G. Hamilton, and B. Detrick (eds), *Manual of Clinical Laboratory Immunology*. ASM Press, Washington, DC, pp. 910–918.

Kurup, V.P. and Grunig, G. (2001). Animal models of allergic bronchopulmonary aspergillosis. *Mycopathologia* 153: 165–177.

Kurup, V.P., Nair, M.P.N., Schwartz, S.A., and Fink, J.N. (1985). Serum antibodies and their role in antibody-dependent cell-mediated cytotoxicity in aspergillosis. *Immunobiology* 169: 362–371.

Kurup, V.P., Mauze, S., Choi, H., Seymour, B.W.P., and Coffman, R.L. (1992). A murine model of allergic bronchopulmonary aspergillosis with elevated eosinophils and IgE. *J. Immunol.* 148: 3783–3788.

Kurup, V.P., Hari, V., Guo, J., Murali, P.S., Resnick, A., Krishnan, M., and Fink, J.N. (1996). *Aspergillus fumigatus* peptides differentially express Th1 and Th2 cytokines. *Peptides* 17: 183–190.

Kurup, V.P., Murali, P.S., Guo, J., Choi, H., Banerjee, B., Fink, J.N., and Coffman, R.L. (1997). Anti-IL-4 and IL-5 antibodies downregulate IgE and eosinophilia in mice exposed to *Aspergillus* antigens. *Allergy* 52: 1215–1221.

Kurup, V.P., Banerjee, B., Murali, P.S., Greenberger, P.A., Krishnan, M., Hari, V., and Fink, J.N. (1998a). Immunodominant peptide epitopes of allergen, Asp f 1 from the fungus *Aspergillus fumigatus*. *Peptides* 19: 1469–1477.

Kurup, V.P., Grunig, G., Knutsen, A.P., and Murali, P.S. (1998b). Cytokines in allergic bronchopulmonary aspergillosis. *73rd Forum in Immunology* 466–477.

Kurup, V.P., Choi, H.Y., Murali, P.S., Xia, J.Q., Coffman, R.L., and Fink, J.N. (1999). Immune responses to *Aspergillus* antigen in IL-4 –/– mice and the effect of eosinophil ablation. *Allergy* 54: 420–427.

Kurup, V.P., Banerjee, B., Hemmann, S., Greenberger, P.A., Blaser, K., and Crameri, R. (2000a). Selected recombinant *Aspergillus fumigatus* allergens bind specifically to IgE in ABPA. *Clin. Exp. Allergy* 30: 988–993.

Kurup, V.P., Shen, H.D., and Banerjee, B. (2000b). Respiratory fungal allergy. *Microbes Infect.* 2: 1101–1110.

Kurup, V.P., Shen, H.D., and Vijay, H. (2002). Immunobiology of fungal allergens. *Int. Arch. Allergy Immunol.* 129: 181–188.

Mathur, M., Herrmann, K., Qin, Y., Gulmen, F., Li, X., Krimins, R., Weinstock, J., Elliot, D., Bluestone, J.A., and Padrid, P. (1999). CD28 interaction with either CD80 or CD86 are sufficient to induce allergic airway inflammation in mice. *Am. J. Respir. Cell Mol. Biol.* 21: 498–509.

Mehlhop, P.D., van de Rijn, M., Goldberg, A.B., Brewer, J.P., Kurup, V.P., Martin, T.R., and Oettgen, H.C. (1997). Allergen-induced bronchial hyperreactivity and eosinophilic inflammation occur in the absence of IgE in a mouse model of asthma. *Proc. Natl. Acad. Sci. USA* 94: 1344–1349.

Menzies-Gow, A., Flood-Page, P., Sehmi, R., Burman, J., Hamid, Q., Robinson, D.S., Kay, A.B., and Denbury, J. (2003). Anti-IL-5 (mepolizumab) therapy induces bone marrow eosinophil maturational arrest and decreases eosinophil progenitors in the bronchial mucosa of atopic asthmatics. *J. Allergy Clin. Immunol.* 111: 714–719.

Nelms, K., Keegan, A.D., Zamorano, J., Ryan, J.J., and Paul, W.E. (1999). The IL-4 receptor: Signaling mechanisms and biologic functions. *Ann. Rev. Immunol.* 17: 701–738.

Patel, A.M., Ryu, J.H., and Reed, C.E. (2001). Hypersensitivity pneumonitis: Current concepts and future questions. *J. Allergy Clin. Immunol.* 108: 661–670.

Rathore, V.B., Johnson, B., Fink, J.N., Kelly, K.J., Greenberger, P.A., and Kurup, V.P. (2001). T cell proliferation and cytokine secretion to T cell epitopes of Asp f 2 in ABPA patients. *Clin. Immunol.* 100: 228–235.

Richter, A., Puddicome, S.M., Lordan, J.L., Bucchieri, F., Wilson, S.J., Djukanovic, R., Dent, G., Holgate, S.T., and Davies, D.E. (2001). The contribution of IL-4 and IL-13 to the epithelial-mesenchymal trophic unit in asthma. *Am. J. Respir. Cell Mol. Biol.* 25: 385–391.

Rothenberg, M.E. (ed.) (2000). *Chemokines in Allergic Diseases*. Marcel Dekker, New York.

Schuyler, M., Gott, K., and Cherne, A. (2002). Is IL-12 necessary in experimental hypersensitivity pneumonitis? *Int. J. Exp. Pathol.* 83: 87–98.

Semenzato, G., Adami, F., Maschio, N., and Agostini, C. (2000). Immune mechanisms in interstitial lung diseases. *Allergy* 55: 1103–1120.

Sousa, A.R., Lane, S.J., Nakhosteen, J.A., Yoshimura, T., Lee, T.H., and Poston, R.N. (1994). Increased expression of the monocyte chemoattractant protein-1 in bronchial tissue from asthmatic subjects. *Am. J. Respir. Cell Mol. Biol.* 10: 142–147.

Suga, M., Yamasaki, H., Nakagawa, K., Kohrogi, H., and Ando, M. (1997). Mechanisms accounting for granulomatous responses in hypersensitivity pneumonitis. *Sarcoidosis Vasc. Diffuse Lung Dis.* 14: 131–138.

Svirshchevskaya, E.V., Alekessva, L.G., Andronova, T.M., and Kurup, V.P. (2001). Do T helpers 1 and 2 recognize different class II MHC molecules? Humoral and cellular immune responses to soluble allergen from *Aspergillus fumigatus* Asp f 2. *Clin. Immunol.* 100: 349–354.

Tang, B., Banerjee, B., Greenberger, P.A., Fink, J.N., Kelly, K.J., and Kurup, V.P. (2000). Antibody binding of deletion mutants of Asp f 2, the major *Aspergillus fumigatus* allergen. *Biochem. Biophys. Res. Comm.* 270: 1128–1135.

Tomee, J.F., Wierenga, A.T.J., Hiemstra, P.S., and Kauffman, H.F. (1997). *Aspergillus fumigatus* induce release of proinflammatory cytokines and cell detachment in airway epithelial lines. *J. Infect. Dis.* 176: 300–303.

Tsitoura, D.C., Verhoef, A., Gelder, C.M., O'Hehir, R.E., and Lamb, J.R. (1996). Altered T cell ligands derived from a major house dust mite allergen enhance IFN-γ but not IL-4 production by human CD4+ T cells. *J. Immunol.* 157: 2160–2165.

Vijay, H., Thaker, A.J., Banerjee, B., and Kurup, V.P. (1998). Mold allergens. In R.F. Lockey and S.C. Bukantz (eds), *Allergens and Allergen Immunotherapy*. Marcel Dekker, New York, pp. 133–154.

Wuethrich, B. (1989). Epidemiology of allergic diseases. Are they really on the increase. *Int. Arch. Allergy Appl. Immunol.* 90: 3–10.

Yamasaki, H., Ando, M., Brazer, W., Center, D.M., and Cruikshank, W.W. (1999). Polarized type 1 cytokine profile in bronchoalveolar lavage T cells of patients with hypersensitivity pneumonitis. *J. Immunol.* 163: 3516–3523.

Zhang, K., Clark, E.A., and Saxon, A. (1991). Stimulation provides an IFN-γ independent and IL-4 dependent differentiation signal directly to human B cells for IgE production. *J. Immunol.* 146: 1836–1842.

Zhang, S., Smartt, H., Holgate, S.T., and Roche, W.R. (1999). Growth factors secreted by bronchial epithelial cells control myofibroblast proliferation: An *in vitro* co-culture model of airway remodeling in asthma. *Lab. Invest.* 79: 395–405.

13

Immunology of Pulmonary *Pneumocystis* Infection: Cell-Mediated Immunity

Judd E. Shellito and James M. Beck

Division of Pulmonary and Critical Care Medicine, Louisiana State Health Sciences Center, New Orleans, LA.
Division of Pulmonary and Critical Care Medicine, University of Michigan Medical School and Department of Veterans Affairs Medical Center, Ann Arbor, MI.

1. Introduction

For many years, pulmonary infection with *Pneumocystis* was an uncommon complication of cytotoxic chemotherapy or severe malnutrition (Gajdusek, 1957; Walzer et al., 1974). However, large outbreaks of *Pneumocystis* pneumonia during the 1980s heralded the beginning of the HIV epidemic and brought *Pneumocystis* to the forefront of medical attention (Masur et al., 1981). For many physicians, *Pneumocystis* pneumonia was (and is) the prototypic manifestation of HIV infection and a hallmark of defective cell-mediated immunity (CMI). Although the incidence of *Pneumocystis* pneumonia has fallen dramatically with the advent of antiretroviral therapy and antimicrobial prophylaxis, *Pneumocystis* pneumonia is still a common AIDS-defining pulmonary illness and remains a routine clinical problem.

CMI is obviously critical to host defense against this pathogen because, in HIV infection, the risk of developing *Pneumocystis* pneumonia can be directly correlated with the numbers of circulating $CD4^+$ T cells (Masur et al., 1981). The greatest risk for subsequent *Pneumocystis* pneumonia is seen at advanced stages of HIV infection, usually when the blood $CD4^+$ T cell count falls below 200/μl. However, the precise mechanisms of cell-mediated and humoral immunity directed against this pathogen are subjects of ongoing investigation. This chapter will consider cell-mediated immune mechanisms that serve to protect the normal host from infection with *Pneumocystis* or, when defective, lead to the acquisition of pulmonary infection.

2. Taxonomy and Transmission

Pneumocystis was traditionally classified as a protozoan, but data for ribosomal RNA sequences more accurately place the organism with the fungi (Edman et al., 1988; Stringer et al., 1989). Genetic studies also show considerable divergence in gene sequence and chromosomes between *Pneumocystis* organisms derived from different animal and human hosts, demonstrating that there are multiple *Pneumocystis* species (Cushion, 1998). These investigations have prompted changes in taxonomy such that the original nomenclature, *Pneumocystis carinii*, is now reserved for organisms that infect the rat. The newer nomenclature, *Pneumocystis jiroveci*, has been adopted for organisms that infect humans (Stringer et al., 2002). In this chapter, the term *Pneumocystis* will be used to indicate all species of the microorganism, unless otherwise specified.

Pneumocystis cannot be reliably cultured in vitro, which has hampered microbiologic research with the pathogen. In clinical and research specimens, two forms of *Pneumocystis* can be identified: the cystic form and the more numerous trophozoite form. Morphologic studies suggest that trophozoite forms mature into cystic forms, but knowledge about the life cycle of *Pneumocystis* is incomplete (Cushion et al., 1991). Electron microscopic studies have shown that *Pneumocystis* has a simple structure with a nucleus, poorly preserved mitochondria, and absent or minimal lysosomes and Golgi apparatus (Bedrossian, 1989).

The ecology and mode of transmission of *Pneumocystis* organisms are also poorly understood. *Pneumocystis* infection is found worldwide in humans and in a variety of mammalian hosts, including rodents, ferrets, rabbits, horses, dogs, and cats (Hughes, 1987). Serologic data suggest that the majority of humans are exposed to the microorganism in childhood (Meuwissen et al., 1977; Pifer et al., 1978; Peglow et al., 1990). However, animal to human transmission of infection has never been demonstrated, and *Pneumocystis* derived from one animal species does not produce infection in another species. Thus, each species of *Pneumocystis* is uniquely adapted to its host.

An environmental reservoir of *Pneumocystis* has not been found, although *Pneumocystis* DNA has been isolated from air samples (Wakefield, 1996).

Most recent investigations suggest that the reservoir of *Pneumocystis* for human infection it is likely to be humans themselves. Attempts to find latent organisms in lung tissue from immunocompetent humans have been generally unsuccessful (Settnes and Genner, 1986; Peters et al., 1992), suggesting that clinical infection is not due to reactivation of latent infection, as with tuberculosis. Moreover, outbreaks of *Pneumocystis* pneumonia among immunocompromised humans support transmission of infection by inhalation (Singer et al., 1975; Chusid and Heyrman, 1978), and a considerable body of animal work supports the idea of airborne transmission of infection among immunocompromised animals (Morris et al., 2002). The relatively small number of HIV-infected or otherwise immunosuppressed patients in the human population has never seemed adequate to explain the almost universal exposure to the organism demonstrated by the serologic data. The answer to this conundrum may involve colonization of the airways/lung tissue of newborns and adults with a very short transit time. Important animal experiments demonstrate that *Pneumocystis* can be transmitted from immunosuppressed animals with pneumonia to normal animals that do not develop infection (Dumoulin et al., 2000). These normal animals can then transmit infection by the airborne route to immunosuppressed animals. This finding suggests that normal hosts without clinical infection might serve as a temporary vector to transmit the organism to susceptible hosts. Additional recent information demonstrates that normal mice, which had not been exposed to *Pneumocystis*, can carry the organism in the respiratory tract and transmit it to other animals (Gigliotti et al., 2003). However, once an immune response developed to *Pneumocystis*, this ability to carry and transmit the organisms was lost. To extend these observations to humans, one can speculate that newborns might be a reservoir for *Pneumocystis*, and that prior to the development of a fully formed immune response, they could transmit the organisms to adults who could then also carry the organisms in their airways for a limited period of time. Clinical disease would then follow when an immunosuppressed individual came into contact with an infant or adult during the limited time that they were carrying organisms in the airways. This idea obviously requires confirmation in humans, but it begins to explain how *Pneumocystis* might persist and be transmitted within the human population.

3. Histopathology

Under the microscope, the histology of *Pneumocystis* pneumonia is that of an alveolar filling process, with little surrounding inflammation that occurs in a patchy distribution. A foamy, eosinophilic exudate fills and expands alveoli accompanied by minimal interstitial infiltration of lymphocytes and proliferation of type II pneumocytes (Watts and Chandler, 1991). At higher magnification using conventional tissue stains, small nuclei of trophozoite forms are visible within the intra-alveolar exudate. Special stains, such as Gomori methenamine silver or toluidine blue, identify the cyst forms of *Pneumocystis*, which are in the shapes of helmets, crescents, or punched-in beach balls. Under the electron microscope, the alveolar exudate is composed of clumps of cystic forms and trophozoite forms in a matrix of cellular debris and fibrin (Huang and Marshall, 1970). Electron microscopy shows that the trophozoite forms of *Pneumocystis* bind tightly to alveolar epithelial cells, but there is no evidence for internalization by epithelial cells (Vavra and Kucera, 1970). Alveolar macrophages ingest *Pneumocystis* organisms, and the role of alveolar macrophages in defense against this pathogen is considered in detail in the following section.

4. Alveolar Macrophages in CMI

Alveolar macrophages are the resident phagocytic cells within lung tissue and are critical to an initial inflammatory response to an inhaled pathogen (Green and Kass, 1964). In animal models of *Pneumocystis* infection, resolution of infection is associated with increased numbers of alveolar macrophages in lung tissue and with microscopic evidence of ingested organisms (Fig. 13.1). This finding has been observed in both the steroid-treated rat model (Barton and Campbell, 1969) and the CD4-depleted mouse model of infection (Shellito et al., 1990). Although numerous investigations have shown that alveolar macrophages can internalize and kill *Pneumocystis* in vitro, the relative importance of this cellular function in host defense against infection compared to other immune effector mechanisms remains uncertain.

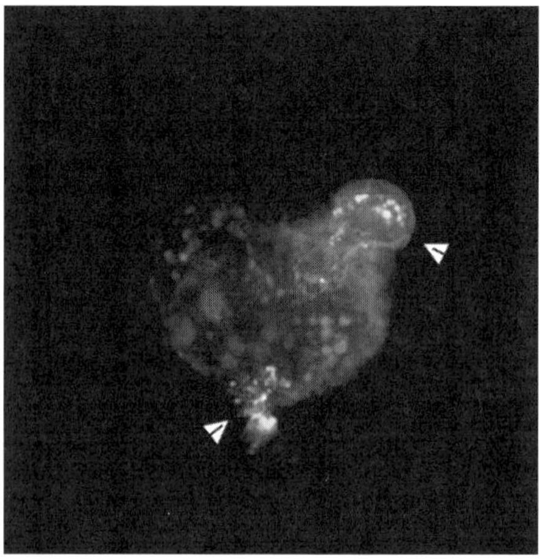

Figure 13.1. Phagocytosis of *Pneumocystis* by a murine alveolar macrophage (deconvolution microscopy, 630×). The DNA-specific dye 4′,6-diamidino-2-phenylindole dihydrochloride (DAPI) was used to stain both alveolar nuclei and fungal DNA. The green indicates surface labeling of both cyst and trophozoite (arrowheads) forms of *Pneumocystis* with fluorescein isothiocyanate (FITC). F-actin filaments within the alveolar cytoskeleton were counterstained with Phalloidin Alexa 568. Copied with permission from Steele, C., Marrero, L., Swain, S., Harmsen, A. G., Zheng, M., Brown, G. D., Gordon, S., Shellito, J. E., and Kolls, J. K. (2003). Alveolar macrophage-mediated killing of *Pneumocystis carinii f. sp. muris* involves molecular recognition by the Dectin-1 beta-glucan receptor. *J. Exp. Med.* 198: 1677–1688.

4.1. Alveolar Macrophage Receptors

Alveolar macrophages are richly endowed with surface receptors that are candidate molecules to facilitate the attachment and internalization of *Pneumocystis* organisms. Early experimental observations demonstrated that phagocytosis of *Pneumocystis* by alveolar macrophages is mediated by Fc immunoglobulin receptors. In these experiments, rat alveolar macrophages cultured with *Pneumocystis* in the absence of serum or with the addition of nonimmune serum show little binding or phagocytosis (Masur and Jones, 1978). However, the addition of rabbit anti-*Pneumocystis* serum to the culture medium markedly enhances attachment and phagocytosis. This response is rapid, with complete ingestion occurring within 20 min. These results are also supported by later experiments (Taylor et al., 1992), showing that rat peritoneal macrophage phagocytosis of *Pneumocystis* was significantly enhanced in a dose-dependent manner with the addition of immune serum.

Considerably more evidence supports interaction of *Pneumocystis* with alveolar macrophage mannose receptors. The major surface glycoprotein of *Pneumocystis* contains mannose residues that interact with macrophage mannose receptors (O'Riordan et al., 1995). Ezekowitz et al. (1991) found that the addition of competitive mannose receptor inhibitors to cultures of human alveolar macrophages almost completely blocks binding of rat *Pneumocystis* organisms. Furthermore, transfection of COS-1 cells that cannot bind *Pneumocystis* with the cDNA for the human mannose receptor endows the cells with the capability to bind and phagocytose the organisms. The importance of these in vitro data have recently been called into question by experiments performed in mannose receptor knockout mice. Surprisingly, mannose receptor-deficient mice clear experimental *Pneumocystis* infection normally and do not show more severe infection during $CD4^+$ T cell depletion (Swain et al., 2003). These observations suggest that additional macrophage receptors are likely to be important in host defense against this pathogen.

β-Glucans comprise a group of glucopyranosyl polymers that are major constituents of fungal cell walls including *Pneumocystis* (De Stefano et al., 1990). Incubation of alveolar macrophages with purified β-glucans from *Pneumocystis* stimulates the release of the proinflammatory cytokine tumor necrosis factor (TNF) (Vassallo et al., 1999). Furthermore, instillation of *Pneumocystis* β-glucan into the lungs of rats stimulates local release of TNF and the chemokine macrophage inflammatory protein-2 (MIP-2) as well as recruitment of neutrophils into the lungs (Vassallo et al., 2000a). These results suggest that alveolar macrophages must have β-glucan receptors on their surface to interact with *Pneumocystis*. Recent work indicates that this receptor is Dectin-1 (Steele et al., 2003). Dectin-1 is a 28 kDa type II transmembrane receptor that has been shown to be important in macrophage binding to the yeast, zymosan (Brown et al., 2001). Dectin-1 on the surface of murine alveolar macrophages colocalizes with adherent *Pneumocystis* organisms, and blockage of Dectin-1 with high concentrations of anti-Dectin-1 antibody inhibits binding and concomitant killing of *Pneumocystis* by alveolar macrophages (Steele et al., 2003).

In addition to receptors that mediate phagocytosis, *Pneumocystis* also binds to receptors on the alveolar macrophage surface that do not appear to initiate internalization or phagocytosis, such as the fibronectin receptor. Binding of *Pneumocystis* to rat alveolar macrophages is inhibited by an antifibronectin antibody or by the addition of the Arg-Gly-Asp-Ser (RGDS) peptide (Pottratz and Martin, 1990). Interestingly, fibronectin binding of *Pneumocystis* in these experiments does not result in phagocytosis. These investigators postulate that fibronectin might serve as a bridge between *Pneumocystis* receptors and receptors on the alveolar macrophage or alveolar epithelial cells. Whether binding to the macrophage surface via fibronectin is helpful or harmful to the organism remains an unanswered question.

Binding without phagocytosis may also occur via receptors for surfactant proteins. The major surface glycoprotein of *Pneumocystis* binds to surfactant protein A (McCormack et al., 1997). This binding has been shown to enhance the adherence of the organisms to alveolar macrophages (Williams et al., 1996). However, addition of exogenous surfactant protein A to cultures of alveolar macrophages and *Pneumocystis* actually inhibits phagocytosis (Koziel et al., 1998). This finding suggests that *Pneumocystis* binding to surfactant protein A, a substance highly concentrated in the alveolar space, may serve to shield the organism from host immune effector mechanisms. It is also of note that surfactant protein A concentrations are increased above control levels in lung tissue from HIV-infected patients with *Pneumocystis* pneumonia (Sternberg et al., 1995). Furthermore, surfactant protein D also increases adherence of *Pneumocystis* to alveolar macrophages without stimulating phagocytosis (O'Riordan et al., 1995; Yong et al., 2003).

4.2. Alveolar Macrophage Killing of *Pneumocystis*

Whether alveolar macrophages are necessary and sufficient for killing of *Pneumocystis* in vivo remains a controversial topic. Short-term (72 h) depletion of alveolar macrophages with liposomal dichloromethylene diphosphonate results in impaired clearance of *Pneumocystis* (Limper et al., 1997). Unfortunately, this technique is not amenable to long-term macrophage depletion, so these results cannot be extrapolated to chronic infection that might be more relevant to human disease. Once internalized, however, *Pneumocystis* stimulates reactive oxygen intermediates as measured by production of hydrogen peroxide (Hidalgo et al., 1992). The role of reactive nitrogen intermediates and nitric oxide in macrophage killing of *Pneumocystis* is unclear. In vitro experiments with rat alveolar macrophages show that exposure to interferon-gamma (IFN-γ) stimulates nitric oxide production and killing of *Pneumocystis* (Downing et al., 1999). However, other investigators were unable to correlate upregulation in alveolar macrophages of nitric oxide synthase, the producer of nitric oxide, with the host response in vivo, either in normal or CD4-depleted mice (Shellito et al., 1996). Thus, the role of nitric oxide compared to reactive oxygen species in alveolar macrophage phagocytosis and killing of *Pneumocystis* in vivo remains unclear.

4.3. Impact of HIV Infection on Alveolar Macrophage Function

HIV infects primarily CD4$^+$ T cells and, as a result, induces profound defects in CMI. However, HIV can also infect macrophages that bear CD4 on their surface, and this includes alveolar macrophages. HIV may infect lung cells either as free virion entering from the blood or through infected lymphocytes or monocytes that are recruited into lung tissue (Agostini et al., 1993). Rather than being killed by HIV, macrophages, including alveolar macrophages (Lebargy et al., 1994), carry the virus in a latent or nonreplicating form with viral replication then initiated upon exposure to a variety of cytokine stimuli. It has been shown that 12% to 58% of alveolar macrophages collected from bronchoalveolar lavages of patients with AIDS express viral antigens (Plata et al., 1987; Autran et al., 1988), but the percentage of alveolar macrophages expressing HIV RNA is very low (Chayt et al., 1986). The viral load in alveolar macrophages is probably similar to that of other tissue macrophage populations in an HIV-infected host (Lewin et al., 1998).

Alveolar macrophages recovered from HIV-infected individuals have altered immunologic functions, but it is unclear how much of this is the result of direct infection with HIV as opposed to exposure to local stimulatory/suppressive signals or altered cellular maturity within the alveolar macrophage population. Macrophages infected with HIV in vitro or exposed to HIV-encoded proteins release a variety of proinflammatory cytokines including TNF, interleukin-1 (IL-1), IL-6, IFN-α, and chemokines, many of which can enhance viral replication (Herbein et al., 2002). Alveolar macrophages lavaged from HIV-infected patients with *Pneumocystis* pneumonia show decreased mannose receptor expression and decreased binding of *Pneumocystis* in vitro in comparison to alveolar macrophages from HIV-infected persons without infection (Koziel et al., 1998). This downregulation of mannose receptors and decreased binding and phagocytosis of *Pneumocystis* can be duplicated in vitro by infecting normal alveolar macrophages with

HIV (Koziel et al., 1998). When alveolar macrophages from patients with *Pneumocystis* infection complicating HIV are compared to the same cells from infected patients with other forms of immunosuppression, alveolar macrophages from the HIV-infected individuals demonstrate less microscopic phagocytosis of *Pneumocystis* organisms (Wehle et al., 1993). Finally, alveolar macrophages from HIV-infected individuals have a decreased oxidative burst response to *Pneumocystis* that correlates directly with severity of HIV infection (Koziel et al., 2000). This macrophage defect is linked to mannose receptor expression and is specific for *Pneumocystis*, in that responses to phorbol myristic acetate and opsonized zymosan are maintained in alveolar macrophages from HIV-infected individuals.

5. CD4$^+$ T Cells in Cell-Mediated Defense

As discussed in the introduction, depletion of CD4$^+$ T cells is a hallmark of HIV infection, and progressive depletion of CD4$^+$ T cells during HIV infection correlates with the risk of developing *Pneumocystis* pneumonia (Phair et al., 1990). Whether the extent of CD4$^+$ T cell depletion correlates with the severity or outcome of *Pneumocystis* pneumonia remains controversial. Reported discrepancies between numbers of peripheral blood CD4$^+$ T cells and numbers of CD4$^+$ T cells in the lung available for defense against *Pneumocystis* further complicate this evaluation. In one such study, numbers of peripheral CD4$^+$ T cells did not predict outcome in AIDS patients with *Pneumocystis* pneumonia, but low numbers of CD4$^+$ T cells in bronchoalveolar lavages did indicate poor prognoses (Agostini et al., 1997). If depletion of CD4$^+$ T cells is the main risk factor for development of *Pneumocystis* pneumonia, it is reasonable to postulate that immunologic reconstitution should decrease the risk of pneumonia. Indeed, the advent of highly active antiretroviral therapy has decreased the incidence of pulmonary infections in HIV-infected individuals dramatically (Kaplan et al., 2000) and successful immune reconstitution significantly decreases the incidence of *Pneumocystis* pneumonia (Yangco et al., 2000).

Despite the convincing association between numbers of CD4$^+$ T cells and risk of *Pneumocystis* infection, the mechanisms by which CD4$^+$ T cells enable elimination of *Pneumocystis* by the host require further study (Vassallo et al., 2000b). As discussed above, exposure in early life to this ubiquitous organism results in antibody formation in the majority of humans (Pifer et al., 1978). The development of CMI in immunocompetent hosts is less well studied. T cells from immunocompetent adults proliferate in response to *Pneumocystis* antigen in vitro, but T cells from the cord blood of neonates do not respond (Herrod et al., 1981). These findings demonstrate that CMI to *Pneumocystis* is likely to be acquired during childhood, as is humoral immunity. Much experimental evidence demonstrates that loss of CMI directed against *Pneumocystis* as HIV infection progresses. For example, peripheral blood mononuclear cells from HIV-infected individuals demonstrate decreased proliferation in response to *Pneumocystis*, in comparison to cells from uninfected individuals (Hagler et al., 1988). The lack of response in cells from HIV-infected individuals is not specific to *Pneumocystis*, because decreased proliferation also occurs in response to antigens such as tetanus toxoid. Additional work demonstrates that proliferative responses of human peripheral blood mononuclear cells to *Pneumocystis* correlates directly with numbers of peripheral CD4$^+$ T cells in HIV-infected individuals (Forte et al., 1992) Therefore, lack of response to *Pneumocystis* probably involves both qualitative and quantitative defects in T cell proliferation.

Because of the inherent difficulties in using human cells to test hypotheses about

$CD4^+$ T cells and their function, much of the recent information about the role of $CD4^+$ T cells have been obtained from animal models (Beck and Harmsen, 1998). Early studies of the host immune response to *Pneumocystis* were performed in rats (Frenkel et al., 1966) and other laboratory animals (Walzer et al., 1979; Stokes et al., 1987) chronically treated with corticosteroids to render them susceptible to infection. These models showed association between the depletion of T cells caused by corticosteroids and susceptibility to *Pneumocystis* pneumonia, as well as improved defense against *Pneumocystis* when corticosteroid administration was discontinued (Walzer and Rutledge, 1981, 1982; Walzer et al., 1984). Furthermore, these studies prepared the field for mouse models by documenting that *Pneumocystis* pneumonia in corticosteroid-immunosuppressed rats resulted in decreased percentages of T helper cells and increased percentages of T suppressor cells in the lung. The diverse effects of corticosteroids on immunity made it difficult to isolate the effects of individual immune effector mechanisms, and led to the development of immunosuppressed mouse models of infection.

Outbreaks of *Pneumocystis* occur sporadically in colonies of athymic mice (which lack T cells) and *scid* mice (which lack T and B cells), indicating that T cell deficiency renders mice susceptible to *Pneumocystis* (Walzer et al., 1989). The use of monoclonal antibodies directed against CD4, which deplete $CD4^+$ T cells in vivo, demonstrates that depletion of $CD4^+$ T cells allows infection, while repopulation with $CD4^+$ T cells clears infection (Harmsen and Stankiewicz, 1990; Shellito et al., 1990). In these models, direct inoculation of mouse-derived *Pneumocystis* is often used to introduce infection at a known time and with known virulence. Similar results have been obtained in rats, demonstrating that both depleting and blocking antibodies directed against CD4 render rats susceptible to *Pneumocystis* infection (Thullen et al., 2003). However, CD4-depleted mice are also susceptible to environmental acquisition of infection.

Scid mice have been used extensively to investigate the roles of $CD4^+$ T cells in defense against *Pneumocystis* (Harmsen and Stankiewicz, 1990; Roths et al., 1990; Beck et al., 1996a). An attractive aspect of these models is the ability to reconstitute *scid* mice with donor T cells. Reconstitution of *scid* mice with $CD4^+$ T cells clears infection (Roths and Sidman, 1992), but depletion of $CD4^+$ T cells from the reconstituting T cells abrogates this effect (Harmsen and Stankiewicz, 1990). It appears that cellular reconstitution completely clears the infection without evidence of latency (Chen et al., 1993a), even during subsequent depletion of $CD4^+$ T cells. Furthermore, $CD4^+$ T cell knockout mice are susceptible to *Pneumocystis* (Hanano et al., 1996; Hanano and Kaufmann, 1998, 1999). Mice lacking conventional $CD4^+$ T cells (H-2I-1β knockout), T cell receptor αβ cells (TCRβ knockout), and all peripheral T and B cells (RAG-1 knockout) are all exquisitely susceptible to *Pneumocystis*.

Many experimental manipulations that result in loss of $CD4^+$ T cell number or function render mice susceptible to infection. For example, ethanol may have a permissive effect by inducing $CD4^+$ T cell dysfunction. Ethanol-fed mice develop *Pneumocystis* infections of low intensity (D'Souza et al., 1995). These investigators subsequently demonstrated that chronic ethanol administration decreases recruitment of $CD4^+$ and $CD8^+$ T cells to the lung, and depletes numbers of splenic lymphocytes (Shellito and Olariu, 1998).

The specific *Pneumocystis* epitopes recognized by $CD4^+$ T cells have not been characterized conclusively in humans, rats, or mice (Garvy, 1998). To determine whether T cells recognize and respond to *Pneumocystis* in a specific manner, most attention has focused on the major surface glycoprotein of

Pneumocystis as a stimulating antigen. T cells from mice immunized with *Pneumocystis* proliferate in response to purified major surface glycoprotein in vitro (Fisher et al., 1991). These specific proliferative responses occur in cells from mice immunized with *Pneumocystis* or with purified major surface glycoprotein, and also occur in cells from reconstituted *scid* mice that had cleared the infection. In rats, proliferation of splenic T cells occurs in response to major surface glycoprotein, but only in T cells obtained from rats previously exposed to *Pneumocystis* (Theus et al., 1993). Further work demonstrates that these specific T cell responses could also be elicited after immunization with a recombinant 55 kDa *Pneumocystis* antigen (Theus et al., 1994). Adoptive transfer experiments have been used to extend these observations in vivo. In vivo, T cells sensitized to the major surface glycoprotein confer resistance to *Pneumocystis* when transferred into corticosteroid-immunosuppressed rats (Theus et al., 1995).

Relatively little is known about the mechanisms of antigen presentation to $CD4^+$ T cells during host defense against *Pneumocystis*. Mice lacking MHC II (H-2I-Aβ knockout mice), which have no conventional $CD4^+$ T cells, are susceptible to *Pneumocystis* (Hanano et al., 1996, 1998). In contrast, mice lacking MHC I (β_2-microglobulin knockout mice), which have no conventional $CD8^+$ T cells are resistant to environmental acquisition (Hanano et al., 1996). In interpreting these data, however, it is difficult to evaluate whether the absence of major histocompatibility complex (MHC) molecules, or the absence of the T cell subsets, confers susceptibility or resistance.

Recent experiments demonstrate a role for antigen presentation in the lung during defense against *Pneumocystis*. Neonatal mice clear *Pneumocystis* more slowly, and manifest less lung inflammation than adult mice. When reconstituted with splenocytes from adult mice, neonatal *scid* mice clear *Pneumocystis* much more slowly than adult *scid* mice (Garvy and Qureshi, 2000). One possible mechanism for this difference is that antigen presentation capabilities are not fully developed in neonatal lungs. Indeed, neonatal lungs contain fewer dendritic cells and Ia^+ ($MHC\ II^+$) cells than adult lungs. When reconstituted with splenocytes from neonatal mice, neonatal and adult mice clear *Pneumocystis* equivalently (Qureshi and Garvy, 2001). These experiments suggest that the immunologic competence of the lung environment, rather than the competence of the transferred splenocytes, determines the outcome of infection. Efficient antigen presentation and clonal proliferation also depends on expression of appropriate surface molecules by the antigen-presenting cell and the responding cell. In fact, recent work demonstrates that mice lacking the T cell costimulatory molecules CD2 and CD28 are susceptible to *Pneumocystis*, despite normal numbers of circulating T cells (Beck et al., 2003). These molecules, which are the ligands for leukocyte function-associated antigen 3 (LFA-3) and B7.1/B7.2, respectively, demonstrate that costimulatory molecule function is critical in determining susceptibility to *Pneumocystis*.

The role of $CD4^+$ T cells in control of lung inflammation during *Pneumocystis* remains much more controversial, and probably depends on the animal model being studied (Hori et al., 2002). In vivo, lymphocytes sensitized to the major surface glycoprotein confer resistance to *Pneumocystis* when transferred into corticosteroid-immunosuppressed rats (Theus et al., 1995). However, transfer of major surface glycoprotein-specific $CD4^+$ T cells produces a severe hyperinflammatory reaction with resultant mortality. $CD4^+$ T cells cause fatal hyperinflammatory reactions after reconstitution of *scid* mice in some models (Roths and Sidman, 1992). Interestingly, this hyperinflammatory response is more pronounced after reconstitution using lymph node-derived cells from mice previously immunized against *Pneumocystis*. Histologic localization of the $CD4^+$ T cells shows that they aggregate in perivascular and peribronchial areas, rather than in the parenchyma. This observation led the authors to speculate that the CD4+ T cells exert their detrimental effects by elaboration of soluble mediators, rather than by direct damage at the alveolus. In later work, these investigators determined that administration of hyperimmune serum prior to the CD4+ T cells resulted in clearance of organisms but prevented the hyperinflammatory reaction (Roths and Sidman, 1993).

Recent work may help to explain why inflammatory responses to *Pneumocystis* have been beneficial in some systems but detrimental in others. Specifically, a better understanding of the phenotype and functional capabilities of the reconstituting cells may determine outcome. For example, a subset of CD4+ regulatory T cells that constitutively express the IL-2 receptor α-chain (CD25) have been shown to prevent autoimmunity (Hori et al., 2002). Transfer of CD25− cells into RAG-2 deficient mice infected with *Pneumocystis* results in lethal pneumonia. However, transfer of CD25+ cells does not produce fatal pneumonitis, and also prevents the inflammation caused by CD4+CD25− cells. Conversely, CD25− cells clear the organisms, but the CD25+ cells inhibit this function of CD25− T cells. Therefore, manipulation of CD4+ T cell phenotypes to cause maximum organism clearance, while minimizing unwanted inflammation, may eventually become possible.

Manipulation of CD4+ T cell subsets to control infection and inflammation has important implications for immunization approaches to *Pneumocystis* infection. Immunization of rats with recombinant *Pneumocystis* p55 antigen reduces organism burden in corticosteroid-immunosuppressed rats (Smulian et al., 2000), and splenocytes from the immunized mice proliferate in response to p55 antigen. The phenotype of the proliferating cells has not been identified, but this work demonstrates that immunization can increase cellular responses. Timing of the immunization, with respect to immunosuppression, also has important consequences (Harmsen et al., 1995). Intact mice were immunized with repeated intratracheal injections of *Pneumocystis*, then were depleted of CD4+ T cells. Rechallenge with *Pneumocystis* results in pneumonia in naive mice, but not in the immunized mice. Immunization prior to T cell depletion protects these mice against *Pneumocystis*, even when the mice are subsequently depleted of CD4+ T cells. In some models, immunologic alterations can overcome persistent lack of CD4+ T cells. For example, bone marrow-derived dendritic cells expressing CD40 ligand were pulsed with *Pneumocystis* antigen in vitro, then administered to CD4 cell-depleted mice (Zheng et al., 2001). Despite the lack of CD4+ T cells, the mice receiving dendritic cells demonstrate significant titers of antibody against *Pneumocystis*, and clear the organisms from their lungs. Because transfer of serum from immunized mice into CD4 cell-depleted, infected mice cleared infection, the investigators conclude that this immunization strategy works primarily by a humoral mechanism. Thus, it is possible that future immunization strategies directed toward humoral immunity can overcome cell-mediated deficits.

6. CD8+ T Cells in Cell-Mediated Defense

The importance of CD8+ T cells in host defense against *Pneumocystis* has not been clearly defined, but recent evidence suggests that CD8+ T cells have both beneficial and detrimental effects for the host during *Pneumocystis* infection. Increased numbers of CD8+ T cells are present in bronchoalveolar lavages obtained from many patients with AIDS, and some of these CD8+ T cells are cytotoxic cells directed against HIV (Autran et al., 1990). It is clear that CD8+ T cells in blood (De Maria et al., 1991) and lung (Semenzato et al., 1995) can be infected with

HIV, and are likely to serve as additional reservoirs. How these CD8+ T cells also participate in defense against *Pneumocystis* in humans requires further study.

In comparison to the role of CD4+ T cells in defense against *Pneumocystis*, the role of CD8+ T cells in decreasing *Pneumocystis* burden in animal models is more controversial (Harmsen and Stankiewicz, 1990; Roths and Sidman, 1992; Beck et al., 1996b). Inoculation of immunologically intact mice with *Pneumocystis* results in accumulation of both CD4+ and CD8+ T cells in the lung, followed by clearance of the organism (Beck et al., 1991b; Ishimine et al., 1995). In mice depleted of CD4+ T cells, inoculation with *Pneumocystis* results in accumulation of CD8+ cells in the lung, although infection progresses (Beck et al., 1991b). The CD8+ T cell response extends to nonhuman primates, as simian immunodeficiency virus (SIV)-infected macaques with *Pneumocystis* pneumonia demonstrate >90% CD8+ T cells in bronchoalveolar lavages during infection (Croix et al., 2002). Because numbers of peripheral CD8+ T cells do not differ in SIV-infected macaques infected with *Pneumocystis* or uninfected, it is likely that the accumulation of CD8+ T cells in these primates was in response to *Pneumocystis*. Importantly, numbers of peripheral CD4+ and CD8+ T cells do not differ in *Pneumocystis*-infected and uninfected mice, demonstrating lung compartmentalization in this species.

The relative contribution of lung CD8+ T cells to defense against *Pneumocystis* remains disputed. In some animal models, CD8+ T cells contribute to defense against *Pneumocystis* during states of CD4+ T cell depletion (Beck et al., 1996b). Specifically, groups of mice were depleted of CD4+ T cells, CD8+ T cells, or both CD4+ and CD8+ T cells. Depletion of CD8+ T cells alone does not result in susceptibility to *Pneumocystis*. However, depletion of both T cell subsets results in more extensive *Pneumocystis* infection than with depletion of only CD4+ T cells. Therefore, in the absence of CD4+ T cells, CD8+ T cells provide partial defense against *Pneumocystis*. A study using the corticosteroid-treated rat model strongly supports a role for CD8+ T cells in host defense against *Pneumocystis* (Theus et al., 1995). Lewis rats, immunosuppressed with corticosteroids and infected with *Pneumocystis*, were reconstituted with CD8+ T cells obtained from the spleens of donor Lewis rats. If reconstitutions are performed with CD8+ T cells from donor rats exposed to *Pneumocystis*, or stimulated in vitro with *Pneumocystis* major surface glycoprotein, the intensity of infection is reduced significantly. In contrast, if reconstitutions are performed with naive CD8+ T cells from unexposed rats, no differences in intensity of infection are observed.

On the other hand, reconstitution experiments performed with *scid* mice do not support an important role for CD8+ T cells in elimination of infection. As discussed above, *scid* mice environmentally exposed to *Pneumocystis* clear organisms from their lungs when given splenocyte infusions (Harmsen and Stankiewicz, 1990). In vivo depletion of CD4+ T cells from the splenocyte preparations abrogates this effect, but depletion of CD8+ T cells still permits clearance. In reconstitution experiments that utilize *scid* mice infected with *Pneumocystis*, the mice do not clear infection when CD8+ T cells are administered, but clear infection when CD4+ T cells are administered (Roths and Sidman, 1992). Furthermore, mice genetically lacking CD8+ T cells (β_2-microglobulin knockout) are not susceptible to *Pneumocystis* (Hanano et al., 1996).

In mice, both CD4+ and CD8+ T cells participate in the development of CMI against *Pneumocystis*, evidenced by the development of delayed-type hypersensitivity (DTH) (Graves et al., 1991). Mice immunized subcutaneously with *Pneumocystis*, then challenged with footpad injections of *Pneumocystis* antigen, demonstrate specific hypersensitivity at the site of challenge. Transfer experiments demonstrate that both

$CD8^+$ T cells and $CD4^+$ T cells must be administered for DTH, and transfer of single subsets does not confer hypersensitivity.

The mechanisms by which $CD8^+$ cells function in control of *Pneumocystis* infection and inflammation in the lung are largely unknown. The lung $CD8^+$ cells that accumulate in the lungs of CD4-depleted mice infected with *Pneumocystis* proliferate in vitro in response to *Pneumocystis* antigen (Beck et al., 1996b). Because this proliferation depends on the presence of macrophages, it is likely that antigen-presenting cells are able to process and present antigen to lung $CD8^+$ T cells. Additionally, these lung $CD8^+$ T cells elaborate IFN-γ in response to *Pneumocystis* antigen, pointing to a possible mechanism by which $CD8^+$ T cells participate in host defense. More recently, a subset of $CD8^+$ T cells that secretes IFN-γ has been shown to demonstrate cytotoxicity for *Pneumocystis* organisms in vitro (Mc Allister et al., 2004). The host defense capabilities of $CD8^+$ T cells against *Pneumocystis* can be augmented by overexpression of IFN-γ, resulting in clearance of infection even with prolonged depletion of $CD4^+$ T cells (Kolls et al., 1999). In these studies, gene transfer has been used to increase lung IFN-γ expression in infected, CD4 cell-depleted mice. This overexpression produces additional recruitment of $CD8^+$ T cells and NK cells to the lung, and results in clearance of infection. Additionally, the presence of $CD8^+$ T cells is required for clearance, because gene transfer into infected *scid* mice, or into mice depleted of both $CD4^+$ and $CD8^+$ T cells, does not result in clearance.

In contrast, several investigations implicate the $CD8^+$ T cell in induction of undesired and detrimental lung inflammation. The experimental literature clearly demonstrates that *Pneumocystis* pneumonia induces surfactant dysfunction. Importantly, *Pneumocystis* reduces levels of the hydrophobic surfactant proteins B and C, leading to increased alveolar surface tension, atelectasis, and hypoxia (Atochina et al., 2000). Other investigators have found no alteration in surfactant biophysical activity in *scid* mice infected with *Pneumocystis* (Wright et al., 2001). When these infected mice are reconstituted with splenocytes, however, the inflammatory response decreases the biophysical activity of surfactant. Importantly, $CD8^+$ T cells drive this response, because reconstitution with CD8-depleted splenocytes abrogates this dysfunction. The same investigators determined that $CD8^+$ T cells, and the resultant lung inflammation they produced, altered lung compliance and oxygenation (Wright et al., 1999b). Mice depleted of $CD4^+$ T cells develop *Pneumocystis* pneumonia with intense inflammation, decreased oxygenation, and decreased lung compliance. In contrast, mice depleted of both $CD4^+$ and $CD8^+$ T cells develop pneumonia, but do not develop physiologic derangements. In this system then the $CD8^+$ T cells recruited in response to *Pneumocystis* induced lung damage.

7. Gamma-Delta T Cells in Cell-Mediated Defense

The roles of $\gamma\delta$ T cells have been less explored than the roles of $CD4^+$ and $CD8^+$ T cells in defense against *Pneumocystis*. TCRδ knockout mice, which lack $\gamma\delta$ T cells, are resistant to *Pneumocystis* infection (Hanano et al., 1996). Furthermore, large numbers of $\gamma\delta$ T cells accumulate in the lungs of mice lacking $\alpha\beta$ T cell receptors (TCRβ knockouts) during *Pneumocystis* infection. Therefore, it is possible that one role of $\gamma\delta$ T cells is an "immunologic salvage" response to *Pneumocystis*, in an effort to compensate for lack of $\alpha\beta$ T cells. Mice lacking both $\alpha\beta$ T cells and $\gamma\delta$ T cells (TCRβxδ knockouts) are extremely susceptible to *Pneumocystis* pneumonia (Hanano and Kaufmann, 1999). The role of $\gamma\delta$ T cells has also been evaluated after intratracheal inoculation with *Pneumocystis* organisms (Steele et al., 2002). In comparison to wild-type controls, $\gamma\delta$ T cell knockout mice demonstrate increased clearance of *Pneumocystis*. Examination of inflammatory responses in the knockout mice shows increased accumulation of $CD8^+$ T cells and increased IFN-γ production. Thus, γδ T cells may limit lung inflammatory responses directed against *Pneumocystis*.

8. Role of Neutrophils in Defense

From an immunologic viewpoint, neutrophils do not appear to play a central role in host defense against *Pneumocystis* infection. Neutrophils have the capacity to phagocytize *Pneumocystis* in vitro (Taylor et al., 1992) and can generate a chemiluminescent response (Taylor and Easmon, 1991). Neutrophils as well as lymphocytes are recruited into lung tissue of animals inoculated with *Pneumocystis*, but enhancement of this response with granulocyte-macrophage colony-stimulating factor (GM-CSF) therapy does not improve host defense (Ieki et al., 1989). Clinically, *Pneumocystis* pneumonia is not associated with immunosuppressive states that cause neutropenia. Interestingly, the presence of lung neutrophils in HIV-infected humans with *Pneumocystis* pneumonia correlates with severe infection and a poor prognosis (Limper et al., 1989; Mason et al., 1989; Bang et al., 2001).

9. Role of Cytokines, Chemokines, and Colony-Stimulating Factors

Cell-mediated immune responses involve local release of a variety of proinflammatory soluble proteins including cytokines, chemokines, and colony-stimulating factors (CSFs). Most of these proteins are released by lung macrophages or monocytes recently recruited into the alveolar spaces, but alveolar epithelial cells are also an important cellular source. Proinflammatory cytokines, which control the influx of inflammatory cells in the lung in response to *Pneumocystis* infection, include IFN-γ, TNF, IL-1, and IL-6. In contrast, the cytokine, IL-10 may serve an anti-inflammatory role.

9.1. Th1 versus Th2 Cytokines

Whether $CD4^+$ T cells induce cytokine responses that are predominantly Th1-like or Th2-like remains under investigation. Recent work suggests that a Th2 response predominates over a Th1 response (Shellito et al., 2000). Cytokine production by lung and lymph node $CD4^+$ T cells after inoculation of immunologically intact mice with *Pneumocystis* was examined. In hilar and paratracheal lymph nodes, $CD4^+$ T cells produced both IFN-γ and IL-4 when examined 1 week after inoculation, and the response diminished over the next 3 weeks. In lung tissue, however, $CD4^+$ T cells producing IL-4 predominated at early time points, followed by cells producing IFN-γ. These data indicate that activation of $CD4^+$ T cells occurs in lymph node prior to the appearance of these cells in the lung. The isotypes of antibody responses to *Pneumocystis* have also been used to determine whether Th1 or Th2 responses predominate (Garvy et al., 1997c). Mice were immunized with *Pneumocystis*, depleted of $CD4^+$ T cells, and then rechallenged with *Pneumocystis* organisms. Despite CD4-depletion, the immunized mice cleared the infectious challenge. Wild-type mice inoculated with *Pneumocystis* mount IgG1 responses, with little production of IgG2a, IgG2b, or Ig3, indicative of a Th2-type response. In contrast, IL-4 knockout mice mount primarily IgG2b responses, indicative of a Th1-type response. Because all groups of mice cleared the inoculum, the investigators argued that either Th1 or Th2 responses are sufficient for protection. Clearly more work is needed to understand the time course and mechanism of Th1 and Th2 $CD4^+$ T cell traffic in response to *Pneumocystis*.

In vitro, major surface glycoprotein stimulation has been used to examine the cytokine repertoire of $CD4^+$ T cells obtained from rats environmentally exposed to *Pneumocystis*. By varying the time course and stimulating antigen, the investigators demonstrated that both Th1 (IFN-γ) and Th2 (IL-4) cytokine production occurred (Theus et al., 1997b). Further cloning of the stimulated cells demonstrated that five clones produced Th1 cytokines (IL-2 and IFN-γ), although one clone also produced small amounts of IL-4 (Theus et al., 1997a).

9.2. IFN-γ

Because of the important role of IFN-γ in Th1 responses, much *Pneumocystis* experimental investigation has focused on this crucial cytokine. In vitro, a specific antigenic component of *Pneumocystis* elicits IFN-γ production from rat T cells (Theus et al., 1994), and T cell clones isolated from rats are of $CD4^+$ phenotype and secreted IL-2 and IFN-.γ (Theus et al., 1997a). IFN-γ, provided as an aerosol, decreases the intensity of *Pneumocystis* infection in CD4-depleted mice, probably by activation of alveolar macrophages (Beck et al., 1991a). More recently, Kolls and coworkers used adenovirus vectors to overexpress IFN-γ in the lungs of mice, decreasing infection (Kolls et al., 1999). IFN-γ also modulates alveolar epithelial defense against *Pneumocystis*, inhibiting the epithelial cells' expression of integrins and decreasing attachment of organisms (Pottratz and Weir, 1997). The beneficial effect of IFN-γ in vivo is controversial. In the *scid* mouse model, neutralization of IFN-γ with a monoclonal antibody does not alter the outcome of *Pneumocystis* infection (Chen et al., 1992a). Furthermore, IFN-γ knockout mice are able to clear *Pneumocystis* organisms from their lungs (Garvy et al., 1997a; Hanano et al., 1998; Rudmann et al., 1998), but IFN-γ may be important in limiting pulmonary inflammation in response to *Pneumocystis* (Garvy et al., 1997a,b).

9.3. TNF

Host release of TNF is a pivotal cytokine in host defense against *Pneumocystis* infection. When exposed to *Pneumocystis* in vitro TNF is released from normal human monocytes (Tamburrini et al., 1991) and alveolar macrophages (Corsini et al., 1992; Hoffman et al., 1993). TNF is also released into lavage fluid in vivo, presumably a product of murine alveolar macrophages (Kolls et al., 1993). Release of TNF in response to *Pneumocystis* in vivo peaks at 3 h and precedes the influx of inflammatory cells into the lung (Kolls et al., 1993). Moreover, *Pneumocystis* induction of TNF appears to be independent of toll-like receptor 4 (TLR4) signaling since TNF can be elicited by an acute challenge of *Pneumocystis* in C3H/HeJ mice. This strain of mice has a point mutation in the cytoplasmic domain, which prevents TLR4 signaling (Poltorak et al., 1998). As mentioned above, TNF may be released as alveolar macrophages bind to β-glucan in the *P. carinii* cyst wall (Vassallo et al., 1999, 2000a).

An enlarging body of evidence supports a protective role for TNF in *Pneumocystis* infection. In HIV-infected patients with *Pneumocystis* pneumonia, TNF is present in the bronchoalveolar lavage fluid and TNF levels inversely correlate with cyst burden (Krishnan et al., 1990). It is not likely that TNF is directly toxic to *Pneumocystis* (Koziel et al., 1993), although data on this point are conflicting (Pesanti, 1991; Pesanti et al., 1991). It is more likely that TNF triggers an inflammatory cytokine cascade in the initial response to infection. TNF is clearly required for adequate host defense against this pathogen in vivo. Chen et al. (1992a) have demonstrated that the use of an anti-TNF antibody delays resolution of murine *Pneumocystis* infection in *scid* mice reconstituted with spleen cells, suggesting that endogenous TNF is critical for resolving the infection (Chen et al., 1992a). Furthermore, neutralization of TNF using a soluble TNF inhibitor delays clearance of murine *Pneumocystis* in CD4⁺ T cell replete mice and exacerbates infection in CD4-depleted mice (Kolls et al., 1997). Moreover, treatment of CD4-depleted, *Pneumocystis*-infected mice with heat-treated *Escherichia coli*, an inducer of TNF, causes near complete resolution of the infection and enhanced resolution of infection in this model could be abrogated with anti-TNF antibodies (Harmsen and Chen, 1992).

TNF is not absolutely essential for host clearance of infection, however. Mice with a homozygous deletion of the two known TNF receptors (TNFRI and TNFRII) can clear an acute challenge with *Pneumocystis* (Rudmann et al., 1998). However, if these mice are crossed to IFN-γ knockout mice, which results in the loss of both TNF and IFN-γ, these mice now become permissive for severe *Pneumocystis* infection (Rudmann et al., 1998). These data suggests that TNF may act in concert with other cytokines to mediate host defense. No single cytokine is the final arbitrator of host defense; clearance of infection requires the coordinated interaction of multiple cytokines interacting locally and over time. Although TNF could be potentially used as therapy for *Pneumocystis*, it carries the risk of potential toxicity. Experimentally, TNF induced in *Pneumocystis*-infected lung tissue in the setting of immune reconstitution in mice and at high tissue concentration may cause lung injury (Wright et al., 1999b). Thus, the same cytokine released to augment clearance in response to a low-level challenge may have a deleterious role in the setting of established infection. Additionally, there is some evidence that the beneficial effects of both pentamidine (Corsini et al., 1992) and corticosteroids (Huang and Eden, 1993) on clinical infection depend, in part, on inhibition of TNF release from alveolar macrophages by these agents.

9.4. IL-1

IL-1 is also an acute-phase cytokine released during infection and plays an important role in the febrile response (Dinarello, 1999, 2000). IL-1 is increased in the bronchoalveolar lavage fluid of HIV-infected patients with *Pneumocystis* pneumonia compared to controls (Perenboom et al., 1997) whereas its antagonist, IL-1 receptor antagonist protein, is elevated in the serum of the same patients. IL-1 activity also increases rapidly in the lungs of reconstituted *scid* mice with *Pneumocystis* infection, and neutralization of IL-1 with an antibody approach completely abrogates resolution of infection after spleen cell reconstitution (Chen et al., 1992b).

9.5. IL-6

IL-6 is released by alveolar epithelial cells in response to *Pneumocystis* (Pottratz et al., 1998), but its role in the inflammatory response to infection is unclear. IL-6 is elevated in lavage fluid in the steroid-treated rat model of *Pneumocystis* infection (Perenboom et al., 1996a). However, it is not detectable in HIV-seronegative patients with *Pneumocystis* pneumonia (Perenboom et al., 1996b). One explanation for this apparent discrepancy may lie in the ability of HIV infection of alveolar macrophages to enhance production of IL-6 in response to *Pneumocystis* (Kandil et al., 1994). In the *scid* mouse reconstitution model, IL-6, which can downregulate IL-1 and TNF, is present in the serum and lungs of infected mice, but administration of an antibody to IL-6 has no effect on the clearance of *Pneumocystis* infection (Chen et al., 1993b). Interestingly, infected mice treated with anti-IL-6 antibody have significantly more inflammatory cells in lung tissue, suggesting that IL-6 might downregulate inflammation associated with *Pneumocystis* infection in mice.

9.6. IL-10

In contrast to the proinflammatory cytokines, IL-10 may function to limit excess inflammation during the host response to infection. IL-10 is released into lavage fluid of mice in response to a *Pneumocystis* challenge, and the concentrations in CD4-depleted mice with heavy infection are higher than in control mice that clear the infection (Ruan et al., 2002). However, gene transfer of IL-10 does not impair clearance of infection. Conversely, other investigators found that clearance was significantly enhanced in IL-10 knockout mice compared to control mice (Qureshi et al., 2003), suggesting that IL-10 serves as a brake on tissue inflammation.

9.7. Chemokines

Chemokines direct migration of leukocytes into infected tissues. The specific type of chemokine released in the tissue as well as the chemokine receptor expressed on the responding cell determines the type of leukocyte that will enter a given tissue and also activates leukocytes at the site of chemokine release. Chemokine classification is based upon the arrangement of cysteine residues in the amino-terminal domains (Luster, 1998). CXC chemokines stimulate migration of neutrophils and T cells, while CC chemokines target monocytes, dendritic cells, eosinophils, and basophils. A variety of cell types have the capacity to release chemokines, but only limited information is available about the types of chemokines released or cellular sources of chemokines in *Pneumocystis* infection.

Pneumocystis stimulates release of CXC chemokines targeting migration of neutrophils in vivo and in vitro. In humans, the CXC chemokine, IL-8 is a major chemoattractant for neutrophils while in mice the same function is served by MIP-2. In HIV-related *Pneumocystis* pneumonia, IL-8 can be detected in lung lavage fluid (Lipschik et al., 1993), and the concentration of lavage fluid IL-8 correlates with more severe infection and increased mortality (Benfield et al., 1995a,b). Furthermore, culture of *Pneumocystis* antigen with monocytes (Benfield et al., 1997) and an alveolar epithelial cell line (Benfield et al., 1999) in vitro results in release of IL-8. The mechanism through which *Pneumocystis* stimulates CXC chemokine release is mediated in part through interactions with β-glucan in the organism cell wall and alveolar macrophages. When purified β-glucan from rat *Pneumocystis* is cultured with alveolar macrophages, there is stimulated release of the CXC chemokine, MIP-2 (Vassallo et al., 2000a). Chemokine release is blocked by incubation of the cells with alpha-mannan, suggesting that the β-glucan is acting through macrophage mannose receptors. MIP-2 production by alveolar macrophages in mice is stimulated through the Dectin-1 glucan receptor (Steele et al., 2003). Components of the *Pneumocystis* cell wall may also stimulate alveolar epithelial cells to release other chemokines. When *Pneumocystis* surface glycoprotein is added to the A549 alveolar epithelial cell line, there is stimulated release of not only the CXC chemokine, IL-8, but also the CC chemokine, MCP-1 (Benfield et al., 1999). Interestingly, glucocorticoids suppress this in vitro chemokine response, which may suggest a mechanism for the beneficial effects of glucocorticoid therapy in severe *Pneumocystis* pneumonia (The National Institutes of Health-University of California Expert Panel, 1990). Similar interactions between *Pneumocystis* cell wall components and lung cells may take place in vivo as well as to recruit neutrophils into lung tissue. In support of this, direct instillation of β-glucan into rat lungs in the absence of intact microorganisms stimulates lung neutrophil influx and tissue inflammation (Vassallo et al., 2000a).

Other investigators assayed lung tissue from infected *scid* mice for mRNA for a battery of chemokines (Wright et al., 1999a). In heavily infected *scid* mice, there was little chemokine mRNA in lung tissue, consistent with the inability of these mice to mount a tissue inflammatory response. However, when these infected mice were immunologically reconstituted with spleen cells from normal mice, mRNA for CC chemokines (RANTES, MCP-1, MIP-1α, MIP-1β), for CXC chemokines (MIP-2), and a C chemokine (lymphotactin) were significantly elevated (Wright et al., 1999a). Presumably, this reconstitution model mimics the host defense mechanisms that permit clearance of infection in normal mice. Interestingly, mRNA for IP-10, which stimulates migration of Th1 cells, was not upregulated in the reconstituted mice, although mRNAs for other chemokines with activity on Th1 cells were increased. It seems clear that local release of chemokines is part of the normal host response to initiate inflammatory cell recruitment into infected lung tissue.

9.8. Colony-Stimulating Factors

CSFs implicated in the host response to *Pneumocystis* pneumonia include GM-CSF, a cytokine that can activate mature macrophages and neutrophils. Paine and coworkers have demonstrated that GM-CSF is a critical regulator of the inflammatory response to *Pneumocystis* in murine lung (Paine et al., 2000). GM-CSF is induced in vivo in response to an acute challenge with *Pneumocystis* and GM-CSF can increase the respiratory burst (as measured by chemiluminescence) of neutrophils that have been exposed to *Pneumocystis* (Taylor and Easmon, 1991). Mice with a homozygous deletion of the GM-CSF gene, which are subsequently CD4 cell-depleted and challenged with *Pneumocystis* develop intense inflammation compared to wild-type control mice. Furthermore local expression of GM-CSF in the lung using a transgene drive by the lung-specific surfactant protein C promoter, reduces the intensity of *Pneumocystis* infection as well as the inflammatory response to the infection (Paine et al., 2000). Additional data show that the systemic administration of GM-CSF protein reduces the intensity of *Pneumocystis* infection in CD4 cell-depleted mice, perhaps through upregulation of TNF production in the lung (Mandujano et al., 1995).

10. Summary

Pneumocystis infections remain a serious cause of morbidity and mortality in immunosuppressed hosts, both in HIV-infected individuals and in other immunosuppressed patients. This chapter reviews cell-mediated immune mechanisms that serve to protect the normal host from infection with *Pneumocystis* or, when defective, lead to the acquisition of pulmonary infection. Alveolar macrophages, $CD4^+$ T cells, $CD8^+$ T cells, and $\gamma\delta$ T cells have important roles in defense against *Pneumocystis*, although their relative contributions require further investigation. Additionally, cytokines and chemokines play vital roles in defense against this organism. Investigations using human cells, as well as animal models and in vitro approaches, have advanced this field recently but many unanswered questions persist. Further investigations examining the roles of these cells and mediators will continue to provide new insights into defense against this important opportunistic pathogen.

References

Agostini, C., Trentin, L., Zambello, R., and Semenzato, G. (1993). HIV-1 and the lung: Infectivity, pathogenic mechanisms and cellular immune responses taking place in the lower respiratory tract. *Am. Rev. Respir. Dis.* 147: 1038–1049.

Agostini, C., Adami, F., Poulter, L.W., Israël-Biet, D., Freitas e Costa, M., Cipriani, A., Sancetta,

R., Lipman, M.C., Juvin, K., Teles-Araujo, A.D., Cadrobbi, P., Masarotto, G., and Semenzato, G. (1997). Role of bronchoalveolar lavage in predicting survival of patients with human immunodeficiency virus infection. *Am. J. Respir. Crit. Care Med.* 156: 1501–1507.

Atochina, E.N., Beers, M.F., Scanlon, S.T., Preston, A.M., and Beck, J.M. (2000). *P. carinii* induces selective alterations in component expression and biophysical activity of lung surfactant. *Am. J. Physiol. Lung Cell Mol. Physiol.* 278: L599–L609.

Autran, B., Mayaud, C.M., Raphael, M., Plata, F., Denis, M., Bourguin, A., Guillon, J.M., Debre, P., and Akoun, G. (1988). Evidence for a cytotoxic T-lymphocyte alveolitis in human immunodeficiency virus-infected patients. *AIDS* 2: 179–183.

Autran, B., Plata, F., Guillon, J.M., Joly, P., Mayaud, C., and Debré, P. (1990). HIV-specific cytotoxic T lymphocytes directed against alveolar macrophages in HIV-infected patients. *Res. Virol.* 141: 131–136.

Bang, D., Emborg, J., Elkjaer, J., Lundgren, J., and Benfield, T. (2001). Independent risk of mechanical ventilation for AIDS-related *Pneumocystis carinii* pneumonia associated with bronchoalveolar lavage neutrophilia. *Respir. Med.* 95: 661–665.

Barton, E. and Campbell, W. (1969). *Pneumocystis carinii* in lungs of rats treated with cortisone acetate. *Am. J. Pathol.* 54: 209–236.

Beck, J.M. and Harmsen, A.G. (1998). Lymphocytes in host defense against *Pneumocystis carinii. Semin. Respir. Infect.* 13: 330–338.

Beck, J.M., Liggitt, H.D., Brunette, E.N., Fuchs, H.J., Shellito, J.E., and Debs, R.J. (1991a). Reduction in intensity of *Pneumocystis carinii* pneumonia in mice by aerosol administration of gamma interferon. *Infect. Immun.* 59: 3859–3862.

Beck, J.M., Warnock, M.L., Curtis, J.L., Sniezek, M.J., Arraj-Peffer, S.M., Kaltreider, H.B., and Shellito, J.E. (1991b). Inflammatory responses to *Pneumocystis carinii* in mice selectively depleted of helper T lymphocytes. *Am. J. Respir. Cell Mol. Biol.* 5: 186–197.

Beck, J.M., Newbury, R.L., and Palmer, B.E. (1996a). *Pneumocystis carinii* pneumonia in *scid* mice induced by viable organisms propagated in vitro. *Infect. Immun.* 64: 4643–4647.

Beck, J.M., Newbury, R.L., Palmer, B.E., Warnock, M.L., Byrd, P.K., and Kaltreider, H.B. (1996b). Role of $CD8^+$ lymphocytes in host defense against *Pneumocystis carinii* in mice. *J. Lab. Clin. Med.* 128: 477–487.

Beck, J.M., Blackmon, M.B., Rose, C.M., Kimzey, S.L., Preston, A.M., and Green, J.M. (2003). T cell costimulatory molecule function determines susceptibility to infection with *Pneumocystis carinii* in mice. *J. Immunol.* 171: 1969–1977.

Bedrossian, C. (1989). Ultrastructure of *Pneumocystis carinii*: A review of internal and surface characteristics. *Semin. Diagn. Pathol.* 6: 212–237.

Benfield, T., Van Steenwuk, R., Nielsen, T., Dichter, J., Lipschik, G., Jensen, B., Shelhamer, J., and Lundgren, J. (1995a). Interleukin-8 and eicosanoid production in the lung during moderate to severe *Pneumocystis carinii* pneumonia in AIDS: A role of interleukin-8 in the pathogenesis of *P. carinii* pneumonia. *Respir. Med.* 89: 285–290.

Benfield, T.L., Vestbo, J., Junge, J., Nielsen, T.L., Jensen, A.B., and Lundgren, J.D. (1995b). Prognostic value of interleukin-8 in AIDS-associated *Pneumocystis carinii* pneumonia. *Am. J. Respir. Crit. Care Med.* 151: 1058–1062.

Benfield, T., Lundgren, B., Levine, S., Kronborg, G., Shelhamer, J., and Lundgren, J. (1997). The major surface glycoprotein of *Pneumocystis carinii* induces release and gene expression of interleukin-8 and tumor necrosis factor alpha in monocytes. *Infect. Immun.* 65: 4790–4794.

Benfield, T.L., Lundgren, B., Shelhamer, J.H., and Lundgren, J.D. (1999). *Pneumocystis carinii* major surface glycoprotein induces interleukin-8 and monocyte chemoattractant protein-1 release from a human alveolar epithelial cell line. *Eur. J. Clin. Invest.* 29: 717–722.

Brown, G., Taylor, P., Reid, D., Wilment, J., Williams, D., Martinez-Pmares, L., Wong, S., and Gordon, S. (2001). Dectin-1 is a major beta-glucan receptor on macrophages. *J. Exp. Med.* 196: 407–412.

Chayt, K.J., Harper, M.E., Marselle, L.M., Lewin, E.B., Rose, R.M., Oleske, J.M., Epstein, L.G., Wong-Staal, F., and Gallo, R.C. (1986). Detection of HTLV-III RNA in lungs of patients with AIDS and pulmonary involvement. *JAMA* 256: 2356–2359.

Chen, W., Havell, E.A., and Harmsen, A.G. (1992a). Importance of endogenous tumor necrosis factor alpha and gamma interferon in host resistance against *Pneumocystis carinii* infection. *Infect. Immun.* 60: 1279–1284.

Chen, W., Havell, E.A., Moldawer, L.L., McIntyre, K.W., Chizzonite, R.A., and Harmsen, A.G. (1992b). Interleukin 1: An important mediator of host resistance against *Pneumocystis carinii. J. Exp. Med.* 176: 713–718.

Chen, W., Gigliotti, F., and Harmsen, A.G. (1993a). Latency is not an inevitable outcome of infection with *Pneumocystis carinii. Infect. Immun.* 61: 5406–5409.

Chen, W., Havell, E.A., Gigliotti, F., and Harmsen, A.G. (1993b). Interleukin-6 production in a murine model of *Pneumocystis carinii* pneumonia: Relation to resistance and inflammatory response. *Infect. Immun.* 61: 97–102.

Chusid, M. and Heyrman, K. (1978). An outbreak of *Pneumocystis carinii* at a pediatric hospital. *Pediatrics* 62: 1031–1035.

Corsini, E., Dykstra, C., Craig, W.A., Tidwell, R.R., and Rosenthal, G.J. (1992). *Pneumocystis carinii* induction of tumor necrosis factor-alpha by alveolar macrophages: Modulation by pentamidine isethionate. *Immunol. Lett.* 34: 303–308.

Croix, D.A., Board, K., Capuano, S. III., Murphey-Corb, M., Haidaris, C.G., Flynn, J.L., Reinhart, T., and Norris, K.A. (2002). Alterations in T lymphocyte profiles of bronchoalveolar lavage fluid from SIV- and *Pneumocystis carinii*-coinfected rhesus macaques. *AIDS Res. Hum. Retrovir.* 18: 391–401.

Cushion, M. (1998). Taxonomy, genetic organization, and life cycle of *Pneumocystis carinii. Semin. Respir. Infect.* 13: 304–312.

Cushion, M., Stringer, J., and Walzer, P. (1991). Cellular and molecular biology of *Pneumocystis carinii. Int. Rev. Cytol.* 131: 59–107.

D'Souza, N.B., Mandujano, J.F., Nelson, S., Summer, W.R., and Shellito, J.E. (1995). Alcohol ingestion impairs host defenses predisposing otherwise healthy mice to *Pneumocystis carinii* infection. *Alcohol Clin. Exp. Res.* 19: 1219–1225.

De Maria, A., Pantaleo, G., Schnittman, S.M., Greenhouse, J.E., Baseler, M., Orenstein, J.M., and Fauci, A.S. (1991). Infection of $CD8^+$ lymphocytes: Requirement for interaction with infected $CD4^+$ cells and induction of infectious virus from chronically infected $CD8^+$ cells. *J. Immunol.* 146: 2220–2226.

De Stefano, J.A., Cushion, M.T., Sleight, R.G., and Walzer, P.D. (1990). Analysis of *Pneumocystis carinii* cyst wall. I. Evidence for an outer surface membrane. *J. Protozool.* 37: 428–435.

Dinarello, C. (1999). Cytokines as endogenous pyrogens. *J. Infect. Dis.* 179: S294–S304.

Dinarello, C. (2000). Proinflammatory cytokines. *Chest* 118: 503–508.

Downing, J.F., Kachel, D.L., Pasula, R., and Martin, W.J. II (1999). Gamma interferon stimulates rat alveolar macrophages to kill *Pneumocystis carinii* by L-arginine- and tumor necrosis factor-dependent mechanisms. *Infect. Immun.* 67: 1347–1352.

Dumoulin, A., Mazars, E., Seguy, N., Gargallo-Viola, D., Vargas, S., Cailliez, J.C., Aliouat, E.M., Wakefield, A.E., and Dei-Cas, E. (2000). Transmission of *Pneumocystis carinii* disease from immunocompetent contacts of infected hosts to susceptible hosts. *Eur. J. Clin. Microbiol. Infect. Dis.* 19: 671–678.

Edman, J., Kovacs, J., Masur, H., Santi, H., and Sogin, M. (1988). Ribosomal RNA sequence shows *Pneumocystis carinii* to be a member of the fungi. *Nature* 334: 519–522.

Ezekowitz, R.A., Williams, D.J., Koziel, H., Armstrong, M.Y., Warner, A., Richards, F.F., and Rose, R.M. (1991). Uptake of *Pneumocystis carinii* mediated by the macrophage mannose receptor. *Nature* 351: 155–158.

Fisher, D.J., Gigliotti, G., Zauderer, M., and Harmsen, A.G. (1991). Specific T-cell response to a *Pneumocystis carinii* surface glycoprotein (gp120) after immunization and natural infection. *Infect. Immun.* 59: 3372–3376.

Forte, M., Maartens, G., Campbell, F., Stubberfield, C., Shahmanesh, M., Kumararatne, D., and Gaston, H. (1992). T-lymphocyte responses to *Pneumocystis carinii* in healthy and HIV-positive individuals. *J. Acquir. Immune Defic. Syndr.* 5: 409–416.

Frenkel, J.K., Good, J.T., and Shultz, J.A. (1966). Latent *Pneumocystis* infection of rats, relapse, and chemotherapy. *Lab. Invest.* 15: 1559–1577.

Gajdusek, D. (1957). *Pneumocystis carinii*: Etiologic agent of interstitial plasma cell pneumonia of premature and young infants. *Pediatrics* 19: 543–565.

Garvy, B. (1998). Host defense to *Pneumocystis carinii*: The missing pieces in the jigsaw. *Trends Microbiol.* 6: 97–98.

Garvy, B.A. and Qureshi, M.H. (2000). Delayed inflammatory response to *Pneumocystis carinii* infection in neonatal mice is due to an inadequate lung environment. *J. Immunol.* 165: 6480–6486.

Garvy, B.A., Ezekowitz, R.A., and Harmsen, A.G. (1997a). Role of gamma interferon in the host immune and inflammatory responses to *Pneumocystis carinii* infection. *Infect. Immun.* 65: 373–379.

Garvy, B.A., Gigliotti, F., and Harmsen, A.G. (1997b). Neutralization of interferon-gamma exacerbates *Pneumocystis*-driven interstitial pneumonitis after bone marrow transplantation in mice. *J. Clin. Invest.* 99: 1637–1644.

Garvy, B.A., Wiley, J.A., Gigliotti, F., and Harmsen, A.G. (1997c). Protection against *Pneumocystis carinii* pneumonia by antibodies generated from either T helper 1 or T helper 2 responses. *Infect. Immun.* 65: 5052–5056.

Gigliotti, F., Harmsen, A.G., and Wright, T.W. (2003). Characterization of transmission of *Pneumocystis carinii f. sp. muris* through immunocompetent BALB/c mice. *Infect. Immun.* 71: 3852–3856.

Graves, D.C., Li, X.H., and Paiva, W.D. (1991). Delayed-type hypersensitivity response in mice to *Pneumocystis carinii*. *J. Protozool.* 38: 49S–52S.

Green, G. and Kass, E. (1964). The role of the alveolar macrophage in the clearance of bacteria from the lung. *J. Exp. Med.* 119: 167–175.

Hagler, D.N., Deepe, G.S., Pogue, C.L., and Walzer, P.D. (1988). Blastogenic responses to *Pneumocystis carinii* among patients with human immunodeficiency (HIV) infection. *Clin. Exp. Immunol.* 74: 7–13.

Hanano, R. and Kaufmann, S.H. (1998). Immune responses to naturally acquired *Pneumocystis carinii* in gene disruption mutant mice. *Res. Immunol.* 149: 429–435.

Hanano, R. and Kaufmann, S.H.E. (1999). *Pneumocystis carinii* pneumonia in mutant mice deficient in both TCRαβ and TCRγδ cells: Cytokine and antibody responses. *J. Infect. Dis.* 179: 455–459.

Hanano, R., Reifenberg, K., and Kaufmann, S.H. (1996). Naturally acquired *Pneumocystis carinii* pneumonia in gene disruption mutant mice: Roles of distinct T-cell populations in infection. *Infect. Immun.* 64: 3201–3209.

Hanano, R., Reifenber, K., and Kaufmann, S.H.E. (1998). Activated pulmonary macrophages are insufficient for resistance against *Pneumocystis carinii*. *Infect. Immun.* 66: 305–314.

Harmsen, A.G. and Chen, W. (1992). Resolution of *Pneumocystis carinii* pneumonia in CD4$^+$ lymphocyte-depleted mice given aerosols of heat-treated *Escherichia coli*. *J. Exp. Med.* 176: 881–886.

Harmsen, A.G. and Stankiewicz, M. (1990). Requirement for CD4$^+$ cells in resistance to *Pneumocystis carinii* pneumonia in mice. *J. Exp. Med.* 172: 937–945.

Harmsen, A.G., Chen, W., and Gigliotti, F. (1995). Active immunity to *Pneumocystis carinii* reinfection in T-cell-depleted mice. *Infect. Immun.* 63: 2391–2395.

Herbein, G., Coaquette, A., Perez-Bercoff, D., and Pancino, G. (2002). Macrophage activation and HIV infection: Can the Trojan horse turn into a fortress? *Curr. Mol. Med.* 2: 723–738.

Herrod, H.G., Valenski, W.R., Woods, D.R., and Pifer, L.L. (1981). The in vitro response of human lymphocytes to *Pneumocystis carinii* antigen. *J. Immunol.* 126: 59–61.

Hidalgo, H.A., Helmke, R.J., German, V.F., and Mangos, J.A. (1992). *Pneumocystis carinii* induces an oxidative burst in alveolar macrophages. *Infect. Immun.* 60: 1–7.

Hoffman, O.A., Standing, J.E., and Limper, A.H. (1993). *Pneumocystis carinii* stimulates tumor necrosis factor-α release from alveolar macrophages through a β-glucan-mediated mechanism. *J. Immunol.* 150: 3932–3940.

Hori, S., Carvalho, T.L., and Demengeot, J. (2002). CD25$^+$CD4$^+$ regulatory T cells suppress CD4$^+$ T cell-mediated pulmonary hyperinflammation driven by *Pneumocystis carinii* in immunodeficient mice. *Eur. J. Immunol.* 32: 1282–1291.

Huang, Z.B. and Eden, E. (1993). Effect of corticosteroids on IL-1 beta and TNF alpha release by alveolar macrophages from patients with AIDS and *Pneumocystis carinii* pneumonia. *Chest* 104: 751–755.

Huang, S. and Marshall, K. (1970). *Pneumocystis carinii* infection: A cytologic, histologic and electron microscopic study of the organism. *Am. Rev. Respir. Dis.* 102: 623–629.

Hughes, W. (1987). Natural occurrences in animals. In *Pneumocystis carinii Pneumonitis*. CRC Press, Boca Raton, pp. 57–70.

Ieki, R., Furuta, T., Asano, S., Mori, S., Kudoh, S., Kimura, H., and Takaku, F. (1989). Effect of recombinant human granulocyte colony-stimulating factor on *Pneumocystis carinii* infection in nude mice. *Jpn. J. Exp. Med.* 59: 51–58.

Ishimine, T., Kawakami, K., Nakamoto, A., and Saito, A. (1995). Analysis of cellular response and gamma interferon synthesis in bronchoalveolar lavage fluid and lung homogenate of mice infected with *Pneumocystis carinii*. *Microbiol. Immunol.* 39: 49–58.

Kandil, O., Fishman, J.A., Koziel, H., Pinkston, P., Rose, R.M., and Remold, H.G. (1994). Human immunodeficiency virus type 1 infection of human macrophages modulates the cytokine response to *Pneumocystis carinii*. *Infect. Immun.* 62: 644–650.

Kaplan, J.E., Hanson, D., Dworkin, M.S., Frederick, T., Bertolli, J., Lindegren, M.L., Holmberg, S., and Jones, J.L. (2000). Epidemiology of human immunodeficiency virus-associated opportunistic infections in the United States in the era of highly active antiretroviral therapy. *Clin. Infect. Dis.* 30: S5–S14.

Kolls, J.K., Beck, J.M., Nelson, S., Summer, W.R., and Shellito, J. (1993). Alveolar macrophage release of tumor necrosis factor during murine *Pneumocystis carinii* pneumonia. *Am. J. Respir. Cell Mol. Biol.* 8: 370–376.

Kolls, J.K., Lei, D.H., Vasquez, C., Odom, G., Summer, W.R., Nelson, S., and Shellito, J. (1997). Exacerbation of murine *Pneumocystis carinii* infection by adenoviral-mediated gene transfer of a TNF inhibitor. *Am. J. Respir. Cell Mol. Biol.* 16: 112–118.

Kolls, J.K., Habetz, S., Shean, M.K., Vazquez, C., Brown, J.A., Lei, D., Schwarzenberger, P., Ye, P., Nelson, S., Summer, W.R., and Shellito, J.E. (1999). IFN-γ and $CD8^+$ T cells restore host defenses against *Pneumocystis carinii* in mice depleted of $CD4^+$ T cells. *J. Immunol.* 162: 2890–2894.

Koziel, H., Armstrong, M., Arena, C., Pelletier, N., Richards, F., and Rose, R. (1993). Tumor necrosis factor-alpha does not affect viability of *Pneumocystis carinii* in vitro. *Am. Rev. Respir. Dis.* 147: A34.

Koziel, H., Eichbaum, Q., Kruskal, B.A., Pinkston, P., Rogers, R.A., Armstrong, M.Y., Richards, F.F., Rose, R.M., and Ezekowitz, R.A. (1998). Reduced binding and phagocytosis of *Pneumocystis carinii* by alveolar macrophages from persons infected with HIV-1 correlates with mannose receptor downregulation. *J. Clin. Invest.* 102: 1332–1344.

Koziel, H., Li, X., Armstron, M., Richards, F., and Rose, R. (2000). Alveolar macrophages from human immunodeficiency virus-infected persons demonstrate impaired oxidative burst response to *Pneumocystis carinii* in vitro. *Am. J. Respir. Cell Mol. Biol.* 23: 452–459.

Krishnan, V.L., Meager, A., Mitchell, D.M., and Pinching, A.J. (1990). Alveolar macrophages in AIDS patients: Increased spontaneous tumour necrosis factor-alpha production in *Pneumocystis carinii* pneumonia. *Clin. Exp. Immunol.* 80: 156–160.

Lebargy, F., Branellec, A., Deforges, L., Bignon, J., and Bernaudin, J. (1994). HIV-1 in human alveolar macrophages from infected patients is latent in vivo but replicates after in vitro stimulation. *Am. J. Respir. Cell Mol. Biol.* 10: 72–78.

Lewin, S.R., Kirihara, J., Sonza, S., Irving, L., Mills, J., and Crowe, S.M. (1998). HIV-1 DNA and mRNA concentrations are similar in peripheral blood monocytes and alveolar macrophages in HIV-1-infected individuals. *AIDS* 12: 719–727.

Limper, A.H., Offord, K.P., Smith, T.F., and Martin, W.J. II. (1989). *Pneumocystis carinii* pneumonia: Differences in lung parasite number and inflammation in patients with and without AIDS. *Am. Rev. Respir. Dis.* 140: 1204–1209.

Limper, A.H., Hoyte, J.S., and Standing, J.E. (1997). The role of alveolar macrophages in *Pneumocystis carinii* degradation and clearance from the lung. *J. Clin. Invest.* 99: 2110–2117.

Lipschik, G.Y., Doerfler, M.E., Kovacs, J.A., Travis, W.D., Andrawis, V.A., Lawrence, M.G., Dichter, J.R., Ognibene, F.P., and Shelhamer, J.H. (1993). Leukotriene B4 and interleukin-8 in human immunodeficiency virus-related pulmonary disease. *Chest* 104: 763–769.

Luster, A. (1998). Chemokines: Chemotactic cytokines that mediate inflammation. *N. Engl. J. Med.* 338: 436–445.

Mandujano, J.F., D'Souza, N.B., Nelson, S., Summer, W.R., Beckerman, R.C., and Shellito, J.E. (1995). Granulocyte-macrophage colony stimulating factor and *Pneumocystis carinii* pneumonia in mice. *Am. J. Respir. Crit. Care Med.* 151: 1233–1238.

Mason, G.R., Hashimoto, C.H., Dickman, P.S., Foutty, L.F., and Cobb, C.J. (1989). Prognostic implications of bronchoalveolar lavage neutrophilia in patients with *Pneumocystis carinii* pneumonia and AIDS. *Am. Rev. Respir. Dis.* 139: 1336–1342.

Masur, H. and Jones, T.C. (1978). The interaction *in vitro* of *Pneumocystis carinii* with macrophages and L-cells. *J. Exp. Med.* 147: 157–170.

Masur, H., Michelis, M., Greene, J., Onorato, I., Vande Stouwe, R., Holzman, R., Wormser, G., Brettman, L., Lange, M., Murray, H., and Cunningham-Rundles, S. (1981). An outbreak of community-acquired *Pneumocystis carinii* pneumonia: Initial manifestation of cellular immune dysfunction. *N. Engl. J. Med.* 305: 1431–1438.

Mc Allister, F., Steele, C., Zheng, M., Young, E., Shellito, J.E., Marrero, L., and Kolls, J.K. (2004). T cytotoxic-1 $CD8^+$ T cells are effector cells against *Pneumocystis* in mice. *J. Immunol.* 172: 1132–1138.

McCormack, F., Festa, A., Andrews, R., Linke, M., and Walzer, P. (1997). The carbohydrate recognition domain of surfactant protein A mediates binding to the major surface glycoprotein of *Pneumocystis carinii. Biochemistry* 36: 8092–8099.

Meuwissen, J., Tauber, I., Leewenberg, A., Beckers, P., and Shiehen, J. (1977). Parasitologic and serologic observations of infection with *Pneumocystis* in humans. *J. Infect. Dis.* 136: 43–49.

Morris, A., Beard, C., and Huang, L. (2002). Update on the epidemiology and transmission of *Pneumocystis carinii. Microbes Infect.* 4: 95–103.

O'Riordan, D.M., Standing, J.E., Kwon, K.Y., Chang, D., Crouch, E.C., and Limper, A.H. (1995). Surfactant protein D interacts with *Pneumocystis carinii* and mediates organism adherence to alveolar macrophages. *J. Clin. Invest.* 95: 2699–2710.

Paine, R. III., Preston, A.M., Wilcoxen, S., Jin, H., Siu, B.B., Morris, S.B., Reed, J.A., Ross, G., Whitsett, J.A., and Beck, J.M. (2000). Granulocyte-macrophage colony-stimulating factor in the innate immune response to *Pneumocystis carinii* pneumonia in mice. *J. Immunol.* 164: 2602–2609.

Peglow, S.L., Smulian, A.G., Linke, M.J., Pogue, C.L., Nurre, S., Crisler, J., Phair, J., Gold, J.W.M., Armstrong, D., and Walzer, P.D. (1990). Serologic responses to *Pneumocystis carinii* antigens in health and disease. *J. Infect. Dis.* 161: 296–306.

Perenboom, R.M., Beckers, P., Van Der Meer, J.W., Van Schijndel, A.C., Oyen, W.J., Corstens, F.H., and Sauerwein, R.W. (1996a). Proinflammatory cytokines in lung and blood during steroid-induced *Pneumocystis carinii* pneumonia in rats. *J. Leukoc. Biol.* 60: 710–715.

Perenboom, R.M., van Schijndel, A.C., Beckers, P., Sauerwein, R., Van Hamersvelt, H.W., Festen, J., Gallati, H., and van der Meer, J.W. (1996b). Cytokine profiles in bronchoalveolar lavage fluid and blood in HIV-seronegative patients with *Pneumocystis carinii* pneumonia. *Eur. J. Clin. Invest.* 26: 159–166.

Perenboom, R.M., Sauerwein, R.W., Beckers, P., van Schijndel, A.C., van Steenwijk, R.P., Borleffs, J.C., van Leusen, R., and van der Meer, J.W. (1997). Cytokine profiles in bronchoalveolar lavage fluid and blood in HIV-seropositive patients with *Pneumocystis carinii pneumonia. Eur. J. Clin. Invest.* 27: 333–339.

Pesanti, E.L. (1991). Interaction of cytokines and alveolar cells with *Pneumocystis carinii* in vitro. *J. Infect. Dis.* 163: 611–616.

Pesanti, E.L., Tomicic, T., and Donta, S.T. (1991). Binding of 125I-labelled tumor necrosis factor to *Pneumocystis carinii* and an insoluble cell wall fraction. *J. Protozool.* 38: 28S–29S.

Peters, S.E., Sinclair, K., Millard, P.R., and Hopkin, J.M. (1992). A search for *Pneumocystis carinii* in post-mortem lungs by DNA amplification. *J. Pathol.* 166: 195–198.

Phair, J., Muñoz, A., Detels, R., Kaslow, R., Rinaldo, C., Saah, A., and the Multicenter AIDS Cohort Study Group (1990). The risk of *Pneumocystis carinii* pneumonia among men infected with human immunodeficiency virus type 1. *N. Engl. J. Med.* 322: 161–165.

Pifer, L.L., Hughes, W.T., Stagno, S., and Woods, D. (1978). *Pneumocystis carinii* infection: Evidence for high prevalence in normal and immunosuppressed children. *Pediatrics* 61: 35–41.

Plata, F., Autran, B., Martins, L.P., Wain-Hobson, S., Raphael, M., Mayaud, C., Denis, M., Guillon, J.M., and Debre, P. (1987). AIDS virus-specific cytotoxic T lymphocytes in lung disorders. *Nature* 328: 348–351.

Poltorak, A., He, X., Smirnova, I., Liu, M., Huffel, C., and Du, X. (1998). Defective LPS signaling in C3H/HeJ and C57BL/10ScCr mice: Mutations in TLR4 gene. *Science* 282: 2085–2088.

Pottratz, S.T. and Martin, W.J. II. (1990). Role of fibronectin in *Pneumocystis carinii* attachment to cultured lung cells. *J. Clin. Invest.* 85: 351–356.

Pottratz, S.T. and Weir, A.L. (1997). Gamma-interferon inhibits *Pneumocystis carinii* attachment to lung cells by decreasing expression of lung cell-surface integrins. *Eur. J. Clin. Invest.* 27: 17–22.

Pottratz, S.T., Reese, S., and Sheldon, J.L. (1998). *Pneumocystis carinii* induces interleukin 6 production by an alveolar epithelial cell line. *Eur. J. Clin. Invest.* 28: 424–429.

Qureshi, M.H. and Garvy, B.A. (2001). Neonatal T cells in an adult lung environment are competent to resolve *Pneumocystis carinii* pneumonia. *J. Immunol.* 166: 5704–5711.

Qureshi, M.H., Harmsen, A.G., and Garvy, B.A. (2003). IL-10 modulates host responses and lung damage induced by *Pneumocystis carinii* infection. *J. Immunol.* 170: 1002–1009.

Roths, J.B. and Sidman, C.L. (1992). Both immunity and hyperresponsiveness to *Pneumocystis carinii* result from transfer of $CD4^+$ but not $CD8^+$ T cells into severe combined immunodeficiency mice. *J. Clin. Invest.* 90: 673–678.

Roths, J.B. and Sidman, C.L. (1993). Single and combined humoral and cell-mediated immunotherapy of *Pneumocystis carinii* pneumonia in immunodeficient *scid* mice. *Infect. Immun.* 61: 1641–1649.

Roths, J.B., Marshall, J.D., Allen, R.D., Carlson, G.A., and Sidman, C.L. (1990). Spontaneous *Pneumocystis carinii* pneumonia in immunodeficient mutant *scid* mice: Natural history and pathobiology. *Am. J. Pathol.* 136: 1173–1186.

Ruan, S., Tate, C., Lee, J.J., Ritter, T., Kolls, J.K., and Shellito, J.E. (2002). Local delivery of the viral interleukin-10 gene suppresses tissue inflammation in murine *Pneumocystis carinii* infection. *Infect. Immun.* 70: 6107–6113.

Rudmann, D.G., Preston, A.M., Moore, M.W., and Beck, J.M. (1998). Susceptibility to *Pneumocystis carinii* in mice depends on simultaneous depletion of interferon-gamma and type 1 and 2 tumor necrosis factor receptor genes. *J. Immunol.* 161: 360–366.

Semenzato, G., Agostini, C., Ometto, L., Zambello, R., Trentin, L., Chieco-Bianchi, L., and De Rossi, A. (1995). $CD8^+$ T lymphocytes in the lung of acquired immunodeficiency syndrome patients harbor human immunodeficiency virus type 1. *Blood* 85: 2308–2314.

Settnes, O. and Genner, J. (1986). *Pneumocystis carinii* in human lungs at autopsy. *Scand. J. Infect. Dis.* 18: 489–496.

Shellito, J.E. and Olariu, R. (1998). Alcohol decreases T-lymphocyte migration into lung tissue in response to *Pneumocystis carinii* and depleted T-lymphocyte numbers in the spleens of mice. *Alcohol Clin. Exp. Res.* 22: 658–663.

Shellito, J., Suzara, V.V., Blumenfeld, W., Beck, J.M., Steger, H.J., and Ermak, T.H. (1990). A new model of *Pneumocystis carinii* infection in mice selectively depleted of helper T lymphocytes. *J. Clin. Invest.* 85: 1686–1693.

Shellito, J.E., Kolls, J.K., Olariu, R., and Beck, J.M. (1996). Nitric oxide and host defense against *Pneumocystis carinii* infection in a mouse model. *J. Infect. Dis.* 173: 432–439.

Shellito, J.E., Tate, C., Ruan, S.B., and Kolls, J. (2000). Murine $CD4^+$ T lymphocyte subsets and host defense against *Pneumocystis carinii.* *J. Infect. Dis.* 181: 2011–2017.

Singer, C., Armstrong, D., Rosen, P., and Schottenfeld, D. (1975). *Pneumocystis carinii* pneumonia: A cluster of eleven cases. *Ann. Intern. Med.* 82: 772–777.

Smulian, A.G., Sullivan, D.W., and Theus, S.A. (2000). Immunization with recombinant *Pneumocystis carinii* p55 antigen provides partial protection against infection: Characterization of epitope recognition associated with immunization. *Microbes Infect.* 2: 127–136.

Steele, C., Zheng, M., Young, E., Marrero, L., Shellito, J., and Kolls, J. (2002). Increased host resistance against *Pneumocystis carinii* pneumonia in γδ T-cell-deficient mice: Protective role of gamma interferon and $CD8^+$ T cells. *Infect. Immun.* 70: 5208–5215.

Steele, C., Marrero, L., Swain, S., Harmsen, A.G., Zheng, M., Brown, G.D., Gordon, S., Shellito, J.E., and Kolls, J.K. (2003). Alveolar macrophage-mediated killing of *Pneumocystis carinii f. sp. muris* involves molecular recognition by the Dectin-1 beta-glucan receptor. *J. Exp. Med.* 198: 1677–1688.

Sternberg, R.I., Whitsett, J.A., Hull, W.M., and Baughman, R.P. (1995). *Pneumocystis carinii* alters surfactant protein A concentrations in bronchoalveolar lavage fluid. *J. Lab. Clin. Med.* 125: 462–469.

Stokes, D.C., Gigliotti, F., Rehg, J.E., Snellgrove, R.L., and Hughes, W.T. (1987). Experimental

Pneumocystis carinii pneumonia in the ferret. *Br. J. Exp. Pathol.* 68: 267–276.
Stringer, S., Stringer, J., Blase, M., Walzer, P., and Cushion, M. (1989). *Pneumocystis carinii*: Sequence from ribosomal RNA implies a close relationship with fungi. *Exp. Parasitol.* 68: 450–461.
Stringer, J.R., Beard, C.B., Miller, R.F., and Wakefield, A.E. (2002). A new name (*Pneumocystis jiroveci*) for *Pneumocystis* from humans. *Emerg. Infect. Dis.* 8: 891–896.
Swain, S.D., Lee, S.J., Nussenzweig, M.C., and Harmsen, A.G. (2003). Absence of the macrophage mannose receptor in mice does not increase susceptibility to *Pneumocystis carinii* infection in vivo. *Infect. Immun.* 71: 6213–6221.
Tamburrini, E., De Luca, A., Ventura, G., Maiuro, G., Siracusano, A., Ortona, E., and Antinori, A. (1991). *Pneumocystis carinii* stimulates in vitro production of tumor necrosis factor-alpha by human macrophages. *Med. Microbiol. Immunol.* 180: 15–20.
Taylor, M.B. and Easmon, C.S. (1991). The neutrophil chemiluminescence response to *Pneumocystis carinii* is stimulated by GM-CSF and gamma interferon. *FEMS Microbiol. Immunol.* 4: 41–44.
Taylor, M.B., Phillips, M., and Easmon, C.S. (1992). Opsonophagocytosis of *Pneumocystis carinii*. *J. Med. Microbiol.* 36: 223–228.
The National Institutes of Health—University of California Expert Panel (1990). Consensus statement on the use of corticosteroids as adjunctive therapy for *Pneumocystis* pneumonia in the acquired immunodeficiency syndrome. *N. Engl. J. Med.* 323: 1500–1504.
Theus, S.A., Linke, M.J., Andrews, R.P., and Walzer, P.D. (1993). Proliferative and cytokine responses to a major surface glycoprotein of *Pneumocystis carinii*. *Infect. Immun.* 61: 4703–4709.
Theus, S.A., Sullivan, D.W., Walzer, P.D., and Smulian, A.G. (1994). Cellular responses to a 55-kilodalton recombinant *Pneumocystis carinii* antigen. *Infect. Immun.* 62: 3479–3484.
Theus, S.A., Andrews, R.P., Steele, P., and Walzer, P.D. (1995). Adoptive transfer of lymphocytes sensitized to the major surface glycoprotein of *Pneumocystis carinii* confers protection in the rat. *J. Clin. Invest.* 95: 2587–2593.
Theus, S.A., Andrews, R.P., Linke, M.J., and Walzer, P.D. (1997a). Characterization of rat CD4 T cell clones specific for the major surface glycoprotein of *Pneumocystis carinii*. *J. Eukaryot. Microbiol.* 44: 96–100.
Theus, S.A., Smulian, A.G., Sullivan, D.W., and Walzer, P.D. (1997b). Cytokine responses to native and recombinant forms of the major surface glycoprotein of *Pneumocystis carinii*. *Clin. Exp. Immunol.* 109: 255–260.
Thullen, T.D., Ashbaugh, A.D., Daly, K.R., Linke, M.J., Steele, P.E., and Walzer, P.D. (2003). New rat model of *Pneumocystis* pneumonia induced by anti-CD4($^+$) T-lymphocyte antibodies. *Infect. Immun.* 71: 6292–6297.
Vassallo, R., Standing, J., and Limper, A. (1999). Beta-glucan from *Pneumocystis carinii* stimulates TNF-alpha release from alveolar macrophages. *J. Eukaryot. Microbiol.* 46: 145S.
Vassallo, R., Standing, J., and Limper, A. (2000a). Isolated *Pneumocystis carinii* cell wall glucan provokes lower respiratory tract inflammatory responses. *J. Immunol.* 164: 3755–3763.
Vassallo, R., Thomas, C.F., Vuk-Pavlovic, Z., and Limper, A.H. (2000b). Mechanisms of defence in the lung: Lessons from *Pneumocystis carinii* pneumonia. *Sarcoidosis Vasc. Diffuse Lung Dis.* 17: 130–139.
Vavra, J. and Kucera, K. (1970). *Pneumocystis carinii*: Its ultrastructure and ultrastructural affinities. *J. Protozool.* 17: 463–472.
Wakefield, A.E. (1996). DNA sequences identical to *Pneumocystis cariniii f. sp. carinii* and *Pneumocystis carinii f. sp. hominis* in samples of air spora. *J. Clin. Microbiol.* 34: 1754–1759.
Walzer, P.D. and Rutledge, M.E. (1981). Humoral immunity in experimental *Pneumocystis carinii* infection. I. Serum and bronchial lavage fluid antibody responses in rats. *J. Lab. Clin. Med.* 97: 820–833.
Walzer, P.D. and Rutledge, M.E. (1982). Serum antibody responses to *Pneumocystis carinii* among different strains of normal and athymic mice. *Infect. Immun.* 35: 620–626.
Walzer, P., Perl, D., Krogstead, D., Rawson, P., and Schultz, M. (1974). *Pneumocystis carinii* pneumonia in the United States: Epidemiologic, diagnostic, and clinical features. *Ann. Intern. Med.* 80: 83–93.
Walzer, P.D., Powell, R.D. Jr., and Yoneda, K. (1979). Experimental *Pneumocystis carinii* pneumonia in different strains of cortisonized mice. *Infect. Immun.* 24: 939–947.

Walzer, P.D., LaBine, M., Redington, T.J., and Cushion, M.T. (1984). Lymphocyte changes during chronic administration of and withdrawal from corticosteroids: Relation to *Pneumocystis carinii* pneumonia. *J. Immunol.* 133: 2502–2508.

Walzer, P.D., Kim, C.K., Linke, M.J., Pogue, C.L., Huerkamp, M.J., Chrisp, C.E., Lerro, A.V., Wixson, S.K., Hall, E., and Shultz, L.D. (1989). Outbreaks of *Pneumocystis carinii* pneumonia in colonies of immunodeficient mice. *Infect. Immun.* 57: 62–70.

Watts, J. and Chandler, F. (1991). Evolving concepts of infection by *Pneumocystis carinii*. In P. Rosen and R. Fechner (eds), *Pathology Annual*. Appleton & Lange, Norwalk, pp. 93–138.

Wehle, K., Schirmer, M., Dunnebacke-Hinz, J., Kupper, T., and Pfitzer, P. (1993). Quantitative differences in phagocytosis and degradation of *Pneumocystis carinii* by alveolar macrophages in AIDS and non-HIV patients in vivo. *Cytopathology* 4: 231–236.

Williams, M., Wright, J., March, K., and Martin, W.I. (1996). Human surfactant protein A enhances attachment of *Pneumocystis carinii* to rat alveolar macrophages. *Am. J. Respir. Cell Mol. Biol.* 14: 232–238.

Wright, T.W., Johnston, C.J., Harmsen, A.G., and Finkelstein, J.N. (1999a). Chemokine gene expression during *Pneumocystis carinii*-driven pulmonary inflammation. *Infect. Immun.* 67: 3452–3460.

Wright, T.W., Gigliotti, F., Finkelstein, J.N., McBride, J.T., An, C.L., and Harmsen, A.G. (1999b). Immune-mediated inflammation directly impairs pulmonary function, contributing to the pathogenesis of *Pneumocystis carinii* pneumonia. *J. Clin. Invest.* 104: 1307–1317.

Wright, T.W., Notter, R.H., Wang, Z., Harmsen, A.G., and Gigliotti, F. (2001). Pulmonary inflammation disrupts surfactant function during *Pneumocystis carinii* pneumonia. *Infect. Immun.* 69: 758–764.

Yangco, B.G., Von Bargen, J.C., Moorman, A.C., and Holmberg, S.D. (2000). Discontinuation of chemoprophylaxis against *Pneumocystis carinii* pneumonia in patients with HIV infection. *Ann. Intern. Med.* 132: 201–205.

Yong, S.J., Vuk-Pavlovic, Z., Standing, J.E., Crouch, E.C., and Limper, A.H. (2003). Surfactant protein D-mediated aggregation of *Pneumocystis carinii* impairs phagocytosis by alveolar macrophages. *Infect. Immun.* 71: 1662–1671.

Zheng, M.Q., Shellito, J.E., Marrero, L., Zhong, Q., Julian, S., Ye, P., Wallace, V., Schwarzenberger, P., and Kolls, J.K. (2001). $CD4^+$ T cell-independent vaccination against *Pneumocystis carinii* in mice. *J. Clin. Invest.* 108: 1469–1474.

14

Antibody-Mediated Immunity to *Pneumocystis* in the Lungs

Beth A. Garvy and Francis Gigliotti

1. Introduction

Pneumocystis (PC) is an opportunistic fungal agent that causes significant pneumonia in mammalian hosts. A newly proposed but as yet not universally accepted system of nomenclature has suggested that *Pneumocystis* infecting different hosts be given distinct species designations based on the host and/or molecular variations of the organisms. Under this proposed system *Pneumocystis jiroveci* would be the species that infects humans, *P. carinii* and *P. ratti* two of the several proposed distinct species that infect rats, and the remainder as yet undesignated (Stringer et al., 2001). We will use the abbreviation PC in this chapter to refer to all organisms identifying the specific host of origin when necessary for clarity. PC can be a significant problem for individuals with compromised cell-mediated immunity (CMI) including those with AIDS. It has been well documented that CD4⁺ T cell function is required for host defense against

Departments of Microbiology, Immunology, and Molecular Genetics and Internal Medicine, University of Kentucky Chandler Medical Center, Lexington, KY 40536-0298.
Departments of Pediatrics and Microbiology and Immunology, University of Rochester Medical Center, Rochester, NY 14642.

PC (Harmsen and Stankiewicz, 1990; Roths and Sidman, 1992; Hanano et al., 1996). However, it is perhaps underappreciated that normal B cell function is also a required component of host defense against PC. This is likely due to the role specific antibody plays in opsonizing and targeting organisms for phagocytosis. Additionally, B cell function other than production of specific antibody, such as interactions with T cells and cytokine production may be quite important in the efficient clearance of PC from the lungs. Recently, animal models have been used to delineate the roles of cellular and humoral immunity to PC. It is clear from these studies that competent B cell and $CD4^+$ T cell functions are crucial for effective host defense against the fungus (Marcotte et al., 1996; Lund et al., 2003). This chapter will focus on the human and animal studies that have addressed the role of specific antibody and B cells in host defense against PC.

2. Immunoreactive Proteins Expressed by *Pneumocystis*

Over the past 15 years it has been recognized that there are at least three to four immunoreactive antigens expressed on the surface of PC organisms. The predominant antigen seen on acrylamide gels is a 95–140-kDa glycoprotein, which varies in size depending on the host species (Gigliotti, 1992). This glycoprotein has been called by various names including gpA and MSG, of which the former will be used here. gpA is a mannosylated protein that is highly variable in both genotype and phenotype. The source of the variability is highly polymorphic and repeated genes that are dispersed throughout the PC genome (Stringer et al., 1993). gpA gene expression is controlled by an upstream conserved sequence (UCS) that is important in determining which gpA variants are expressed (Wada et al., 1995).

Western blot analysis indicates that there are both shared and unique gpA epitopes expressed on PC isolated from different mammalian species (Gigliotti, 1992). Expression of multiple gpA variants have been shown to be expressed in a single host suggesting that variation of surface gpA antigens may be important in evading host defenses (Angus et al., 1996). We found that monoclonal antibody pressure eliminated specific gpA phenotypes from a population of murine PC allowing other phenotypes to predominate (Gigliotti et al., 1996). However, unlike antigenic variation seen in other organisms such as trypanosomes, new phenotypes were not rapidly introduced into the population (Gigliotti et al., 1996). These studies suggest that PC uses the genotypic and phenotypic variations of gpA to evade selective antibody pressure by the host. The advantage to the organisms may simply be allowing more time to find new hosts.

In addition to gpA, other potentially immunostimulatory antigens have been identified on PC. These include a 55-kDa protein identified in rat PC that has antibody and T cell epitopes (Theus et al., 1994). An immunodominant protein of about the same molecular weight was also found localized to the surface of mouse PC (Gigliotti et al., 1998a), however it is not clear whether these are the same proteins. The mouse 55-kDa protein was found to be immunodominant in that 91% of B cell hybridomas generated from the draining lymph nodes of PC-infected severe combined immunodeficiency (SCID) mice reconstituted with immunocompetent splenocytes were specific for proteins in the 50–100 kDa range, but not gpA (Gigliotti et al., 1998a). Interestingly, in a previous study it was shown that 89% of splenic B cell hybridomas produced antibodies specific for gpA (Gigliotti and McCool, 1996) suggesting that in mice natural infection and immunization results in different types of antibody responses. In humans, seroprevalence of gpA-specific antibodies is highly variable and may differ in individuals from different world regions (Smulian et al., 1993a; Chatterton et al., 1999). In one study antibodies against a 30–40 kDa protein were shown to be relatively abundant (40–60%) in sera regardless of geographic location of the individuals (Smulian et al., 1993a). In contrast, others have found higher seroprevalence in a 50–60 kDa protein, agreeing with data in mice (Gigliotti et al., 1998a; Chatterton et al., 1999).

A host of PC-specific monoclonal antibodies (mAb) have been generated, which generally do not react across PC species. However, there are some mAb that react with gpA from multiple species and recently a screen of cross-reactive antibodies identified a protein similar to fungal proteases known as kexins (Lee et al., 2000). Antibodies to this protease (KEX-1) were shown to confer some control of PC growth when passively transferred to the lungs of infected SCID mice (Gigliotti et al., 2002). It is apparent that there are multiple potential epitopes that are targeted by antibody responses to PC. However, as will be elaborated on in subsequent sections of this chapter, antibody responses to these specific proteins do not always equate to protective immunity.

3. Specific Antibodies to *Pneumocystis* in Human Lungs

It has been known for some time that *Pneumocystis* pneumonia (PCP) is a characteristic illness in individuals with defects in humoral immunity such as hypogammaglobulinemia (Saulsbury et al., 1979; Rao and Gelfand, 1983). It is evident from serological data that humans encounter PC early in life because it has been reported that most individuals have circulating antibodies to the organisms by 4 years of life (Peglow et al., 1990). Interestingly, PCP was originally known as interstitial plasma cell pneumonia due to the predominance of plasma cells in the interstitial spaces of patients with epidemic infection such as infants living in orphanages (Burke and Good, 1973). These individuals with "epidemic" PCP are generally premature or 2- to 4-month-old infants with marasmus or malnutrition (Burke and Good, 1973). In contrast, the lung infiltrates of immunocompromised individuals with PCP are generally composed of lymphocytes and macrophages with rare polymorphonuclear cells (Burke and Good, 1973). Undoubtedly, the characteristics of the lung cellular infiltrates in persons with PCP reflect the immunodeficiency disease that has predisposed them to infection. Unfortunately, very little is known regarding the immune response to human PC in immunocompetent individuals since it is rarely diagnosed. Recent studies have indicated that primary infection may occur in immunocompetent infants, a concept that will be addressed in a later section of this chapter.

It may be inferred that humoral immunity is important for *P. jiroveci* lung infections because most individuals seroconvert to *Pneumocystis* by 2 years of age (Meuwissen et al., 1977). However, individuals with hypogammaglobulinemia are susceptible to developing PCP even though it has been reported that T cell function in these patients is normal as determined by delayed-type hypersensitivity (DTH) and responsiveness to mitogenic stimulation (Saulsbury et al., 1979; Rao and Gelfand, 1983). Although not a direct measure of T cell responses to PC, these observations imply that specific antibody is needed for protections against PCP.

Since nearly all individuals seroconvert to PC, the presence of antibodies is not diagnostic for active disease. However, in a small study, it was shown that there was an increase in serum IgG antibodies specific for a PC gpA in three individuals with atypical pneumonia, one known to have PCP (Lundgren et al., 1993). The authors suggested that increased PC-specific antibody levels could be indicative of active disease (Lundgren et al., 1993). However, in HIV-infected patients with PCP, there does not seem to be a consistent change in organism-specific antibody in the lungs (Jalil et al., 2000; Laursen et al., 2003). In fact, in many HIV-infected individuals with PCP PC-specific antibody levels in the lungs decrease during active disease (Laursen et al., 1994, 2003; Laursen and Anderson, 1998). This may make one speculate that the loss of specific antibody predisposes individuals to PC infection. However, this is very difficult to prove in humans particularly since there are often T cell losses or defects associated with the underlying immunodeficiency disease.

PC-specific IgM, IgG, and IgA have all been identified in the bronchoalveolar lavage fluid of individuals with PCP (Lundgren et al., 1993; Jalil et al., 2000). It is not specifically known whether these different isotypes contribute significantly to the clearance of PC in vivo. However, it has been recently shown that opsonization of PC cysts with specific human IgG or IgA and complement stimulated a respiratory burst in both human neutrophils and monocytes (Laursen et al., 2003). Interestingly, PC-specific IgM and complement stimulated activation of neutrophils but not monocytes (Laursen et al., 2003). Although the in vivo significance of this is unknown, it is consistent with the fact that individuals with hyper-IgM syndrome are susceptible to developing PCP possibly due to the lack of class-switched antibody (Jain et al., 1999). These patients with hyper-IgM syndrome also have defects in T cell activation due to a disruption in the CD40–CD40L interaction, making it difficult to determine whether it is antibody or T cell insufficiency that predisposes to PCP (Jain et al., 1999). However murine studies, as shown in Fig. 14.1, have suggested that interruption of the CD40–CD40L interaction disrupts both antibody and T cell-mediated immunity to PC (Wiley and Harmsen, 1995; Lund et al., 2003). It is very difficult to tease apart the roles of antibody and T cells in host defense against PC, particularly in humans. Therefore, over the past 20 years, animal models have been utilized to examine the various components to host defense against PC. These models have significantly advanced our understanding of the contributions that B cells make to the control of PC infection.

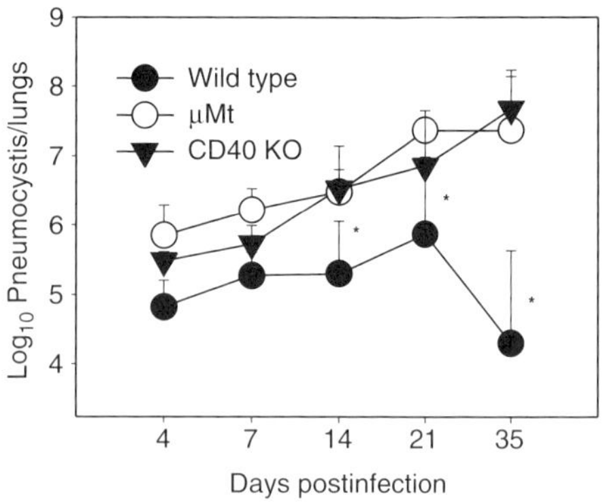

Figure 14.1. Mice deficient in CD40 (CD40 KO) or B cells (μMT) are susceptible to PC. Mice were given intratracheal inoculations of PC and lung burden quantitated microscopically over time. Reprinted with permission from *J. Immunol.* 2003; 171: 1423–1430. Copyright 2003, The American Association of Immunologists.

4. Animal Models of PCP

Some of the earliest studies examining antibody responses to PC were performed in immunosuppressed rat models. Walzer and Rutledge (1981) used corticosteroid-treated rats to determine that serum antibody titers specific for PC increased over time as corticosteroid was tapered off (Walzer and Rutledge, 1981). Furthermore, these experiments demonstrated that rats housed together or acquired from different vendors acquired serum PC-specific antibodies as they aged without evidence of active disease (Walzer and Rutledge, 1981). Recently it was shown that PC could be transmitted among immunocompetent BALB/c mice by cohousing infected with uninfected animals (Gigliotti et al., 2003). Seroconversion corresponded with clearance of the organisms as has been found in models in which mice were infected with an intratracheal bolus of organisms (Garvy and Harmsen, 1996; An et al., 2003; Lund et al., 2003). Since the appearance of antibody either in the sera or lungs does not precede clearance of PC, it is not clear from these studies whether the antibody response contributes significantly to control the infection, particularly in a primary response (Garvy and Harmsen, 1996; An et al., 2003; Gigliotti et al., 2003; Lund et al., 2003). Several strategies have been used to address the importance of specific antibody in control of PC infection and these will be discussed in the following sections.

4.1. Passive Immunization against PC

Early studies addressed the importance of antibody in host defense against PC by transferring either immune sera or monoclonal antibodies specific for PC into immunosuppressed animals. Not only is this a logical approach for identifying components of the immune system critical for host defense, but also passive immunization is used commonly in treatment and prevention of infectious diseases in the form of infusing intravenous immunoglobulin (IVIG) or monoclonal antibodies (Burns et al., 1990; Zeitlin et al., 1999). In fact, in a human trial in which renal transplant patients were treated with hyperimmune anti-cytomegalovirus (CMV) to prevent CMV infections, patients also experienced significant decreases in invasive fungal infections, including PCP (Snydman et al., 1987). This study provided at least a proof of principle in humans that passive immunization can be effective against PC.

Initial studies found that a mAb specific for gpA caused a 50–90% reduction in PC burden in the lungs of corticosteroid-suppressed rats and ferrets (Gigliotti and Hughes, 1988). This is a striking result considering that corticosteroids have known broad-spectrum immunosuppressive properties including suppressing T cell and macrophage function. Interestingly, injection of mAb (2B5) specific for an epitope of gpA into SCID mice with active infection also resulted in reduced lung PC burden but not sterilizing clearance (Gigliotti et al., 1996). The PC that remained in the lungs did not express the 2B5 epitope, however, gpA was detected on organisms using mAb for a different epitope. These findings indicate that the variation in gpA may allow organisms to evade complete eradication by the host humoral immune responses.

More recently, it has been shown that passive immunoprophylaxis via an intranasal route can be effective in reducing lung burden in immunodeficient mice exposed to PC-infected SCID mice (Gigliotti et al., 2002). Previous studies had mostly injected antibodies intraperiotoneally, however, an intranasal route of antibody transfer is attractive in that the antibodies are placed at the mucosal surfaces where PC first enters the host. In these experiments intranasal administration of mAbs directed against a kexin-like molecule, KEX1, on the first day of exposure of SCID mice to infected source mice resulted in none of the treated mice having detectable organisms in the lungs 6 to 7 weeks after treatment and withdrawal of the "seed" mice (Gigliotti et al., 2002). Interestingly, it was shown that antibodies specific for antigens other than gpA were most effective in preventing PC infection in SCID mice. These experiments demonstrated that mAb, particularly when used in combination, have the capacity of protecting mice against PC in the absence of T or B cells.

Polyclonal antiserum has also been used in vivo to protect mice against PC infection. Intraperioneal injections of hyperimmune serum into PC-infected SCID mice resulted in an 80% decrease in lung organism burden without inducing significant lung inflammation (Roths and Sidman, 1992). In contrast, transfer of immune $CD4^+$ lymphocytes resulted in clearance of organisms but also in increased morbidity due to a hyperimmune response in the lungs. However, when

SCID mice were treated with a short course of immune sera prior to transfer of $CD4^+$ cells, complete and lasting elimination of the organisms occurred without the complication of an intense immune response (Roths and Sidman, 1993). Presumably, the specific antibody opsonized the organisms targeting them for phagocytosis and destruction by resident alveolar macrophages. The presence of $CD4^+$ T cells in addition to hyperimmune serum was a key for inducing a sterilizing response. This is an interesting observation that suggests the presence of specific antibody early during a secondary response is critical for reducing the potential for lung pathology.

4.2. Active Immunization against PCP

Active immunization against PC requires B–T cell interactions, resulting in specific antibody production. Mice that lack B cells, either due to a targeted mutation in the μ chain of immunoglobulin or to depleting antibody treatment, have been shown to be susceptible to PCP (Fig. 14.1) (Harmsen and Stankiewicz, 1991; Marcotte et al., 1996; Macy et al., 2000; Lund et al., 2003). Moreover, interruption of the CD40–CD40L interaction between B and T cells, respectively, has been shown to result in the inability of murine B cells to produce class-switched PC-specific IgG (Wiley and Harmsen, 1995; Lund et al., 2003). Using a model of splenocyte reconstitution of PC-infected SCID mice, Wiley and Harmsen demonstrated that treatment with anti-CD40L monoclonal antibodies resulted in the inability to clear the infection within 21 days (Wiley and Harmsen, 1995). However, in a model in which chimeric mice were generated so that only B cells were deficient in CD40, mice were able to clear PC infection, although with a delayed kinetics, even though they did not produce class-switched antibody (Lund et al., 2003). In addition, mice deficient in Fcγ receptors also cleared PC infection but with the same delayed kinetics as demonstrated with the CD40-deficient chimeric mice (Lund et al., 2003). Together these studies suggest that class-switched antibody production is not required for clearance of PC infection. Although not specifically demonstrated by these studies, it is possible that PC-specific IgM was sufficient for clearance of infection. However, this may not be an adequate explanation for these results since we have shown that passive immunization with a PC-specific murine monoclonal IgM did not result in complete eradication of organisms (Gigliotti and Hughes, 1988; Gigliotti et al., 1996). As mentioned previously, humans with hyper-IgM syndrome produce IgM but are susceptible to PCP suggesting that IgM is not sufficient for clearance of the organisms (Jain et al., 1999). However, B cells are required for clearance, which raises the question of what specific functions are required of B cells if production of class-switched antibody is optional? This is a difficult question to answer because, as will be discussed below, specific antibody can be quite effective at facilitating clearance of PC. It is very difficult to separate antibody-producing functions from other B cell functions in vivo. However, possibilities include antigen presentation to T cells, costimulation of T cells, and/or cytokine production.

Several studies have been performed that demonstrate that specific antibody production positively impacts protection against PCP. In one study, normal immunocompetent mice were immunized with live PC and allowed to resolve the infection (Harmsen et al., 1995). After documenting that an antibody response had taken place, mice were depleted of T cells and rechallenged with PC organisms. Immunized mice were completely resistant to infection, whereas T cell depletion of naïve mice rendered them susceptible to PCP (Harmsen et al., 1995). This same strategy was used in IL-4 or

IFN-γ knockout mice to demonstrate that the IgG isotype, whether a Th1-biased IgG2a or a Th2-biased IgG1 response, was irrelevant for facilitating clearance of PC (Fig. 14.2) (Garvy et al., 1997). Both IL-4 and IFN-γ-deficient mice resolved infection utilizing different predominant IgG isotypes. Interestingly, we also found that wild-type mice generated a Th2-like antibody response that was primarily IgG1, though a T cell bias in the pulmonary response to PC has not been reported (Garvy et al., 1997).

These results, in which immunosuppressed mice were protected from developing PCP if they were immunized against whole organisms prior to T cell suppression, have led to further studies examining the potential for immunotherapy for at-risk humans. These could include individuals who are slated for chemotherapy susceptible to PC infection for a limited period of time. A whole cell vaccine is unlikely, since we are unable to propagate PC in culture systems. Therefore, some effort has been made in identifying target antigens expressed by PC. In an effort to identify the repertoire of PC antigens recognized by antibody-secreting B cells, monoclonal antibody-secreting hybridomas were produced from draining lymph node cells isolated from PC-infected and splenocyte-reconstituted SCID mice (Gigliotti et al., 1998a). This strategy yielded 54 hybridomas that secreted monoclonal antibodies specific for PC. Of these, 91% were specific for antigens other than gpA. Most of these, 55%, reacted with a 50–65 kDa antigen. Similarly, Pascale et al. (1999) demonstrated that intranasal immunization with soluble PC antigens resulted in a strong antibody response to a 55–65 kDa antigen. This could be a homolog of the 55 kDa PC antigen that has been shown to elicit a protective immune response in rats (Smulian et al., 1993b). Interestingly, these data suggest that gpA may be immunodominant when PC is used as a vaccine, however, the antigenic targets for a protective response are quite different when PCP is acquired by a more natural route in the lungs. To confirm this hypothesis, mice were immunized intraperitoneally with gpA or whole PC, resulting in comparable specific IgG responses and then depleted of CD4 T cells and challenged with live organisms in the lungs (Gigliotti et al., 1998b). Interestingly, mice immunized with gpA were not protected from subsequent PC challenge while mice immunized with whole PC were (Gigliotti et al.,

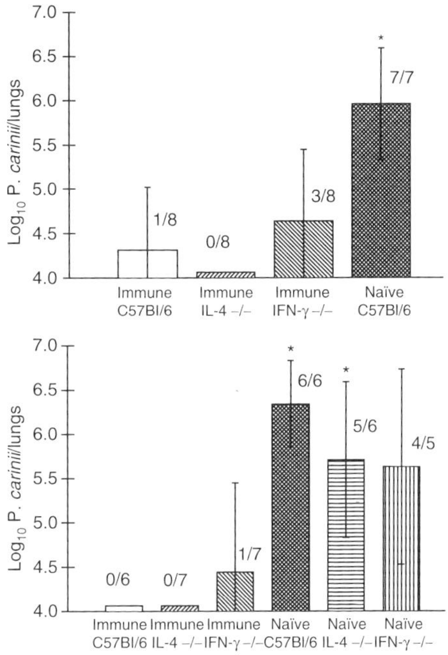

Figure 14.2. PC-specific antibody facilitates clearance of organisms in the absence of CD4 T cells. Wild type (C57Bl/6), IL-4 deficient (IL-4 –/–), and IFN-γ deficient (IFN-γ –/–) mice were infected with PC and allowed to resolve the infection. Mice were then depleted of CD4 T cells using a monoclonal antibody and rechallenged with PC organisms. Lung PC burdens were determined at day 21 postreinfection. CD4-depleted naïve mice are shown for comparison. Numbers over the bars represent the number of mice without detectable lung PC burden/total number of mice. Reprinted with permission from *Infect. Immun.* 1997; 65: 5052–5056.

1998b). This is consistent with passive immunization data that demonstrated that monoclonal antibodies specific for gpA have some role in controlling the growth of PC organisms, but are unable to facilitate complete eradication of the organisms (Gigliotti and Hughes, 1988; Gigliotti et al., 1996).

An important theme that continues to emerge regarding the humoral immunity to PC is that competent $CD4^+$ T cells are required for generating effective primary and secondary antibody responses. This means that even though we can identify the antigens needed for effective vaccination, unless a strategy is adopted that bypasses the need for competent helper T cells, long-term protection from PCP is not possible. Recently this issue was addressed by vaccinating $CD4^+$ T cell-deficient mice with bone marrow-derived dendritic cells expressing CD40L and pulsed with PC antigen (Zheng et al., 2001). This strategy resulted in a protective humoral response to PC characterized by IgG reactivity predominantly against a 55-kDa antigen of PC (Zheng et al., 2001). This non-gpA antigen is possibly the same antigen reported previously to be immunodominant in protective responses to PC in mice and rats (Smulian et al., 1993b; Gigliotti et al., 1998a; Pascale et al., 1999). Notably, vaccination was only effective if dendritic cells were transduced with a CD40L-expressing adenoviral vector (Zheng et al., 2001) confirming that the ligation of CD40 on B cells is critical for generation of PC-specific class-switched antibody.

5. Humoral Responses to PC in Neonates

Exposure to PC occurs early in life as evidenced by the fact that most individuals have PC-specific serum antibodies by the age of 4 years (Peglow et al., 1990). PCP was originally identified in malnourished infants (Burke and Good, 1973). More recently, it has been recognized that a significant proportion of otherwise healthy young children carry PC organisms and may acquire primary infections which are asymptomatic or mildly symptomatic and indistinguishable from other mild respiratory infections so common in young children (Vargas et al., 1999, 2001). This could be because even the developing immune system is able to mount an effective immune response to PC, which limits the extent of infection, although there is very little data in human infants regarding the development of the host response to PC.

5.1. Maternal Antibody

Very young infants acquire antibody in utero as well as through suckling and so it is thought that infants are protected from a number of infectious agents as long as they have maternal antibody. Maternal antibody begins to wane in human infants by about 6 months of age. In this regard, it was reported that a foal with hypogammaglobulinemia presumably due to the lack of colostrum from the dam, developed PCP and died at 46 days of age (Tanaka et al., 1994). In a murine model of PC infection, dams were immunized with the organisms prior to breeding and during gestation in order to develop high PC-specific antibody levels in both the blood and milk of the dams (Garvy and Harmsen, 1996). Offspring from the immunized dams were infected with PC within 72 h of birth. Neonatal mice from immunized dams had elevated serum PC-specific antibody at day 2 postinfection compared to neonates from naïve dams (Garvy and Harmsen, 1996). Moreover, significant levels of PC-specific IgG were found in the bronchial alveolar lavage fluids of neonatal mice born to immunized mothers (B.A. Garvy, unpublished observations). Elevated antibody levels corresponded to a 90% reduction of lung PC burden between days 15 and 20 postinfection whereas there was no reduction on lung burden over that time in mice from naïve dams (Garvy and Harmsen, 1996).

Even though maternal antibody facilitated expedited clearance of PC, the response was still slower than seen in immunized adult mice and was similar to the kinetics of clearance of adult naïve mice. This may have been due to the lack of responsiveness of neonatal alveolar macrophages to opsonized organisms, an issue that has yet to be resolved. These studies clearly show that maternal antibody can play a significant role in clearance of PC in neonates.

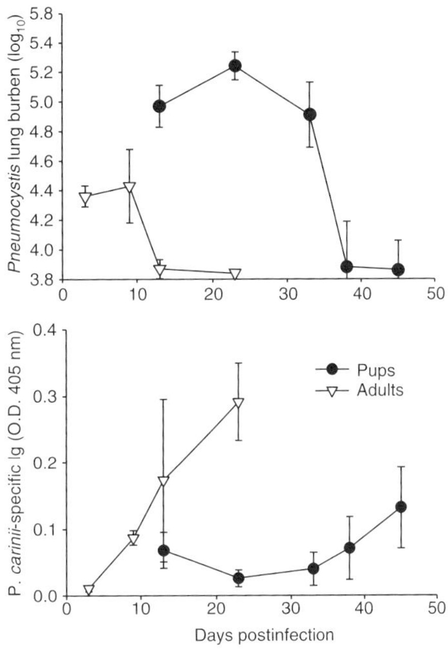

Figure 14.3. Clearance of PC precedes appearance of PC-specific antibodies in the serum of neonatal mice. Mice were infected with PC and lung organism burden and sera PC-specific antibody levels determined at the indicated time points. Adapted with permission from Garvy, B.A. and Harmsen, A.G. (1996). *Infect. Immun.* 64: 3987–3992.

5.2. B Lymphocytes and Antibody

Soulez et al. (1989) reported that weanling rabbits develop spontaneous infection with PC and that when they develop a humoral response the organisms are cleared. Consistent with this observation, serum antibody levels are very low in PC-infected neonatal mice as compared to infected adults through about 5 weeks postinfection (Garvy and Harmsen, 1996). Similarly, we found PC-specific antibody secreting cells in the draining lymph nodes of adult mice between days 9 and 15 postinfection whereas these cells were present at very low frequencies in mice infected as newborns until day 35 postinfection (B.A. Garvy and A.G. Harmsen, unpublished observations). Moreover, our attempts at generating PC-specific antibody-secreting hybridomas from draining lymph nodes isolated from PC-infected neonatal mice have not been successful perhaps indicative of slow development of B cell responses in neonates (B.A. Garvy and F. Gigliotti, unpublished observations).

The appearance of PC-specific antibody in mice infected as infants corresponds to clearance of the organisms (Fig. 14.3) (Garvy and Harmsen, 1996). This antibody response was shown to be protective even when 6-weeks-old mice infected as neonates were depleted of $CD4^+$ cells and rechallenged with PC. These animals had high levels of PC-specific IgG in the sera and cleared a second challenge with PC in the absence of T cells (B.A. Garvy and A.G. Harmsen, unpublished observations). These studies are consistent with the known importance of B cells and antibody for protection against PC in adults, however, it is still not clear as to why there is a delay in the appearance of antibody and antibody-secreting cells in neonatal mice. One possibility is the lack of appropriate costimulatory signals such as CD40L expressed on T cells as discussed above. It is also possible that migration of B cells to the site of infection is delayed. This could be due to the lack of chemokine production or the inability to upregulate adhesion molecules. These issues are currently being examined.

References

An, C.L., Gigliotti, F., and Harmsen, A.G. (2003). Exposure of immunocompetent adult mice to *Pneumocystis carinii* f. sp. muris by cohousing: Growth of *P. carinii* f. sp. muris and host immune response. *Infect. Immun.* 71: 2065–2070.

Angus, C.W., Tu, A., Vogel, P., Qin, M., and Kovacs, J.A. (1996). Expression of variants of the major surface glycoprotein on *Pneumocystis carinii*. *J. Exp. Med.* 183: 1229–1234.

Burke, B.A. and Good, R.A. (1973). *Pneumocystis carinii* infection. *Medicine* 52: 23–52.

Burns, S.M., Read, J.A., Yap, P.L., and Brettle, R.P. (1990). Reduced concentrations of IgG antibodies to *Pneumocystis carinii* in HIV-infected patients during active *Pneumocystis carinii* infection and the possibility of passive immunisation. *J. Infect.* 20: 33–39.

Chatterton, J.M.W., Joss, A.W.L., Pennington, T.H., and Ho-Yen, D.O. (1999). Usefulness of rat-derived antigen in the serodiagnosis of *Pneumocystis carinii* infection. *J. Med. Microbiol.* 48: 681–687.

Garvy, B.A. and Harmsen, A.G. (1996). Susceptibility to *Pneumocystis carinii* infection: Host responses of neonatal mice from immune or naive mothers and of immune or naive adults. *Infect. Immun.* 64: 3987–3992.

Garvy, B.A., Wiley, J.A., Gigliotti, F., and Harmsen, A.H. (1997). Protection against *Pneumocystis carinii* pneumonia by antibodies generated from either T helper 1 or T helper 2 responses. *Infect. Immun.* 65: 5052–5056.

Gigliotti, F. (1992). Host species-specific antigenic variation of a mannosylated surface glycoprotein of *Pneumocystis carinii*. *J. Infect. Dis.* 165: 329–336.

Gigliotti, F. and Hughes, W.T. (1988). Passive immunoprophylaxis with specific monoclonal antibody confers partial protection against *Pneumocystis carinii* pneumonitis in animal models. *J. Clin. Invest.* 81: 1666–1668.

Gigliotti, F. and McCool, T. (1996). Glycoprotein A is the immunodominant antigen of *Pneumocystis carinii* in mice following immunization. *Parasitol. Res.* 82: 90–91.

Gigliotti, F., Garvy, B.A., and Harmsen, A.G. (1996). Antibody-mediated shift in the profile of glycoprotein A phenotypes observed in a mouse model of *Pneumocystis carinii* pneumonia. *Infect. Immun.* 64: 1892–1899.

Gigliotti, F., Garvy, B.A., Haidaris, C.G., and Harmsen, A.G. (1998a). Recognition of *Pneumocystis carinii* antigens by local antibody-secreting cells following resolution of *P. carinii* pneumonia in mice. *J. Infect. Dis.* 178: 235–242.

Gigliotti, F., Wiley, J.A., and Harmsen, A.G. (1998b). Immunization with *Pneumocystis carinii* gpA is immunogenic but not protective in a mouse model of *P. carinii* pneumonia. *Infect. Immun.* 66: 3179–3182.

Gigliotti, F., Haidaris, C.G., Wright, T.W., and Harmsen, A.G. (2002). Passive intranasal monoclonal antibody prophylaxis against murine *Pneumocystis carinii* pneumonia. *Infect. Immun.* 70: 1069–1074.

Gigliotti, F., Harmsen, A.G., and Wright, T.W. (2003). Characterization of transmission of *Pneumocystis carinii* f. sp. muris through immunocompetent BALB/c mice. *Infect. Immun.* 71: 3852–3856.

Hanano, R., Reifenberg, K., and Kaufmann, S.H.E. (1996). Naturally acquired *Pneumocystis carinii* pneumonia in gene disruption mutant mice: Roles of distinct T-cell populations in infection. *Infect. Immun.* 64: 3201–3209.

Harmsen, A.G. and Stankiewicz, M. (1990). Requirement for $CD4^+$ cells in resistance to *Pneumocystis carinii* pneumonia in mice. *J. Exp. Med.* 172: 937–945.

Harmsen, A.G. and Stankiewicz, M. (1991). T cells are not sufficient for resistance to *Pneumocystis carinii* pneumonia in mice. *J. Protozool.* 38: 44S–45S.

Harmsen, A.G., Chen, W., and Gigliotti, F. (1995). Active immunity to *Pneumocystis carinii* reinfection in T-cell-depleted mice. *Infect. Immun.* 63: 2391–2395.

Jain, A., Atkinson, T.P., Lipsky, P.E., Slater, J.E., Nelson, D.L., and Strober, W. (1999). Defects of T-cell effector function and post-thymic maturation in X-linked hyper-IgM syndrome. *J. Clin. Invest.* 103: 1151–1158.

Jalil, A., Moja, P., Lambert, C., Perol, M., Cotte, L., Livrozet, J.M., Boibieux, A., Vergnon, J.M., Lucht, F., Tran, R., Contini, C., and Genin, C. (2000). Decreased production of local immunoglobulin A to *Pneumocystis carinii* in bronchoalveolar lavage fluid from human immunodeficiency virus-positive patients. *Infect. Immun.* 68: 1054–1060.

Laursen, A.L. and Anderson, P.L. (1998). Low levels of IgG antibodies against *Pneumocystis carinii* among HIV-infected patients. *Scand. J. Infect. Dis.* 30: 495–499.

Laursen, A.L., Jensen, B.N., and Andersen, P.L. (1994). Local antibodies against *Pneumocystis carinii* in bronchoalveolar lavage fluid. *Eur. Respir. J.* 7: 679–685.

Laursen, A.L., Obel, N., Holmskov, U., Jensenius, J.C., Aliouat, E.M., and Anderson, P.L. (2003). Activation of the respiratory burst by *Pneumocystis carinii*. Efficiency of different antibody isotypes, complement, lung surfactant protein D, and mannan-binding lectin. *APMIS* 111: 405–415.

Lee, L.H., Gigliotti, F., Wright, T.W., Simpson-Haidaris, P.J., Weinberg, G.A., and Haidaris, C.G. (2000). Molecular characterization of KEX1, a kexin-like protease in mouse *Pneumocystis carinii*. *Gene* 242: 141–150.

Lund, F.E., Schuer, K., Hollifield, M., Randall, T.D., and Garvy, B.A. (2003). Clearance of *Pneumocystis carinii* in mice is dependent on B cells but not on *P. carinii*-specific antibody. *J. Immunol.* 171: 1423–1430.

Lundgren, B., Lebech, M., Lind, K., Nielson, J.O., and Lundgren, J.D. (1993). Antibody response to a major human *Pneumocystis carinii* surface antigen in patients without evidence of immunosuppression and in patients with suspected atypical pneumonia. *Eur. J. Microbiol. Infect. Dis.* 12: 105–109.

Macy, J.D., Weir, E.C., Compton, S.R., Shlomchik, M.J., and Brownstein, D.G. (2000). Dual infection with *Pneumocystis carinii* and *Pasturella pneumotropica* in B cell-deficient mice: Diagnosis and therapy. *Lab. Animal Sci.* 50: 49–55.

Marcotte, H., Levesque, D., Delanay, K., Bourgeault, A., de la Durantaye, R., Brochu, S., and Lavoie, M.C. (1996). *Pneumocystis carinii* infection in transgenic B cell-deficient mice. *J. Infect. Dis.* 173: 1034–1037.

Meuwissen, J.H.E.T., Tauber, I., Leeuwenberg, A.D.E.M., Beckers, J.J.A., and Siebe, M. (1977). Parasitologic and serologic observations of infection with *Pneumocystis* in humans. *J. Infect. Dis.* 136: 43–49.

Pascale, J.M., Shaw, M.M., Durant, P.J., Amador, A.A., Bartlett, M.S., Smith, J.W., Gregorty, R.L., and McLaughlin, G.L. (1999). Intranasal immunization confers protection against murine *Pneumocystis carinii* lung infection. *Infect. Immun.* 67: 805–809.

Peglow, S.L., Smulian, A.G., Linke, M.J., Pogue, C.L., Nurre, S., Crisler, J., Phair, J., Gold, J.W., Armstrong, D., and Walzer, P.D. (1990). Serologic responses to *Pneumocystis carinii* antigens in health and disease. *J. Infect. Dis.* 161: 296–306.

Rao, C.P. and Gelfand, E.W. (1983). *Pneumocystis carinii* pneumonitis in patients with hypogammaglobulinemia and intact T cell immunity. *J. Pediatr.* 103: 410–412.

Roths, J.B. and Sidman, C.L. (1992). Both immunity and hyperresponsiveness to *Pneumocystis carinii* result from transfer of $CD4^+$ but not $CD8^+$ T cells into severe combined immunodeficiency mice. *J. Clin. Invest.* 90: 673–678.

Roths, J.B. and Sidman, C.L. (1993). Single and combined humoral and cell-mediated immunotherapy of *Pneumocystis carinii* pneumonia in immunodeficient SCID mice. *Infect. Immun.* 61: 1641–1649.

Saulsbury, F.T., Bernstein, M.T., and Winkelstein, J.A. (1979). *Pneumocystis carinii* pneumonia as the presenting infection in congenital hypogammaglobulinemia. *J. Pediatr.* 95: 559–561.

Smulian, A.G., Sullivan, D.W., Linke, M.J., Halsey, N.A., Quinn, T.C., MacPhail, A.P., Hernandez Avila, M.A., Hong, S.T., and Walzer, P.D. (1993a). Geographic variation in the humoral response to *Pneumocystis carinii*. *J. Infect. Dis.* 167: 1243–1247.

Smulian, A.G., Theus, S.A., Denko, N., Walzer, P.D., and Stringer, J.R. (1993b). A 55 kDa antigen of *Pneumocystis carinii*: Analysis of the cellular immune response and characterization of the gene. *Mol. Microbiol.* 7: 745–753.

Snydman, D.R., Werner, B.G., Heinze-Lacey, B., Berardi, V.P., Tilney, N.L., Kirkman, R.L., Milford, E.L., Cho, S.I., Bush, H.L., and Levey, A.S. (1987). Use of cytomegalovirus immune globulin to prevent cytomegalovirus disease in renal-transplant recipients. *N. Engl. J. Med.* 317: 1049–1054.

Soulez, B., Dei-Cas, E., Charet, P., Mougeot, G., Caillaux, M., and Camus, D. (1989). The young rabbit: A nonimmunosuppressed model for *Pneumocystis carinii* pneumonia. *J. Infect. Dis.* 160: 355–356.

Stringer, S.L., Garbe, T., Sunkin, S.M., and Stringer, J.R. (1993). Genes encoding antigenic surface glycoproteins in *Pneumocystis carinii* from humans. *J. Eukaryot. Microbiol.* 40: 821–826.

Stringer, J.R., Cushion, M.T., and Wakefield, A. (2001). New nomenclature for the genus *Pneumocystis*. *J. Eukaryot. Microbiol.* Suppl: 184S–189S.

Tanaka, S., Kaji, Y., Taniyama, H., Matsukawa, K., Ochiai, K., and Itakura, C. (1994). *Pneumocystis carinii* pneumonia in a thoroughbred foal. *J. Vet. Med. Sci.* 56: 135–137.

Theus, S.A., Sullivan, D.W., Walzer, P.D., and Smulian, A.G. (1994). Cellular responses to a 55-kilodalton recombinant *Pneumocystis carinii* antigen. *Infect. Immun.* 62: 3479–3484.

Vargas, S.L., Ponce, C.A., Hughes, W.T., Wakefield, A.E., Weitz, J.C., Donoso, S., Ulloa, A.V., Madrid, P., Gould, S., Latorre, J.J., Ávila, R., Benveniste, S., Gallor, M., Belletti, J., and López, R. (1999). Association of primary *Pneumocystis carinii* infection and sudden infant death syndrome. *Clin. Infect. Dis.* 29: 1489–1493.

Vargas, S.L., Hughes, W.T., Santolaya, M.E., Ulloa, A.V., Ponce, C.A., Cabrera, C.E., Cumsille, F., and Gigliotti, F. (2001). Search for primary infection by *Pneumocystis carinii* in a cohort of normal, healthy infants. *Clin. Infect. Dis.* 32: 855–861.

Wada, M., Sunkin, S.M., Stringer, J.R., and Nakamura, Y. (1995). Antigenic variation by positional control of major surface glycoprotein gene expression in *Pneumocystis carinii*. *J. Infect. Dis.* 171: 1563–1568.

Walzer, P.D. and Rutledge, M.E. (1981). Humoral immunity in experimental *Pneumocystis carinii* infection I. Serum and bronchial lavage fluid antibody responses in rats. *J. Lab. Clin. Med.* 97: 820–833.

Wiley, J.A. and Harmsen, A.G. (1995). CD40 ligand is required for resolution of *Pneumocystis carinii* pneumonia in mice. *J. Immunol.* 155: 3525–3529.

Zeitlin, L., Cone, R.A., and Whaley, K.J. (1999). Using monoclonal antibodies to prevent mucosal transmission of epidemic infectious diseases. *Emerg. Infect. Dis.* 5: 66.

Zheng, M., Shellito, J.E., Marrero, L., Zhong, Q., Julian, S., Ye, P., Wallace, V., Schwarzenberger, P., and Kolls, J.K. (2001). $CD4^+$ T cell-independent vaccination against *Pneumocystis carinii* in mice. *J. Clin. Invest.* 108: 1469–1474.

15

Innate and Adaptive Immunity against *Candida* spp. Infections in the Gastrointestinal Tract

Robert D. Wagner

1. Introduction

The *Candida* species lead dual lives as commensal passengers and as potential agents of disease in the gastrointestinal (GI) tracts of mammalian hosts. Their dual nature has intrigued medical science for many decades. Now, in the twenty-first century, a better understanding of intestinal ecology and mucosal immunology is starting to piece together the puzzle of these opportunistic pathogenic fungi.

Mucosal candidiasis in humans usually occurs in the oral and vaginal cavities, while

National Center for Toxicological Research, Microbiology Division, Jefferson, Arkansas, USA.

systemic infections occur from contamination of medical devices or invasion from the microflora of the alimentary tract. Infections restricted to GI tract tissues, which lead to apparent morbidity, are not commonly reported; however, humans can get intestinal candidiasis when the endogenous microflora is depleted by antimicrobial drug therapy (Ruiz-Sánchez et al., 2002). Germfree mice are also more susceptible to GI tract infections by *Candida albicans* than mice with a conventional intestinal microflora (Wagner et al., 1997). These studies agree with the concept of colonization resistance by an intestinal microflora that prevents infections by enteric pathogens. In this report, intestinal infection by *Candida* spp. will be defined as invasion of the intestinal epithelium and induction of inflammation, as apposed to colonization, which is the persistence of fungus in the GI tract.

Animal models of infection have been very helpful in gaining an understanding of the pathogenic mechanisms that may be at work in human candidiasis (Wiesner et al., 2001; Bendel et al., 2002). Like humans, mice do not typically get severe intestinal infections with *Candida* spp., but they are susceptible to esophageal and gastric candidiasis, especially in the keratinized gastric antrum (Wagner et al., 1997). The human stomach does not have a keratinized epithelium and gastric candidiasis is not generally found in humans. However, candidiasis is often described in the keratinized esophageal epithelium of immunodeficient humans.

Apart from intestinal infections, the presence of *Candida* spp. in the GI tract may induce other forms of disease. Human celiac disease may be triggered by *C. albicans* (Nieuwenhuizen et al., 2003). The *C. albicans* hyphal wall protein 1 (HWP1) is homologous to T cell epitopes involved in celiac disease, which can initiate autoimmune disease by molecular mimicry. Although *Candida* spp. have been found to be involved in a variety of disorders collectively named "*Candida* hypersensitivity syndrome," analysis of accumulated research has found no evidence in support of this concept (Lacour et al., 2002).

The following sections of this chapter will explore the host defense and microbial ecological reasons why intestinal *Candida* spp. infections in humans are rare, why intestinal colonization by *Candida* spp. is associated with many systemic infections, and what is now known about host defenses against *Candida* spp. in the GI tract.

2. Interactions of *Candida* spp. with the GI Tract Environment

When a *Candida* sp. yeast cell enters the intestinal lumen, it interacts with the preexisting intestinal microflora, it may adhere to the mucous layer that coats the epithelium, or it may interact with cells of the host epithelium and mucosal immune system. These interactions may lead to several outcomes for the yeast; it may pass on through the GI tract without host cell contact, it may interact with the immune system of the host and establish either a defensive or tolerance response, or it may be stimulated to germinate into a hyphal morphology.

Various reports suggest that *C. albicans* is a commensal in the GI tracts of 3% to 88% of normal immunocompetent people (Lacour et al., 2002). Considering a median incidence of 45% of people colonized with *Candida* spp., obviously, the GI tract is a significant point of contact between the fungus and the host defenses. Even though *Candida* spp. are often found in the GI tracts of humans, confirmed mucosal infections are rarely reported. Immunocompetent humans are rarely diagnosed with intestinal *Candida* sp. infections because of the difficulty in obtaining a diagnosis by endoscopic biopsy (Lacour et al., 2002). Presumably, intestinal candidiasis is not usually severe enough to require an endoscopic examination.

A corollary to the previous statement is intestinal candidiasis resulting from disruption of the barrier to *Candida* colonization by the intestinal microflora after broad-spectrum antibiotic treatments. In a recent report, Ruiz-Sánchez et al. (2002) described the case of an 8-year-old girl treated with antimicrobials for a respiratory infection, who developed a confirmed case of intestinal candidiasis. Subsequent nystatin treatment eliminated the infection.

Several steps appear to predispose a host to GI tract candidiasis. The first step necessary for GI tract candidiasis or intestinal colonization is adhesion of the fungus to mucous or epithelial cells. The mucous layer is probably the first point of contact for a *Candida* cell in the GI tract. The capacity for binding of *Candida* spp. to intestinal mucin correlates with colonization and virulence (de Repentigny et al., 2000). In the latter report, the more virulent strains, *C. albicans*, *C. tropicalis*, and *C. dublinensis*, adhered better to mucous than the less virulent *C. lusitaniae*, *C. krusei*, and *C. glabrata*. Mucous binding by *Candida* spp. appears to be mediated by hydrophobic interactions, rather than by specific mannose receptors, which are used for adherence to epithelial cells (de Repentigny et al., 2000).

Another factor in colonization and virulence is the ability of *Candida* cells to separate from bound mucin and attach to epithelial cells. *C. albicans* produces a secreted aspartic protease 2 (SAP2), which degrades mucous and facilitates penetration of the intestinal mucous layer to the epithelium (Colina et al., 1996; de Repentigny et al., 2000). Untreated AIDS patients usually develop mucocutaneous candidiasis, but the therapeutic introduction of antiviral HIV protease inhibitors serendipitously prevents candidiasis, apparently by inhibition of the SAP proteases secreted by *C. albicans* (Bektic et al., 2001).

After mucous binding and penetration, cells of *Candida* spp. can adhere to intestinal epithelial cells (IEC). Several mechanisms are used by *C. albicans* to adhere to IEC; in one mechanism, *C. albicans* adheres to IEC with the β-1,2-mannosides located on their surfaces, which differ from the α-1,2-mannosides present on most enteric commensal bacteria (Dromer et al., 2002). Another mechanism for adherence of *C. albicans* to IEC is mediated by 15.7 kDa receptors on the *C. albicans* cell surface that can adhere to glycosphingolipids similar to human H and A blood group antigens (Cameron and Douglas, 1996). Adherence of *Candida* spp. to epithelial cells or to artificial surfaces is also proportional to the hydrophobicity of the surface (Panagoda et al., 2001).

In mammalian immune systems, leukocytes migrate from one tissue to another under the control of surface adhesion receptors called integrins. Integrin-like adhesion molecules expressed on the surface of *C. albicans* cells were first observed in a complement-binding effect similar to the E-rosetting of sheep erythrocytes, a test for integrins (Hostetter, 1999). The *C. albicans* *INT*1 gene product, which enhances binding in the presence of bacterial endotoxin, mediates colonization of the cecum in mice (Bendel et al., 2000). The latter study suggests that the presence of the indigenous microflora can enhance the ability of *Candida* spp. to colonize and infect the intestinal tract. In contrast, germfree immunocompetent mice are more susceptible to lethal candidiasis of endogenous origin than mice with bacteria in their GI tracts (Wagner et al., 1996). This contrast indicates that the specific roles of the indigenous microflora still need to be elucidated.

After adhesion of *Candida* sp. to IEC, the next step is tissue invasion, which may occur by physical disruption of the epithelial barrier by the fungus or by receptor-mediated endocytosis across the epithelial monolayer (Drago et al., 2000). A long debated concept that *C. albicans* is a more invasive pathogen in the hyphal form than the yeast form continues, but invasiveness by both forms has been observed and discussed (Gow et al., 2002). Both yeast and hyphal forms appear to bind to the surface of enterocytes equally well, mediated by the *INT*1 gene product (Wiesner et al., 2002). In contrast, other studies reported hyphae were more invasive, requiring expression of the *CDC*24 gene product for morphogenesis (Bassilana et al., 2003). In the latter study, *CDC*24 gene-deficient mutants of *C. albicans* were unable to transform from blastospores to hyphae and were also less invasive (Bassilana et al., 2003). The debate will continue until the pathogenic mechanisms of *C. albicans* are more fully characterized.

3. Recruitment of Host Defenses

If the host's epithelial surface has been breached and the immune system has been challenged by *Candida* spp., a process is set in motion to recruit the resources needed for an effective protective immune response. The first step in initiation of an immune response is detection of *Candida* sp. antigens and host cell-secreted molecules that indicate the presence of damage to the epithelial monolayer. Early recruitment of inflammatory and immune responses is mediated by chemokines and other molecules. Enterocytes are the primary source of the C–C chemokine macrophage inhibitory protein-3α (MIP-3α) for the recruitment of mononuclear cells (Fig. 15.1) to an intestinal infection (Kwon et al., 2002). Interleukin-15 (IL-15) secretion by antigen-presenting cells (APC) is an essential activation signal for innate immune responses, where it is essential for the development and inhibition of apoptosis in natural killer (NK) and natural killer T (NKT) cells, TCR$\gamma\delta^+$ intestinal intraepithelial lymphocytes (IEL), and macrophage and dendritic cells (DC) maturation (Fig. 15.1) (Ohteki, 2002).

Complement-dependent anti-*Candida* activation occurs, in part, by a lectin-activated complement pathway. The mannans present on the *Candida* sp. cell surface may be bound by initiators of the complement cascade. The collectin family member, mannose-binding lectin-C (MBL), is produced by IEC in mice and can activate the complement cascade (Fig. 15.1) after binding to *Candida* sp. surface mannans (Wagner et al., 2003).

After enterocytes, macrophages and DC in the GI tract are among the first members of the mucosal immune system to recognize *Candida* spp. antigens and recruit other immunological assets. DC are the predominant APC of *Candida* sp. antigens to mucosal helper T cells (Fig. 15.1). DC phagocytose *Candida* spp. via a mannose–fucose receptor, without the need for opsonization (Newman and Holly, 2001).

A fascinating phenomenon has been reported for the ability of DC on the basolateral side of an epithelial cell monolayer to push dendrites or lammelapodia between epithelial cell tight junctions in vitro, and sample antigens on the apical side of the monolayer (Rescigno et al., 2001). Studies in vivo with mice have shown that DC do not need to be associated with formally organized lymphoid tissue to sample luminal antigens (Alpan et al., 2001).

Besides DC, the major type of cells that sample antigens from the intestinal lumen is the specialized Peyer's patch microfold (M) cell. Particles transported by M cells into the subepithelial domes of Peyer's patches are readily engulfed by $CD11c^+$ $CD11b^-$ $CD8\alpha^-$ (myeloid) DC. These DC are induced by antigens to migrate to the B cell follicles and parafollicular T cell zones within the Peyer's patches (Shreedhar et al., 2003). The lamina propria of the human colon contains about 0.6% immature ($CD11^+$ $HLA\text{-}DR^-$ lin^- $CD40^+$ $CD83^{low}$ $CD86^{low}$ $CD80^-$ $CD25^-$) DC that spontaneously mature in vitro to a $CD40^{high}$ $CD83^{high}$ $CD86^{high}$ $CD80^{high}$ phenotype (Bell et al., 2001). These matured cells have low endocytic activity, but they can stimulate mixed leukocyte reactions in vitro.

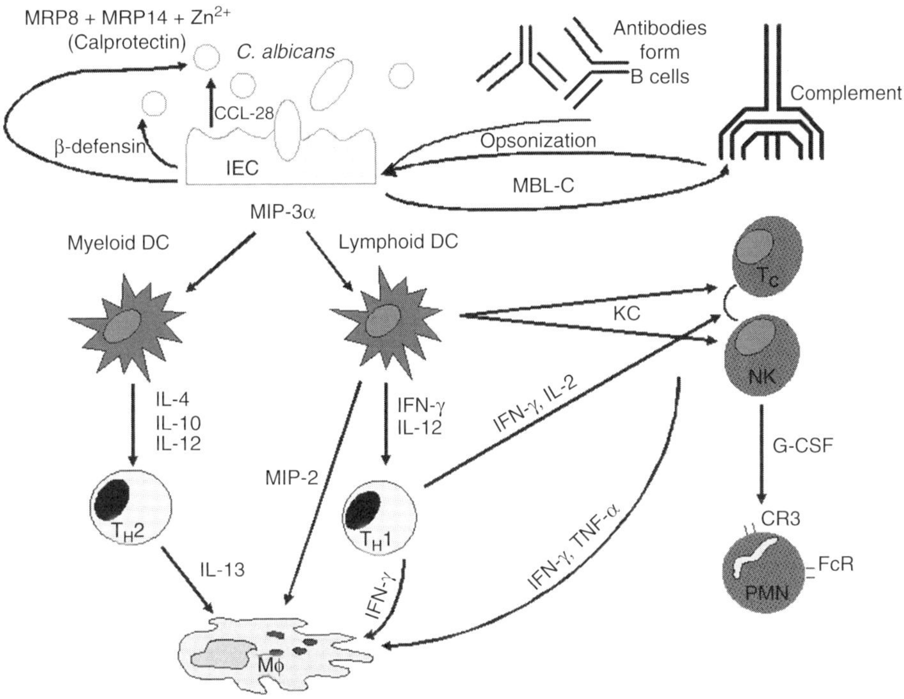

Figure 15.1. Recruitment and activation of immune effectors to GI tract *Candida* sp. infections. Invasion of intestinal epithelial cells (IEC) by *Candida* sp. initiates a cascade of activation that mobilizes innate and adaptive immune cells and production of protective molecules. Abbreviations: ADCC, antibody-dependent cell-mediated cytotoxicity (ADCC); CCL; cathepsin-L; CR3, complement receptor 3; DC, dendritic cell; FcR, Fc receptor; G-CSF, granulocyte-colony-stimulating factor; IFN, interferon; IL, interleukin; MBL, mannose-binding lectin; Mϕ, macrophage; MIP, migration inhibitory protein; MRP, migration inhibitory binding protein related; NK; natural killer; PMN, polymorphonuclear cell; T_C, cytotoxic T cell; T_H, helper T cell.

Viable *C. albicans* blastospores, but not hyphae, induce DC adoptively transferred into mice to direct a systemic T_H1-type cytokine response (d'Ostiani et al., 2000). Fungal RNA from blastospores also induces DC to elicit a protective immune response (Bacci et al., 2002). One of the integrins that help lymphocytes home to gut tissue is integrin α4β7, which binds to the MAdCAM-1 receptor in the intestinal tissue. DC from the Peyer's patches induce high expression of integrin α4β7 on lymphocytes, regardless of where in the body (of the mouse) they came from (Stagg et al., 2002). This activity keeps recruited lymphocytes in the Peyer's patches long enough to become activated by *Candida* spp. antigens.

4. Inducing the Immune Response to *Candida* spp. in the Intestines

The DC appears to play a central role in the recruitment and activation of effector cells in the immune response to *Candida* spp.

infection. Of the numerous toll-like receptors (TLR) expressed on DC, some of the receptors confer a more protective effect against pathogens than others. Each type of TLR recognizes a different type of microbial surface antigen. DC expressing TLR4 present *C. albicans* antigens (Fig. 15.1), as shown by increased susceptibility of TLR4 knockout mice to experimental candidiasis (Netea et al., 2002). These DC also produce the CXC chemokines KC and MIP-2, which recruit macrophages and polymorphonuclear cells (PMN) to sites of *Candida* infections (Fig. 15.1).

When *Candida* antigens are detected by DC and other APC, many other cells involved in the immune response are activated. A large proportion of IEL in mice (40–80%) express the CD8αα homodimer on their surfaces (Marsal et al., 2002). These cells also express either TcRαβ or TcRγδ on their surfaces, as well. Most of them develop extrathymically, perhaps in the intestines, and they express the CCR9 chemokine receptor that binds chemokine CCL25 (Marsal et al., 2002). The CCL25 chemokine appears to be important for the development and activation of these cells (Fig. 15.1).

Costimulatory molecules involved in antigen presentation to T cells, B7.1 (CD80), B7.2 (CD86) on the APC and CD28 on the T cell, have been evaluated for their roles in resistance to intestinal candidiasis (Montagnoli et al., 2002). Mice deficient in CD86 and CD28 were less susceptible to reinfection than CD80-deficient mice. The expansion of $CD4^+$ $CD25^+$ regulatory T cells in mesenteric lymph nodes (MLN) was inhibited in the CD86- and CD28-deficient mice. IL-10-producing DC activated by *C. albicans* antigens were necessary for the maturation of murine regulatory T cells, which corresponded with reduced interferon gamma (IFN-γ) production in the MLN. These results imply that modulation of T_H1-mediated protective responses against *Candida* spp. is an important part of the protective immune response. The latter results complicate the generally accepted understanding that effective acquired cell-mediated immunity (CMI) to GI tract candidiasis is induced by T_H1-type helper T cells (Bistoni et al., 1993). Future studies of regulation at the initiation stages of acquired GI tract immunity to *Candida* spp. will be helpful in clarifying this apparent contradiction.

5. The Coalition of Host Defenses Activated against *Candida* spp. in the GI Tract

5.1. Dendritic Cells

Although DC are very important as initiators of immune responses and for recruitment of resources, they also function as effector cells for fungal killing and regulatory cells to suppress and modulate the IR. The β-D-glucans of *C. albicans* induce activation and IL-12 production by DC to levels comparable with lipopolysaccharide activation (Kikuchi et al., 2002). The C-type lectin DC-SIGN (CD209), which is involved in viral binding by DC, is also capable of binding to *C. albicans* (Cambi et al., 2003). Human DC and mouse DC kill *Candida* cells by different mechanisms (Newman and Holly, 2001). Human DC kill phagocytosed *Candida* cells without dependence on superoxide or nitric oxide mechanisms (Newman and Holly, 2001).

Some DC are derived from the peripheral blood monocyte population. Human monocyte-derived DC stimulated 48 h with IL-13 had increased phagocytic and candidacidal activity against *C. albicans* blastoconidia than at 2 h after IL-13 treatment (Katsifa et al., 2001). Whether a DC responds to *Candida* spp. antigens by initiating an immune response or tolerance may be determined by the environment it develops in after being recruited from the blood circulation.

At least three populations of DC are recognized in the Peyer's patches and given the names myeloid if they are $CD11b^+$ $CD8\alpha^-$, lymphoid if they are $CD11b^-$ $CD8\alpha^+$, and double negative (DN) if they are $CD11b^-$ $CD8\alpha^-$ (Iwasaki and Kelsall, 2001). The DN DC are found predominantly in mucosal lymphoid sites, especially the follicle-associated epithelium of the Peyer's patches. The myeloid DC secrete IL-4 and IL-10, but lymphoid and DN DC secrete IFN-γ (Fig. 15.1). Antigen stimulates expression of IL-12p70 secretion by all three subsets. The cytokine expression profiles suggest that myeloid DC activate T_H2-type and lymphoid DC stimulate T_H1-type mucosal immune responses (Iwasaki and Kelsall, 2001).

A long debate in fungal pathogenesis circles has ensued about whether hyphal morphotypes are more virulent than yeast morphotypes. It is now becoming clearer that the switch between yeast and hyphal morphotypes affect whether DC mount an immune response or induce tolerance of the fungus' presence (Romani et al., 2002). There is a subset of DC in lymphoid organs that are $B220^+$ and have a toleragenic activity profile, but they can be stimulated by some antigens to rapidly induce expression of major histocompatibility complex (MHC) and costimulatory molecules, and produce IL-12 and IL-10 in a proinflammatory manner (Martin et al., 2002). Further study is needed to work out the relationship between fungal morphotypes and tissue location with respect to activation of immunity or tolerance mediated by DC.

5.2. NK Cells

NK cells are cytotoxic lymphocytes that are part of the innate immune response. In general, NK cells appear to be important parts of the intestinal mucosal immune system. One study reports that intestinal intraepithelial NK cells respond to IL-15 produced by distressed IEC (Fig. 15.1) to induce apoptosis in the IEC, with a measurable increase in NK cell production of Ly-49, NKG2, and perforin effector molecules (Kinoshita et al., 2002). The human intestinal epithelium contains a subset of IEL that are $CD3^-$ and express IFN-γ, tumor necrosis factor alpha (TNF-α), and IL-2 that have NK cell activity (León et al., 2003). Some of these cells are $CD8\alpha\alpha^+$, which is a possible marker of extrathymic intestinal ontogeny often seen in the IEL compartment. NK cells are important initiators of immune responses by their prodigious production of IFN-γ (Kawakami et al., 2001).

Natural killer T cells (NKT cells) restricted by the class I MHC antigen CD1d recognize glycolipid antigens on the surfaces of microorganisms early in an infection. Their role in early innate immune recognition of *Candida* infections in the GI tract has not yet been reported, but CD1d-restricted NKT cells recognize antigens similar to α-galactylceramide on the fungus *Cryptococcus neoformans* (Kawakami et al., 2001). Early in vitro studies suggested that NK cells were not fungicidal (Zumino and Hudig, 1988). Later studies that evaluated cytokine activation of NK cells suggested that NK cells have antifungal activity in vitro. When activated by IL-2, $NK1.1^+$ lymphocytes secrete IFN-γ, which is associated with antifungal activity, but only on blastospores (Mathews and Witek-Janusek, 1998). Most of the studies of NK antifungal activity have been done with antibody depletions of NK cells in vitro or with immunodeficient mouse strains. Transgenic epsilon 26 mice, lacking NK and T cell functions, were susceptible to oroesophageal candidiasis, despite functional PMN and macrophages (Balish et al., 2001). Specific studies of NK cell antifungal activity in the GI tract remain to be done.

5.3. Macrophages and PMN

Macrophages are more plentiful in the lamina propria than DC, and their antifungal activity is enhanced by granulocyte-macrophage colony-stimulating factor (GM-CSF) (Gioulekas et al., 2001) and IL-13 (Katsifa et al., 2001). They are also stimulated to higher anti-*Candida* activity by IFN-γ, TNF-α, IL-12, and MIP-2 (Fig. 15.1) (Major et al., 2002; Mansour and Levitz, 2002).

When a macrophage phagocytoses a *C. albicans* cell, TLR in the macrophage cell membrane are mobilized to mediate signals that induce secretion of proinflammatory cytokines. TNF-α expression by macrophages is optimized by the activation of TLR4 (Li and Cherayil, 2003). An adapter protein, myeloid differentiation factor 88 (MyD88), is involved in this signal transduction pathway, as determined in studies with MyD88$^{-/-}$ mice (Marr et al., 2003). The TNF-α expressed by macrophages promotes influx of other inflammatory cells.

When a *C. albicans* blastospore is engulfed by a macrophage, it may change into a pseudohyphal form and escape the phagolysosome and burst out of the macrophage as it grows. This process appears to be initiated by nutrient starvation of the yeast in the phagolysosome, which activates glyoxylate cycle enzymes in a search for alternate carbon sources (Lorenz and Fink, 2002). When this happens, other inflammatory cells recruited by TNF-α, are needed to combat the fungus. Fungal survival within the phagolysosomes of DC or macrophages appears to be dependent upon whether internalization occurred by way of mannose or CR3 receptors, with the latter mechanism favoring survival (Romani *et al.*, 2002). However, these observations contrast with the role of complement opsonization long considered to enhance phagocytosis and killing of *Candida* sp. by macrophages and PMN.

The primary phagocytic/cytotoxic cells involved in host defense against systemic *Candida* infections are the PMN cells. However, the importance of PMN for resistance to GI tract infections is not clear. For example, mice with the "beige" defect are immunodeficient in macrophage and PMN function, but do not succumb to lethal candidiasis after GI tract challenge (Cantorna and Balish, 1991). The author has observed increasing severity of gastric lesions in *C. albicans* monoassociated beige mice over a period of 14 days, suggesting that PMN are important for reduced morbidity (Fig. 15.2). Since

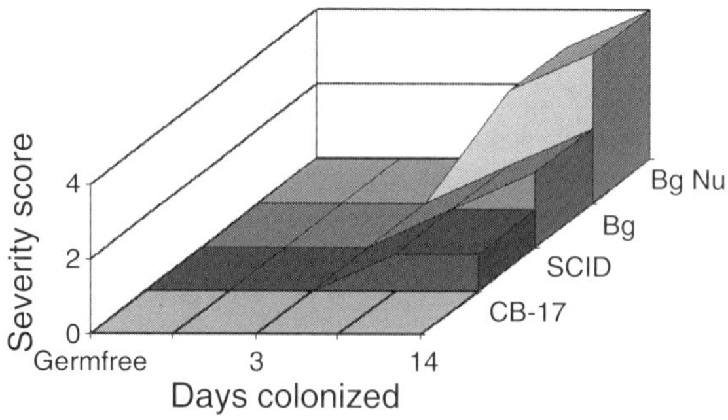

Figure 15.2. Severity of gastric candidiasis in immunodeficient mouse strains monoassociated with *Candida albicans*. Mice were monoassociated with *C. albicans* and groups of four mice of each strain were euthanized and scored for severity of gastric lesions at each time point ($n = 80$). The average severity scores are represented, with 0, no signs of disease to 4, most severe lesions with inflammation and fungal tissue invasion. The CB-17 mice were immunocompetent controls, SCID mice have T cell-mediated immune defects, Bg, beige defect mice have deficient phagocytic cell functions and Bg Nu, beige-nude mice are athymic beige defect mice lacking T cell and phagocytic cell functions.

little work on GI infections in PMN-deficient mice has been done, further study is needed to assess the contributions of all the defensive components present during an infection.

PMN conduct their antifungal activity by an antibody-dependent cytotoxic mechanism. *C. albicans* cells opsonized with antibody and complement are readily phagocytosed and killed by PMN, especially when costimulated with granulocyte colony-stimulating factor (G-CSF) (Fig. 15.1) (van Spriel et al., 2001). PMN also produce defensins that are candidacidal (Tran et al., 2002). PMN granules containing oxidative and nonoxidative molecules attack *C. albicans* pseudohyphae at the cell membrane and on the cellular DNA early in the candidacidal process (Christin et al., 1997). *C. albicans* excretes a protease that prevents opsonization of its cellular surface by complement and antibodies, which reduces the ability of PMN to destroy the fungus by antibody-dependent cell-mediated cytotoxicity (ADCC) (dos Santos et al., 2002). How the host immune system copes with the consequences of these defensive proteases is a fertile area for further research.

5.4. T Cells

Studies in T cell-deficient mice showed that T cells were essential for protection from mucosal candidiasis (Balish et al., 1990). Acquired mucosal immunity to *Candida* sp. is regulated by helper T cells (T_H) and appears to also involve $CD8^+$ T cells (Fig. 15.1). The $CD8^+$ population is partially thymic-derived $CD8\alpha\beta^+$ T cells, and partially extrathymic (probably intestinal in origin) $CD8\alpha\alpha^+$, $TCR\alpha\beta^+$, and $TCR\gamma\delta^+$ T cells (Mysorekar et al., 2002). The mechanism of action for the $CD8^+$ T cells is unclear, but appears to be activated by IL-2 and involve a non-MHC restricted growth inhibition of *Candida* hyphae (as shown with splenic T cells) (Beno et al., 1995).

When the T_H1/T_H2 helper T cell paradigm was popularized, initial studies indicated that protective CMI to mucosal candidiasis was promoted by T_H1 cells derived from the periphery or Peyer's patches that express IFN-γ and IL-2, but not T_H2 cells that express IL-4 and IL-10 (Bistoni *et al.*, 1993). More recently, the T_H1/T_H2 paradigm has become an inadequate description of protective immunity regulation in candidiasis. Although IL-4 tends to drive T_H2 type mucosal immune responses, the lack of the cytokine in IL-$4^{-/-}$ mice prevented complete $CD4^+$ lymphocyte activation and IFN-γ and IL-12 production for a candidacidal T_H1 response (Mencacci et al., 1998).

A new class of T cell, the regulatory T cell (T_R), has been identified that may also be involved in immunity to *Candida* sp., especially in the role of limiting immune responsiveness. A T cell subset in the lamina propria and T_R1 cells in the IEL express the CCR9 chemokine receptor and are $CD4^+$. They respond to anti-CD2 or anti-CD3 stimulation by producing IFN-γ and IL-10 (Papadakis et al., 2003). These cells act as T-regulating cells that support antibody production by naïve $CD19^+$ B cells without exogenous cytokines. These cells are present in the peripheral blood of humans and may exist as a link between the mucosal and systemic immune systems (Papadakis et al., 2003). A new regulatory paradigm will need to be established that incorporates the roles of T-regulatory cells and T_H3 (TGF-β expressing cells), which modulate immune responses. We will then gain a better understanding of the conditions and mechanisms that determine tolerance and response to *Candida* sp. colonization and infection of the GI tract.

5.5. Humoral Immunity

There has been a debate over the importance and role of humoral immunity in protection against candidiasis. B cell-deficient mice that lack specific antibody production are susceptible to disseminated candidiasis of endogenous (intestinal tract) origin, but resistant to mucosal candidiasis (Wagner et al., 1996). We concluded that CMI was necessary for protection of mucosal surfaces, but humoral immunity was necessary for resistance to systemic infections. This was a surprising finding, since antibody-dependent cytotoxic cell activity has traditionally been considered to be the main mucosal defense against *Candida* sp.

Vaccination induces humoral immunity against candidiasis, but only certain epitopes of *Candida* sp. antigens elicit protective antibodies (Casadevall et al., 2002). Antibodies have numerous effects in defense against candidiasis. Using monoclonal antibodies, Moragues et al. (2003) determined that antibodies block *Candida* sp. binding to epithelial cells, inhibit germination of blastospores to pseudohyphae, and also directly mediate fungal killing.

Antibodies are produced by B cells in the lamina propria and are bound by receptors on the basolateral surfaces of IEC (Rojas and Apodoca, 2002). The receptor pIgR binds dimeric IgA and FcRn binds IgG. The immunoglobulins are intracellularly transcytosed for secretion into the intestinal lumen at the apical (intestinal lumen) surfaces of the cells. Immunoglobulins can then bind to *Candida* spp. cells and inhibit their attachment to the epithelial cells. In support of this mechanism, using B cell knockout mice we observed enhanced fungal binding to IEC in vivo, compared with immunocompetent mice (Wagner et al., 1996). Since those mice were more susceptible to disseminated candidiasis of endogenous origin, it appears that antibodies are important for resistance to IEC invasion.

5.6. Other Defense Mechanisms

Small peptides produced by IEC and myeloid cells called defensins (Fig. 15.1) have antimicrobial activity against *C. albicans* blastospores (Porter et al., 1997). Murine β-defensin-3 (homologous to human β-defensin-2) is produced by IEC and has inhibitory activity on the growth of *C. albicans* in vitro (Burd et al., 2002). The CC chemokine CCL28 (Fig. 15.1) is expressed in the colons, small intestines, and Peyer's patches of mice and is a ligand for the CCR10 and CCR3 receptors on T cells. The peptide itself is also candidacidal (Hieshima et al., 2003). Migration-inhibitory factor-related proteins MRP8 and MRP14 dimerize to form calprotectin (Fig. 15.1), a dipeptide produced by myeloid and epithelial cells that inhibits *C. albicans* growth in a zinc-dependent manner (Sohnle et al., 2000).

New defensins and other antifungal molecules secreted by host cells continue to be discovered. These molecules provide exciting opportunities for mechanistic research and biotechnology products that may compliment or replace current antifungal drug therapy.

6. The Indigenous Intestinal Microbiota affects *Candida* spp. Colonization and the Host Response to Fungal Antigens

The mammalian host has numerous allies in the defense against invasive *Candida* spp. in the form of approximately 400 or more species of the indigenous intestinal microflora that collectively restrict colonization by exogenous microorganisms (Jenkinson and Douglas, 2002). Candidiasis of endogenous origin is the title given to systemic *C. albicans* infections that start from gut-colonizing fungi. We have been able to induce candidiasis of endogenous origin in immunocompetent gnotobiotic mice that lack an intestinal microflora (Wagner et al., 1997). Prior colonization of gnotobiotic mice with pure cultures of probiotic bacteria reduced the incidence of candidiasis of endogenous origin. Treatment of conventional mice with broad-spectrum antibiotics can also induce candidiasis of endogenous origin (Wiesner et al., 2001; Bendel et al., 2002). These and many other studies demonstrate that the intestinal microflora is an important ally in a host's resistance to mucosal and systemic candidiasis.

The composition of the intestinal microflora is modulated by host dietary habits. Experiments with nondigestible (by the host) oligosaccharides (NDO) of different compositions show selective advantages for some species of bacteria and fungi over others (Hopkins and MacFarlane, 2003). It is believed that feeding of NDO, also known as prebiotics, can modify the composition of the intestinal microflora to favor growth of microbes with increased capacities for colonization resistance.

There are several likely mechanisms that contribute to colonization resistance against *Candida* spp. One mechanism is direct antimicrobial activity by bacteria against *Candida* cells. For example, although not generally considered part of the indigenous intestinal microflora, *Pseudomonas aeruginosa* forms biofilms on *C. albicans* hyphae, but not blastospores in in vitro experiments (Hogan and Kolter, 2002). In the latter study, virulence factor deficient mutants of *P. aeruginosa* exhibited decreased candidacidal activity. These results indicate that some bacteria can play a distinct and direct role in control of *C. albicans*.

Another mechanism for the indigenous microflora to affect host resistance to *Candida* spp. is by immunomodulation. It is not clear how commensal bacteria enhance host defenses against *Candida* spp., since many immunological parameters do not appear to change with the presence of bacteria. For example, when germfree mice are colonized with intestinal bacteria, the peripheral $CD3\beta^+$ $CD8^+$ cytotoxic T cell repertoire does not change (Bousso et al., 2000). Also, lactic acid bacteria fed to mice were not shown to change the proportions of splenic or Peyer's patch $CD8^+$, $B220^+$, or IgA^+, and IgM^+ cells (Pestka et al., 2001). However, another report claims that in germfree mice, intestinal IEL with Thy 1.2^- $CD3^+$ $CD8^+$ $CD4^-$ phenotypes expand after colonization with lactic acid bacteria (Link et al., 1995). Lymphoproliferative activities and production of antibodies to *C. albicans* antigens are enhanced by the presence of antigens from heat-killed probiotic bacteria in immunocompetent mice (Wagner et al., 2000b).

The intestinal microflora have an anti-inflammatory influence on the mucosal immune system that appears to reduce the host response to *Candida* spp. under commensal conditions. This immunomodulation requires direct contact between some bacteria species and the mucosal epithelium (Neish et al., 2000). Microflora-associated immunomodulation affects the IκB/NFκB intracellular signaling pathways that are involved in activation of proinflammatory cytokine expression by IEC. The interaction of bacteria and mucosal epithelium inhibits the ubiquitination of IκB, preventing proteolytic degradation of the inhibitor for activation if NFκB and inhibits the cytokine expression cascade that it initiates.

Since many of the effects of the intestinal microflora appear to inhibit immune responses, it is tempting to conclude that bacteria promote immunological tolerance of *C. albicans* rather than a strong immune response. It is still unclear why the intestinal microflora can induce host immune tolerance to *Candida* spp. and also prevent enteric *Candida* infections. However, we recently reported that the presence of probiotic bacteria in the GI tracts of mice-modulated total antibody production to *C. albicans* antigens, but increased the production of some antibodies to specific *C. albicans* antigens (Wagner et al., 2000a). Much more study is needed to understand the interactions between the indigenous microflora, the host immune system, and *Candida* spp.

7. Modulation of the Immune Response and Repair of Damaged Intestinal Tissues

7.1. Regulation of Effector Mechanisms

Once an immune response has been initiated and the presence of *Candida* spp. in the tissue has been eliminated, the immune response must be terminated and tissue repaired. Some signals come from the IEC. For example, purified membranes from IEC suppress T_H1 and T_H2 cytokine production and proliferation of stimulated $\alpha\beta$ and $\gamma\delta$ T cells in vitro (Yamamoto et al., 1998). Such suppressive signals are important to maintain the homeostasis that prevents immunity from becoming self-destructive.

Microbial surface molecules are recognized by receptors on macrophages and activate inflammatory responses as part of the innate immune system by signal transduction with the Janus kinase-signal transducer and activator of transcription (JAK-STAT) signal transduction pathway. This pathway of signal transduction is modulated by suppressor of cytokine signaling molecule-1 (SOCS-1) in the signal cascade (Nakagawa et al., 2002). When IL-6 is encountered by activated macrophages, SOCS-3 is expressed, which inhibits inflammatory cytokine expression through the JAK-STAT signaling pathways (Lang et al., 2003).

The role of transforming growth factor-beta (TGF-β1) produced by T_H3 and T-regulatory (T_R1) cells is to inactivate the antigen-activated T cells without subsequent apoptosis. The inactivated T cells can become memory cells for reactivation in subsequent immune responses to *Candida* sp. infections. Not all T cells respond to TGF-β1 with the same sensitivity (Kunzmann et al., 2003).

Antigens sampled from the intestinal lumen may enter the lamina propria and are presented to $CD4^+$ cells residing there. Many T_R1 type (IL-10 secreting) regulatory T cells in the lamina propria prevent inappropriate inflammatory and autoimmune responses occurring in the intestinal tract prompted by microbial antigens from the intestinal lumen (Cong et al., 2002). A $CD4^+$ $CD25^+$ subset of regulatory T cells, appear to be reactive to self-antigens and inhibit accumulation of $CD134L^+$ DC, suggesting that they are involved in suppressing autoimmunity and inflammatory processes (Singh et al., 2001). Responses of T_R1 cells to *Candida* sp. antigens need to be evaluated for their role in maintaining the commensal state.

Whether the mucosal immune system responds to *Candida* antigens with a protective response or with anergy appears to be a function of the APC involved. Human duodenal epithelial cells express MHC Class II antigens that are capable of presenting antigen to lymphocytes; however, they do not express the important costimulatory molecules CD40, CD80, or CD86 (Byrne et al., 2002). The result of this type of antigen presentation develops into a suppressive response with the development of a T_H3-type of regulatory response, characterized by $CD4^+$ cells that express TGF-β (Mowat, 2003).

7.2. Regulation of Tissue Repair

After a *Candida* sp. has invaded tissue, initiated an immune response, and the infection has been eliminated, the damaged intestinal tissue must be repaired. Part of the repair process is the normal rapid turnover of epithelial cells in the intestines, and part of the process requires specific tissue regeneration mechanisms. One of the ways that homeostasis of intestinal monolayer integrity is maintained is by the constant movement of new enterocytes along the extracellular matrix from the crypts to the villus tips. This process involves a coordination of integrin molecules on the cell surfaces and E-cadherin–actin cytoskeletal complexes (Schreider et al., 2002). For tissue repair, enterocytes must detach from each other and the basement membrane. This is accomplished in part by release of β-catenin from α-catenin and E-cadherin molecules after tyrosine phosphorylation (Guo et al., 2002).

Macrophages direct the repair process in response to tissue damage. They phagocytose damaged, necrotic, and apoptotic IEC and secrete cytokines and chemokines to attract the necessary support systems (Wilson, 1997). Macrophage migration inhibitory factor (MIF), involved in delayed-type hypersensitivity (DTH) reactions and macrophage activation, is also involved in chemotaxis of keratinocytes and fibroblasts for wound healing (Nishihira, 2000).

An inflammatory process must occur before tissue damage can be repaired. Studies with IL-6 knockout mice show that the secretion of IL-6 in the vicinity of the wound is necessary in the early initiation of the repair process (Gallucci et al., 2000). Surgical anastomosis of bowel sections has been a useful model to study the role of immune effectors in the healing process. The presence of activated macrophages improves the tensile strength of the anastomoses, indicating that they influence the quality of intestinal tissue healing (Compton et al., 1996). In the latter study, improved healing was observed in the presence of macrophages with suppressed expression of TGF-β and platelet-derived growth factor (PDGF) cytokines, indicating that some cytokines are not conducive to the healing process.

In keratinized tissues, such as the gastric antrum of the mouse, keratinocytes at a site of tissue damage by *Candida* sp. infection produce macrophage chemoattractant protein-1 (MCP-1) and later, macrophage inflammatory protein-1 (MIP-1) that attract macrophages to the damaged tissue (Jackman et al., 2000). Keratinocytes also secrete IL-18, which attracts PMN to a wound site (Kämpfer et al., 2000). The PMN secrete TNF-α that inhibits further IL-18 production by the keratinocytes.

Restitution of the epithelial monolayer after damage in an infection is enhanced by IL-2 and IFN-γ secreted by PMN that migrate into the damaged tissue (Cario et al., 1999). These latter cells also secrete TGF-β and TNF-α, neither of which appears to enhance restitution of the epithelium.

Activated lymphocytes are primed with a time bomb of apoptosis, so that they will expire when their services are no longer needed following an immune response. This mechanism prevents autoimmunity and chronic inflammatory problems. An activated T cell requires constant stimulation by cytokines that signal through the IL-2Rγ chain (Crowston et al., 1997). In the presence of fibroblasts, a 30 kDa soluble factor inhibits T cell death to maintain an immune response during tissue repair and healing (Crowston et al., 1997). An example of the ability of fibroblasts to overcome the normal tendency of activated T cells to succumb to apoptosis is revealed in rheumatoid arthritis, where synovial fibroblasts can prevent apoptosis of T cells, even though the T cells have low intracellular Bcl-2 and high Bcl-X_L expression, which is a proapoptotic phenotype (Crowston et al., 1997). Many components of the immune system are involved in the secondary role of tissue restitution after a *Candida* sp. infection. These secondary functions of immunity are vital to recovery of health, but they have not been adequately considered as part of host defense. Future therapeutic approaches to mucosal candidiasis should consider the enhancement of repair processes as a valid objective.

8. Conclusions

Although *Candida* spp. are rarely implicated as etiological agents of enteritis, the high frequency of colonization in the human population suggests that *Candida* spp. in the GI tract interact frequently with the indigenous microflora and the defense systems of the host. Infection of the human

GI tract by *Candida* spp. is rare, because these factors maintain a balance that favors commensalism. Antimicrobial drug perturbation of colonization resistance or severe immunodeficiency can result in intestinal candidiasis. Innate and acquired immune systems function uniquely in the gut-associated lymphoid tissue (GALT), which includes the Peyer's patches, IEL, and lamina propria compartments, to maintain a balance between immunity and tolerance of *Candida* cells present in the GI tract. Recent studies reveal the importance of DC and regulatory T cells for control of the host response to the presence of *Candida* spp. in the GI tract, adding them to the list of immunological assets involved in anti-*Candida* host defense. As more is learned about the functions of these components (DC, regulatory T cells, the intestinal microflora) of the host response to *Candida* spp., the contradictory reports regarding immune regulation will be clarified. Further study of the immune regulatory systems will also clarify the long-standing debate over the role of humoral immunity in antifungal defense. Future studies of the interactions of *Candida* spp., the indigenous microflora, and the host in animal models will increase our understanding of mucosal immunity and how it maintains the balance between activation of immune responses and tolerance toward *Candida* spp.

Acknowledgments

The author would like to thank Edward Balish for his mentorship and for passing on the torch after his long years of expertise in fungal immunology. Thanks also go to Virginia Taylor for work on the illustrations.

References

Alpan, O., Rudomen, G., and Matzinger, P. (2001). The role of dendritic cells, B cells, and M cells in gut-oriented immune responses. *J. Immunol.* 166: 4843–4852.

Bacci, A., Montagnoli, C., Peruccio, K., Bozza, S., Gaziano, R., Pitzurra, L., Velardi, A., d'Ostiani, C.F., Cutler, J.E., and Romani, L. (2002). Dendritic cells pulsed with fungal RNA induce protective immunity to *Candida albicans* in hematopoietic transplantation. *J. Immunol.* 168: 2904–2913.

Balish, E., Filutowicz, H., and Oberly, T.D. (1990). Correlates of cell-mediated immunity in *Candida albicans*-colonized gnotobiotic mice. *Infect. Immun.* 58: 107–113.

Balish, E., Warner, T., Pierson, C.J., Bock, D.M., and Wagner, R.D. (2001). Oroesophageal candidiasis is lethal for transgenic mice with combined natural killer and T-cell defects. *Med. Mycol.* 39: 261–268.

Bassilana, M., Blyth, J., and Arkowitz, R. (2003). Cdc24, the GDP-GTP exchange factor for Cdc42, is required for invasive hyphal growth of *Candida albicans*. *Eukaryot. Cell* 2: 9–18.

Bektic, J., Lell, C.P., Fuchs, A., Stoiber, H., Speth, C., Lass-Flörl, C., Borg-von Zepelin, M., Dierich, M.P., and Würzner, R. (2001). HIV protease inhibitors attenuate adherence of *Candida albicans* to epithelial cells *in vitro*. *FEMS Immunol. Med. Microbiol.* 31: 65–71.

Bell, S.J., Rigby, R., English, N., Mann, S.D., Knight, S.C., Kamm, M.A., and Stagg, A.J. (2001). Migration and maturation of human colonic dendritic cells. *J. Immunol.* 166: 4958–4967.

Bendel, C.M., Kinneberg, K.M., Jechorek, R.P., Erlandsen, S.L., Sahar, D.E., and Wells, C.L. (2000). The *Candida albicans INT*1 gene facilitates cecal colonization in endotoxin-treated mice. *Shock* 13: 453–458.

Bendel, C.M., Wiesner, S.M., Garni, R.M., Cebelinski, E., and Wells, C.L. (2002). Cecal colonization and systemic spread of *Candida albicans* in mice treated with antibiotics and dexamethasone. *Pediatr. Res.* 51: 290–295.

Beno, D.W.A., Stöver, A.G., and Mathews, H.L. (1995). Growth inhibition of *Candida albicans* hyphae by $CD8^+$ lymphocytes. *J. Immunol.* 154: 5273–5281.

Bistoni, F., Cenci, E., Mencacci, A., Schiafella, E., Mosci, P., Puccetti, P., and Romani, L. (1993). Mucosal and systemic T helper cell function after intragastric colonization of adult mice with *Candida albicans*. *J. Infect. Dis.* 168: 1449–1457.

Bousso, P., Lemaître, F., Laouini, D., Kanellopoulos, J., and Kourilsky, P. (2000). The peripheral CD8 T cell repertoire is largely independent of the presence of intestinal flora. *Int. Immunol.* 12: 425–430.

Burd, R.S., Furrer, J.L., Sullivan, J., and Smith, A. (2002). Murine β-defensin-3 is an inducible peptide with limited tissue expression and broad-spectrum antimicrobial activity. *Shock* 18: 461–464.

Byrne, B., Madrigal-Estebas, L., McEvoy, A., Carton, J., Doherty, D.G., Whelan, A., Feighery, C., O'Donoghue, D.P., and O'Farrelly, C. (2002). Human duodenal epithelial cells constitutively express molecular components of antigen presentation but not costimulatory molecules. *Hum. Immunol.* 63: 977–986.

Cambi, A., Gijzen, K., de Vries, I.J.M., Torensma, R., Joosten, B., Adema, G.J., Netea, M.G., Kullberg, B.-J., Romani, L., and Figdor, C.G. (2003). The C-type lectin DC-SIGN (CD209) is an antigen-uptake receptor for *Candida albicans* on dendritic cells. *Eur. J. Immunol.* 33: 532–538.

Cameron, B.J. and Douglas, L.J. (1996). Blood group glycolipids as epithelial cell receptors for *Candida albicans*. *Infect. Immun.* 64: 891–896.

Cantorna, M.T. and Balish, E. (1991). Acquired immunity to systemic candidiasis in immunodeficient mice. *J. Infect. Dis.* 164: 936–943.

Cario, E., Becker, A., Sturm, A., Goebell, H., and Dignass, A.U. (1999). Peripheral blood mononuclear cells promote intestinal epithelial restitution in vitro through an interleukin-2/interferon-γ-dependent pathway. *Scand. J. Gastroenterol.* 34: 1132–1138.

Casadevall, A., Feldmesser, M., and Pirofski, L.-A. (2002). Induced humoral immunity and vaccination against major human fungal pathogens. *Curr. Opin. Microbiol.* 5: 386–391.

Christin, L., Wysong, D.R., Meshulam, T., Wang, S., and Diamond, R.D. (1997). Mechanisms and target sites of damage in killing of *Candida albicans* hyphae by human polymorphonuclear neutrophils. *J. Infect. Dis.* 176: 1567–1578.

Colina, A.-R., Aumont, F., Deslauriers, N., Belhumeur, P., and de Repentigny, L. (1996). Evidence of degradation of gastrointestinal mucin by *Candida albicans* secretory aspartyl proteinase. *Infect. Immun.* 64: 4514–4519.

Compton, R., Williams, D., and Browder, W. (1996). The beneficial effect of enhanced macrophage function on the healing of bowel anastomoses. *Am. Sur.* 62: 14–18.

Cong, Y., Weaver, C.T., Lazenby, A., and Elson, C.O. (2002). Bacterial-reactive T regulatory cells inhibit pathogenic immune responses to the enteric flora. *J. Immunol.* 169: 6112–6119.

Crowston, J.G., Salmon, M., Khaw, P.T., and Akbar, A.N. (1997). T-lymphocyte–fibroblast interactions. *Biochem. Soc. Trans.* 25: 529–531.

dos Santos, A.A., de Sá, E.A.C., Gaziri, L.C.J., and Felipe, I. (2002). Treatment of serum with supernatants from cultures of *Candida albicans* reduces its serum-dependent phagocytosis. *Braz. J. Microbiol.* 33: 79–83.

Drago, L., Mombelli, B., Vecchi, E.D., Bonaccorso, C., Fassina, M.C., and Gismondo, M.R. (2000). *Candida albicans* cellular internalization: A new pathogenic factor? *Int. J. Antimicrob. Agents* 16: 545–547.

Dromer, F., Chevalier, R., Sendid, B., Improvisi, L., Jouault, T., Robert, R., Mallet, J.M., and Poulain, D. (2002). Synthetic analogues of β-1,2 oligomannosides prevent intestinal colonization by the pathogenic yeast *Candida albicans*. *Antimicrob. Agents Chemother.* 46: 3869–3876.

Gallucci, R.M., Simeonova, P.P., Matheson, J.M., Kommineni, C., Guriel, J.L., Sugawara, T., and Luster, M.I. (2000). Impaired cutaneous wound healing in interleukin-6-deficient and immunosuppressed mice. *FASEB J.* 14: 2525–2531.

Gioulekas, E., Goutzioulis, M., Farmakis, C., Drossou, V., Kremenopoulos, G., Tsiouris, J., and Roilides, E. (2001). Effects of macrophage colony-stimulating factor on antifungal activity of neonatal monocytes against *Candida albicans*. *Biol. Neonate* 80: 251–256.

Gow, N.A.R., Brown, A.J.P., and Odds, F. (2002). Fungal morphogenesis and host invasion. *Curr. Opin. Microbiol.* 5: 366–371.

Guo, X., Rao, J.N., Liu, L., Rizvi, M., Turner, D.J., and Wang, J.-Y. (2002). Polyamines regulate β-catenin tyrosine phosphorylation via Ca^{2+} during intestinal epithelial cell migration. *Am. J. Physiol. Cell Physiol.* 283: C722–C734.

Hieshima, K., Ohtani, H., Shibano, M., Izawa, D., Nakayama, T., Kawasaki, Y., Shiba, F., Shiota, M., Katou, F., Saito, T., and Yoshie, O. (2003). CCL28 has dual roles in mucosal immunity as a chemokine with broad-spectrum antimicrobial activity. *J. Immunol.* 170: 1452–1461.

Hogan, D.A. and Kolter, R. (2002). *Pseudomonas–Candida* interactions: An ecological role for virulence factors. *Science* 296: 2229–2232.

Hopkins, M.J. and MacFarlane, G.T. (2003). Nondigestible oligosaccharides enhance bacterial colonization resistance against *Clostridium difficile in vitro. Appl. Environ. Microbiol.* 69: 1920–1927.

Hostetter, M.K. (1999). Integrin-like proteins in *Candida* spp. and other microorganisms. *Fungal Genet. Biol.* 28: 135–145.

Iwasaki, A. and Kelsall, B.L. (2001). Unique functions of CD11b$^+$, CD8α^+, and double-negative Peyer's patch dendritic cells. *J. Immunol.* 166: 4884–4890.

Jackman, S.H., Yoak, M.B., Keerthy, S., and Beaver, B.L. (2000). Differential expression of chemokines in a mouse model of wound healing. *Ann. Clin. Lab. Sci.* 30: 201–207.

Jenkinson, H.F. and Douglas, L.J. (2002). Interactions between *Candida* species and bacteria in mixed infections. In K.A. Bogden and J.M. Guthmiller (eds), *Polymicrobial Diseases*, Vol. 1. ASM Press, Washington, DC, pp. 357–373.

Kämpfer, H., Mühl, H., Manderscheid, M., Kalina, U., Kauschat, D., Pfeilschifter, J., and Frank, S. (2000). Regulation of interleukin-18 (IL-18) expression in keratinocytes (HaCaT): Implications for early wound healing. *Eur. Cytokine Netw.* 11: 626–633.

Katsifa, H., Tsaparidou, S., Diza, E., Gil-Lamaignere, C., Walsh, T.J., and Roilides, E. (2001). Effects of interleukin-13 on antifungal activity of human monocytes against *Candida albicans. FEMS Immunol. Med. Microbiol.* 31: 211–217.

Kawakami, K., Kinjo, Y., Yara, S., Koguchi, Y., Uezu, K., Nakayama, T., Taniguchi, M., and Saito, A. (2001). Activation of vα14$^+$ natural killer T cells by α-galactylceramide results in development of Th1 response and local host resistance in mice infected with *Cryptococcus neoformans. Infect. Immun.* 69: 213–220.

Kikuchi, T., Ohno, N., and Ohno, T. (2002). Maturation of dendritic cells induced by *Candida* β-D-glucan. *Int. Pharmacol.* 2: 1503–1508.

Kinoshita, N., Hiroi, T., Ohta, N., Fukuyama, S., Park, E.J., and Kiyono, H. (2002). Autocrine IL-15 mediates intestinal epithelial cell death via the activation of neighboring intraepithelial NK cells. *J. Immunol.* 169: 6187–6192.

Kwon, J.H., Keates, S., Bassani, L., Mayer, L.F., and Keates, A.C. (2002). Colonic epithelial cells are a major site of macrophage inflammatory protein 3α (MIP-3α) production in normal colon and inflammatory bowel disease. *Gut* 51: 818–826.

Kunzmann, S., Wohlfahrt, J.G., Itoh, S., Asao, H., Komada, M., Akdis, C.A., Blaser, K., and Schmidt-Weber, C.B. (2003). SARA and Hgs attenuate susceptibility to TGF-β1-mediated T cell suppression. *FASEB J.* 17: 194–202.

Lacour, M., Zunder, T., Huber, R., Sander, A., Daschner, F., and Frank, U. (2002). The pathogenetic significance of intestinal *Candida* colonization—a systematic review from an interdisciplinary and environmental medical point of view. *Int. J. Hyg. Environ. Health* 205: 257–268.

Lang, R., Pauleau, A.-L., Parganas, E., Takahashi, Y., Mages, J., Ihle, J.N., Rutschman, R., and Murray, P.J. (2003). SOCS3 regulates the plasticity of gp130 signaling. *Nat. Immunol.* 6: 546–550.

León, F., Roldán, E., Sanchez, L., Camarero, C., Bootello, A., and Roy, G. (2003). Human small-intestinal epithelium contains functional natural killer lymphocytes. *Gastroenterology* 125: 345–356.

Li, Q. and Cherayil, B.J. (2003). Role of toll-like receptor 4 in macrophage activation and tolerance during *Salmonella enterica* serovar Typhimurium infection. *Infect. Immun.* 71: 4873–4882.

Link, H., Rochat, F., Saudan, K.Y., and Schiffrin, E. (1995). Immunomodulation of the gnotobiotic mouse through colonization with lactic acid bacteria. In J. Mestecky, M.W. Russell, S. Jackson, S.M. Michalek, H.T. Hoganová, and J. Sterzl (eds), *Advances in Mucosal Immunology* Plenum Press, New York, pp. 465–467.

Lorenz, M.C. and Fink, G.R. (2002). Life and death in a macrophage: Role of the glyoxylate cycle in virulence. *Eukaryot. Cell* 1: 657–662.

Major, J., Fletcher, J.E., and Hamilton, T.A. (2002). IL-4 pretreatment selectively enhances cytokine production in lipopolysaccharide-stimulated mouse peritoneal macrophages. *J. Immunol.* 168: 2456–2463.

Mansour, M.K. and Levitz, S.M. (2002). Interactions of fungi with phagocytes. *Curr. Opin. Microbiol.* 5: 359–365.

Marr, K.A., Balajee, S.A., Hawn, T.R., Ozinsky, A., Pham, U., Akira, S., Aderem, A., and Liles, W.C. (2003). Differential role of MyD88 in macrophage-mediated responses to opportunistic fungal pathogens. *Infect. Immun.* 71: 5280–5286.

Marsal, J., Svensson, M., Ericsson, A., Iranpour, A.H., Carramolino, L., Márquez, G., and Agace, W.W. (2002). Involvement of CCL25 (TECK) in the generation of the murine small-intestinal CD8αα^{+}Cd3^{+} intraepithelial lymphocyte compartment. *Eur. J. Immunol.* 32: 3488–3497.

Martin, P., del Hoyo, G.M., Anjuère, F., Arias, C.F., Vargas, V.H., Fernández, L.A., Parrillas, V., and Ardavin, C. (2002). Characterization of a new subpopulation of mouse CD8α^{+} B220^{+} dendritic cells endowed with type 1 interferon production capacity and tolerogenic potential. *Blood* 100: 383–390.

Mathews, H.L. and Witek-Janusek, L. (1998). Antifungal activity of interleukin-2-activated natural killer (NK1.1^{+}) lymphocytes against *Candida albicans. J. Med. Microbiol.* 47: 1007–1014.

Mencacci, A., Del Soro, G., Cenci, E., d'Ostiani, C., Bacci, A., Montagnoli, C., Kopf, M., and Romani, C. (1998). Endogenous interleukin 4 is required for development of protective CD4+ T helper type 1 cell responses to *Candida albicans. J. Exp. Med.* 187: 307–317.

Montagnoli, C., Bacci, A., Bozza, S., Gaziano, R., Mosci, P., Sharpe, A.H., and Romani, L. (2002). B7/CD28-dependent CD4^{+}CD25^{+} regulatory T cells are essential components of the memory-protective immunity to *Candida albicans. J. Immunol.* 169: 6298–6308.

Moragues, M.D., Omaetxebarria, M.J., Elguezabal, N., Sevilla, M.J., Conti, S., Polonelli, L., and Pontón, J. (2003). A monoclonal antibody directed against a *Candida albicans* cell wall mannoprotein exerts three anti-*C. albicans* activities. *Infect. Immun.* 71: 5273–5279.

Mowat, A.M. (2003). Anatomical basis of tolerance and immunity to intestinal antigens. *Nat. Rev. Immunol.* 3: 331–341.

Mysorekar, I.U., Lorenz, R.G., and Gordon, J.I. (2002). Gnotobiotic transgenic mouse model for studying interactions between small intestinal enterocytes and intraepithelial lymphocytes. *J. Biol. Chem.* 277: 37811–37819.

Nakagawa, R., Naka, T., Tsutsui, H., Fujimoto, M., Kimura, A., Abe, T., Seki, E., Sato, S., Takeuchi, O., Takeda, K., Akira, S., Yamanishi, K., Kawase, I., Nakanishi, K., and Kishimoto, T. (2002). SOCS-1 participates in negative regulation of LPS responses. *Immunity* 17: 677–687.

Neish, A.S., Gewirtz, A.T., Zeng, H., Young, A.N., Hobert, M.E., Karmali, V., Rao, A.S., and Madara, J.L. (2000). Prokaryotic regulation of epithelial responses by inhibition of IκB-α ubiquitination. *Science* 289: 1560–1563.

Netea, M.G., Van der Graaf, C.A.A., Vonk, A.G., Verschuren, I., van der Meer, J.W.M., and Kullberg, B.J. (2002). The role of toll-like receptor (TLR) 2 and TLR4 in the host defense against disseminated candidiasis. *J. Infect. Dis.* 185: 1483–1489.

Newman, S.L. and Holly, A. (2001). *Candida albicans* is phagocytosed, killed, and processed for antigen presentation by human dendritic cells. *Infect. Immun.* 69: 6813–6822.

Nishihira, J. (2000). Macrophage migration inhibitory factor (MIF): Its essential role in the immune system and cell growth. *J. Interferon Cytokine Res.* 20: 751–762.

Nieuwenhuizen, W.F., Pieters, R.H.H., Knippels, L.M.J., Jansen, M.C.J.F., and Koppelman, S.J. (2003). Is *Candida albicans* a trigger in the onset of coeliac disease? *Lancet* 361: 2152–2154.

Ohteki, T. (2002). Critical role for IL-15 in innate immunity. *Curr. Mol. Med.* 2: 371–380.

d'Ostiani, C.F., Del Sero, G., Bacci, A., Montagnoli, C., Spreca, A., Mencacci, A., Ricciardi-Castagnoli, P., and Romani, L. (2000). Dendritic cells discriminate between yeasts and hyphae of the fungus *Candida albicans*: Implications for initiation of T helper cell immunity *in vitro* and *in vivo. J. Exp. Med.* 191: 1661–1673.

Panagoda, G.J., Ellepola, A.N.B., and Samaranayake, L.P. (2001). Adhesion of *Candida parapsilosis* to epithelial and acrylic surfaces correlates with cell surface hydrophobicity. *Mycoses* 44: 29–35.

Papadakis, K.A., Landers, C., Prehn, J., Kouroumalis, E.A., Moreno, S.T., Gutierrez-Ramos, J.-C., Hodge, M.R., and Targan, S.R. (2003). CC chemokine receptor 9 expression defines a subset of peripheral blood lymphocytes with mucosal T cell phenotype and Th1 or T-regulatory 1 cytokine profile. *J. Immunol.* 171: 159–165.

Pestka, J.J., Ha, C.-L., Warner, R.W., Lee, J.H., and Ustunol, Z. (2001). Effects of ingestion of yogurts containing *Bifidobacterium* and *Lactobacillus acidophilus* on spleen and Peyer's patch lymphocyte populations in the mouse. *J. Food Protect.* 64: 392–395.

Porter, E.M., van Dam, E., Valore, E.V., and Ganz, T. (1997). Broad-spectrum antimicrobial activity of human intestinal defensin 5. *Infect. Immun.* 65: 2396–2401.

de Repentigny, L., Aumont, F., Bernard, K., and Belhumeur, P. (2000). Characterization of binding of *Candida albicans* to small intestinal mucin and its role in adherence to mucosal epithelial cells. *Infect. Immun.* 68: 3172–3179.

Rescigno, M., Urbano, M., Valzasina, B., Francolini, M., Rotta, G., Bonasio, R., Granucci, F., Kraehenbuhl, J.-P., and Ricciardi-Castagnoli, P. (2001). Dendritic cells express tight junction proteins and penetrate gut epithelial monolayers to sample bacteria. *Nat. Immunol.* 2: 361–367.

Rojas, R. and Apodaca, G. (2002). Immunoglobulin transport across polarized epithelial cells. *Nat. Rev. Mol. Cell Biol.* 3: 944–955.

Romani, L., Bistoni, F., and Puccetti, P. (2002). Fungi, dendritic cells and receptors: A host perspective of fungal virulence. *Trends Microbiol.* 10: 508–514.

Ruiz-Sánchez, D., Calderón-Romero, L., Sánchez-Vega, J.T., and Tay, J. (2002). Intestinal candidiasis. A clinical report and comments about this opportunistic pathology. *Mycopathologia* 156: 9–11.

Schreider, C., Peignon, G., Thenet, S., Chambaz, J., and Pinçon-Raymond, M. (2002). Integrin-mediated functional polarization of Caco-2 cells through E-cadherin–actin complexes. *J. Cell Sci.* 115: 543–552.

Shreedhar, V.K., Kelsall, B.L., and Neutra, M.R. (2003). Cholera toxin induces migration of dendritic cells from the subepithelial dome region to T- and B-cell areas of Peyer's patches. *Infect. Immun.* 71: 504–509.

Singh, B., Read, S., Asseman, C., Malmström, V., Mottet, C., Stephens, L.A., Stepankova, R., Tlaskalova, H., and Powrie, F. (2001). Control of intestinal inflammation by regulatory T cells. *Immunol. Rev.* 182: 190–200.

Sohnle, P.G., Hunter, M.J., Hahn, B., and Chazin, W.J. (2000). Zinc-reversible antimicrobial activity of recombinant calprotectin (migration inhibitory factor-related proteins 8 and 14). *J. Infect. Dis.* 182: 1272–1275.

Stagg, A.J., Kamm, M.A., and Knight, S.C. (2002). Intestinal dendritic cells increase T cell expression of $\alpha 4\beta 7$ integrin. *Eur. J. Immunol.* 32: 1445–1454.

Tran, D., Tran, P.A., Tang, Y.-Q., Yuan, J., Cole, T., and Selsted, M.E. (2002). Homodimeric θ-defensins from *Rhesus macaque* leukocytes. *J. Biol. Chem.* 277: 3079–3084.

van Spriel, A.B., van den Herik-Oudijk, I.E., and van de Winkel, J.G.J. (2001). Neutrophil FcγRI as target for immunotherapy of invasive candidiasis. *J. Immunol.* 166: 7019–7022.

Wagner, R.D., Vazquez-Torres, A., Jones-Carson, J., Warner, T., and Balish, E. (1996). B cell knockout mice are resistant to mucosal and systemic candidiasis of endogenous origin but susceptible to experimental systemic candidiasis. *J. Infect. Dis.* 174: 589–597.

Wagner, R.D., Pierson, C., Warner, T., Dohnalek, M., Farmer, J., Roberts, L., Hilty, M., and Balish, E. (1997). Biotherapeutic effects of probiotic bacteria on candidiasis in immunodeficient mice. *Infect. Immun.* 65: 4165–4172.

Wagner, R.D., Dohnalek, M., Hilty, M., Vezquez-Torres, A., and Balish, E. (2000a). Effects of probiotic bacteria on humoral immunity to *Candida albicans* in immunodeficient *bg/bg-nu/nu* and *bg/bg-nu/*$^+$ mice. *Rev. Iberoam. Micol.* 17: 55–59.

Wagner, R.D., Pierson, C., Warner, T., Dohnalek, M., Hilty, M., and Balish, E. (2000b). Probiotic effects of feeding heat-killed *Lactobacillus casei* to *Candida albicans*-colonized immunodeficient mice. *J. Food Protect.* 63: 638–644.

Wagner, S., Lynch, N.J., Walter, W., Schwaeble, W.J., and Loos, M. (2003). Differential expression of the murine mannose-binding lectins A and C in lymphoid and nonlymphoid organs and tissues. *J. Immunol.* 170: 1462–1465.

Wilson, K. (1997). Wound healing: The role of macrophages. *Nurs. Crit. Care* 2: 291–296.

Wiesner, S.M., Jechorek, R.P., Garni, R.M., Bendel, C.M., and Wells, C.L. (2001). Gastrointestinal colonization by *Candida albicans* mutant strains in antibiotic-treated mice. *Clin. Diagn. Lab. Immunol.* 8: 192–195.

Wiesner, S.M., Bendel, C.M., Hess, D.J., Erlandsen, S.L., and Wells, C.L. (2002). Adherence of yeast and filamentous forms of *Candida albicans* to cultured enterocytes. *Crit. Care Med.* 30: 677–683.

Yamamoto, M., Fujihashi, K., Kawabata, K., McGhee, J.R., and Kiyono, H. (1998). A mucosal intranet: Intestinal epithelial cells down-regulate intraepithelial, but not peripheral, T lymphocytes. *J. Immunol.* 160: 2188–2196.

Zumino, S.J. and Hudig, D. (1988). Interactions between human natural killer (NK) lymphocytes and yeast cells: human NK cells do not kill *Candida albicans,* although *C. albicans* blocks NK lysis of K562 cells. *Infect. Immun.* 56: 564–569.

16

Innate and Adaptive Cell-Mediated Immunity against Vaginal Candidiasis

Paul L. Fidel, Jr.

1. Introduction

Vulvovaginal candidiasis (VVC) is a common mucosal infection caused by *Candida* species that affects a significant number of women predominantly in their reproductive years (Kent, 1991; Sobel, 1992, 2002). In fact, up to 75% of all women will experience at least one lifetime episode of acute VVC (Sobel, 1992, 2002). In 2002 alone women in the US spent US$500 million in medications to treat VVC, half of which was over the counter medications (Consumer Health Care Products Association, 2003). *Candida albicans* is the causative agent in approximately 85% to 90% of VVC cases, followed by *C. glabrata* and *C. tropicalis* as a distant third. A host of other *Candida* species cause VVC even less frequently (Sobel, 1992, 2002).

Acute VVC has several known predisposing factors including antibiotic and high estrogen oral contraceptive usage, hormone replacement therapy, pregnancy, and uncontrolled diabetes mellitus (Sobel, 1988, 1992).

Department of Microbiology, Immunology, and Parasitology, Louisiana State University Health Sciences Center, New Orleans, LA.

Recurrent VVC (RVVC) occurs in a small subset of women (5–10%) and is defined as having three or more episodes annually. There are two forms of RVVC. Primary RVVC is idiopathic with no known predisposing factors such as those identified for acute VVC (Sobel, 1992). Secondary RVVC is simply frequent episodes of acute VVC because certain women cannot avoid certain predisposing factors (i.e., diabetes mellitus, hormone replacement therapy) (Vanden-Bossche et al., 1992). Women with RVVC generally respond to antifungal regimens adequately with no resistance, but these regimens do not prevent recurrence (Sobel, 1992). A summary of the epidemiology of VVC and RVVC is shown in Table 16.1. There is little evidence that antifungal resistance plays a role in the pathogenesis of primary RVVC (Lynch et al., 1996). Instead, susceptibility to primary RVVC is postulated to be immune-based that until recently embraced the concept that these women experience repeated symptomatic episodes as a result of some immunological deficiency. However, host defense mechanisms functioning at the vaginal mucosa are poorly understood, not to mention those specifically acting against *C. albicans*. Accordingly, animal models of experimental vaginal candidiasis have been employed to investigate vaginal host defense mechanisms against *C. albicans*. To date, much of these data have come from both a mouse and rat model, although recently a nonhuman primate model has also been explored. Interestingly, the most recent data is beginning to challenge some of the previous concepts for susceptibility to infection.

Protective immunity against pathogenic organisms may occur in the form of adaptive or acquired immunity. The protection can be long-lived from as little as one exposure to antigen or short-lived requiring repeated antigen exposures, depending on the strength of the memory response, and can be induced by vaccination or in response to the live organism. Protective immunity may also only be partial, allowing the organism to colonize mucosal surfaces, but not invade or cause disease. This graded protection can be in the form of innate or adaptive

Table 16.1. Epidemiology and Factors Affecting *Candida albicans* Infection at the Vaginal Mucosa

Percent of healthy individuals asymptomatically colonized by yeast species in the vagina	5–20%
Lifetime occurrence of at least one episode of vaginal candidiasis in healthy women	50–75%
Candida albicans as causative agent	85–90%
Predisposing factors for infection (acute VVC, secondary RVVC)	
Antibiotics	+++
High estrogen contraceptive therapy	+
Steroids	+
Chronic mucocutaneous candidiasis	+/–
Chemotherapy	
Lymphoma/hematologic malignancy	+/–
Transplantation (allogeneic)	+/–
AIDS	+
Prevalence of recurrent infection in healthy women (HIV-negative)—primary RVVC (idiopathic)	5%
Antifungal resistance	Rare

immunity. Innate responses must be activated at each exposure since memory does not exist. The adaptive response must be tightly controlled by positive immunity and tolerance or immunoregulation to allow for asymptomatic colonization. If either of these immune mechanisms (which may not be mutually exclusive) is overwhelmed or even dysfunctional, symptomatic infection will ensue. Yet another mechanism is a hyperresponse to the organism that overwhelms the normal protection resulting in symptoms. In such cases the infection is actually host-mediated (synonomous with autoimmunity) rather than organism mediated. Protection against, or susceptibility to, *C. albicans* vaginal infection falls into these latter categories. This chapter will review the innate and adaptive cell-mediated host defense mechanisms acting at the vaginal mucosa against *C. albicans*, including both systemic and local mechanisms generated from animal models as well as clinical studies. The chapter will conclude by exploring interesting new hypotheses regarding mechanisms of resistance and susceptibility to vaginitis from a recently established live challenge model in humans.

2. Cell-Mediated Host Defense against Vaginal Candidiasis

Mucosal candidiasis includes oropharyngeal, esophageal, gastrointestinal, and vaginal infections. Prior to the AIDS epidemic, all mucosal sites were grouped together and as such considered equally susceptible to infection. Thus, early hypotheses for studies involving susceptibility to primary RVVC were borne from this broad definition. Accordingly, since mucosal candidiasis occurred most frequently in those with T cell immunosuppression (Clift, 1984; Klein et al., 1984; Samaranayake, 1992) and experimental models also showed a strong role for T cells against candidal infections (Romani et al., 1996; Mathews and Witek-Janusek, 2002; Sohnle et al., 2002), cell-mediated immunity (CMI) became the center of all hypotheses to explain RVVC. The following is a history of the evolution of the studies to uncover the innate and adaptive cell-mediated host defenses against vaginitis and the proposed immune deficiencies/dysfunctions in those with primary RVVC.

2.1. Role of Adaptive CMI

2.1.1. Early Clinical Studies

The majority of early clinical studies tested women with primary RVVC and normal healthy women for systemic *Candida*-specific CMI, but these studies have not been without controversy. In a comprehensive study from our laboratory, we showed that although some primary RVVC patients may experience a loss in *Candida*-specific cutaneous skin test reactivity, the majority of RVVC patients, both during symptomatic infections and infection-free periods of remission, had normal levels of *Candida*-specific systemic CMI detected by both peripheral blood lymphocyte (PBL) proliferation and cytokine expression (Fidel et al., 1993a). Interestingly, not only was the systemic CMI response present in RVVC patients, the cytokine expression was identified as the $CD4^+$ Th1-type (IL-2, IFN-γ, and IL-12) known to be associated with resistance to candidiasis (Romani et al., 1991, 1993; Cenci et al., 1995). We concluded from these results that the immune dysfunction/deficiency, if present in RVVC patients, was at the local rather than systemic level and that the loss of *Candida*-specific skin test reactivity was the result rather than a cause of infection (Fidel et al., 1993a). However, studies previous to this examined solely delayed cutaneous skin test responses and/or PBL proliferative responses showed that women with RVVC had some form of impairment of systemic CMI (Hobbs et al.,

1977; Witkin, 1986; Witkin et al., 1986; Fong et al., 1992) either at the T cell or macrophage level, or had no detectable defect (Syverson et al., 1979; Fong et al., 1992; Mendling and Koldovsky, 1996). The controversy continues into the present with a limited number of additional studies that examined *Candida*-specific CMI (lymphocyte proliferation, cytokine production). One described a dysfunction in proliferation and interferon gamma (IFN-γ) and tumor necrosis factor alpha (TNF-α) production during acute episodes of RVVC that was restored in remission (Nawrot et al., 2000). A second reported reduced responsiveness in RVVC patients during the follicular phase of the menstrual cycle (least influence of hormones) (Corrigan et al., 1998). While it is unclear what significance the latter study carries since most women with RVVC do not show a pattern of episodic recurrences during the follicular stage of the menstrual cycle, it does emphasize that stage of the menstrual cycle should be taken into account when examining local or systemic immune reactivity to *C. albicans*. These data also confirm the systemic cytokine profile in response to *Candida* antigen, that in all studies to date show that control women and RVVC patients have some level of Th1-type responses in the virtual absence of Th2-type responses (Fidel et al., 1993a, 1997a; Corrigan et al., 1998). Our results specifically showing that most episodes of RVVC occur in the presence of normal levels of *Candida*-specific Th1-type CMI correlate with two relevant clinical observations; women with RVVC are generally not susceptible to oral, esophageal, or other forms of cutaneous candidiasis (Sobel, 1988), and women with CMC are rarely susceptible to RVVC (Odds, 1988). Based on this information, we postulated that the proposed immune deficiency in RVVC patients is primarily localized to the vaginal mucosa and does not involve systemic CMI.

The lack of effects of systemic CMI at the vaginal mucosa appears to extend as well to the HIV patient although again the studies are not without controversy. Some reports have suggested both that vaginitis is more common in the HIV patient and the incidence of infection increases as the CD4 cell counts decrease (Spinillo et al., 1994; Burns et al., 1997; Duerr et al., 1997). In contrast, other reports have suggested that vaginitis is not more common in the HIV$^+$ or AIDS patients than in HIV$^-$ women (Clark et al., 1995; White, 1996; Schuman et al., 1998; Leigh et al., 2001), or at least does not correlate with decreased CD4 cell counts if present (Rhoads et al., 1987; Imam et al., 1990). These discordant results likely stem from the lack of appropriate control groups. For example, comparing parameters between HIV$^+$ and HIV$^-$ individuals require several matched groups, including age and associated behavioral risk factors. However, the design of too many studies failed to also include an unmatched control group that can be used to identify true baseline levels. Additionally, the lack of knowledge of host defense mechanisms important for protection against vaginal candidiasis has hampered our ability to adequately interpret data from the clinical studies. Nevertheless, the controversy itself indicated that the effects of HIV and systemic immunocompromising conditions on the vaginal mucosa is different from that observed at the oral mucosa where it is quite clear that reduced blood CD4 cell counts correlate with increased incidence of oropharyngeal and esophageal candidiasis (Knight and Fletcher, 1971; Klein et al., 1984; Imam et al., 1990; Samaranayake, 1992). A study conducted in our laboratory that examined *Candida*-specific systemic CMI in HIV$^+$ women with or without VVC showed that although delayed cutaneous skin test reactivity to *Candida* antigen was reduced in HIV$^+$ women with <200 CD4 cells/μl, there was no correlation of reduced skin test reactivity to VVC. Furthermore, PBL proliferation and Th1/Th2 cytokine production in response to *Candida* antigens was relatively similar in HIV^{+} women with or without symptomatic VVC with the exception of one cytokine, IFN-γ, that was reduced in $HIV^{+}VVC^{+}$ women compared to HIV^{-} women (Leigh et al., 2001). This provides yet another example for the virtual lack of any role for *Candida*-specific systemic CMI against vaginal *C. albicans* infections.

2.1.2. Early Studies in Animal Models

The majority of studies to date have employed rodent models of experimental vaginitis. These models require that the animals be in a state of pseudoestrus to obtain a persistent infection that can be studied for immunological or therapeutic purposes (Ryley and McGregor, 1986; Fidel et al., 1993b; Valentin et al., 1993). Estrogen converts vaginal columnar epithelium to thick stratified squamous epithelium and increases glycogen content and growth substrates, all of which increase the avidity of the yeast for the tissue and enhances growth of the yeast (Kinsman and Collard, 1986). Animals are usually treated subcutaneously with estradiol (0.2–0.5 mg/rodent) 48–72 h before vaginal inoculation although a similar infection can be achieved if estrogen is administered several days postinoculation (Fidel et al., 2000). The inoculum consists of a stationary phase *C. albicans* culture given intravaginally in a small volume of phosphate-buffered saline (PBS). The vaginal infection resulting from this pseudoestrus state is usually persistent in mice ($>10^{4}$ CFU) lasting for weeks as long as the hormonal condition is maintained (Fidel et al., 2000). In rats, however, the infection spontaneously resolves ($<10^{3}$ CFU) in 3 to 4 despite the maintenance of pseudoestrus (De Bernardis et al., 2000). The experimental infection is usually monitored by quantitative vaginal lavage culture or micropipet culture (Fidel et al., 1993b; Cassone et al., 1995). The vaginal fungal burden in colony-forming units (CFU) is then used as a measure of the level of infectivity. Animals can be sampled independently over time or longitudinally. One interesting caveat of the rodents is their general resistance to yeast colonization and subsequent lack of *C. albicans*-derived immune sensitization (delayed-type hypersensitivity (DTH), lymphocyte responses) to *C. albicans* antigen in the naïve state. Additionally, the vaginal pH of rodents is significantly higher (7–9) compared to that of the human vagina (4–4.5).

Because of the apparent limitations of the rodent model, nonhuman primates have been considered as an alternative model to study pathogenesis of human *C. albicans* vaginal infection. As in humans, both rhesus and pigtailed macaques were found to have detectable yeast colonization at mucosal sites and evidence of positive immune sensitization at both the local mucosal and systemic levels (*Candida*-specific PBL responses, *Candida*-specific vaginal antibody expression, and vaginal-associated cytokine expression) (Steele et al., 1999b). However, only the rhesus macaques were susceptible to an experimental *C. albicans* vaginal infection, either untreated, after antibiotic-mediated reduction of normal vaginal flora, or following the induction of a state of estrus. In each case, although the experimental vaginal infection resolved spontaneously in some animals, most had to be treated with topical antifungal agents. Figure 16.1 shows a typical progression of an experimental *C. albicans* vaginal infection in mice, rats, and macaques.

Animal studies were initially designed and conducted to evaluate the role of systemic CMI against vaginal candidiasis. In our laboratory, recognizing that a systemic Th1-type response was generated in mice as a result of a vaginal *C. albicans* infection and that this response had also been reported to be associated with protection against systemic and mucosal *C. albicans* infection (Romani et al., 1991, 1993; Cenci et al., 1995), preinduced *Candida*-specific systemic CMI was evaluated with regard to

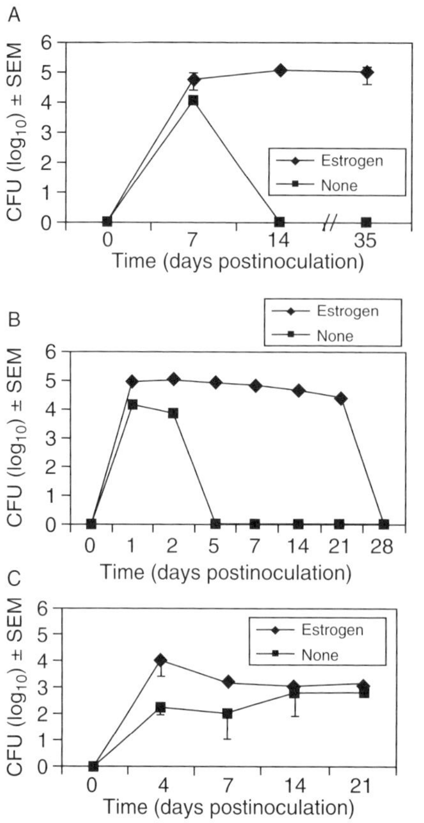

Figure 16.1. Experimental *C. albicans* vaginitis in mice (A), rats (B), and primates (C). Mice, oophorectomized rats, and rhesus macaques were inoculated intravaginally with *C. albicans* blastoconidia with or without exogenous estrogen treatment. Quantitative vaginal lavages were used to quantify the vaginal fungal burden over time. Rats and primates were tested longitudinally, while separate mice were tested at each time interval. Reproduced with the permission of ASM Press.

impact on vaginal *Candida* burden during experimental *Candida* vaginitis. Results showed, however, that in this model system, neither $CD4^+$ Th1-type CMI nor the presence of *Candida*-specific suppressor T cells that suppressed the infection-induced DTH reactivity had any effect on vaginal fungal titers (Fidel et al., 1994). These results were the first experimental evidence that systemic CMI expressed in the peripheral circulation may not represent a dominant host defense mechanism at the vaginal mucosa. Partial protection against vaginitis was, however, achieved in animals given a second inoculation of *C. albicans* following the spontaneous resolution of a primary infection in the absence of estrogen (Fidel et al., 1995b). Interestingly, although anamnestic DTH occurred during the secondary infection, suppression of this systemic Th1-type reactivity, either by *Candida*-specific suppressor T cells or depletion of all systemic $CD4^+$ cells, had no effect on the protection against vaginitis (Fidel et al., 1995b), providing additional evidence that systemic CMI had a limited role in protection against vaginal candidiasis. Also in support of this, we showed that mice either resistant or susceptible to systemic *C. albicans* infection (Hector et al., 1982) were equally susceptible to vaginitis and could equally be partially protected against a second vaginal infection (Fidel et al., 1995a). This was supported further by another study that employed six different strains of mice representing four haplotypes (Black et al., 1999a). We concluded from these studies that some form of locally acquired mucosal immunity, T cell and/or antibody-mediated, was responsible for protecting mice against vaginal *C. albicans* infection and that the vaginal mucosa had some level of immunological independence or immune compartmentalization. In support of the concept of immune compartmentalization, complement-fixing antibodies specific for T cells given intravenously to mice-depleted T cells in the periphery, but not in the vagina, whereas intravaginal administration of the same antibodies depleted T cells in both the vagina and the periphery (Fidel et al., 1997b). Additionally, adoptive transfer of *Candida*-sensitized T cells into T cell-deficient (nude) mice had no effect on vaginitis (Black et al., 1999b). Despite this overwhelming evidence for a lack of effects of systemic responses against a vaginal *C. albicans* infection, a group has recently described T cell-mediated protection against vaginitis by systemic immunization in a particular strain of mice (Mulero-Marchese et al., 1998, 1999). Although it is unclear what type of immunity was generated (Th1/Th2), this suggests that under some circumstances (i.e., genetic background, antigen), systemic responses may have some effect on the vaginal mucosa. These studies, however, reflect a minority view of the protective role of systemic CMI.

In light of little evidence suggesting a role for systemic CMI against *C. albicans* vaginal infection, subsequent studies focused on the presence of T cell subpopulations at the vaginal mucosa and the role of local CMI against vaginal *C. albicans* infection. The murine vaginal mucosa, while not containing organized lymphoid areas as that in the gastrointestinal (GI) tract (i.e., Peyer's patches, tonsils), nevertheless has all the necessary components for competent adaptive immune responses. This includes immunoglobulin expression, T cells, and major histocompatibility complex (MHC) class II^+ cells (i.e., Langerhan's cells, macrophages, epithelial cells) to serve as antigen-presenting cells (Parr and Parr, 1990; Parr et al., 1991). Of critical importance, several investigators report that vaginal lymphocytes in mice are phenotypically distinct from those in the periphery (Itohara et al., 1990; Nandi and Allison, 1991; Ibraghimov et al., 1995; Fidel et al., 1996). Similar observations have been made in humans (Inghirami et al., 1990; Hladik et al., 1999; Johansson et al., 2000). In mice, flow cytometric data showed that although $CD4^+$, α/β TCR^+ cells predominate the T cell repertoire at the vaginal mucosa in a manner similar to lymph node cells or PBLs, there exists a 5- to 40-fold higher percentage of γ/δ TCR^+ cells (15–50%) (Itohara et al., 1990; Nandi and Allison, 1991; Ibraghimov et al., 1995; Fidel et al., 1996) and very few if any $CD8^+$ cells (normally 20% in blood) (Fidel et al., 1996). In humans, the ratio of α/β and γ/δ T cells are similar to mice (Inghirami et al., 1990; Hladik et al., 1999), but there are abundant $CD8^+$ T cells (Hladik et al., 1999) that have cytotoxic T lymphocytes (CTL) function (White et al., 1997). Similar findings have been reported in nonhuman primates (Miller et al., 1992; Lohman et al., 1995). These observations further support the concept of immunological independence or compartmentalization of vaginal T cells.

Through several independent studies (i.e., flow cytometry, immunohistochemistry, and RT-PCR), our laboratory has evidence suggesting that murine vaginal $CD4^+$ T cells atypically express the CD4 protein compared to their systemic counterparts in peripheral blood or lymph nodes. This was first observed by the differential recognition of epitope-distinct anti-CD4 antibodies under nondenatured conditions (Fidel et al., 1996). A similar atypical expression of the CD4 protein on the vaginal cells was observed in situ using the intravaginal administration of complement-fixing antibodies (Fidel et al., 1996). Evidence for the masking of the N-terminus epitope of the CD4 protein, or rather the absence of the epitope, came from positive and negative immunohistochemical staining of collagenase-treated vaginal cells under denatured and nondenatured conditions, respectively, using anti-CD4 antibodies directed to the N-terminus (Wormley et al., 2000). The uniqueness of the murine vaginal CD4 protein was also found to extend to the level of transcription (Wormley et al., 2000). The inability to amplify CD4 mRNA from a purified population of the unique $CD4^+$ vaginal lymphocytes confirmed the absence of CD4 mRNA in the cells. Possibilities for the presence of the atypical CD4 protein on vaginal $CD4^+$ T cells include differential splicing or a passive acquisition from a source or soluble CD4 in the tissue.

The ultimate question then became whether this unique CD4 protein was specific to the vagina as opposed to other mucosal tissues, and whether or not a similar unique CD4 protein is present in human vaginal tissue. Unfortunately, the expression was found to be unique to the murine vagina and possibly to mice alone as the unique expression of CD4 has not been observed on human vaginal CD4$^+$ T cells (Fidel et al., 2001).

During the same time interesting properties were being uncovered for vaginal γ/δ T cells. In contrast to γ/δ T cells at other mucosal sites, the γ/δ T cells in the vaginal mucosa of mice express a homogenous Vγ4/Vδ1 TCR lacking N-region junctional diversity (Nandi and Allison, 1991; Rakasz et al., 1997). Although all γ/δ T cells share a limited repertoire of antigenic recognition, the site-specific phenotype of the vaginal γ/δ T cells implies compartmentalization and the potential for unique function(s). Furthermore, the murine vaginal γ/δ T cells lack both CD2 and CD28, two potent costimulatory signals, but show an effector phenotype with the expression of CD44, CD45RB, and LFA-1 (Rakasz et al., 1996, 1997). These cells too can be expanded by the intravenous injection of pan anti-γδ TCR antibodies (Rakasz et al., 1996). Taken together, it appears that both types of T cells in the murine vaginal mucosa are phenotypically and potentially functionally distinct from their peripheral and other mucosal tissue counterparts.

2.1.3. Later Animal Studies

In light of the vaginal mucosal of mice and humans showing significant independence and compartmentalization, the next series of studies were designed to evaluate potential changes in vaginal T cells during a *C. albicans* experimental infection. Previous to this, the only studies that examined the role of local T cells during vaginitis were by Balish and coworkers. In these studies, immunodeficient mice were used to study the natural history of *Candida* vaginal infections (Cantorna et al., 1990). The nude strain of mice deficient in T cells (*nu*/*nu*) showed no increase in susceptibility to vaginitis compared to the immunocompetent controls. However, since the animals were not maintained in a state of pseudoestrus and vaginal T cells were not evaluated, it is difficult to interpret these findings. Recently, however, these studies were repeated under pseudoestrus conditions with similar findings (Black et al., 1999b; Wormley et al., 2003). With regard to the role of γ/δ T cells, a study showed that mice depleted of γ/δ T cells had an increased susceptibility to vaginitis, suggesting a potential role for these cells as a first-line defense mechanism (Jones-Carson et al., 1995). In stark contrast to this, however, δ-chain TCR knockout mice are more resistant to vaginitis suggesting a tolerance role for vaginal γ/δ T cells (Wormley et al., 2001b). Clearly more investigation is required to fully understand the role of these vaginal T cells against *Candida*.

Studies to examine changes in vaginal T cells using flow cytometry, immunohistochemistry, and RT-PCR, all showed little evidence for modulation of α/β or γ/δ vaginal T cells during either primary or secondary experimental vaginal *C. albicans* infections, and no evidence for systemic T cell infiltration during a vaginal *Candida* infection (Fidel et al., 1999). These results are consistent with those from the immunodeficient or knockout mice (Cantorna et al., 1990; Black et al., 1999b) as well as the systemic immune studies in immunocompetent mice (Fidel et al., 1994, 1995a–c). This lack of responsiveness to *Candida* infection is in direct contrast to comprehensive studies conducted in a murine model of a genital *Chlamydia trachomatis* or herpes simplex virus (HSV)-2 infection where significant activity by CD4$^+$ T cells has been reported (Kelly and Rank, 1997; Parr and Parr, 1997, 1998). Interestingly, a study examining a dual infection with *Candida* and *Chlamydia* showed a complete independence of "responsiveness" in the upper genital tract (*Chlamydia*) and "lack of responsiveness" in the lower tract (*Candida*) (Kelly et al., 2001), revealing the complexity of genital tract immunity.

Experimental studies that followed focused on local cytokines and chemokines during infection to better understand the lack of vaginal responsiveness to *C. albicans*. Examination of chemokines showed that MCP-1 (chemotactic for macrophages and T cells) was increased in the vaginal mucosa during infection and MIP-2 (chemotactic for neutrophils) was constitutively expressed at high levels in the vagina (Saavedra et al., 1999). Furthermore, in vivo neutralization of MCP-1 with anti-MCP-1 antibodies resulted in increased vaginal fungal burden suggesting some role for the chemokine in the host response. However, elevated levels of MCP-1 did not result in any demonstrable increases in T cells or macrophages in vaginal lavage fluid (previously well shown in vaginal tissue (Fidel et al., 1999)). Thus, either MCP-1 was playing a role independent of chemotaxis or it was being regulated such that a stronger function was prohibited. When local Th1/Th2 cytokines were evaluated, high constitutive levels of transforming growth factor-beta (TGF-β) were found whereas other Th1/Th2 cytokines (i.e., IL-2, IFN-γ, IL-12, IL-4, IL-10) were low or undetectable (Taylor et al., 2000). During pseudoestrus and/or infection, TGF-β, but not the other cytokines, was transiently increased. Furthermore, TGF-β was significantly higher in the lower genital tract than in the upper genital tract. These results suggested a possible Th3-type condition where TGF-β contributes to immunoregulation or tolerance in the tissue. This represented a possible explanation for the lack of responsiveness in the vagina during a *Candida* infection. Furthermore, since TGF-β inhibits chemokine receptors (Sallusto et al., 1998), its presence may also explain the lack of stronger effects by MCP-1 during infection (Saavedra et al., 1999).

A final series of studies in mice evaluated adhesion molecules on the vaginal epithelium and T cells in the draining lymph nodes. Results showed that while the appropriate adhesion molecules (mucosal addressin cell adhesion molecule (MAdCAM), vascular adhesion molecule (VCAM-1)) were upregulated as expected on the surface on the vaginal epithelium following infection, the T cells with the reciprocal homing receptors ($\alpha_4\beta_1$, $\alpha_4\beta_7$) were being decreased in the lymph nodes, possibly by circulating out or apoptosis (Wormley et al., 2001a). This served as an explanation for the lack of any T cell infiltration into the vagina during infection. Interestingly, the draining lymph nodes of infected mice contained a considerable number of $CD4^+CD25^+$ T cells, that although once considered activated T cells, are now considered to be regulatory T (T_{reg}) cells with profound suppressive capabilities (Baecher-Allan et al., 2001; Ermann et al., 2001; Jonuleit and Schmitt, 2003), potentially involving TGF-β (Yamagiwa et al., 2000; Nakamura et al., 2001). Thus, the overwhelming conclusion from the animal model studies is that CMI is not protective against *C. albicans* at the vaginal mucosa due to local and systemic immunoregulation.

In contrast to these results in mice, a recent study in the rat model revealed quite different findings. Although the rat model has been used predominantly to study the role of humoral immunity against vaginal *C. albicans* infection, the same model was most recently used to examine the role of T cells during an infection (De Bernardis et al., 2000; Santoni et al., 2002). As mentioned earlier, an important difference between the rat and mouse model is the fact that under a state of pseudoestrus, the infection in rats resolves spontaneously over a 2 to 3-week period (De Bernardis et al., 2000), while the infection in mice remains persistent for several weeks (Fidel et al., 1993b,c) (Fig. 16.1). With this fact in mind, although the relative percentages of vaginal-associated T cells was similar in rats and mice (infected or uninfected), significant numbers of $CD8^+$ T cells were identified in the rat vagina similar to humans (Hladik et al., 1999). During successive infections, the protection was enhanced indicative of a secondary response together with a change in the ratio of CD4:CD8 cells with increases in $CD4^+$ α/β T cells. Additionally, Th1-type cytokines (IL-12, IL-2, and IFN-γ) in vaginal lavage fluid increased as well during the infections and vaginal lymphocytes, but not draining lymph nodes, from infected rats proliferated in vitro to *Candida* antigen (De Bernardis et al., 2000). Finally, vaginal $CD4^+$ and to a lesser extent $CD8^+$ T cells, but not lymph node cells, transferred protection to naïve animals (Santoni et al., 2002) indicating an extremely restricted local response compared to the predominant systemic responsiveness with little evidence for a local CMI response in mice (Fidel et al., 1999; Saavedra et al., 1999; Taylor et al., 2000). These results are consistent with the relative outcomes for each. Furthermore, based on these results it would not appear that the immunoregulation or tolerance predicted in mice and humans is operative in the rat.

In uninfected nonhuman primates, a Th2-type cytokine profile was observed in vaginal secretions (cervicovaginal lavage fluid) predominated by IL-4 and IL-10 (Steele et al., 1999b). Under estrogen and infected conditions (rhesus) the vaginal-associated cytokines declined, suggesting a potential protective role of Th2-type cytokines. However, a similar profile was observed in pigtailed macaques that were resistant to infection (Steele et al., 1999b). Clearly, these models are quite distinct with respect to local immunity during an infection. Although disparate, each may serve in their own right to elucidate aspects of the host response(s) to vaginal *C. albicans* infection.

2.1.4. Later Clinical Studies

Subsequent clinical studies evaluated the presence of cytokines/chemokines in vaginal secretions. In keeping with the general view that $CD4^+$ Th1- and Th2-type cellular reactivity was associated with resistance and susceptibility, respectively, to *Candida* infection at other mucosal sites (i.e., oral, gastrointestinal) (Romani et al., 1991, 1993; Cenci et al., 1995), we evaluated Th1-(IL-2, IL-12, IFN-γ) and Th2-type (IL-4, IL-5, IL-10) cytokines in vaginal lavage fluid from women with primary RVVC (Fidel et al., 1997a). Interestingly, we found a constitutive presence of Th1-type, but not Th2-type, cytokines in cervicovaginal lavage fluid of normal healthy control women that might reflect a natural immune homeostasis, possibly in response to normal flora, including *C. albicans*. With respect to patients in the study, although some differences in cytokine expression were detected between fluids collected from control women and RVVC patients with or without a symptomatic infection, we did not detect any characteristic pattern of cytokine changes that would reflect a major deviation or shift from the profile in control women. There is some recent evidence for the presence of heat shock proteins in vaginal secretions and/or sera of women with RVVC that are postulated to downregulate local Th1-type CMI, creating susceptibility to primary RVVC (Giraldo et al., 1999a,b). However, there is little evidence, based on data in the above study, that vaginal cytokines are vastly affected in RVVC if such proteins are present. In a more recent study many of these same cytokines were evaluated over the menstrual cycle in normal control women (Fidel et al., 2003). Results showed that the Th2-type cytokines tended to increase under more hormonal influence during the menstrual cycle. This included TGF-β, which while constitutively present, increased during the ovulatory and luteal phases of the menstrual cycle and was equally present in the homogenates of vaginal cuff tissue from nondiseased hysterectomy surgeries. Interestingly, although not yet identified in vaginal secretions, a T cell-derived antigen-binding molecule (TABM) has been identified in serum of RVVC patients, and to a lesser extent in control women that can become associated with TGF-β and inhibit *Candida*-specific PBL proliferation and cytokine production (Little et al., 2000). Taken together, clinical studies evaluating local immunity in women with or without RVVC show evidence for immunoregulatory mechanisms against more profound adaptive CMI similar to the mouse model.

2.2. Role of Innate Cellular Immunity

Innate cellular immunity may also play a significant role in protection against vaginitis. This was initially predicted based on a leukocytic infiltrate of predominantly polymorphonuclear neutrophils (PMNs) that is often observed in vaginal lavage fluid of infected animals. These leukocytic cells are usually associated with or attached to the hyphae and/or sheets of epithelial cells. On the other hand, when this infiltrate is present during infection it does not correlate with lower vaginal fungal titers (Fidel et al., 1999; Saavedra et al., 1999). Although PMNs and macrophages (two types of leukocytes with considerable effector function against *C. albicans*) (Odds, 1988; Candida and Candidiasis, 2002) are potential candidates for anti-*Candida* innate resistance and are present at or near the vaginal mucosa, Balish and coworkers showed that animals with the beige mutation and immunodeficient in *phagocytic* cells (*bg/bg*) were not more susceptible to a natural *C. albicans* infection under nonestrogenized conditions (Cantorna et al., 1990). Several additional studies have been conducted since. Although one early study showed increased susceptibility to infection in the absence of PMNs (Fulurija et al., 1996), more recently two studies showed no effect of neutropenia (Black et al., 1998; Fidel et al., 1999). In one study depletion of PMNs under pseudoestrus conditions had no effect on vaginal fungal burden, although microabscesses within the tissue were significantly reduced (Black et al., 1998). Although no differences in fungal titers were observed, the authors nevertheless speculated that PMNs may in fact play a significant role against *C. albicans* in the vagina, but they cannot consistently be deployed in high enough numbers during pseudoestrus to be effective. We tested this hypothesis by examining the effects of PMN depletion both in estrogen and nonestrogen-treated mice. Results similarly showed that depletion of PMNs had no effect on vaginal fungal burden under either hormonal condition (Fidel et al., 1999), suggesting that PMNs do not in fact appear to play a significant role against *C. albicans* in the vagina despite their presence in the vaginal lumen during some experimental infections. Perhaps this reflects their inability to function against *C. albicans* in the vaginal microenvironment compared to blood or tissue culture as a result of putative immunoregulatory mechanisms or other environmental conditions in the vagina. In support of this, Calderone and coworkers recently showed that a mutant strain of *Candida* that was killed more readily by PMNs in vitro and was avirulent in a systemic model of candidiasis, was as virulent as the wild-type strain in the vaginal candidiasis model (Torosantucci et al., 2002).

Natural killer (NK) cells may represent another potential innate resistance mechanism against *C. albicans* at the vaginal mucosa. However, most studies have shown little or no role for NK cells against *C. albicans* (Djeu and Blanchard, 1987; Arancia et al., 1995). Furthermore, NK cells do not appear to be resident cells in the vaginal mucosa (Parr and Parr, 1991). Thus, although NK cells may have the potential to be recruited into the vaginal mucosa in response to *C. albicans*, it is unlikely that NK cells play a major role in innate resistance against *C. albicans* at the vaginal mucosa.

Epithelial cells now appear to represent another form of innate cellular immunity. Our laboratory found that vaginal epithelial cells from mice, humans, and macaques have the ability to inhibit the growth of *C. albicans* in vitro, potentially representing an innate host defense mechanism localized to the vaginal mucosa (Steele et al., 1999a,b; Barousse et al., 2001). This seemed reasonable since epithelial cells are the primary cells that *Candida* interacts with at mucosal sites. Subsequent studies on the physical properties showed that the activity involves a strict requirement for cell contact with no known role for any soluble factor, no phagocytosis, and no role for microtubules or microfilaments (Steele et al., 1999a; Nomanbhoy et al., 2002; Yano et al., 2004). Studies on the mechanism showed no oxidative or nonoxidative killing (Nomanbhoy et al., 2002). In fact, the activity is static rather than cidal and noninflammatory (Nomanbhoy et al., 2002). We postulate that this may represent a noninflammatory means to control *C. albicans* on the tissue surface as a commensal. Studies to identify the effector moiety showed that the activity was resistant to inhibitors of surface proteins (proteinase K) and phospholipids (phospholipase A_2), but sensitive to an inhibitor of carbohydrates (periodic acid). However, a putative carbohydrate moiety was not identified with inhibitors of specific carbohydrates (Nomanbhoy et al., 2002). The most recent studies show that the effector moiety cannot be regenerated or reattached and cannot competitively inhibit the activity of fresh epithelial cells (Yano et al., 2004). Furthermore, the antifungal activity is not dependent on the amount of carbohydrate released (Yano et al., 2004) and can be abrogated in the presence of several other acids (Yano et al., 2004). Together these results suggest that the activity is acid-labile rather than dependent on an effector carbohydrate. Finally, the partial or full resistance of the activity by epithelial cell fixation or irradiation together with viability evaluation with trypan blue and propidium iodide/fluorescein diacetate revealed that the activity is dependent on intact (trypan blue impermeable), but not necessarily live epithelial cells (Yano et al., 2005). Interestingly, oral epithelial cells function similarly but with greater inhibition (Steele et al., 2000, 2001). Figure 16.2 shows the comparison between vaginal epithelial cell antifungal activity in various species and

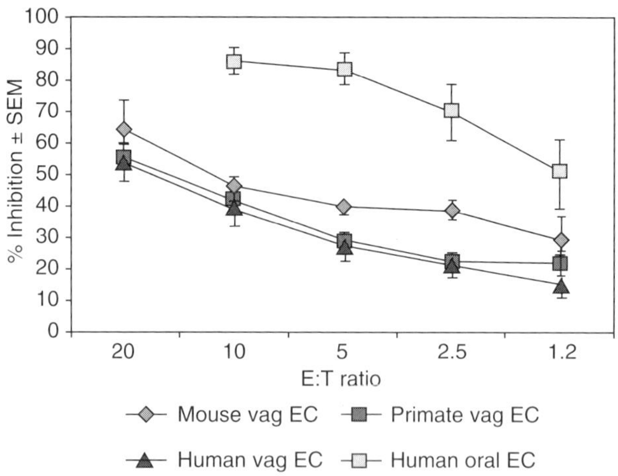

Figure 16.2. Vaginal and oral epithelial cell anti-*Candida* activity. Vaginal epithelial cells from humans (vaginal lavage), nonhuman primates (vaginal lavage), and mouse (vaginal tissue extraction) and oral epithelial cells (collected from saliva) were cocultured with *C. albicans* at various effector to target (E:T) ratios for 9 h. Controls included epithelial cells and *Candida* cultured alone. Growth of *Candida* was determined by ^{3}H-glucose uptake and percent inhibition in the coculture was determined.

human oral epithelial cell antifungal activity. In a study comparing vaginal epithelial cell antifungal activity between women with primary RVVC and normal healthy women, while there was no difference in activity by control women at different stages of the menstrual cycle, a significant reduction of vaginal epithelial cell antifungal activity was detected in those with RVVC at low effector to target ratios (10:1, 1:1) (Barousse et al., 2001). We contend, however, that while this may represent a contributing factor to RVVC, the level of activity where these differences were observed was modest (<10%). Thus, we believe there are other innate factors that are important for protection against vaginitis.

3. Development of a Human Live Challenge Model

The clinical studies and animal models to date strongly suggest that adaptive immunity is not likely involved in protection against infection and innate resistance is moderate at best. A summary is illustrated in Table 16.2. Although informative, these studies failed to reveal any cellular protective mechanisms or primary immune factors associated with susceptibility to VVC. Accordingly, either one assumes there are little to no active cellular protective mechanisms (possibly due to immunoregulatory mechanisms), or alternatively, that the models and clinical studies have not been able to reveal them adequately. Support for the latter came from a recent study evaluating adolescents for vaginal yeast colonization and local and systemic immune sensitization (Barousse et al., 2003). Interestingly, adolescents were found to be asymptomatically colonized with yeast in the vagina at a rate of 26%, which is at the high end of the normal range for adults (Table 16.1). These adolescents had the same species distribution of *Candida* in the vagina (90% *C. albicans*), and were sensitized to *Candida* systemically (peripheral blood responses

Table 16.2. Protective Host Defenses against Vaginal Candidiasis[a]

	Local	Systemic
T cell		
CD4	–[b]	–[b]
CD8	–[c]	–[c]
Antibody	+/–[d]	–[c]
Innate		
PMN	N/A	–[c]
NK	–[c]	–[c]
Macrophage	?[e]	?
DC/LC[b]	?	?
Epithelial	+	N/A

[a]*Abbreviations*: PMN, polymorphonuclear neutrophil; NK, natural killer cell, DC/LC, dendritic cells/Langerhans cells; N/A, not applicable.
[b]Possible immunoregulation precludes immune responsiveness.
[c]No known role.
[d]Controversial.
[e]Unknown.

and antibodies) similar to adults. However, what set the adolescents apart from the adults was an extremely high vaginal fungal burden in those asymptomatically colonized (50% had between 200 and 1000 CFUs compared to 95% of adults having <200 CFUs). Probably most intriguing was that the attack rate of acute VVC in this population (in a longitudinal study over 3 years) was <3%. Thus, the adolescents could maintain large numbers of *Candida* vaginally without symptomatic infection, suggesting strong protective activity/responsiveness.

In light of all the findings to date, we reasoned that the design that was likely to provide valuable information on putative vaginal protective host defenses against *C. albicans* was a controlled challenge with *Candida* that offers the ability to properly monitor the responses. The initial design involved the intravaginal administration of *Candida* antigen with immune reactivity detected in vaginal lavages collected pre- and post-intravaginal antigen challenge. A pilot study using commercial soluble skin test antigen in a small number of women revealed a Th1-type cytokine response (Fidel et al., 1997a). However, results from a formal study with large numbers of women tested during each of the three stages of the menstrual cycle did not reproduce those original observations (Fidel et al., 2003). We next embarked on an intravaginal challenge with live *C. albicans*. Live challenge models in humans are not new. Currently there are live challenge models for *Haemophilus ducreyi*, *Neissaria gonorrhoeae*, and Norwalk virus (Cohen et al., 1994; Al-Tawfig et al., 1999; Lindesmith et al., 2003). The primary rationale for these models is the inability of the organism to colonize or easily infect animals. There is considerable risk with these models since the organisms/virus have pathogenic potential. Nevertheless, the ability to treat the infections successfully provided confidence that a well-constructed experimental design would have minimal risk to the subject. Vaginal *C. albicans* infections are similarly treated with a high level of success, providing a high level of confidence for use of *Candida* organisms in a live challenge. Furthermore, the fact that *C. albicans* is a commensal organism of the vaginal mucosa with no known migration to extravaginal sites make *C. albicans* an excellent organism for a live challenge model with minimal risk.

The results of these studies to date evaluating the natural history following intravaginal inoculation of live *C. albicans* into healthy women have completely reshaped our hypotheses relative to host defense against vaginitis and susceptibility to infection. In a very conservative initial approach testing women with no history of vaginitis and inoculating small numbers (yet bolus) of *Candida*, few women became symptomatic with vaginitis (~15%). Broadening the inoculating condition to include higher numbers of *Candida*, inoculating women at different stages of the menstrual cycle, and inclusion of growth promoting supplements in the inoculum vehicle (growth media, glucose, estrogen) had very little effect as well. In fact, a high percentage of women did not even become asymptomatically colonized. In contrast, inclusion of women with documented infrequent episodes of VVC (antibiotic usage, oral contraceptive usage, pregnancy, etc.) had higher rates of symptomatic infection (~55%) with the majority of the remaining women becoming asymptomatically colonized (Fidel et al., 2004). Interestingly, in either design, protection occurred in the absence of any evidence of inflammation or an inflammatory response, whereas those with symptomatic infection had a heavy vaginal cellular infiltrate consisting almost entirely of PMNs. Furthermore, a high PMN infiltration score in those with symptomatic infection correlated with higher fungal burdens. Although the more pathogenic hyphal form of *Candida* was present along with blastoconidia in those with symptomatic infection, hyphae were also detected in some of those asymptomatically colonized.

Based on these data, we hypothesize that VVC is associated with signals following *Candida*–vaginal epithelial cell interactions that promote a nonprotective inflammatory PMN response and concomitant clinical symptoms, while resistance to VVC is associated with a lack of signals and/or the presence of the appropriate local milieu of innate mediators that is noninflammatory. The association of symptomatic infection with PMNs is further supported by the fact that VVC is rare in neutropenic women (J. Sobel, personal communication). The resistance may also include vaginal epithelial cell antifungal activity that was found to be significantly increased in those who would become colonized or not colonized compared to those that would become infected (P.L. Fidel, unpublished observations). We also postulate that a threshold number of organisms in the vagina following inoculation (not inocula itself) is crucial to the signal(s) in the face of T cell immunoregulation, and this threshold is different for different groups of women. For example, women with primary RVVC inevitably acquire an infection shortly after completing a regimen of antifungal therapy. In these women, the threshold of *Candida* required to signal the PMN infiltration would be extremely low. Women with an infrequent history of VVC or secondary RVVC have a higher threshold of *Candida* required to signal the PMNs. In these women the threshold is usually met when the population numbers of *Candida* increase following antibiotic therapy or hormone replacement therapy (HRT), high estrogen oral contraceptives, during pregnancy, or due to diabetes mellitus. In women with no history of VVC, the threshold number of *Candida* is extremely high (levels rarely attainable). Thus, although the population numbers of *Candida* can increase with reduced bacterial flora during antibiotic therapy or increased estrogen from oral contraceptives, they never reach the threshold numbers to signal the PMN migration and hence symptoms of vaginitis rarely occur. We can extend this concept also to adolescents whose threshold of *Candida* is expected to be high (similar to adults with no history of vaginitis). This would explain the extremely high population numbers of *Candida* in the vaginas of adolescents with few symptomatic infections observed. A schematic diagram of this hypothesis is shown in Fig. 16.3. A study designed to identify ranges of vaginal fungal burden in the different groups of women under conditions of a symptomatic infection with specific correlates to PMN infiltration will be required to formally test this hypothesis.

In considering this hypothesis, it is interesting that the pathogenesis of VVC is now being considered host-mediated rather than organism-mediated that has been the longstanding paradigm for VVC. However, this newly found PMN hyperresponse is quite distinct to the hyper-IgE syndrome that appears to occur in a small population of women with primary RVVC (Rigg et al., 1990; Witkin, 1991; Fidel et al., 1997a). Yet in either case, it would appear that most, if not all, the symptomatology associated with

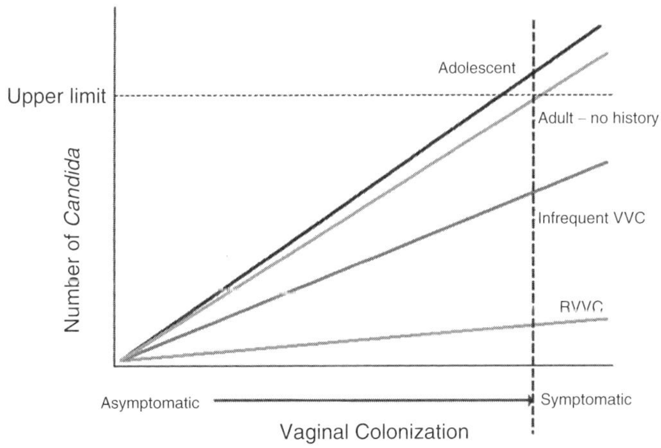

Figure 16.3. Hypothesis for acquisition of symptomatic vulvovaginal candidiasis. The hypothesis centers on the acquisition of vulvovaginal candidiasis by achieving a threshold of *Candida* organisms in the vagina. Under the threshold the vaginal presence of *Candida* is considered commensal and asymptomatic. Once the threshold is crossed (vertical dotted line), the signals are initiated that allow for migration of PMNs into the vagina that cause the symptoms associated with vaginitis. Accordingly, there is a different threshold for different groups of women. For women with RVVC the threshold is very low and increases incrementally in those with infrequent episodes of VVC, no history of VVC, and adolescents. The upper limit is an arbitrary level of organism number that would be considered unattainable.

VVC is indeed host-mediated. This concept is supported by a limited number of reports suggesting a genetic predisposition to VVC in animals and humans (Chaim et al., 1997; Mulero-Marchese et al., 1998; Calderon et al., 2003), although there have been as many studies suggesting the contrary (Fidel et al., 1995a; Black et al., 1999a). Another interesting point to consider is that the vaginal presence of the PMNs during the live challenge is consistent with the presence of PMNs in the mouse model of vaginitis (Fulurija et al., 1996; Black et al., 1998; Fidel et al., 1999). While these PMNs in most animal studies were not found to have any demonstrable effects on vaginitis, it is possible that the presence of PMNs in the mouse vaginal cavity too is a sign of symptomatology. While PMNs are not a hallmark of clinical cases of VVC, it is possible that they are present and that they fail to be seen because of their short halflife or that the tools used to diagnose infections (i.e., KOH smears) kill the PMNs. Finally, taking into account the *Candida* threshold theory for the initiation of PMN infiltration and concomitant symptoms it is interesting to postulate that women with primary RVVC and VVC are distinct populations only by virtue of their tolerability to *Candida* and resulting frequency of infectious episodes rather than by distinct predisposing factors (i.e., immune deficiency, hormone imbalance).

4. Conclusions

From experimental studies using the animal model of vaginal candidiasis as well as clinical studies and observations, it is clear that the local immune response is more relevant than the systemic response in protecting the vaginal mucosa against *C. albicans* infection. In addition, the mechanisms responsible for protection against *Candida* vaginitis are different than those that protect against candidal infections at other mucosal surfaces (e.g., oral mucosa) due to immunoregulation that inhibit adaptive, and possibly innate, cell-mediated immune mechanisms. This is probably an evolutionary property of the commensal *Candida* at a reproductive site where chronic inflammatory responses are unwanted. A key then to effective adaptive immune protection may be to provide the necessary immunomodulators (cytokines/chemokines) to overcome the immunoregulatory mechanisms (i.e., upregulate adhesion molecules and initiate the systemic infiltration of CMI) at a time when it is needed the most. Clearly the rat appears to have these factors based on the fairly rigorous response observed during a vaginal infection. Therefore, the rat model appears more valuable to understand what a protective adaptive response against the vaginal infection should be, while the value of the mouse model has been in the ability to better understand the apparent vaginal immunoregulation/tolerance predicted in humans.

With the extensive history of studies to understand the pathogenesis of VVC and RVVC through clinical studies and animal models, it has been the live challenge in humans that has finally advanced our understanding of the natural history of infection with the potential of identifying factors associated with protection and susceptibility to infection. This live challenge appears safe with conditions identified (history of VVC) where symptomatic infection can be predicted with some reliability. This represents a unique situation in humans where the pathogenesis of an infectious disease can be studied systemically and in real-time. To this end, instead of susceptibility to infection being associated with a deficient or missing adaptive immune component and protection associated with a T cell inflammatory response, it is now being suggested that susceptibility to infection is associated with an aggressive inflammatory response, while resistance to infection is noninflammatory. Thus, both resistance and susceptibility appears to be associated with innate immunity recognizing the immunoregulation against adaptive cellular immunity. And finally, the symptoms associated with vaginitis appear to be caused by the neutrophil response (host) rather than the organism. This effectively renews the possible role for a genetic predisposition to infection. In any event, the task now will be to identify the mechanism(s) of the protection and susceptibility to infection (i.e., signal associated with PMN infiltration, noninflammatory innate mediators associated with protection (if any), role of epithelial cells in protection against infection, and genetic and/or environmental factors associated with resistance and susceptibility to infection). Other interesting questions center on the concept of the PMN infiltration as a contributor to the symptoms. Once these questions are answered definitive new immunotherapeutic strategies can be developed that may reduce or prevent the incidence of VVC and RVVC. But if indeed the PMNs are the main instigator of the symptoms associated with vaginitis, immunotherapy to eliminate the signals associated with the PMN infiltration may be used to alleviate the symptoms associated with vaginitis, leaving the organism to exist as the harmless commensal it began as.

Acknowledgments

The author would like to thank Floyd L. Wormley, Chad Steele, Brad Taylor, Michael Saavedra, Karen Wozniak, Melissa Barousse, Junko Yano, Mace Scott, Wei Luo, Vitali Lounev, and Marc Baker of Louisiana State University Health Sciences, New Orleans, and Norbert Wolf and Jessica Cutright of Wayne State University School of Medicine, for their scientific contributions in the mouse and nonhuman primate models of experimental vaginitis as well as clinical studies described in the manuscript. The author also wishes to thank Antonio Cassone and Flavia De Bernardis of Rome, Italy, for their scientific contributions in the rat model of *Candida* vaginitis. Finally, the author wishes to acknowledge the National Institute of Allergy and Infectious Disease for supporting a considerable portion of the work summarized in this chapter (AI-32556; AI-41693).

References

(2002). *Candida and Candidiasis*. R. Calderone (ed.), ASM Press, Washington, DC.

Consumer Health Care Products Association. (2003). www.chpa.info.org

Al-Tawfig, J.A., Palmer, K.L., Chen, C., Haley, J.C., Katz, B.P., Hood, A.F., and Spinola, S.M. (1999). Experimental infection of human volunteers with *Haemophilus decreyi* does not confer protection against subsequent challenge. *J. Infect. Dis* 179: 1283–1287.

Arancia, G., Molinari, A., Crateri, P., Stringaro, A., Ramoni, C., Dupuis, M.L., Gomez, M.J., Torosantucci, A., and Cassone, A. (1995). Noninhibitory binding of human interleukin-2-activated natural killer cells to the germ tube forms of *Candida albicans*. *Infect. Immun.* 63: 280–288.

Baecher-Allan, C., Brown, J.A., Freeman, G.J., and Hafler, D.A. (2001). $CD4^{+}CD25^{high}$ regulatory cells in human peripheral blood. *J. Immunol.* 167: 1245–1253.

Barousse, M., Steele, C., Dunlap, K., Espinosa, T., Boikov, D., Sobel, J.D., and Fidel, P.L. Jr. (2001). Growth inhibition of *Candida albicans* by human vaginal epithelial cells. *J. Infect. Dis.* 184: 1489–1493.

Barousse, M., Van Der Pol, B.J., Fortenberry, D., Orr, D., and Fidel, P.L. Jr. (2003). Vaginal yeast colonization, prevalence of vaginitis, and associated local immunity in adolescents. *Sex. Trans. Infect.* 80: 48–53.

Black, C.A., Eyers, F.M., Russell, A., Dunkley, M.L., Clancy, R.L., and Beagley, K.W. (1998). Acute neutropenia decreases inflammation associated with murine vaginal candidiasis but has no effect on the course of infection. *Infect. Immun.* 66: 1273–1275.

Black, C.A., Eyers, F.M., Dunkley, M.L., Clancy, R.L., and Beagley, K.W. (1999a). Major histocompatibility haplotype does not impact the course of experimentally induced murine vaginal candidiasis. *Lab. Animal Sci.* 49: 668–672.

Black, C.A., Eyers, F.M., Russell, A., Dunkley, M.L., Clancy, R.L., and Beagley, K.W. (1999b). Increased severity of *Candida* vaginitis in

BALB/c *nu/nu* mice versus the parent strain is not abrogated by adoptive transfer of T cell enriched lymphocytes. *J. Reprod. Immunol.* 45: 1–18.

Burns, D.N., Tuomala, R., Chang, B.H., Hershow, R., Minkoff, H., Rodriquez, E., Zorrilla, C., Hammill, H., and Regan, J. (1997). Vaginal colonization or infection with *Candida albicans* in human immunodeficiency virus-infected women during pregnancy and during postpartum period. *Clin. Infect. Dis.* 24: 201–210.

Calderon, L., William, R., Martinez, M., Clemons, K.V., and Stevens, D.A. (2003). Genetic susceptibility to vaginal candidiasis. *Med. Mycol.* 41: 143–147.

Cantorna, M.T., Mook, D., and Balish, E. (1990). Resistance of congenitally immunodeficient gnotobiotic mice to vaginal candidiasis. *Infect. Immun.* 58: 3813–3815.

Cassone, A., Boccanera, M., Adriani, D.A., Santoni, G., and De Bernardis, F. (1995). Rats clearing a vaginal infection by *Candida albicans* acquire specific, antibody-mediated resistance to vaginal infection. *Infect. Immun.* 63: 2619–2624.

Cenci, E., Mencacci, A., Spaccapelo, R., Tonnetti, L., Mosci, P., Enssle, K.H., Puccetti, P., Romani, L., and Bistoni, F. (1995). T helper cell type 1 (Th1)- and Th2-like responses are present in mice with gastric candidiasis but protective immunity is associated with Th1 development. *J. Infect. Dis.* 171: 1279–1288.

Chaim, W., Foxman, B., and Sobel, J.D. (1997). Association of recurrent vaginal candidiasis and secretory ABO and Lewis phenotype. *J. Infect. Dis.* 176: 828–830.

Clark, R.A., Blakley, S.A., Rice, J., and Brandon, W. (1995). Predictors of HIV progression in women. *J. Acquir. Immune Defic. Syndr. Hum. Retrovir.* 9: 43–50.

Clift, R.A. (1984). Candidiasis in the transplant patient. *Am. J. Med.* 77 (Suppl. 4D): 34–38.

Cohen, M.S., Cannon, J.G., Jerse, A.E., Charniga, L.M., Isbey, S.F., and Whicker, L.G. (1991). Human experimentation with *Neissaria gonorrhoeae*: rationale, methods, and implications for the biology of infection and vaccine development. *J. Infect. Dis.* 169: 532–537.

Corrigan, E.M., Clancy, R.L., Dunkley, M.L., Eyers, F.M., and Beagley, K.W. (1998). Cellular immunity in recurrent vulvovaginal candidiasis. *Clin. Exp. Immunol.* 111: 574–578.

De Bernardis, F., Santoni, G., Boccanera, M., Spreghini, E., Adriana, D., Morelli, L., and Cassone, A. (2000). Local anticandidal immune responses in a rat model of vaginal infection by and protection against *Candida albicans*. *Infect. Immun.* 68: 3297–3304.

Djeu, J.Y. and Blanchard, D.K. (1987). Regulation of human polymorphonuclear neutrophil (PMN) activity against *Candida albicans* by large granular lymphocytes via release of a PMN-activating factor. *J. Immunol.* 139: 2761–2767.

Duerr, A., Sierra, M.F., Feldman, J., Clarke, L.M., Ehlich, I., and Dehovitz, J. (1997). Immune compromise and prevalence of *Candida* vulvovaginitis in human immunodeficiency virus-infected women. *Obstet. Gynecol.* 90: 252–256.

Ermann, J., Szanya, V., Ford, G.S., Paragus, V., Fathman, C.G., and Lejon, K. (2001). $CD4^{+}CD25^{+}$ T cells facilitate the induction of T cell anergy. *J. Immunol.* 167: 4271–4275.

Fidel, P.L. Jr., Lynch, M.E., Redondo-Lopez, V., Sobel, J.D., and Robinson, R. (1993a). Systemic cell-mediated immune reactivity in women with recurrent vulvovaginal candidiasis (RVVC). *J. Infect. Dis.* 168: 1458–1465.

Fidel, P.L. Jr., Lynch, M.E., and Sobel, J.D. (1993b). *Candida*-specific cell-mediated immunity is demonstrable in mice with experimental vaginal candidiasis. *Infect. Immun.* 61: 1990–1995.

Fidel, P.L. Jr., Lynch, M.E., and Sobel, J.D. (1993c). *Candida*-specific Th1-type responsiveness in mice with experimental vaginal candidiasis. *Infect. Immun.* 61: 4202–4207.

Fidel, P.L. Jr., Lynch, M.E., and Sobel, J.D. (1994). Effects of preinduced *Candida*-specific systemic cell-mediated immunity on experimental vaginal candidiasis. *Infect. Immun.* 62: 1032–1038.

Fidel, P.L. Jr., Cutright, J.L., and Sobel, J.D. (1995a). Effects of systemic cell-mediated immunity on vaginal candidiasis in mice resistant and susceptible to *Candida albicans* infections. *Infect. Immun.* 63: 4191–4194.

Fidel, P.L. Jr., Lynch, M.E., Conaway, D.H., Tait, L., and Sobel, J.D. (1995b). Mice immunized by primary vaginal *C. albicans* infection develop acquired vaginal mucosal immunity. *Infect. Immun.* 63: 547–553.

Fidel, P.L. Jr., Lynch, M.E., and Sobel, J.D. (1995c). Circulating CD4 and CD8 T cells have little impact on host defense against experimental vaginal candidiasis. *Infect. Immun.* 63: 2403–2408.

Fidel, P.L. Jr., Wolf, N.A., and KuKuruga, M.A. (1996). T lymphocytes in the murine vaginal mucosa are phenotypically distinct from those in the periphery. *Infect. Immun.* 64: 3793–3799.

Fidel, P.L. Jr., Ginsburg, K.A., Cutright, J.L., Wolf, N.A., Leaman, D., Dunlap, K., and Sobel, J.D. (1997a). Vaginal-associated immunity in women with recurrent vulvovaginal candidiasis: Evidence for vaginal Th1-type responses following intravaginal challenge with *Candida* antigen. *J. Infect. Dis.* 176: 728–739.

Fidel, P.L. Jr., Luo, W., Chabain, J., Wolf, N.A., and Van Buren, E. (1997b). Use of cellular depletion analysis to examine circulation of immune effector function between the vagina and the periphery. *Infect. Immun.* 65: 3939–3943.

Fidel, P.L. Jr., Luo, W., Steele, C., Chabain, J., Baker, M., and Wormley, F.L. (1999). Analysis of vaginal cell populations during experimental vaginal candidiasis. *Infect. Immun.* 67: 3135–3140.

Fidel, P.L. Jr., Cutright, J.L., and Steele, C. (2000). Effects of reproductive hormones on experimental vaginal candidiasis. *Infect. Immun.* 68: 651–657.

Fidel, P.L. Jr., Wormley, F.L. Jr., Chaiban, J., Chesson, R.R., and Lounev, V. (2001). Analysis of the CD4 protein on human vaginal CD4+ T cells. *Am. J. Reprod. Immunol.* 45: 200–204.

Fidel, P.L. Jr., Barousse, M., Espinosa, T., Chesson, R.R., and Dunlap, K. (2003). Local immune responsiveness following intravaginal challenge with *Candida* antigen in adult women at different stages of the menstrual cycle. *Med. Mycol.* 41: 97–109.

Fidel, P.L. Jr., Barousse, M., Espinosa, T., Camaratti, C., Ficarra, M., Martin, D.H., Quayle, A.J., and Dunlap, K. (2004). A live intravaginal *Candida* challenge in humans reveals new hypotheses for the immunopathogenesis of vulvovaginal candidiasis. *Infect. Immun.* 72: 2939–2946.

Fong, I.W., McCleary, P., and Read, S. (1992). Cellular immunity of patients with recurrent or refractory vulvovaginal moniliasis. *Am. J. Obstet. Gynecol.* 166: 887–890.

Fulurija, A., Ashman, R.B., and Papadimitriou, J.M. (1996). Neutrophil depletion increases susceptibility to systemic and vaginal candidiasis in mice, and reveals differences between brain and kidney in mechanisms of host resistance. *Microbiology* 142: 3487–3496.

Giraldo, P., Neuer, A., Korneeva, I.L., Ribeiro-Filho, A., Simoes, J.A., and Witkin, S.S. (1999a). Vaginal heat shock protein expression in symptom-free women with a history of recurrent vulvovaginitis. *Am. J. Obstet. Gynecol.* 180: 524–529.

Giraldo, P.C., Ribeiro-Filho, A.D., Simoes, J.A., Neuer, A., Feitosa, S.B., and Witkin, S.S. (1999b). Circulating heat shock proteins in women with a history of recurrent vulvovaginitis. *Infect. Dis. Obstet. Gynecol.* 7: 128–132.

Hector, R.F., Domer, J.E., and Carrow, E.W. (1982). Immune responses to *Candida albicans* in genetically distinct mice. *Infect. Immun.* 38: 1020–1028.

Hladik, F., Lentz, G., Delpit, E., McElroy, A., and McElrath, M.J. (1999). Coexpression of CCR5 and IL-2 in human genital but not blood cells: Implications for the ontogeny of the CCR5+ Th1 phenotype. *J. Immunol.* 163: 2306–2313.

Hobbs, J.R., Briden, D., Davidson, F., Kahan, M., and Oates, J.K. (1977). Immunological aspects of candidal vaginitis. *Proc. R. Soc. Med.* 70: 11–14.

Ibraghimov, A.R., Sacco, R.E., Sandor, M., Iakoubov, Z., and Lynch, R.G. (1995). Resident CD4+ αβ T cells of the murine female genital tract: A phenotypically distinct T cell lineage that rapidly proliferates in response to systemic T cell activation stimuli. *Int. Immunol.* 7: 1763–1769.

Imam, N., Carpenter, C.C.J., Mayer, K.H., Fisher, A., Stein, M., and Danforth, S.B. (1990). Hierarchical pattern of mucosal *Candida* infections in HIV-seropositive women. *Am. J. Med.* 89: 142–146.

Inghirami, G., Zhu, B.Y., Chess, L., and Knowles, D.M. (1990). Flow cytometric and immunohistochemical characterization of the gamma/delta T-lymphocyte population in normal human lymphoid tissue and peripheral blood. *Am. J. Pathol.* 136: 357–367.

Itohara, S., Farr, A.G., Lafaille, J.J., Bonneville, M., Takagaki, Y., Haas, W., and Tonegawa, S. (1990). Homing of a gamma/delta thymocyte subset with homogenous T-cell receptors to mucosal epithelia. *Nature* 343: 754–757.

Johansson, E.-L., Rudin, A., Wassen, L., and Holmgren, J. (2000). Distribution of lymphocytes and adhesion molecules in human cervix and vagina. *Immunology* 96: 272–277.

Jones-Carson, J., Vazquez-Torres, A., van der Heyde, H.C., Warner, T., Wagner, R.D., and

Balish, E. (1995). γ/δ T cell-induced nitric oxide production enhances resistance to mucosal candidiasis. *Nat. Med.* 6: 552–557.

Jonuleit, H. and Schmitt, E. (2003). The regulatory T cell family: Distinct subsets and the interrelations. *J. Immunol.* 171: 6323–6327.

Kelly, K.A. and Rank, R.G. (1997). Identification of homing receptors that mediate the recruitment of CD4 T cells to the genital tract following intravaginal infection with *Chlamydia trachomatis. Infect. Immun.* 65: 5198–5208.

Kelly, K.A., Gray, H.L., Walker, J.C., Rank, R.G., Wormley, F.L., and Fidel, P.L. Jr. (2001). *Chlamydia trachomatis* infection does not enhance local cellular immunity against concurrent *Candida albicans* vaginal infection. *Infect. Immun.* 69: 3451–3454.

Kent, H.L. (1991). Epidemiology of vaginitis. *Am. J. Obstet. Gynecol.* 165: 1168–1175.

Kinsman, O.S. and Collard, A.E. (1986). Hormonal factors in vaginal candidiasis in rats. *Infect. Immun.* 53: 498–504.

Klein, R.S., Harris, C.A., Small, C.B., Moll, B., Lesser, M., and Friedland, G.H. (1984). Oral candidiasis in high-risk patients as the initial manifestation of the acquired immunodeficiency syndrome. *N. Engl. J. Med.* 311: 354–357.

Knight, L. and Fletcher, J. (1971). Growth of *Candida albicans* in saliva: Stimulation by glucose associated with antibiotics, corticosteroids and diabetes mellitus. *J. Infect. Dis.* 123: 371–377.

Leigh, J.E., Barousse, M., Swoboda, R.K., Myers, T., Hager, S., Wolf, N.A., Cutright, J.L., Thompson, J., Sobel, J.D., and Fidel, P.L. Jr. (2001). *Candida*-specific systemic cell-mediated immune reactivities in HIV-infected persons with and without mucosal candidiasis. *J. Infect. Dis.* 183: 277–285.

Lindesmith, L., Moe, C., Marionneau, S., Ruvoen, N., Jiang, X., Lindblad, L., Stewart, P., LePendu, J., and Baric, R. (2003). Human susceptibility and resistance to Norwalk virus infection. *Nat. Med.* 9: 548–553.

Little, C.H., Georgiou, G.M., Marceglia, A., Ogedgebe, H., Cone, R.E., and Mazza, D. (2000). Measurement of T-cell-derived antigen binding molecules and immunoglobulin G specific to *Candida albicans* mannan in sera of patients with recurrent vulvovaginal candidiasis. *Infect. Immun.* 68: 3840–3847.

Lohman, B., Miller, C.J., and McChesney, M.B. (1995). Antiviral cytotoxic T lymphocytes in vaginal mucosa of simian immunodeficiency virus-infected rhesus macaques. *J. Immunol.* 155: 5855–5860.

Lynch, M.E., Sobel, J.D., and Fidel, P.L. Jr. (1996). Role of antifungal drug resistance in the pathogenesis of recurrent vulvovaginal candidiasis. *J. Med. Veter. Mycol.* 34: 337–339.

Mathews, H.L. and Witek-Janusek, L. (2002). Host defense against oral, esophageal, and gastrointestinal candidiasis. In R.A. Carderone (ed.), *Candida and Candidiasis*. ASM Press, Washington, DC, pp. 179–192.

Mendling, W. and Koldovsky, U. (1996). Investigations by cell-mediated immunologic tests and therapeutic trials with thymopentin in vaginal mycoses. *Infect. Dis. Obstet. Gynecol.* 4: 225–231.

Miller, C.J., McChesney, M., and Moore, P.F. (1992). Langerhans cells, macrophages, and lymphocyte subsets in the cervix and vagina of rhesus macaques. *Lab. Invest.* 67: 628–634.

Mulero-Marchese, R.D., Blank, K.J., and Sieck, T.G. (1998). Genetic basis for protection against experimental vaginal candidiasis by peripheral immunization. *J. Infect. Dis.* 178: 227–234.

Mulero-Marchese, R.D., Blank, K.J., and Sieck, T.G. (1999). Strain-dependent migration of lymphocytes to the vaginal mucosa after peripheral immunization. *Immunogenetics* 49: 973–980.

Nakamura, K., Kitani, A., and Strober, W. (2001). Cell contact-dependent immunosuppression by $CD4^+CD25^+$ regulatory T cells is mediated by cell surface-bound transforming growth factor B. *J. Exp. Med.* 194: 629–644.

Nandi, D. and Allison, J.P. (1991). Phenotypic analysis and gamma/delta-T cell receptor repertoire of murine T cells associated with the vaginal epithelium. *J. Immunol.* 147: 1773–1778.

Nawrot, U., Grzybek-Hryncewicz, K., Zielska, U., Czarny, A., and Podwinska, J. (2000). The study of cell-mediated immune response in recurrent vulvovaginal candidiasis. *FEMS Immunol. Med. Microbiol.* 29: 89–94 [in process citation].

Nomanbhoy, F., Steele, C., Yano, J., and Fidel, P.L. Jr. (2002). Vaginal and oral epithelial cell anti-*Candida* activity. *Infect. Immun.* 70: 7081–7088.

Odds, F.C. (1988). Chronic mucocutaneous candidiasis. In F.C. Odds (ed.), *Candida and Candidosis*. University Park Press, Baltimore, MD, pp. 104–110.

Parr, M.B. and Parr, E.L. (1990). Antigen recognition in the female reproductive tract. I. Uptake of intraluminal protein tracers in the mouse vagina. *J. Reprod. Immunol.* 17: 101–114.

Parr, M.B. and Parr, E.L. (1991). Langerhans cells and T lymphocyte subsets in the murine vagina and cervix. *Biol. Reprod.* 44: 491–498.

Parr, M.B. and Parr, E.L. (1997). Protective immunity against HSV-2 in the mouse vagina. *J. Reprod. Immunol.* 36: 77–92.

Parr, M.B. and Parr, E.L. (1998). Mucosal immunity to herpes simplex virus type 2 infection in the mouse vagina is impaired by in vivo-depletion of T lymphocytes. *J. Virol.* 72: 2677–2685.

Parr, M.B., Kepple, L., and Parr, E.L. (1991). Antigen recognition in the female reproductive tract. II. Endocytosis of horseradish peroxidase by Langerhans cells in murine vaginal epithelium. *Biol. Reprod.* 45: 261–265.

Rakasz, E., Sandor, M., Hagen, M., and Lynch, R.G. (1996). Activation features of intraepithelial γδ T-cells of the murine vagina. *Immunol. Lett.* 54: 129–134.

Rakasz, E., Hagen, M., Sandor, M., and Lynch, R.G. (1997). γδ T cells of the murine vagina: T cell response in vivo in the absence of the expression of CD2 and CD28 molecules. *Int. Immunol.* 9: 161–167.

Rhoads, J.L., Wright, D.C., Redfield, R.R., and Burke, D.S. (1987). Chronic vaginal candidiasis in women with human immunodeficiency virus infection. *JAMA* 257: 3105–3107.

Rigg, D., Miller, M.M., and Metzger, W.J. (1990). Recurrent allergic vulvovaginitis. Treatment with *Candida albicans* allergen immunotherapy. *Am. J. Obstet. Gynecol.* 162: 332–336.

Romani, L., Mocci, S., Bietta, C., Lanfaloni, L., Puccetti, P., and Bistoni, F. (1991). Th1 and Th2 cytokine secretion patterns in murine candidiasis: Association of Th1 responses with acquired resistance. *Infect. Immun.* 59: 4647–4654.

Romani, L., Mencacci, A., Cenci, E., Spaccapelo, R., Mosci, P., Puccetti, P., and Bistoni, F. (1993). $CD4^+$ subset expression in murine candidiasis. *J. Immunol.* 150: 925–931.

Romani, L., Puccetti, P., and Bistoni, F. (1996). Biological role of Th cell subsets in candidiasis. In S. Romagnani (ed.), *Th1 and Th2 Cells in Health and Disease*. Karger, Farmington, CT, pp. 114–137.

Ryley, J.F. and McGregor, S. (1986). Quantitation of vaginal *Candida albicans* infections in rodents. *J. Med. Vet. Mycol.* 24: 455–460.

Saavedra, M., Taylor, B., Lukacs, N.W., and Fidel, P.L. Jr. (1999). Local production of chemokines during experimental vaginal candidiasis. *Infect. Immun.* 67: 5820–5829.

Sallusto, F., Lanzavecchia, A., and Mackay, C.R. (1998). Chemokines and chemokine receptors in T-cell priming and Th1/Th2-mediated responses. *Immunol. Today* 19: 568–574.

Samaranayake, L.P. (1992). Oral mycoses in HIV infection. *Oral Surg. Oral Med. Oral Pathol.* 73: 171–180.

Santoni, G., Boccanera, M., Adriani, D., Lucciarini, R., Amantini, C., Morrone, S., Cassone, A., and De Bernardis, F. (2002). Immune cell-mediated protection against vaginal candidiasis: Evidence for a major role of vaginal $CD4(^+)$ T cells and possible participation of other local lymphocyte effectors. *Infect. Immun.* 70: 4791–4797.

Schuman, P., Sobel, J.D., Ohmit, S., Mayer, K.H., Rompalo, A., Duerr, A., Smith, D.K., Warren, D., and Klein, R.S. (1998). Mucosal candidal colonization and candidiasis in women with or at risk for human immunodeficiency virus infection. *Clin. Infect. Dis.* 27: 1161–1167.

Sobel, J.D. (1988). Pathogenesis and epidemiology of vulvovaginal candidiasis. *Ann. NY Acad. Sci.* 544: 547–557.

Sobel, J.D. (1992). Pathogenesis and treatment of recurrent vulvovaginal candidiasis. *Clin. Infect. Dis.* 14: S148–S153.

Sobel, J.D. (2002). Pathogenesis of recurrent vulvovaginal candidiasis. *Curr. Inf. Dis. Rep.* 4: 514–519.

Sohnle, P.G., Bhatti, M., and Wagner, D.K. (2002). Immunology of cutaneous candidiasis. In R. Calderone (ed.), *Candida and Candidiasis*. ASM Press, Washington, DC, pp. 211–221.

Spinillo, A., Michelone, G., Cavanna, C., Colonna, L., Capuzzo, E., and Nicola, S. (1994). Clinical and microbiological characteristics of symptomatic vulvovaginal candidiasis in HIV-seropositive women. *Genitourin. Med.* 70: 268–272.

Steele, C., Ozenci, H., Luo, W., Scott, M., and Fidel, P.L. Jr. (1999a). Growth inhibition of

Candida albicans by vaginal cells from naive mice. *Med. Mycol.* 37: 251–260.

Steele, C., Ratterree, M., and Fidel, P.L. Jr. (1999b). Differential susceptibility to experimental vaginal candidiasis in macaques. *J. Infect. Dis.* 180: 802–810.

Steele, C., Leigh, J.E., Swoboda, R.K., and Fidel, P.L. Jr. (2000). Growth inhibition of *Candida* by human oral epithelial cells. *J. Infect. Dis.* 182: 1479–1485.

Steele, C., Leigh, J.E., Swoboda, R.K., Ozenci, H., and Fidel, P.L. Jr. (2001). Potential role for a carbohydrate moiety in anti-*Candida* activity of human oral epithelial cells. *Infect. Immun.* 69: 7091–7099.

Syverson, R.A., Buckley, H., Gibian, J., and Ryan, J.J.M. (1979). Cellular and humoral immune status in women with chronic *Candida* vaginitis. *Am. J. Obstet. Gynecol.* 134: 624–627.

Taylor, B.N., Saavedra, M., and Fidel, P.L. Jr. (2000). Local Th1/Th2 cytokine production during experimental vaginal candidiasis. *Med. Mycol.* 38: 419–431.

Torosantucci, A., Chiani, P., De Bernardis, F., Cassone, A., Calera, J.A., and Calderone, R. (2002). Deletion of the two-component histidine kinase gene (*CHK1*) of *Candida albicans* contributes to enhanced growth inhibition and killing by human neutrophils in vitro. *Infect. Immun.* 70: 985–987.

Valentin, A., Bernard, C., Mallie, M., Huerre, M., and Bastide, J.M. (1993). Control of *Candida albicans* vaginitis in mice by short-duration butoconazole treatment in situ. *Mycoses* 36: 379–384.

Vanden-Bossche, H., Marichal, P., Odds, F.C., LeJeune, L., and Coene, M.C. (1992). Characterization of an azole-resistant *Candida glabrata* isolate. *Antimicrob. Agents Chemother.* 36: 2602–2610.

White, M.H. (1996). Is vulvovaginal candidiasis an AIDS-related illness. *Clin. Infect. Dis.* 22 (Suppl. 2): S124–S127.

White, H.D., Crassi, K.M., Givan, A.L., Stern, J.E., Gonzalez, J.L., Memoli, V.A., Green, W.R., and Wira, C.R. (1997). $CD3^+CD8^+$ CTL activity within the human female reproductive tract: Influence of stage of the menstrual cycle and menopause. *J. Immunol.* 158: 3017–3027.

Witkin, S.S. (1986). Inhibition of *Candida*-induced lymphocyte proliferation by antibody to *Candida albicans. Obstet. Gynecol.* 68: 696–699.

Witkin, S.S. (1991). Immunologic factors influencing susceptibility to recurrent candidal vaginitis. *Clin. Obstet. Gynecol.* 34: 662–668.

Witkin, S.S., Hirsch, J., and Ledger, W.J. (1986). A macrophage defect in women with recurrent *Candida* vaginitis and its reversal in vitro by prostaglandin inhibitors. *Am. J. Obstet. Gynecol.* 155: 790–795.

Wormley, F.L., Scott, M., Luo, W., Baker, M., Chaiban, J., and Fidel, P.L. Jr. (2000). Evidence for a unique expression of CD4 on murine vaginal $CD4^+$ cells. *Immunology* 100: 300–308.

Wormley, F.L. Jr., Chaiban, J., and Fidel, P.L. Jr. (2001a). Cell adhesion molecule and lymphocyte activation marker expression during experimental vaginal candidiasis. *Infect. Immun.* 69: 5072–5079.

Wormley, F.L., Jr., Steele, C., Wozniak, K., Fujihashi, K., McGhee, J.R., and Fidel, P.L. Jr. (2001b). Resistance of TCR δ-chain knock-out mice to experimental *Candida* vaginitis. *Infect. Immun.* 69: 7162–7164.

Wormley, F.L. Jr., Cutright, J.L., and Fidel, P.L. Jr. (2003). Multiple experimental designs to evaluate the role of T-cell-mediated immunity against experimental vaginal *Candida albicans* infection. *Med. Mycol.* 41: 401–410.

Yamagiwa, S., Gray, J.D., Hashimoto, S., and Horwitz, D.A. (2000). A role for TGF-B in the generation and expansion of $CD4^+CD25^+$ regulatory T cells from human peripheral blood. *J. Immunol.* 166: 7282–7289.

Yano, J., Lilly, E., Cutler, J.E., and Fidel, P.L. Jr. (2005). Mucosal epithelial cell anti-*Candida* activity: Evidence against a role for carbohydrates. *Oral Microbial. Immunol.* (in press).

17

The Role of Humoral Immunity against Vaginal Candida Infection

Flavia De Bernardis, Maria Boccanera, and Antonio Cassone

1. Introduction

Vulvovaginal candidiasis (VVC) is a widespread mucosal infection caused by *Candida* species that affects a significant number of childbearing women and it is a prime reason for physician consultation (Sobel, 1989, 1992; Fidel and Sobel, 1996). Acute VVC has several predisposing factors including antibiotic and oral contraceptive usage, pregnancy, uncontrolled diabetes mellitus, immunosuppressive therapy, and HIV infection (Sobel, 1992; Fidel and Sobel, 1996, 1998). Recurrent vulvovaginal candidiasis (RVVC) is usually defined as idiopathic with no known predisposing factors and seems to affect around 5% of all women (Sobel, 1989). Antifungal therapy is highly effective for individual symptomatic attacks but does not prevent subsequent recurrences; in fact there is little evidence that antifungal resistance plays a role in the pathogenesis of RVVC (Sobel, 1989). Susceptibility to RVVC has been postulated to be due to some immune dysfunction, and some women experience repeated symptomatic episodes as a result of immunological deficiencies. However, the pathogenesis of

Department of Infectious, Parasitic and Immune-Mediated Diseases, Istituto Superiore di Sanità, Rome, Italy.

RVVC remains unknown. Fidel and collaborators have suggested that local rather than systemic cell-mediated immunity (CMI) is an important host defense mechanism of the vaginal mucosa (1993a,b, 1994, 1995a–c; 1996), and this is clearly strengthened by some of our recent observations in the rat vaginitis model (De Bernardis et al. 2000, Santoni et al. 2002). Clinical studies conducted by Fidel and collaborators (1997a,b) in women with RVVC showed that the majority of patients had normal levels of *Candida*-specific systemic CMI. The authors suggest that if women with RVVC have immune defects, they are local rather than systemic. This is supported by the evidence that women with idiopathic RVVC rarely experience oral, esophageal, or cutaneous candidiasis (Sobel, 1992; Fidel and Sobel, 1996).

The nature of host defense mechanisms functioning at the vaginal mucosa are undefined particularly those specifically acting against *C. albicans*. Therefore, understanding the components of the host–fungus interaction at the mucosal level can lead to a better understanding of the pathogenesis of mucosal candidiasis and result in the optimization of preventive and therapeutic antifungal strategies. Both humoral and cellular factors have been suggested to confer protection.

This chapter summarizes the salient features of the humoral immune responses to *Candida* at the vaginal level with emphasis on the role of antibodies (Abs) and molecular interaction involved in their secretion. It also focuses on the humoral response mechanisms characterized in several animal models of candidiasis. In fact, animal models have provided an important contribution to the study of various aspects of the host's immune response against *C. albicans* at the vaginal level. Finally, we also discuss experimental approaches, which could have potential therapeutic effects on human vaginal candidiasis such as the use of Abs against cell surface mannoprotein or enzymes, the idiotypic vaccination, and the production of therapeutic vaccines and immunomodulators.

2. Immune Response to *Candida* in the Vaginal Mucosa

The female reproductive tract mucosa has been shown to comprise all the cell populations required for initiating an immune response. HLA-DR$^+$ Langerhans cells with elevated antigen presentation capability have been identified in the vaginal and cervical epithelia, being most abundant in the vulval epithelium (Czerkinnsky et al., 1999). Intraepithelial T cells have been found at all sites and comprise a majority of CD8$^+$ cells (Czerkinnsky et al. 1999). A significant proportion of these cells express perforin and TIA-1, suggestive of cytolytic capacity. In contrast, CD4$^+$ T cells are rarely found in these epithelia but predominate in the submucosal vaginal, cervix, and fallopian tube tissues (Czerkinnsky et al., 1999). Remarkably, the proportion of CD4$^+$ and CD8$^+$ T cells may vary much substantially in the tissue districts. Although all components of the mucosal immune system are present in the female reproductive tract, the precise sites of induction of secretory immune responses in this organ are largely unknown. Moreover, even large differences in the cellular composition and distinct phenotypes have been reported in the same genital district of the different mammals. An example is the very different proportion of CD4$^+$ and CD8$^+$ T lymphocytes in the subepithelial layers of mouse and rat vagina (Fidel et al., 1999, De Bernardis et al., 2000). Interestingly, such an immunologically essential parameter as the CD4$^+$/CD8$^+$ T cell ratio in healthy women is much more similar to the rat than to the mouse (Elitsur et al., 1998).

Colonization of vaginal mucosa by *C. albicans* induces both antibody (Ab) and CMI. *C. albicans* can persist on the vaginal mucosal of healthy women despite demonstrable adaptive anti-*Candida* immunity. After antigen stimulation, locally induced specific secretory IgA^+ B cells and T cells migrate to mucosal effector tissues in the lamina propria regions of the genitourinary tract via a common mucosal immune pathway (Scicchitano et al., 1988). T cells in the intestinal lamina propria represent 30% to 40% of the total lymphocytes with a $CD4^+/CD8^+$ ratio of about 2 to 3. Both $CD4^+$ T helper cells (Th1 and Th2) are present in the lamina propria. In response to antigen stimulation, Th cells secrete a number of cytokines capable of activating B cells. Th2 cells produce interleukin (IL-4, IL-5, IL-6), and TGF-β that act directly on secretory IgA^+ B cells and induce them to differentiate into IgA^- producing cells (McGhee et al., 1989). Thus, an adequate number of functioning T cells is essential for the development of a normal secretory immune response to *Candida*. The mucosal tissues of humans and animals reveal a remarkable preponderance of IgA-producing plasma cells, which are generated by precursors in the organized gut-associated lymphoid tissues (GALT) and bronchus-associated lymphoid tissues (BALT) as demonstrated in animal models (Czerkinnsky et al., 1999).

Patients with disorders of the sIgA immune system (deficiency of the secretory component or decreased production of sIgA) are prone to develop recurrent mucosal candidiasis without an increased susceptibility to disseminated candidiasis (Marodi, 1997).

The transition of *C. albicans* from commensal to invasive pathogen is primarily the consequence of a defective host cellular immune response, but the virulence of *C. albicans* strains may also be relevant (De Bernardis et al., 1990, 1995; Cutler, 1991; Greenfield, 1992). The virulence factors of *Candida* that play a role in vaginal candidiasis and can induce the immune system to generate a neutralizing, protective response are adherence, morphogenesis, antigenic variation, enzyme production, especially proteinase secretion, and cell surface composition (Ghannoum and Abu-Elteen, 1990; Cutler, 1991, Calderone and Fonzi 2001). In particular, the ability of this fungus in vivo to grow in different forms (yeast, hyphae, and pseudohyphae), is associated with its evasion to the host clearance mechanisms either by mechanical obstacles imposed on phagocytes or by more subtle mechanisms of immune evasion, such as antigenic variations, secretion of immunoinhibitory factors, and other factors (Cassone and Torosantucci, 1991; Cassone et al., 1998). In such cases, *C. albicans* is able to modify the nature of some cell wall constituents under the selective pressure of the host and to adapt its growth to invasion in different tissues, each with its own environmental triggers. An example of *C. albicans* adaptation is the expression of pH-regulated proteins, in relation to the environment of the vaginal canal (low pH) versus the pH of the bloodstream and tissues (De Bernardis et al., 1998).

3. Role of Humoral Immunity in Vaginal Candidiasis

Vaginal colonization with *C. albicans* induces humoral responses. A positive effect of Abs against candidiasis was first suggested in the 1960s by Mourad and Friedman (1961, 1968). In subsequent studies conducted in the 1970s and 1980s the importance of anti-*Candida*-specific Abs was largely dismissed. Clinical and experimental data led to conclusion that Abs do not protect against various forms of candidiasis. Two important features supporting this conclusion are that *Candida* vaginitis is not frequent in subjects with immunoglobulin disorders and that subjects with candidiasis often have high titers of anti-*Candida* Abs. Additionally, there are no reports showing that patients with congenital or acquired B cell deficiencies are susceptible to mucosal or systemic *Candida* infections

(Rogers and Balish, 1980). In fact, the presence of Abs do not preclude development of disseminated or mucosal candidiasis (Kirkpatrick et al., 1971; Aronson and Soltani, 1976; GarciaRuiz et al., 1997). CMI as the primary host defense against candidiasis was much more supported, and the majority of the authors tended to be dismissive about the role of Abs. However, literature contains many observations about the possible role of anti-*Candida* Abs having a protective role at the mucosal level. For instance, Roger and Balish (1980) showed that serum Ab and complement can kill *C. albicans* in vitro. Walker and Urbaniak (1980) reported that Abs specific for *C. albicans* inhibit in vitro phagocytosis of the fungus.

The controversial role of humoral immunity has been reviewed by Casadevall and colleagues (Casadevall, 1995, Casadevall et al., 1998), who postulated that protective, nonprotective, and immunologically indifferent Abs exist in the repertoire of Abs present during an infection. A plethora of irrelevant Abs raised against irrelevant fungal constituents could obscure protective epitopes.

In the studies which suggested anti-*Candida* Abs were not protective, the specificity and isotype of the elicited Ab have not been established. Now, it is quite clear that the above qualifications are essential factors for a protective Ab response. As reviewed by Cutler et al. (2002) the cell wall of *Candida* cells contains an enormous number of epitopes and only Abs elicited to specific epitopes can be protective. People who are exposed to *C. albicans* do not necessarily respond by producing protective Abs contrasting the development of candidiasis, but this hypothesis does not exclude a possible role of Abs in host defense against various forms of candidiasis. It is important that Ab responses are being analyzed with respect to predominant antigenic specificities, isotypes, and titers. Regarding the specificity, it has been shown that Ab response against *Candida* elicits protective, nonprotective, and also disease-enhancing Abs similar to that for anti-cryptococcal Abs (Cassone et al., 1995, Han et al., 1997; Bromuro et al,. 1998). Ig isotype may also be critical for the protective role of Abs, where IgM IgG1 and IgG3 are generally most protective (Han et al. 1997, 2000). Finally, if *Candida* colonization induces the secretion of Abs with the correct specificity and Ig isotype, the titer of these Abs is also important for protective activity.

3.1. Experimental Vaginal Candidiasis

Animal models have been employed to study various aspects of the immune response in *Candida* vaginitis under conditions possibly mimicking human infection. In these models *Candida* infections may be established under controlled and reproducible conditions. Experimental *Candida* vaginitis has been reproduced especially in mice and rats, and more recently a primate model has also been explored (Steele et al., 1999).

In the mouse model of *Candida* vaginitis Fidel and collaborators (1994, 1995a,b) were the first to show that local rather than systemic CMI is an important host defense mechanism of the vaginal mucosa. They have also suggested some level of immunological independence or immune compartmentalization.

Jones-Carson et al. (1995) observed an enhanced susceptibility to *Candida* vaginitis in mice depleted of γ/δ T cells and suggested a potential role of γ/δ T cells in the protective response in the vaginal mucosa. In the studies of Mulero-Marchese et al. (1998) protection from vaginal candidiasis was transferred to BALB/c mice by adoptive transfer of *C. albicans* immune splenic T cells. Depletion of $CD3^+$ or $CD4^+$, but not $CD8^+$ T cells before transfer, completely abrogated protection. These results demonstrate a significant role for $CD4^+$ T lymphocytes in the resistance to vaginal candidiasis.

Little information exists on the role of Abs in resistance to mucosal vaginal candidiasis, and the results are somewhat controversial. We investigated the efficacy of Abs in the protection against *C. albicans* vaginal infection using a rat vaginitis model. The induction and the maintenance of "pseudoestrus" in rats requires oophorectomy and estrogen administration (Kinsman and Collard, 1986; Kinsman et al., 1986). Under estrogen administration, the vaginal epithelium is fully keratinized and *C. albicans* colonization is greatly facilitated. Germ-tube (hyphal) formation, adherence, and secretion of aspartyl proteinase activity are also induced by the production of the keratin layer. In addition, the estrogens reduce leukocyte infiltration, which helps fungal growth and the establishment of infection. After clearing the primary *C. albicans* infection, rats were highly resistant to a second vaginal challenge with the fungus (Cassone et al. 1995). We assumed that if adherence, germ tube formation, and secretion of aspartyl proteinase play a role in vaginal infection, it is conceivable that specific Abs against these factors could be protective. Thus, we investigated the potential protective effect of specific Abs against a well-defined immunogenic cell-wall antigen (mannoprotein) and against a well-established virulence factor of *Candida* such as aspartyl proteinase (Sap). Animals receiving vaginal fluids from *C. albicans*-infected rats and containing anti-mannan (MP) and anti-aspartyl proteinase (Sap) Abs were significantly protected against vaginitis compared to animals given Ab-free vaginal fluid from noninfected rats (De Bernardis et al., 1997). Preabsorption of the Ab-containing fluids with either one or both proteins MP and Sap sequentially reduced or abolished, respectively, the amount of protection. A degree of protection from a vaginal infection with *C. albicans* was also conferred by postinfectious administration of anti-Sap and anti-Mp monoclonal Abs and by intravaginal or intranasal immunization with MP or Sap preparations (De Bernardis et al., 1997, 2002). As shown in Fig. 17.1 immu-

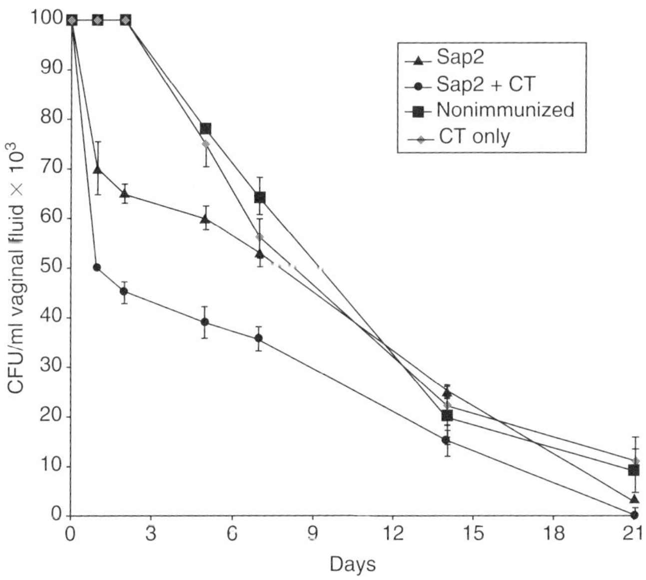

Figure 17.1. Outcome of vaginal infection by *C. albicans* in rats intravaginally immunized with proteinase (Saps) 2 plus or minus mucosal adjuvant cholera toxin (CT). Each curve represents the mean (± standard error of the mean) of the number of fungal CFU for five rats. Statistical significance was assessed by Student's *t* test (two tailed).

nization with a preparation of Sap2 resulted in statistically significant acceleration of fungal clearance from the vagina within the first week of infection and more significantly when a mucosal adjuvant, cholera toxin (CT) was coadministered with Sap 2 compared with controls (nonimmunized animals or only CT-treated rats). The immunized animals elicited anti-Sap Abs in the vaginal fluids. In order to investigate whether the protection conferred by Ab response was T-dependent, we reproduced *Candida* vaginitis in congenitally athymic nude rats. The animals showed a primary infection not dissimilar in extent and duration to that observed in euthymic rats but they were not protected against a secondary fungal challenge. No anti-Mp or anti-Sap Abs was elicited in the vaginal fluids of athymic rats during both the first and the second *Candida* infections (De Bernardis et al. 1997). These results demonstrated that the induction of Ab response was T cell-dependent and also evidenced a link between cell-mediated and humoral immunity in vaginal infection with *C. albicans*. (De Bernardis et al. 1997, 2000, 2002, 2004). Overall, the results of our studies evidenced the protective role in *Candida* vaginitis of specific Abs against mannoprotein or proteinase of *C. albicans*. The recombinant forms of these antigens (65 kDa mannoprotein and Sap 2) have been investigated as active immunogens in vaginal candidiasis. (De Bernardis et al., manuscript in preparation).

The mechanisms by which anti-mannan and anti-proteinase Abs protect against candidiasis are unclear. The hypotheses are that anti-Sap Abs act by neutralizing the proteinase activity of *C. albicans* and inhibiting adherence to the vaginal mucosa and consequent colonization. In addition the binding of Abs to cell wall may facilitate phagocytosis of the fungus. More investigations are required for a clear undestanding of how Abs can help the host resolve vaginal candidiasis.

Cutler and coworkers (Han et al., 1998), in a murine model of vaginitis, demonstrated that immunization with a mannan liposome preparation (L-mann) enhanced resistance against *Candida* vaginal infection. The same authors (Han et al., 1997) purified two monoclonal Abs from splenocytes of L-mann immunized mice. Both Abs were IgM, agglutinated *C. albicans* yeast cells, and were specific for cell wall mannan. However, MAb B6 is specific for an epitope located in the acid stable part of phosphomannan and MAb B61 is specific for a B-1,2 mannotriose, which is acid-labile component of phosphomannan. Intravaginal administration of MAb 6.1 resulted in a highly effective reduction of vaginal colonization by *C. albicans* compared to the same treatment with MAb B6. These results indicated that there are indeed cell surface-located epitopes on *C. albicans* that lead to production of protective and nonprotective Abs. Interestingly, the protective MAb used in these studies had the same specificity of the protective anti-B-mannan MAb (MAb AF1) used in our studies (De Bernardis et al., 1997), indicating the relevance of mannan epitopes.

Further investigations conducted by Cutler and collaborators (Caesar-TonThat and Cutler, 1997) on the mechanisms by which Abs protect against candidiasis suggested that the protection seems to be dependent on complement activation. In fact, mouse neutrophils were able to kill more *C. albicans* yeast cells in the presence of MAb B6.1 and complement addition than without complement in vitro. On the basis of these results the authors hypothesized that MAb B6.1 induce a deposition of complement on the *Candida* surface, which favor *Candida* phagocytosis by neutrophils. A direct effect of Abs on *C. albicans* cells was previously reported by Casanova et al. (1990). In this study, Fab fragments of a MAb specific for a hyphal cell wall moiety inhibited germ tube formation. San Millan et al. (1996) demonstrated the inhibition of *C. albicans* adherence to polystyrene by two MAbs directed against cell wall antigens of *C. albicans*.

Undoubtedly, the use of animal models has been invaluable to investigate and understand the humoral host defense mechanisms that protect against *C. albicans* at the vaginal mucosal surface. Overall, several studies have evidenced the protective role of Abs directed against a specific immunogenic antigen of the *Candida* cell wall (mannan) or against specific virulence factors of *C. albicans* (adhesins, proteinase, germ tube). Although the mechanisms by which these Abs exert protection during vaginal infection is not completely understood (inhibition of adhesion or germ tube formation, opsonization and neutralization of proteolytic enzymes are the mechanisms hypothesized), these observations provide a valuable approach to the potential therapeutic use of some Abs or their engineered derivatives in the treatment of *Candida* vaginal infections refractory to antimycotic therapy.

3.2. The Role of Killer-Toxin Antiidiotypic Abs in Protection against Vaginal Candidiasis

Killer toxins (KTs) are proteins secreted by yeasts, which are able to kill other microorganisms presenting specific cell wall receptors (KTR) (Tipper and Bostian, 1984, Magliani et al. 1997). Killer factors have been described to be produced by *Saccharomyces* sp. (Bevan et al. 1973), *Ustilago* sp., *Kluveromyces* sp., *Pichia* sp., *Hansenula* sp., *Candida* sp., (Polonelli and Morace, 1986, Polonelli et al., 1997). Polonelli et al. (1986, 1993) have suggested the potential use of a KT produced by *Pichia anomala* in the treatment of fungal disease. Subsequently, because KT was of no practical use for its instability, antigenicity, and toxicity, a KT-neutralizing monoclonal Ab MAb (MAb KT4) was used to produce antiidiotypic (anti-Id) Abs possessing the internal image of KT-active domain (KT-IdAb), a functional mimick. These antiidiotypic Abs were able to exert a direct candidacidal activity in vitro like the KT by interacting with a specific KT cell wall receptor (Polonelli and Morace, 1987; Polonelli et al., 1991). The KTR has recently been identified as a B-glucan (Guyard et al., 2002).

In collaboration with Polonelli and coworkers we have evidenced the KT antiidiotypic monoclonal Ab (MAb KT4) and its recombinant single-chain fragment (KT-scFV) exert a therapeutic activity in *Candida* vaginal infection (Polonelli et al., 1994, 1997; Cassone et al., 1997; Magliani et al., 2002). Oophorectomized and estradiol-treated rats were vaccinated by the intravaginal administration (day 0–7 to 14–21) of MAb KT4 or KT-scFV before *C. albicans* vaginal challenge. The Id-vaccinated animals showed a highly significant decrease of vaginal *Candida* colony-forming unit (CFU) compared with controls (nonimmunized or irrelevant MAb-immunized animals). The protection was associated with rising vaginal titres of antiidiotypic Abs, predominantly of the IgA isotype. The Id-Ab containing vaginal fluids taken from MAb KT4-immunized animals were able to passively transfer the anti-*Candida* protection to nonimmunized rats and to kill *Candida* in vitro. The killing was neutralized by the MAb KT4. Thus, secretory Id-Abs, elicited by intravaginal Id vaccination with MAb KT4, protected the rats from the infectious challenge with *C. albicans* by molecular mimicking KT activity as its internal image (Polonelli et al., 1994). KT-Id-Abs were also found in significant titres in the vaginal fluids of women with *Candida* vaginitis. These Abs were candidacidal in vitro and were also able to confer protection to naïve rats as those raised in the rat vagina by Id-vaccination (Polonelli et al. 1996). These results suggested that KT-Abs represent part of the immune response elicited against microorganisms bearing a KT-receptor. Whether they have a role in natural *Candida* infections is still unclear.

The KT-sc-FV was cloned and expressed in the human commensal *Streptococcus gordonii* as a secreted or surface-displayed molecule. Engineered *S. gordonii* strain was able to colonize the mucosal surfaces and when intravaginally injected in rats exerted a strong therapeutic effect on *Candida* vaginal infection (Beninati et al., 2000; Oggioni et al., 2001).

Thus, to obtain standardizable, active fragments for therapeutic use we have sequenced KT-sc-FV and synthesized a decapeptide derived from the sequence of the variable region and containing part of KT-scFv light chain. We demonstrated that this peptide exerts a potent anti-*Candida* activity in vitro and in vivo in vaginal infection (Polonelli et al., 2003; Oggioni et al., 2001).

Overall, the mimicry of the yeast killer phenomenon through the Id-Abs has led to the development of the Id-vaccination and anti-Id therapy, which could represent new approaches to the control of mucosal candidiasis.

4. Conclusions

Candida is essentially an extracellular organism and, as such, Abs against critical antigens for virulence are expected to play a role. This has been dismissed in the light of evidence that cell-mediated immune dysfunctions favor candidiasis. However, this does not exclude any additional or even replacing role of Abs in defined settings. There is now clear experimental evidence that some Abs may indeed be therapeutic; the experiments also suggest that under natural conditions, protective Abs may be obscured by the plethora of irrelevant if not disease-enhancing Abs. The time has now come that not only have Abs been shown to play more than a likely protective role against vaginitis, more importantly, these Abs or their engineered fragments should be used therapeutically. Our findings with protective Abs at the vaginal level may constitute the basis for such a clinical development.

Acknowledgments

We would like to thank Daniela Adriani and Antonietta Girolamo for their contribution to the work described. We are also grateful to Dr. G. Mandarino for her valuable help in manuscript preparation.

References

Aronson, I.K. and Soltani, K. (1976). Chronic mucocutaneous candidosis: A review. *Mycopathologia* 60: 17–25.

Beninati, C., Oggioni, M.R., Boccanera, M., Spinosa, M.R., Maggi, T., Conti, S., Magliani W., De Bernardis, F., Teti, G., Cassone, A., Pozzi, G., and Polonelli, L. (2000). Therapy of experimental mucosal candidiasis by engineered human commensal bacteria expressing a microbicidal recombinant anti-idiotype. *Nat. Biotechnol.* 8: 1060–1064.

Bevan, E.A., Herring, A.J., and Mitchell, D.J. (1973). Preliminary characterization of two species of dsRNA in yeast and their relationship to the "Killer" character. *Nature* 142: 81–86.

Bromuro, C., La Valle, R., Sandini, S., Urbani, F., Ausiello, C.M., Morelli, L., Fe d'Ostiani, C., Romani, L., and Cassone, A. (1998). A 70-kilodalton recombinant heat shock protein of *Candida albicans* is highly immunogenic and enhances systemic murine candidiasis. *Infect. Immun.* 66: 2154–2162.

Caesar-TonThat, T.C. and Cutler, J.E. (1997). A monoclonal antibody to *Candida albicans* enhances mouse neutrophil candidacidal activity. *Infect. Immun.* 65: 5354–5357.

Calderone, R. and Fonzi, W. (2001). Virulence factors of *Candida albicans*. *Trends Microbiol.* 9: 327–335.

Casadevall, A. (1995). Antibody immunity and invasive fungal infections. *Infect. Immun.* 63: 4211–4218.

Casadevall, A., Cassone, A., Bistoni, F., Cutler, J.E., Magliani, W., Murphy, J.W., Polonelli, L., Romani, L. (1998). Antibody and/or cell-mediated immunity, protective mechanisms in fungal disease: An ongoing dilemma or an unnecessary dispute? *Med. Mycol.* 36(S1): 95–105.

Casanova, M., Martinez, J.P., Chaffin, W.L. (1990). Fab fragments from a monoclonal antibody against a germ tube mannoprotein block the yeast- to mycelium transition in *Candida albicans*. *Infect. Immun.* 58: 3810–3812.

Cassone, A. and Torosantucci, A. (1991). Immunological moieties of the cell wall. In R. Prasad (ed.), *Candida albicans*. Springler-Verlag, Berlin, pp. 89–107.

Cassone, A., Boccanera, M., Adriani, D., Santoni, G., and De Bernardis, F. (1995). Rats clearing a vaginal infection by *Candida albicans* acquire specific, antibody-mediated resistance to vaginal reinfection. *Infect. Immun.* 63: 2619–2624.

Cassone, A., Corti, S., De Bernardis, F., and Polonelli, L. (1997). Antibodies killer toxins and antifungal immunoprotection: A lesson from nature? *Immunol. Today* 18: 163–169.

Cassone, A., De Bernardis, F., Ausiello, C.M., Gomez, M.J., Boccanera, M., La Valle, R., and Torosantucci, A. (1998). Immunogenic and protective *Candida albicans* constituents. *Res. Immunol.* 149: 289–299.

Cutler, J. (1991). Putative virulence factors of *Candida albicans*. *Annu. Rev. Microbiol.* 45: 187–218.

Cutler, J.E., Granger, B.L., and Han, Y. (2002). Vaccines, antibodies and passive immunity in candidiasis. In R.A. Calderone and R.L. Cihlar (eds), *Fungal Pathogenesis*. Marcel Dekker, New York, pp. 243–251.

Czerkinnsky, C., Anjuere, F., McGhee, J.R., George-Chandy, A., Holmgren, J., Kieny, M.P., Fujiyashi, K., Mestecky, J.F., Pierrefite-Carle, V., Rask, C., and Sun, J.B. (1999). Mucosal immunity and tolerance: Relevance to vaccine development. *Immun. Rev.* 170: 197–222.

De Bernardis, F., Agatensi, L., Ross, I.K., Emerson, G.W., Lorenzini, R., Sullivan, P.A., and Cassone, A. (1990). Evidence for a role for secreted aspartate proteinase of *Candida albicans* in vulvovaginal candidiasis. *J. Infect. Dis.* 161: 1276–1283.

De Bernardis, F., Cassone, A., Sturtevant, J., and Calderone, R. (1995). Expression of *Candida albicans* SAP1 and SAP2 in experimental vaginitis. *Infect. Immun.* 6: 1887–1892.

De Bernardis, F., Boccanera, M., Adriani, D., Spreghini, E., Santoni, G., and Cassone, A. (1997). Protective role of antimannan and anti-aspartyl proteinase antibodies in an experimental model of *Candida albicans* vaginitis in rats. *Infect. Immun.* 65: 3399–3405.

De Bernardis, F., Muhlschlegel, F.A., Cassone, A., and Fonzi, W.A. (1998). The pH of the host niche controls gene expression in and virulence of *Candida albicans*. *Infect. Immun.* 66: 3317–3325.

De Bernardis, F., Santoni, G., Boccanera, M., Spreghini, E., Adriani, D., Morelli, L., and Cassone, A. (2000). Local anticandidal immune responses in a rat model of vaginal infection by and protection, *Candida albicans*. *Infect. Immun.* 68: 3297–3304.

De Bernardis, F., Boccanera, M., Adriani, D., Girolamo, A., and Cassone, A. (2002). Intravaginal and intranasal immunization are equally effective in inducing vaginal antibodies and conferring protection against vaginal candidiasis. *Infect. Immun.* 70: 2725–2729.

De Bernardis, F., Boccanera, M., Amantini, C., and Santoni, G. (2004). T and B lymphocytes in mucosal candidiasis. In G. San-Blas and R. Calderone (eds), *Pathogenic Fungi: Host Interaction and Emerging Strategies for Control*, Caister Academic Press, UK.

Elitsur, Y., Jackman, S., Neace, C., Keerthy, S., Liu, S., Dosescu, J., and Mosheir, J.A. (1998). Human vaginal mucosa Immune system: Characterization and function. *Gen. Diagn. Pathol.* 143: 271–277.

Fidel, P.L. Jr. and Sobel, J.D. (1996). Immunopathogenesis of recurrent vulvovaginal candidiasis. *Clin. Microbiol. Rev.* 9: 335–348.

Fidel, P.L. Jr. and Sobel, J.D. (1998). Protective immunity in experimental *Candida* vaginitis. *Res. Immunol.* 146: 361–373.

Fidel, P.L. Jr. and Sobel, J.D. (2002). Host defense against vaginal candidiasis. In: R.A. Calderone (ed.), *Candida and Candidosis*, ASM Press, Washington, pp. 193–209.

Fidel, P.L., Lynch, M.E., and Sobel, J.D. (1993a). *Candida*-specific Th1-type responsiveness in mice with experimental vaginal candidiasis. *Infect. Immun.* 61: 4202–4207.

Fidel, P.L., Jr., Lynch, M.E., and Sobel, J.D. (1993b). *Candida*-specific cell-mediated immunity is demonstrable in mice with experimental vaginal candidiasis. *Infect. Immun.* 61: 1990–1995.

Fidel, P.L. Jr., Lynch, M.E., and Sobel, J.D. (1994). Effects of preinduced *Candida*-specific systemic cell-mediated immunity on experimental vaginal candidiasis. *Infect. Immun.* 62: 1032–1038.

Fidel, P.L., Cutright, J.L., and Sobel, J.D. (1995a). Effects of systemic cell-mediated immunity on vaginal candidiasis in mice resistant and susceptible to *Candida albicans* infections. *Infect. Immun.* 63: 4191–4194.

Fidel, P.L. Jr., Lynch, M.E., Conaway, D.H., Tait, L., and Sobel, J.D. (1995b). Mice immunized by primary vaginal *Candida albicans* infection develop acquired vaginal mucosal immunity. *Infect. Immun.* 63: 547–553.

Fidel, P.L., Lynch, M.E., and Sobel, J.D. (1995c). Circulating CD4 and CD8 T-cells have little impact on host defence against experimental vaginal candidiasis. *Infect. Immun.* 63: 2403–2408.

Fidel, P.L., Wolf, N.A., and Kukuruga, M.A. (1996). T lymphocytes in the murine vaginal mucosa are phenotypically distinct from those in the periphery. *Infect. Immun.* 64: 3793–3799.

Fidel, P.L., Ginsburg, K.A., Cutright, J.L., Wolf, N.A., Leaman, D., Dunlops, K., and Sobel, J.D. (1997a). Vaginal-associated immunity in women with recurrent vulvovaginal candidiasis: Evidence for vaginal Th1-type responses following intravaginal challenge with Candida antigen. *J. Infect. Dis.* 176: 728–739.

Fidel, P.L., Luo, W., Chabain, J., Wolf, N.A., and Vanburen, E. (1997b). Use of cellular depletion analysis to examine circulation of immune effector function between the vagina and the periphery. *Infect. Immun.* 65: 3939–3943.

Fidel, P.L. Jr., Luo, W., Steele, C., Chabain, J., Baker, M., and Wormley, F. Jr. (1999). Analysis of vaginal cell populations during experimental vaginal candidiasis. *Infect. Immun.* 67: 3135–3140.

Garcia-Ruiz, J.C., Del Carmen Arilla, M., Regulez, P., Quindos, G., Alvarez, A., and Ponton, J. (1997). Detection of antibodies to *Candida albicans* germ tubes for diagnosis and therapeutic monitoring of invasive candidiasis inpatients with hematologic malignancies. *J. Clin. Microbiol.* 35: 3284–3287.

Ghannoum, M.A. and Abu-Elteen, K.H. (1990). Pathogenicity determinant of *Candida. Mycoses* 33: 265–282.

Greenfield, R.A. (1992). Host defense system interaction with *Candida. J. Med. Vet. Mycol.* 30: 89–104.

Guyard, C., Dehecq, E., Tissier, J.P., Polonelli, L, Dei-Cas, E., Cailliez, J.C., and Menozzi, F.D. (2002). Involvement of beta-glucan in the wide spectrum antimicrobial activity Williopsis saturnus var mrakii MUCL 41968 killer toxin. *Mol. Med.* 8: 686–694.

Han, Y., Kanbe, T., Cherniak, R., and Cutler, J. (1997). Biochemical characterization of *Candida albicans* epitopes that can elicit protective and nonprotective antibodies. *Infect. Immun* 65: 4100–4107.

Han, Y., Morrison, R.P., and Cutler, J.E. (1998). A vaccine and monoclonal antibodies that enhance mouse resistance to *Candida albicans* vaginal infection. *Infect. Immun.* 66: 5771–5776.

Han, Y., Riesselman, M., and Cutler, J.E. (2000). Protection against candidiasis by an immunoglobulin G3 (IgG3) monoclonal antibody specific for the same mannotriose as an IgM protective antibody. *Infect. Immun.* 68: 1649–1654.

Jones-Carson, J., Vazquez-Torres, A., van der Heyde, T., Warner, T., Wagner, R.D., and Balish, E. (1995). $\gamma\delta$ T cell-induced nitric oxide production enhances resistance to mucosal candidiasis. *Nat. Med.* 6: 552–557.

Kinsman, O.S. and Collard, A.E. (1986). Hormonal factors in vaginal candidiasis in rats. *Infect. Immun.* 53: 498–504.

Kinsman, O.S., Collard, A.E., and Savage, T.J. (1986). Ketoconazole in experimental vaginal candidosis in rats. *Antimicrob. Agents Chemother.* 30: 771–773.

Kirkpatrick, C.H., Rich, R.R., and Bennett, J.E. (1971). Chronic mucocutaneous candidiasis: Model-building in cellular immunity. *Ann. Intern. Med.* 74: 955–978.

Magliani, W., Conti, S., De Bernardis, F., Gerloni, M., Bertolotti, D, Mozzoni, P., Cassone, A., and Polonelli, L. (1997). Therapeutic activity of single chain fragment variable yeast-killer toxin-like candidacidal recombinant antiidiotypic antibodies. *Nat. Biotechnol.* 15: 155–158.

Magliani, W., Conti, S., De Bernardis, F., Cassone, A., and Polonelli, L. (2002). New immunotherapeutic strategies to control vaginal candidiasis. *Trends Mol. Med.* 8: 121–126.

Marodi, L. (1997). Local and systemic host defence mechanisms against *Candida*: Immunopathology of candidal infections. *Pediatr. Infect. Dis.* 16: 795–801.

McGhee, J.R., Mestecky, J., Elson, C.O., and Kiyono, H. (1989). Regulation of IgA synthesis and immune response by T cells and interleukins. *J. Clin. Immun.* 9: 175–180.

Mourad, S. and Friedman, L. M. (1961). Active immunization of mice against *Candida albicans*. *Proc. Soc. Exp. Biol. Med.* 106: 570–572.

Mourad, S. and Friedman, L. M. (1968). Passive immunization of mice against *Candida albicans*. *Sabouradia* 6: 103–105.

Mulero-Marchese, R.D., Blank, K.J., and Siek, T.G. (1998). Genetic basis for protection against experimental vaginal candidiasis by peripheral immunization. *J. Infect. Dis.* 178: 227–234.

Oggioni, M.R., Beninati, C., Boccanera, M., Medaglini, D., Spinosa, M.R., Maggi, T., Conti, S., Magliani, W., De Bernardis, F., Teti, G., Cassone, A., Pozzi, G., and Polonelli, L. (2001). Recombinant *Streptococcus gordonii* for mucosal delivery of a scFv microbicidal antibody. *Intern. Rev. Immunol.* 20: 267–279.

Polonelli, L. and Morace, G. (1986). Re-evaluation of the yeast killer phenmenon. *J. Clin. Microbiol.* 24: 866–869.

Polonelli, L. and Morace, G. (1987). Production and characterization of yeast killer toxin monoclonal antibodies. *J. Clin. Microbiol.* 25: 460–462.

Polonelli, L., Conti, S., Gerloni, M., Magliani, W., Chezzi, C., and Morace, G. (1991). Interfaces of the yeast killer phenomenon. *Crit. Rev. Microbiol.* 18(1): 47–87.

Polonelli, L., Lorenzini, R., De Bernardis, F., Gerloni, M., Conti, S., Morace, G., Magliani, W., and Chezzi, C. (1993). Idiotypic vaccination immunoprotection mediated by anti-idiotypic antibodies with antibiotic activity. *Scand. J. Immunol.* 37: 105–110.

Polonelli, L., De Bernardis, F., Conti, S., Boccanera, M., Gerloni, M., Morace, G., Magliani, W., Chezzi, C., and Cassone, A. (1994) Idiotypic intravaginal vaccination to protect against candidal vaginitis by secretory, yeast killer toxin-like anti-idiotypic antibodies. *J. Immunol.* 152: 3175–3182.

Polonelli, L., De Bernardis, F., Conti, S., Boccanera, M., Magliani, W., Gerloni, M., Cantelli, C., and Cassone, A. (1996). Human natural yeast killer toxin-like, candidacidal antibodies. *J. Immunol.* 156: 1880–1885.

Polonelli, L., De Bernardis, F., Conti, S., Gerloni, M., and Cassone, A. (1997). Yeast killer toxin-like antibodies in experimental and clinical candidiasis. In Y. Shoenfeld, R.C. Kennedy, and S. Ferrone (eds), *Idiotypes in Medicine: Autoimmunity, Infection and Cancer*. Elsevier Science, Amsterdam, pp. 369–380.

Polonelli, L., Magliani, W., Conti, S., Bracci, L., Lozzi , L., Neri, P., Adriani, D., De Bernardis, F., and Cassone, A. (2003). Therapeutic activity of an engineered synthetic killer antiidiotypic antibody fragment against experimental mucosal and systemic candidiasis. *Infect. Immun.* 71: 6205–6212.

Rogers, T.J. and Balish, E. (1980). Immunity to *Candida albicans*. *Microbiol. Rev.* 44: 660–682.

San Millan, R., Ezkurra, P.A., Quindòs, G., Robert, R., Senet, J.M., and Pontòn J. (1996). Effect of monoclonal antibodies directed against *Candida albicans* cell wall antigens on the adhesion of the fungus to polystyrene. *Microbiology* 142: 2271–2277.

Santoni, G., Boccanera, M., Adriani, D., Lucciarini, R., Amantini, C., Morrone, S., Cassone, A., and De Bernardis, F. (2002). Immune cell-mediated protection against vaginal candidiasis: Evidence for a mayor role of vaginal CD4+ T cells and possible participation of other local lymphocyte effectors. *Infect. Immun.* 70: 4791–4797.

Scicchitano, R., Stanisz, A., Ernst, P.B., and Bunenstock, J. (1988). A common mucosal immune system revised. In A.J. Husband (ed.), *Migration and Homing of Lymphoid Cells*, Vol. 2. CRC Press, Boca Raton, FL, pp. 1–34.

Sobel, J.D. (1989). Pathogenesis of *Candida* vulvovaginitis. In M.R. Mc Ginnis and M. Borges (eds), *Current Topics in Medical Mycology*. Springer-Verlag, Stuttgart, pp. 86–108.

Sobel, J.D. (1992). Pathogenesis and treatment of recurrent vulvovaginal candidiasis. *Clin. Infect. Dis.* 14: S148–S153.

Steele, C., Ratteree, M., Harrison, R., and Fidel, P.L. Jr. (1999). Differential susceptibility to experimental vaginal candidiasis in macaque. *J. Infect. Dis.* 180: 802–810.

Tipper, D.J. and Bostian, K.A. (1984). Double-stranded ribonucleic acid killer system in yeasts. *Microbiol. Rev.* 48: 125–156.

Walker, S.M. and Urbaniak, S.J. (1980). A serum-dependent defect of neutrophil function in chronic mucocutaneous candidiasis. *J. Clin. Pathol.* 33: 370–372.

18

Role of Complement in Fungal Infections

Thomas R. Kozel

1. Introduction

The complement system is a component of host resistance where innate and adaptive immunity intersect. Innate resistance is invoked when a microbe activates the alternative pathway or when mannan-binding lectin binds to a microbe and activates the classical pathway. The adaptive immune system utilizes the complement system when an IgG or IgM antibody binds to a microbial surface and activates the classical pathway.

Department of Microbiology and Immunology, University of Nevada School of Medicine, Reno, NV 89557.

Regardless of the manner of activation, the consequences of activation of the complement system include deposition of opsonic serum proteins on a microbial surface that facilitate phagocytosis by macrophages and neutrophils, attraction of inflammatory cells to the site of infection through the release of chemotactic peptides, and activation of a cascade of proteins that comprise the membrane attack complex that may produce damage to membranes on the surface of cells on which complement activation occurs. Fungi are surrounded by thick carbohydrate cell walls, which likely restrict complement-mediated killing, but opsonization and promotion of an inflammatory response are critical components of host resistance to fungal infection.

Fungi have served as model targets for the study of complement activation for over 100 years. von Dungern reported in 1900 that treatment of serum with yeast cells inactivates a heat-sensitive component of serum that is normally destructive to bacteria (von Dungern, 1900). This report was confirmed in 1902 in a study by Ehrlich and Sachs (1902). Zymosan, a cell wall product of *Saccharomyces cerevisiae*, which is rich in glucan content, has been a prototype for study of the alternative complement pathway and mechanisms of opsonization (Pillemer and Ecker, 1941; Fizpatrick and DiCarlo, 1964). Indeed, zymosan led to the discovery of the alternative pathway (Pillemer et al., 1954). Studies of complement activation by pathogenic fungi have built on this legacy of prior work.

Production of many disseminated fungal infections requires that the fungus, usually a yeast cell, spend a portion of its time in the bloodstream. Since serum is rich in proteins of the complement cascade, there is a high probability that the consequences of interaction between a yeast cell and the complement system will have a major impact on the course of disease. This chapter focuses primarily on complement activation by *Cryptococcus neoformans* and *Candida albicans*, two fungi that rely on hematogenous dissemination for spread from sites of initial infection to target organs.

2. Activation of the Complement System by Pathogenic Fungi

2.1. Experimental Systems for Study of Complement Activation

Several experimental approaches have been used to study complement activation by pathogenic fungi. In the first approach, microbes are incubated in serum and the biological consequences of complement activation are assessed. As discussed in a later section, the two most commonly studied biological consequences of complement activation are opsonization and release of inflammatory mediators. The second approach is measurement of the depletion of complement proteins as a consequence of complement activation. The standard complement fixation assay is an example of a complement depletion assay. The third approach is immunochemical evaluation of the release of cleavage products of complement proteins via complement activation. Typically, supernatant fluids are examined for fragments of C3 or factor B following incubation of fungi in serum. Finally, complement activation can be assessed by measurement of the deposition of cleavage fragments of C3 onto the fungal surface. Two methods for measurement of C3 deposition are: use of radiolabeled C3 and immunofluorescence. Radiolabeled C3 is advantageous because it allows for a quantitative assessment of C3 binding. Staining for C3 binding by immunofluorescence is valuable because it identifies the sites of C3 binding. Given the critical role of C3 fragments in opsonization, both quantitative and qualitative examination of C3 binding are needed to fully assess the manner of interaction of fungi with the complement system.

Activation of the complement system can occur via three pathways. Binding of antibody to the fungal surface can activate the classical pathway. Binding of mannan-binding lectin (MBL) to the cell can also activate the classical pathway. Finally, fungi can activate the alternative pathway. The reader is referred to a standard immunology text for a more detailed discussion of the pathways for complement activation.

There are several experimental tools that can be used to identify mechanisms of complement activation. Some complement proteins are heat labile. As a consequence, one of the most common methods to identify a role for the complement system in a biological process is heating of serum for 30 min at 56°C. An alternative approach is treatment of serum with EDTA. Such treatment chelates the Ca^{2+} needed for activation of the classical pathway and the Mg^{2+} that is critical to both the classical and alternative pathways. Since the classical pathway is activated by the presence of antibody or MBL in serum, the classical pathway can be blocked by absorption of serum to remove such initiators. Addition of antibody or MBL back to the absorbed serum confirms the role of these proteins in complement activation. It should be noted that antibody also contributes to activation of the alternative pathway, so interpretation of results from experiments using absorbed serum requires rigorous controls and should be interpreted with caution. Another approach to identification of pathways of activation is treatment of serum with EGTA. Ca^{2+} is required for the classical pathway but not the alternative pathway. The high affinity of EGTA for Ca^{2+} and its relatively low affinity for Mg^{2+} allows for selective blockade of the classical pathway while leaving the alternative pathway intact (Fine et al., 1972; Platts-Mills and Ishizaka, 1974). Finally, the complement system can be studied by experimental reconstitution of the complement system from isolated proteins.

2.2. *C. albicans*

Evidence for activation of the complement system by *C. albicans* is based on several lines of study. First, treatment of yeast cells with serum leads to enhanced phagocytosis (Ferrante and Thong, 1979; Morrison and Cutler, 1981). Second, chemotactic peptides are produced by incubation of yeast cells with serum (Ray and Wuepper, 1976; Thong and Ferrante, 1978). Finally, incubation of *Candida* spp. in human serum results in conversion of C3 and factor B as measured by immunoelectrophoresis (Ray and Wuepper, 1976).

There are multiple mechanisms by which *C. albicans* activates the complement system. Activation of the classical pathway is the primary mechanism for deposition of C3 when the yeast is incubated in serum from normal adult donors. The classical pathway is initiated by an antimannan IgG that is found in the serum of most adults (Jones, 1980; Lehmann and Reiss, 1980). Antimannan IgM is also found in sera from adult donors, but the levels of antibody are much lower than levels of antimannan IgG (Lehmann and Reiss, 1980; Kozel et al., 2004). Normal serum also contains the lectin MBL. MBL binds to *C. albicans* (Neth et al., 2000) and MBL deficiencies have been associated with yeast infection (Summerfield et al., 1995). MBL is a potent activator of the classical pathway (Lu et al., 1990; Ohta et al., 1990) and likely contributes to complement activation by *C. albicans*. However, the relative contributions of antimannan IgG and MBL to activation of the classical pathway have not been rigorously studied.

There are several characteristic features of C3 deposition on *C. albicans* via the classical pathway (Kozel et al., 1996). Some of these features are illustrated in Fig. 18.1.

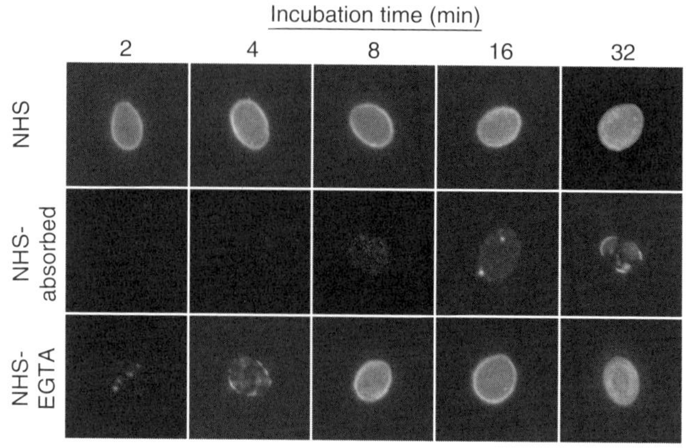

Figure 18.1. Sites and kinetics for deposition of C3 on *C. albicans*. *C. albicans* blastoconidia were incubated for the indicated times in (i) normal human serum (NHS), (ii) NHS that had been absorbed with *C. albicans* to remove antibody (NHS-absorbed), or (iii) NHS that had been treated with Mg-EGTA to block the alternative pathway (NHS-EGTA). Sites of C3 binding were identified by use of FITC-labeled antibody specific for human C3. Photomicrographs courtesy of Marcellene Gates.

Deposition of C3 is very rapid. C3 is readily detectable on the yeast by either immunofluorescence or by the use of radiolabeled C3 after 2 min incubation in normal serum. The process is largely complete after 4 min. In contrast to yeast cells, the rate of C3 deposition is somewhat slower on germ tubes. C3 that is deposited via the classical pathway is uniformly distributed over the surface of both yeast cells and germ tubes.

The antibody in normal human serum that is responsible for activation of the classical pathway by *C. albicans* is specific for *Candida* mannan (Kozel et al., 1996; Zhang et al., 1997). Absorption of serum to remove antimannan antibody markedly delays the kinetics for early deposition of C3 that characterizes the classical pathway. This antibody is removed by absorption with *C. albicans* yeast cells, but not by absorption with *S. cerevisiae*, encapsulated *C. neoformans* or acapsular *C. neoformans*. The antibody is removed by absorption with purified *Candida* mannan, and antimannan IgG that is affinity purified from normal human serum restores early C3 deposition kinetics to absorbed serum.

Monoclonal antibodies specific for *Candida* mannan also activate the classical pathway (Han et al., 2001). Such activation is dependent on antibody concentration; suboptimal activation and binding of C3 fragments occurs if too little or too much antibody is present. Importantly, a functional complement system is needed if passive immunization with mannan mAb is to be protective. Monoclonal antibodies that are protective in complement-normal mice fail to protect in C3-deficient mice.

C. albicans yeast cells and germ tubes also activate the alternative pathway leading to deposition of C3 on the yeast surface. Activation of the alternative pathway is complex, occurring via antibody-dependent and antibody-independent pathways (Kozel et al., 1996; Zhang et al., 1997; Zhang and Kozel, 1998). Antibody-dependent activation of the alternative pathway is shown by C3 binding in the presence of EGTA to chelate the Ca^{2+} required to activate the classical pathway (see Fig. 18.1 for an example). Antibody-independent activation is demonstrated by binding of C3 in serum that has been absorbed with mannan to remove antimannan antibody and MBL.

The pattern and kinetics for deposition of C3 onto *C. albicans* in the presence of EGTA differ markedly from what is observed with an intact classical pathway (Kozel et al., 1996; Zhang et al., 1997). There is a delay of 2–4 min before readily measurable deposition of C3 occurs (Fig. 18.1). In addition, the pattern of C3 binding is asynchronous and focal, in contrast to the relatively uniform early deposition that occurs when the classical pathway is intact. C3 deposition appears to be a nucleation event in which a small focal site of early C3 binding spreads in a centripetal fashion. The sites of early C3 foci appear to be randomly distributed over the yeast surface. As foci of bound C3 expand, they eventually coalesce to cover the yeast surface.

Antibody-independent activation of the alternative pathway is observed when yeast cells are incubated in serum that has been absorbed to remove antimannan antibody or MBL (Zhang and Kozel, 1998). Antibody-independent activation of the alternative pathway follows the asynchronous, focal pattern of deposition observed with antibody-dependent activation of the alternative pathway; however, the kinetics for deposition via antibody-independent activation are dramatically delayed (Fig. 18.1). Focal binding sites are observed after 16 min incubation, and incubation times of greater than 30 min are required to coat the cells with C3. Even with extended incubation times, the amount of C3 bound via antibody-independent activation is markedly less than the amounts that accumulate via the classical pathway or the antibody-dependent alternative pathway.

2.3. *C. neoformans*

The encapsulated yeast *C. neoformans* is a potent activator of the complement system. Incubation of encapsulated cryptococci in human serum leads to the binding of 10^7–10^8 C3 molecules per yeast cell (Young and Kozel, 1993). The numbers of C3 molecules binding to encapsulated cryptococci are much greater than that are observed with other fungi, e.g., 2×10^6 per *C. albicans* cell (Kozel et al., 1996), 4×10^6 per zymosan particle (Kozel et al., 1991), or 2×10^6 per acapsular *C. neoformans* yeast cell (Kozel et al., 1991). The binding capacity of *C. neoformans* for C3 likely reflects the large capsular volume that is presented by the three-dimensional capsular matrix. Remarkably, the yeast is such a powerful activator of the complement system that some patients with disseminated cryptococcosis exhibit depletion of the complement system (Macher et al., 1978).

2.3.1. Activation of the Alternative Pathway

Incubation of encapsulated cryptococci in human serum leads to activation of the complement system entirely via the alternative pathway. Unlike antimannan antibodies and *C. albicans*, normal human serum typically lacks the amounts of anticapsular antibody needed for activation of the classical pathway. Evidence for activation of the alternative pathway is derived from three lines of study. First, treatment of serum with EGTA to chelate the Ca^{2+} needed for activation of the classical pathway does not block the ability of the yeast to activate the complement system (Kozel et al., 1991). Second, the ability of the yeast to activate the complement system is lost if serum is heated at 50°C (Diamond et al., 1974). Factor B of the alternative pathway is quite heat labile; consequently, heating of serum at 50°C is a means to selectively block the action of the alternative pathway (Götze and Müller-Eberhard, 1971). Finally, activation and binding of C3 occurs when the yeast is incubated in an alternative pathway that is reconstituted from the six purified proteins of the alternative pathway (Kozel et al., 1989b). Both the kinetics and sites of C3 binding are identical when cryptococci are treated with normal human serum or an experimentally constructed alternative pathway.

Activation of the alternative pathway by encapsulated cryptococci resembles the kinetics and cellular pattern of C3 deposition found with antibody-dependent activation of the alternative pathway by *C. albicans* (Kozel et al., 1991). Little binding of C3 is apparent after 2–4 min incubation (Fig. 18.2). This lag is followed by a phase of rapid accumulation of C3 on the cell. This rapid accumulation terminates abruptly after 16 min incubation. Presumably the termination of accumulation occurs because available sites for C3 binding have been filled and/or because the bound C3b has been completely converted to iC3b, which cannot support further amplification.

The patterns of C3 binding shown by immunofluorescence resemble the asynchronous focal nature of initiation and amplification found with antibody-dependent activation of the alternative pathway by *C. albicans*. The critical difference between the nucleation events that occur on *C. albicans* and *C. neoformans* is that the expansion phase likely occurs in two dimensions on the surface of *C. albicans*, whereas expansion occurs in three dimensions within the cryptococcal capsule. A kinetic analysis of C3 accumulation during the amplification phase with encapsulated cryptococci found that accumulation of C3 follows the kinetics predicted by an expanding sphere (Kozel et al., 1992).

2.3.2. Sites of C3 Binding

The capsule itself is the site for binding of C3 fragments to encapsulated cryptococci. An examination of the sites for C3 binding by transmission electron microscopy (TEM) found C3 to be bound throughout the capsule (Kozel et al., 1989b). The early studies of C3 binding to encapsulated cryptococci utilized cells that were grown under standard laboratory culture conditions. Two recent reports of cryptococci that were grown under conditions that lead to induction of large capsules similar to

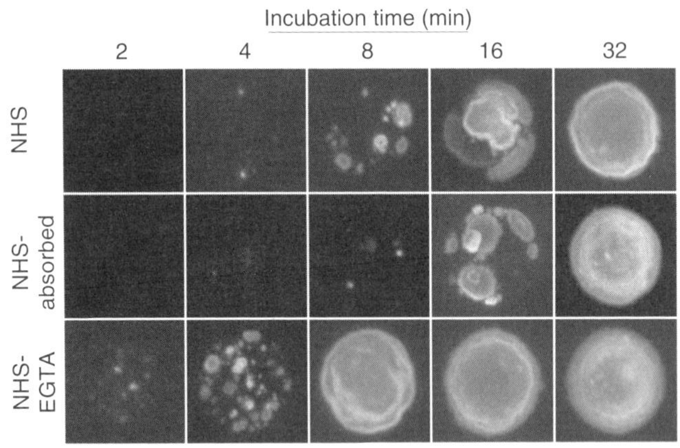

Figure 18.2. Sites and kinetics for deposition of C3 on encapsulated *C. neoformans*. Yeast cells were incubated for the indicated times in (i) normal human serum (NHS), (ii) NHS that had been absorbed with encapsulated cryptococci to remove antibody (NHS-absorbed), or (iii) NHS that had been treated with Mg-EGTA to block the alternative pathway (NHS-EGTA). Sites of C3 binding were identified by use of FITC-labeled antibody specific for human C3. Photomicrographs courtesy of Marcellene Gates.

capsules produced in vivo suggest that factors determining the sites of C3 binding are more complex than were found with cells grown in the absence of capsule induction conditions. Zaragoza et al. (2004) found that the location of C3 binding in the capsule was a function of capsule diameter. Incubation of small-capsule cryptococci in normal mouse serum led to C3 binding to the capsule edge. In contrast, large-capsule cryptococci bound C3 beneath the capsule surface but not at the capsule edge. These results led to the conclusion that large-capsule cryptococci avoid surveillance by the complement system by directing C3 deposition to a site where the C3 fragments would not be available for interaction with phagocyte complement receptors.

Capsule size also influences the extent to which complement activation penetrates to the capsule interior (Gates et al., 2004). Incubation of small-capsule cryptococci in serum leads to deposition of C3 throughout the capsule. In contrast, C3 binding does not occur in the deep capsule interior of cryptococci grown in vitro for production of large capsules or of cryptococci harvested from infected brain tissue. The failure of C3 to bind to the deep capsule interior is due to molecular sieving that prevents penetration of high molecular weight complement proteins to the capsule interior.

2.3.3. Mechanism for Binding of C3 to the Capsule

C3b can bind to target cells via ester or amide linkages. Studies of model compounds found that ester bonds formed between C3b and hydroxyl groups are sensitive to hydrolysis with hydroxylamine, whereas amide bonds are resistant to hydrolysis (Law and Levine, 1977; Law et al., 1979; Hostetter et al., 1982). The capsule is rich in hydroxyl groups that would be available for formation of ester bonds. C3 fragments bound to the cryptococcal capsule are resistant to elution with detergents or chaotropes, but bound C3 is completely removed by treatment with hydroxylamine, indicating that C3 is bound to the capsule via ester linkages (Kozel and Pfrommer, 1986).

2.3.4. Molecular forms of Bound C3

C3 that is bound to the cryptococcal capsule is almost entirely in the form of iC3b (Kozel and Pfrommer, 1986). iC3b is a highly opsonic protein that is formed by the cleavage of C3b by factor I with the assistance of factor H as a cofactor. C3b bound to the cryptococcal capsule has a uniformly high susceptibility to conversion to iC3b by factors H and I (Pfrommer et al., 1993). Rapid conversion of C3b to iC3b suggests that the expanding sphere of bound C3 in the capsule consists of C3b on the surface of the sphere that supports amplification, but the C3b in the interior of the sphere is rapidly converted to iC3b as the sphere expands. The fact that most of the C3 bound to the cryptococcal capsule is in the form of iC3b suggests that receptors with a high affinity for iC3b, such as CR3 and CR4, will be the primary phagocyte receptors involved in phagocytosis of cryptococci that are opsonized by incubation in normal serum.

2.3.5. Effects of Anticapsular mAbs on Complement Activation

The lag in activation of the complement system by encapsulated cryptococci is greatly reduced if anticapsular antibody is present for activation of the classical pathway. However, the ability of an anticapsular antibody to activate the classical pathway is dramatically influenced by the epitope specificity of the antibody. For example, mAbs that are reactive with a capsular epitope found on cryptococci of serotypes A, B, C, and D activate the classical pathway with cells of serotype A (Kozel et al., 1998). In contrast, mAbs reactive with an epitope found only on cryptococcal serotypes A and D fails to activate the classical pathway. This differential interaction with the complement system has been demonstrated with two distinct mAbs of each specificity class. The molecular mechanism that allows for one antibody to activate the classical pathway whereas another antibody with a different epitope specificity fails to activate is not known.

Unlike *C. albicans*, anticapsular antibodies do not appear to contribute to activation of the alternative pathway. However, studies of anticapsular mAbs found an unexpected result. In an epitope-specific manner, some mAbs have no effect on activation of the alternative pathway that would normally occur on incubation of encapsulated cryptococci with normal serum (Kozel et al., 1998). Other anticapsular mAbs suppress the overall rate and amount of C3 binding via the alternative pathway. Those mAbs that suppress overall rates of C3 accumulation are the same mAbs that support activation of the classical pathway. Those mAbs that have no effect on alternative pathway activation are the antibodies that fail to activate the classical pathway. A critical difference between antibodies that suppress rates of overall C3 accumulation and antibodies that have no effect is the ability of the former class of mAbs to cross-link the capsular surface (MacGill et al., 2000). Such cross-linking likely blocks penetration of complement proteins to the capsular interior, thus accounting for suppression of overall rates and amounts of C3 binding.

2.3.6. Molecular Basis for Regulation of Complement Activation by Encapsulated Cryptococci

Limited information is available regarding the molecular nature of the cryptococcal capsule that accounts for either its ability to activate the alternative pathway or to regulate rapid conversion of capsule-bound C3b to iC3b. The primary constituent of the cryptococcal capsule is glucuronoxylomannan (GXM). GXM consists of a (1б3)-linked linear α-D-mannopyran with single β-D-xylopyranosyl, β-D-glucuronopyranosyl, and 6-*O*-acetyl substituents. The polysaccharide occurs as four primary serotypes, which differ in the degrees of substitution with xylopyranosyl and *O*-acetyl groups. Production of GXM is critical to the patterns of complement activation described above. Acapsular mutants produce a markedly different pattern of complement activation (see below). Notably, complementation of the capsular mutation in an acapsular strain restores the pattern of complement activation to the pattern observed with encapsulated strains (Chang et al., 1997).

Paradoxically, purified GXM shows little ability to activate the complement system, even when used in high concentrations (Laxalt and Kozel, 1979). Any explanation for the complement-activating properties of the cryptococcal capsule must account for this dichotomous behavior in which GXM assembled in the form of a capsule is a potent activator, whereas soluble GXM fails to activate. One possible explanation is the random and infrequent formation of activation foci, e.g., Fig. 18.2. The massive activation and binding of C3 to the capsule appears to be highly dependent on amplification of bound C3 from a limited number of foci. The lifetime of the reactive site of metastable C3b that is formed during complement activation has been estimated at 60 μs, during which time it could diffuse approximately 40 nm (Hughes-Jones, 1986). If the metastable C3b fails to bind to a reactive site, it is inactivated and can no longer support amplification. In the case of capsular GXM, a limited number of initiation sites can easily expand to fill the capsule through amplification to adjacent capsular sites. In the case of soluble GXM, the molecular distances between soluble molecules may be too great to allow for amplification. As a consequence, initiation could occur on a limited number of soluble molecules, but there would be a failure to amplify.

Xylose residues that decorate the mannan backbone appear to play a complex role in activation of the alternative pathway. A study of the attachment efficiency for C3b binding to a variety of model compounds found a high degree of attachment efficiency to xylose (Sahu et al., 1994). This same study found a hierarchy for efficiency of binding of C3b to cryptococci of different serotypes that paralleled the xylose content of each serotype: serotype C > serotype B > serotype A > serotype D. This result suggests that xylosylation should favor activation.

In contrast to the high efficiency of binding of C3b to cryptococcal strains having a high xylose content, xylose-negative strains exhibit an accelerated kinetics for C3 deposition compared to wild-type parents (Kozel et al., 2003). This latter result indicates that factors other than efficiency in binding of C3b are the dominant force in determining kinetics of complement activation when xylose-positive and xylose-negative cells are compared. One explanation is the possibility that the presence or absence of xylose influences the affinity of factor B or factor H for capsule-bound C3b. Particles that favor binding of factor B and discourage binding of factor H are activators of the alternative pathway, whereas particles that encourage binding of factor H are nonactivators (Horstmann et al., 1985). It is quite possible that xylose residues in the cryptococcal capsule increase the efficiency with which factor H can function as a cofactor for factor I thus leading to a reduction in alternative pathway activation. Accelerated kinetics for activation and binding of C3 to xylose-negative mutants is consistent with the relative kinetics observed with cells of different serotypes (Young and Kozel, 1993). There is a greater rate of accumulation of C3 on cells of serotypes A and D (low xylose content) than serotypes B and C (high xylose content). Taken together, studies of the contribution of the xylosyl residue to complement activation suggest that xylosylation may have multiple and independent effects on initiation, amplification, and regulation.

O-acetylation is another structural feature of the cryptococcal capsule that impacts activation and binding of C3 to encapsulated cryptococci. *O*-acetylation is not necessary for activation of the alternative pathway (Young and Kozel, 1993; Kozel et al., 2003), but de-*O*-acetylation of encapsulated cells leads to a significant increase in the amount of C3 binding to encapsulated cryptococci. One explanation for this increased binding is the possibility that *O*-acetyl groups occupy or sterically block potential sites on GXM for binding of metastable C3b.

2.3.7. Acapsular *C. neoformans*

Acapsular cryptococci activate the complement system leading to deposition of C3 on the cell surface and opsonization for phagocytosis. However, the features of activation closely resemble activation produced by *C. albicans* and differ markedly from patterns found with encapsulated cryptococci (Fig. 18.3). Incubation of acapsular cryptococci in normal human serum leads to a rapid and largely synchronous deposition of C3 similar to classical pathway activation by *C. albicans* (Kozel et al., 1991). Chelation of serum with EGTA to block the classical pathway produces a delay in activation, and accumulation of C3 follows the asynchronous, focal pattern observed with encapsulated cryptococci, or *C. albicans* incubated in EGTA-treated serum.

Rapid, synchronous accumulation of C3 and susceptibility of rapid binding to acapsular cryptococci to inhibition by EGTA indicate that antibody-mediated activation of the classical pathway is the primary mechanism for activation of the complement

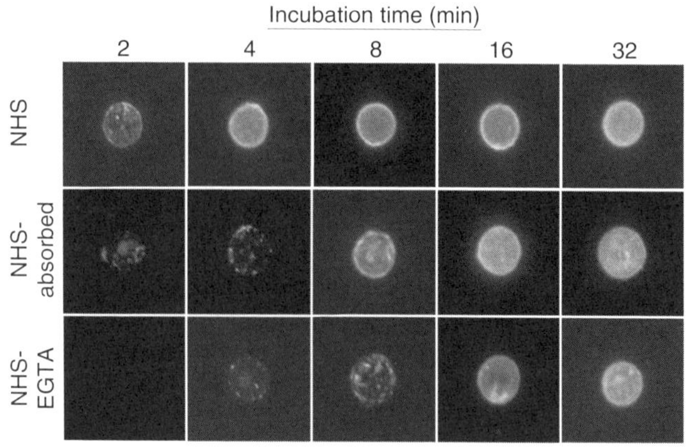

Figure 18.3. Sites and kinetics for deposition of C3 on acapsular *C. neoformans*. Yeast cells were incubated for the indicated times in (i) normal human serum (NHS), (ii) NHS that had been absorbed with acapsular cryptococci to remove antibody (NHS-absorbed), or (iii) NHS that had been treated with Mg-EGTA to block the alternative pathway (NHS-EGTA). Sites of C3 binding were identified by use of FITC-labeled antibody specific for human C3. Photomicrographs courtesy of Marcellene Gates.

system when acapsular cryptococci are incubated in normal serum. A potential role for antibody in normal serum in initiating the classical pathway was confirmed by absorption of antibody from normal serum (Wilson and Kozel, 1992). Absorbed serum showed the delayed, asynchronous, focal pattern of binding that was found in EGTA-treated serum. The fact that early activation kinetics can be restored to absorbed serum by addition of purified IgG indicates that normal sera contain antibodies reactive with the cell wall of acapsular cryptococci. Unlike *C. albicans*, there is no evidence of a role for antibody in activation of the alternative pathway by acapsular cryptococci.

Further study of antibodies to acapsular cryptococci in normal human serum found that the antibodies are of the IgG2 class (Keller et al., 1994), a result that is in agreement with numerous reports that human antibodies to microbial polysaccharides are predominantly IgG2. Antibodies reactive with acapsular cryptococci are blocked by treatment with isolated yeast glucan but not mannan or chitin. The antibodies are removed by absorption with zymosan but not *C. albicans* or *S. cerevisiae*. Zymosan consists of ghosts of *S. cerevisiae* that have been treated in a manner that likely exposes internal glucan (DiCarlo and Fiore, 1958). Taken together, comparative studies of initiation of the classical pathway by *C. albicans* and acapsular cryptococci indicate that the pathways to activation are similar, but activation by *C. albicans* utilizes antimannan IgG found in normal human serum, whereas acapsular cryptococci utilize antiglucan IgG.

Complement activation by acapsular cryptococci differs in several additional respects from activation by encapsulated cryptococci. First, C3b on encapsulated cryptococci is much more susceptible to conversion to iC3b by factors H and I than C3b found to acapsular cells (Pfrommer et al., 1993). Second, the ratio of iC3b:C3b on encapsulated cryptococci is much higher than on acapsular cryptococci. Finally, the rate of accumulation of C3 fragments on encapsulated cryptococci is much higher than the rate of accumulation on acapsular cells (Kozel et al., 1992).

2.4. *Blastomyces dermatitidis* and *Aspergillus fumigatus*

Activation of the complement system by *Blastomyces dermatitidis* yeast cells follows the paradigms described above for *C. albicans* and acapsular cryptococci. Incubation of *B. dermatitidis* in serum from normal adults leads to rapid binding of C3 via the classical pathway (Zhang and Klein, 1997; Zhang et al., 2001). The antibody in normal serum that mediates classical pathway activation is specific for β-glucan. The classical pathway can also be activated by antibodies specific for BAD1, an immunodominant antigen of *B. dermatitidis*. If the classical pathway is blocked by treatment of serum with EGTA or by removal of antibody, delayed activation occurs via the alternative pathway. Most, but not all, C3 fragments are bound via ester bonds, and the molecular forms of the C3 fragments are a mixture of C3b and iC3b.

Optimal phagocytosis of *A. fumigatus* conidia is dependent on opsonization by complement proteins (Sturtevant et al., 1992). A comparative study of activation and binding of C3 to resting conidia, swollen conidia, and hyphae showed that complement activation by resting conidia is mediated by the alternative pathway; however, there is a progressive dependence on the classical pathway as the fungal particles mature into swollen conidia and then hyphae (Kozel et al., 1989a). Despite the use of different activation pathways, the three particles are similar in utilizing ester bonds for linkage of C3 fragments. The C3 fragments bound to the three particles are a mixture of C3b and iC3b indicating that opsonized cells have the potential for interaction with receptors for both fragments.

3. Direct Binding of Complement Proteins to Fungi

In addition to covalent binding of C3 fragments to fungi as a consequence of complement activation, several laboratories have reported direct binding of complement proteins to putative receptors on the fungal surface. The best studied of the complement receptors are those for iC3b and C3d. These receptors were discovered serendipidously in two separate laboratories where, in one instance, yeast cells contaminating a lymphoblastoid culture reacted with complement-coated sheep erythrocytes (Heidenreich and Dierich, 1985). In the second instance, an experiment was done to induce expression of complement receptors on endothelial cells by infecting the cells in vitro with *C. albicans*. When complement-coated erythrocytes were added as a measure of receptor expression, the erythrocytes bound to the yeast cells rather than to the endothelial cells (Edwards et al., 1986). Further studies found that *C. albicans* and its closely related species *C. stellatoidea*, but not other yeast species, bound erythrocytes that were coated with C3d and iC3b. Binding of complement-coated erythrocytes was prominent with germ tubes and pseudohyphae, whereas there was little binding to blastoconidia.

A great deal has been learned about the candidal receptor for iC3b since its original discovery, and the receptor has been shown to have functional and structural homology to the α-subunit of the leukocyte adhesion glycoproteins CD11b/CD18 and CD11c/CD18. Murine monoclonal antibodies that recognize CD11b and CD11c cross-react with surface proteins of *C. albicans* (Edwards, et al., 1986; Bendel and Hostetter, 1993; Bendel et al., 1995). Binding of iC3b to *C. albicans* is specific, saturable, and reversible, indicating the presence of a true receptor (Gilmore et al., 1988). The integrin-like protein of *Candida* spp. has been proposed as a means for evasion of innate immunity by the use of molecular mimicry to avoid phagocytosis (Gilmore et al., 1988), but a more important function may be that of adhesion. Candidal cells bind to HeLa cells that express iC3b and fibronectin in a process that is inhibited by RGD peptides encompassing the RGD site and surrounding amino acids in iC3b (Bendel and Hostetter, 1993). The gene encoding the candidal integrin, *INT1*, has been cloned and sequenced (Gale et al., 1996). Expression of Int1p in *S. cerevisiae* allows for adhesion of this normally nonadherent yeast to human cervical epithelial cells, whereas disruption of *INT1* in *C. albicans* reduces epithelial cell adhesion (Gale et al., 1998). Finally, disruption of both alleles markedly reduces virulence in an intravenous murine model of candidiasis (Gale et al., 1998; Bendel et al., 1999).

Many microbes bind complement regulatory proteins in a process of immune evasion and downregulation of complement activation. *Streptococcus pyogenes*, *Streptococcus pneumoniae*, *Neisseria gonorrhoeae*, *Borrelia burgdorferi*, and human immunodeficiency virus bind factor H and/or FHL-1. These proteins act as cofactors for factor I in cleavage of C3b and compete with factor B in binding to cell-bound C3b. As a consequence, binding of factor H or FHL-1 may attenuate or terminate activation of the complement cascade. A recent study by Meri et al. (2002) found that factor H and FHL-1 also bind to *C. albicans*. Factor H and FHL-1 that bind to the candidal surface retain their regulatory activities and facilitate factor I-mediated cleavage of C3b.

4. Functional Consequences of Complement Activation

The complement system can contribute to host resistance through a number of effector systems. Activation of the complement system can also contribute to a diverse array of disease processes by production and amplification of inflammation. The primary means by which the complement system contributes to host resistance include opsonization, stimulation of inflammation, and cytolysis.

Opsonization occurs when activation of the complement cascade leads to deposition of potentially opsonic fragments of C3 onto the fungal surface. The primary opsonic fragments of C3 are C3b and iC3b. The primary cellular receptor for C3b is complement receptor type 1 (CR1; CD35). CR1 is present on erythrocytes, macrophages, monocytes neutrophils, and B cells. The primary receptors for iC3b are complement receptor type 3 (CR3; CD11b/18) and complement receptor type 4 (CR4; CD11c/18). CR3 and CR4 are found on phagocytic cells such as macrophages, monocytes and neutrophils, and mediate phagocytosis of target cells coated with iC3b.

Several studies have identified the fragments of C3 found on fungal surfaces after incubation with human serum. C3 fragments bound to zymosan particles are primarily in the form of C3b (Law and Levine, 1977). Similarly, C3 fragments bound to the surface of *C. albicans* yeast cells are almost entirely C3b (Kozel et al., 1987). The molecular form of C3 binding to *A. fumigatus* varies with the target cell (Kozel et al., 1989a). C3 fragments bound to resting conidia are primarily iC3b, whereas C3 bound to swollen conidia or hyphae are a mixture of C3b and iC3b. The presence of high proportions of C3b on the surface of many fungi after incubation in human serum suggests a role for CR1 in phagocytosis of these cells when opsonized with normal serum.

The presence of large amounts of iC3b on encapsulated cryptococci suggests a key role for CR3 and CR4 in phagocytosis of cryptococci opsonized by incubation in human serum. Levitz and Tabuni (1991) found that mAbs directed against CR1, CR3, and CR4 profoundly inhibited phagocytosis of normal-serum-opsonized cryptococci by monocyte-derived macrophages. Similarly, serum-opsonized cryptococci bound to CHO cells that were transfected with human CR1, CR3, or CR4 (Levitz et al., 1997). The substantial roles for CR3 and CR4 in phagocytosis are not surprising given the massive presence of iC3b in the cryptococcal capsule. The contribution of CR1 could be due to the limited C3b found in the capsule that has not been converted to iC3b.

The second mechanism by which the complement system can contribute to host resistance is the release of mediators of inflammation. Activation of the complement system leads to the release of C4a, C3a, and C5a. These peptides have properties that include chemotaxis and chemokinesis for neutrophils, stimulation of the respiratory burst, and targeting of vascular endothelial cells to increase vascular permeability. Generation of chemotactic peptides following incubation of various fungi in serum has been demonstrated for *C. neoformans* (Laxalt and Kozel, 1979; Diamond and Erickson, 1982), *C. albicans* (Ray and Wuepper, 1976; Thong and Ferrante, 1978), *A. fumigatus* (Budzko and Negroni, 1975), *Trichophyton* spp. (Dahl and Carpenter, 1986), and *C. immitis* (Galgiani et al., 1978). Finally, C5a contributes to killing by neutrophils. Lovchik and Lipscomb (1993) found that killing of encapsulated cryptococci by neutrophils was largely absent if done in the presence of C5-deficient serum. This deficiency was restored by the addition of recombinant C5a.

An important biological activity of the complement system is the ability to assemble a membrane attack complex (MAC) leading to cytolysis of the target cell. Microbes having thick external cell walls such as gram-positive bacteria are generally regarded as resistant to complement-mediated bacteriolysis (Joiner et al., 1983; Brown, 1985). Moreover, there has not been convincing evidence of complement-mediated lysis or killing of fungi. However, these paradigms have recently been called into question by a report of antibody-dependent bacteriolysis of the gram-positive *Bacillus anthracis* (Rhie et al., 2003). Lukasser-Vogl et al. (2000) recently reported that incubation of *C. albicans* in normal serum leads to the binding of terminal complement proteins on the yeast surface. Such deposition did not occur if the serum was treated with EDTA or preactivated with zymosan, indicating that deposition of the MAC was not due to nonspecific binding of proteins. Binding of terminal complement proteins to *C. albicans* has functional consequences for the yeast because treatment with normal serum produces decreased fungal growth and an alteration in fungal mitochondrial activities (Triebel et al., 2003). The effects of terminal complement proteins and the complement MAC on fungal cell surface signaling, metabolism, and viability are areas that merit further study.

5. Role of the Complement System In Vivo

The in vitro studies described above clearly demonstrate that exposure of pathogenic fungi to the complement system has functional consequences that are likely to influence the course of fungal infection in vivo. As a complement to these in vitro studies, there are numerous reports of the effects of complement deficiency on the course of fungal infection in vivo. The model system that has received the greatest amount of study is the C5-deficient mouse. C5-deficient mice have decreased resistance to disseminated cryptococcosis (Rhodes, 1985; Lovchik and Lipscomb, 1993), disseminated candidiasis (Morelli and Rosenberg, 1971; Lyon et al., 1986; Hector et al., 1990; Ashman et al., 2003), cutaneous candidiasis (Wilson and Sohnle, 1988), and aspergillosis (Hector et al., 1990).

The critical role of C5 in host resistance to disseminated fungal infection is illustrated by the course of infection following intravenous administration of *S. cerevisiae*. This weakly pathogenic yeast is not lethal in immunocompetent mice (Clemons et al., 1994), but produces a lethal infection in C5-deficient mice (Byron et al., 1995). Tissue census studies following intravenous administration of yeast cells showed higher numbers of yeast cells in spleen, liver, kidney, and lung of C5-deficient mice than in congenic C5-normal mice. The greatest differences were found in lung and kidney.

A seminal report by Lovchik and Lipscomb provides a potential explanation for the role of C5a in hematogenously disseminated fungal infection. Mice were infected intravenously with encapsulated cryptococci and clearance of the yeast in the lung was assessed. The results showed rapid accumulation of yeast cells in the lungs of C5-sufficient mice 30 min after infection, but the lungs were largely free of cryptococci after 24 h. Histopathological and TEM examination of lung tissue showed a marked accumulation of polymorphonuclear neutrophil leukocytes (PMN) in the vicinity of cryptococci within the lumina of capillaries or venules, and there was considerable phagocytosis of the yeast. In contrast, the number of PMN in the lungs of C5-deficient mice was not increased over normal levels, and there was no evidence of phagocytosis of cryptococci 30 min after inoculation. However, by 24 h after infection, cryptococci had replicated within the pulmonary vessels, but there was still no accumulation of PMN. These results indicate that C5 facilitates removal of cryptococci from the bloodstream within pulmonary vessels. The authors suggested that this mechanism could prevent development of foci of lung infection during extrapulmonary dissemination and reduce the number of yeasts that disseminate to other organs. Importantly, there was no difference between C5-sufficient and C5-deficient mice in clearance of encapsulated cryptococci inoculated via the intratracheal route.

A second approach to study the role of the complement system in vivo is administration of cobra venom factor (CVF) to experimental animals. Treatment with CVF leads to temporary depletion of C3 and C5 (Van den Berg et al., 1991). Studies of pathogenic fungi have shown increased susceptibility of CVF-treated experimental animals to disseminated cryptococcosis (Diamond et al., 1973; Graybill and Ahrens, 1981) and candidiasis (Gelfand et al., 1978).

Finally, the increasing availability of transgenic mice and mice with targeted gene disruptions offer powerful new means to study the role of the complement system in fungal infections. Although only a limited number of studies have been done, the promise of this approach has been clearly established. In one example, the acute phase production of MBL in response to systemic challenge with *C. albicans* was studied in transgenic mice bearing the human MBL gene (Tabona et al., 1995). The results showed an initial reduction in serum MBL levels that was followed by a slow recovery of MBL levels. In another example, the susceptibility of MBL-$A^{-/-}$ mice to disseminated candidiasis was examined (Lee et al., 2002). The results showed no differences in the survival rates and fungal burdens of wild-type and MBL-$A^{-/-}$ mice. This negative result should be interpreted with caution because MBL in mice is encoded by two genes, the MBL-A and the MBL-C genes, whose gene products are found in serum in comparable amounts and have similar complement activating activities (Hansen et al., 2000). Finally, as noted above, Han et al. (2001) found that antimannan IgM and IgG3 mAbs that are protective in complement-normal mice fail to protect $C3^{-/-}$ mice from a hematogenous challenge. In contrast, murine IgG1, IgG2a, and IgG2b mAbs that are reactive with the capsular polysaccharide of *C. neoformans* are protective in a murine model of disseminated cryptococcosis in $C3^{-/-}$ mice (Shapiro et al., 2002). Surprisingly, a IgG3 anticapsular mAb that was not protective in complement-normal mice was protective against intravenous challenge in $C3^{-/-}$ mice. This latter result suggests a previously unrecognized complexity for the role of the complement system in acquired immunity. The use of genetically modified mice to study the contribution of individual complement proteins to host resistance will likely increase dramatically as mice become more readily available and as new strains are generated.

6. Conclusions

Disseminated infection exposes fungi to proteins of the complement system. Every pathogenic fungus that has been studied to date has been shown to activate the complement system using a combination of the classical and alternative complement pathways. Studies of fungal infections in animals with a variety of induced or genetic complement deficiencies have shown that the complement system contributes greatly to host defense. The biological activities of the complement system that likely contribute to host defense include opsonization and generation of an inflammatory response. Serum from most normal adults contains variable and often high levels of antibodies directed against glucans and mannans found on fungal surfaces. As a consequence, incubation of fungi that display surface glucan and/or mannan, e.g., *C. albicans*, *B. dermatitidis*, or acapsular *C. neoformans*, in human serum leads to rapid activation of the classical pathway and deposition of opsonic fragments of C3 on the fungal surface. If sera lack antibodies or surface glucan or mannan is occluded, e.g., encapsulated *C. neoformans*, activation of the complement system proceeds via the alternative pathway, however, the kinetics for such alternative pathway activation are much slower than occurs via the classical pathway.

References

Ashman, R.B., Papadimitriou, J.M., Fulurija, A., Drysdale, K.E., Farah, C.S., Naidoo, O., and Gotjamanos, T. (2003). Role of complement C5 and T lymphocytes in pathogenesis of disseminated and mucosal candidiasis in susceptible DBA/2 mice. *Microb. Pathog.* 34: 103–113.

Bendel, C.M. and Hostetter, M.K. (1993). Distinct mechanisms of epithelial adhesion for *Candida albicans* and *Candida tropicalis*. Identification of the participating ligands and development of inhibitory peptides. *J. Clin. Invest.* 92: 1840–1849.

Bendel, C.M., St Sauver, J., Carlson, S., and Hostetter, M.K. (1995). Epithelial adhesion in yeast species: Correlation with surface expression of the integrin analog. *J. Infect. Dis.* 171: 1660–1663.

Bendel, C.M., Kinneberg, K.M., Jechorek, R.P., Gale, C.A., Erlandsen, S.L., Hostetter, M.K., and Wells, C.L. (1999). Systemic infection following intravenous inoculation of mice with *Candida albicans* int1 mutant strains. *Mol. Genet. Metab.* 67: 343–351.

Brown, E.J. (1985). Interaction of gram-positive microorganisms with complement. *Curr. Top. Microbiol. Immunol.* 121: 159–187.

Budzko, D.B. and Negroni, R. (1975). Hemolytic, cytotoxic and complement inactivating properties of extracts of different species of *Aspergillus*. *Mycopathologia* 57: 23–26.

Byron, J.K., Clemons, K.V., McCusker, J.H., Davis, R.W., and Stevens, D.A. (1995). Pathogenicity of *Saccharomyces cerevisiae* in complement factor five-deficient mice. *Infect. Immun.* 63: 478–485.

Chang, Y.C., Cherniak, R., Kozel, T.R., Granger, D.L., Morris, L.C., Weinhold, L.C., and Kwon-Chung, K.J. (1997). Structure and biological activities of acapsular *Cryptococcus neoformans* 602 complemented with the CAP64 gene. *Infect. Immun.* 65: 1584–1592.

Clemons, K.V., McCusker, J.H., Davis, R.W., and Stevens, D.A. (1994). Comparative pathogenesis of clinical and nonclinical isolates of *Saccharomyces cerevisiae*. *J. Infect. Dis.* 169: 859–867.

Dahl, M.V. and Carpenter, R. (1986). Polymorphonuclear leukocytes, complement, and *Trichophyton rubrum*. *J. Invest. Dermatol.* 86: 138–141.

Diamond, R.D. and Erickson, N.F. III. (1982). Chemotaxis of human neutrophils and monocytes induced by *Cryptococcus neoformans*. *Infect. Immun.* 38: 380–382.

Diamond, R.D., May, J.E., Kane, M., Frank, M.M., and Bennett, J.E. (1973). The role of late complement components and the alternate complement pathway in experimental cryptococcosis. *Proc. Soc. Exp. Biol. Med.* 144: 312–315.

Diamond, R.D., May, J.E., Kane, M.A., Frank, M.M., and Bennett, J.E. (1974). The role of the classical and alternate complement pathways in host defenses against *Cryptococcus neoformans* infection. *J. Immunol.* 112: 2260–2270.

DiCarlo, F.J. and Fiore, J.V. (1958). On the composition of zymosan. *Science* 127: 756–757.

Edwards, J.E. Jr., Gaither, T.A., O'Shea, J.J., Rotrosen, D., Lawley, T.J., Wright, S.A., Frank, M.M., and Green, I. (1986). Expression of specific binding sites on *Candida* with functional and antigenic characteristics of human complement receptors. *J. Immunol.* 137: 3577–3583.

Ehrlich, P. and Sachs, H. (1902). Ueber die vielheit der complemente des serums. *Berlin. Klin. Wochschr.* 39: 297–299.

Ferrante, A. and Thong, Y.H. (1979). Requirement of heat-labile opsonins for maximal phagocytosis of *Candida albicans*. *Sabouraudia* 17: 293–297.

Fine, D.P., Marney, S.R. Jr., Colley, D.G., Sergent, J.S., and Des Prez, R.M. (1972). C3 shunt activation in human serum chelated with EGTA. *J. Immunol.* 109: 807–809.

Fizpatrick, F.W. and DiCarlo, F.J. (1964). Zymosan. *Ann. N Y Acad. Sci.* 118: 235–261.

Gale, C., Finkel, D., Tao, N., Meinke, M., McClellan, M., Olson, J., Kendrick, K., and Hostetter, M. (1996). Cloning and expression of a gene encoding an integrin-like protein in *Candida albicans*. *Proc. Natl. Acad. Sci. USA* 93: 357–361.

Gale, C.A., Bendel, C.M., McClellan, M., Hauser, M., Becker, J.M., Berman, J., and Hostetter, M.K. (1998). Linkage of adhesion, filamentous growth, and virulence in *Candida albicans* to a single gene, *INT1*. *Science* 279: 1355–1358.

Galgiani, J.N., Isenberg, R.A., and Stevens, D.A. (1978). Chemotaxigenic activity of extracts from the mycelial and spherule phases of *Coccidioides immitis* for human polymorphonuclear leukocytes. *Infect. Immun.* 21: 862–865.

Gates, M.A., Thorkildson, P., and Kozel, T.R. (2004). Molecular architecture of the *Cryptococcus neoformans* capsule. *Mol. Microbiol.* 52: 13–24.

Gelfand, J.A., Hurley, D.L., Fauci, A.S., and Frank, M.M. (1978). Role of complement in host defense against experimental disseminated candidiasis. *J. Infect. Dis.* 138: 9–16.

Gilmore, B.J., Retsinas, E.M., Lorenz, J.S., and Hostetter, M.K. (1988). An iC3b receptor on *Candida albicans*: Structure, function, and correlates for pathogenicity. *J. Infect. Dis.* 157: 38–46.

Götze, O. and Müller-Eberhard, H.J. (1971). The C3-activator system: An alternate pathway of complement activation. *J. Exp. Med.* 134: 90s–108s.

Graybill, J.R. and Ahrens, J. (1981). Immunization and complement interaction in host defence against murine cryptococcosis. *J. Reticuloendothel. Soc.* 30: 347–357.

Han, Y., Kozel, T.R., Zhang, M.X., MacGill, R.S., Carroll, M.C., and Cutler, J.E. (2001). Complement is essential for protection by an IgM and an IgG3 monoclonal antibody against experimental hematogenously disseminated candidiasis. *J. Immunol.* 167: 1550–1557.

Hansen, S., Thiel, S., Willis, A., Holmskov, U., and Jensenius, J.C. (2000). Purification and characterization of two mannan-binding lectins from mouse serum. *J. Immunol.* 164: 2610–2618.

Hector, R.F., Yee, E., and Collins, M.S. (1990). Use of DBA/2N mice in models of systemic candidiasis and pulmonary and systemic aspergillosis. *Infect. Immun.* 58: 1476–1478.

Heidenreich, F. and Dierich, M.P. (1985). *Candida albicans* and *Candida stellatoidea*, in contrast to other *Candida* species, bind iC3b and C3d but not C3b. *Infect. Immun.* 50: 598–600.

Horstmann, R.D., Pangburn, M.K., and Müller-Eberhard, H.J. (1985). Species specificity of recognition by the alternative pathway of complement. *J. Immunol.* 134: 1101–1104.

Hostetter, M.K., Thomas, M.L., Rosen, F.S., and Tack, B.F. (1982). Binding of C3b proceeds by a transesterification reaction at the thiolester site. *Nature* 298: 72–75.

Hughes-Jones, N.C. (1986). The classical pathway. In G.D. Ross (ed.), *Immunobiology of the Complement System: An Introduction for Research and Clinical Medicine*. Academic Press, Orlando, pp. 21–44.

Joiner, K., Brown, E., Hammer, C., Warren, K., and Frank, M. (1983). Studies on the mechanism of bacterial resistance to complement-mediated killing. III. C5b-9 deposits stably on rough and type 7 *S. pneumoniae* without causing bacterial killing. *J. Immunol.* 130: 845–849.

Jones, J.M. (1980). Quantitation of antibody against cell wall mannan and a major cytoplasmic antigen of *Candida* in rabbits, mice, and humans. *Infect. Immun.* 30: 78–89.

Keller, R.G., Pfrommer, G.S.T., and Kozel, T.R. (1994). Occurrences, specificities, and functions of ubiquitous antibodies in human serum that

are reactive with the *Cryptococcus neoformans* cell wall. *Infect. Immun.* 62: 215–220.
Kozel, T.R. and Pfrommer, G.S.T. (1986). Activation of the complement system by *Cryptococcus neoformans* leads to binding of iC3b to the yeast. *Infect. Immun.* 52: 1–5.
Kozel, T.R., Brown, R.R., and Pfrommer, G.S.T. (1987). Activation and binding of C3 by *Candida albicans*. *Infect. Immun.* 55: 1890–1894.
Kozel, T.R., Wilson, M.A., Farrell, T.P., and Levitz, S.M. (1989a). Activation of C3 and binding to *Aspergillus fumigatus* conidia and hyphae. *Infect. Immun.* 57: 3412–3417.
Kozel, T.R., Wilson, M.A., Pfrommer, G.S.T., and Schlageter, A.M. (1989b). Activation and binding of opsonic fragments of C3 on encapsulated *Cryptococcus neoformans* by using an alternative complement pathway reconstituted from six isolated proteins. *Infect. Immun.* 57: 1922–1927.
Kozel, T.R., Wilson, M.A., and Murphy, J.W. (1991). Early events in initiation of alternative complement pathway activation by the capsule of *Cryptococcus neoformans*. *Infect. Immun.* 59: 3101–3110.
Kozel, T.R., Wilson, M.A., and Welch, W.H. (1992). Kinetic analysis of the amplification phase for activation and binding of C3 to encapsulated and nonencapsulated *Cryptococcus neoformans*. *Infect. Immun.* 60: 3122–3127.
Kozel, T.R., Weinhold, L.C., and Lupan, D.M. (1996). Distinct characteristics of initiation of the classical and alternative complement pathways by *Candida albicans*. *Infect. Immun.* 64: 3360–3368.
Kozel, T.R., deJong, B.C.H., Grinsell, M.M., MacGill, R.S., and Wall, K.K. (1998). Characterization of anti-capsular monoclonal antibodies that regulate activation of the complement system by the *Cryptococcus neoformans* capsule. *Infect. Immun.* 66: 1538–1546.
Kozel, T.R., Levitz, S.M., Dromer, F., Gates, M.A., Thorkildson, P., and Janbon, G. (2003). Antigenic and biological characteristics of mutant strains of *Cryptococcus neoformans* lacking capsular *O* acetylation or xylosyl side chains. *Infect. Immun.* 71: 2868–2875.
Kozel, T.R., MacGill, R.S., Percival, A., and Zhou, Q. (2004). Biological activities of naturally occurring antibodies reactive with *Candida albicans* mannan. *Infect. Immun.* 72: 209–218.
Law, S.K. and Levine, R.P. (1977). Interaction between the third complement protein and cell surface macromolecules. *Proc. Natl. Acad. Sci. USA* 74: 2701–2705.
Law, S.K., Lichtenberg, N.A., and Levine, R.P. (1979). Evidence for an ester linkage between the labile binding site of C3b and receptive surfaces. *J. Immunol.* 123: 1388–1394.
Laxalt, K.A. and Kozel, T.R. (1979). Chemotaxigenesis and activation of the alternative complement pathway by encapsulated and non-encapsulated *Cryptococcus neoformans*. *Infect. Immun.* 26: 435–440.
Lee, S.J., Gonzalez-Aseguinolaza, G., and Nussenzweig, M.C. (2002). Disseminated candidiasis and hepatic malarial infection in mannose-binding-lectin-A-deficient mice. *Mol. Cell Biol.* 22: 8199–8203.
Lehmann, P.F. and Reiss, E. (1980). Comparison by ELISA of serum anti-*Candida albicans* mannan IgG levels of a normal population and in diseased patients. *Mycopathologia* 70: 89–93.
Levitz, S.M. and Tabuni, A. (1991). Binding of *Cryptococcus neoformans* by human cultured macrophages: Requirements for multiple complement receptors and actin. *J. Clin. Invest.* 87: 528–535.
Levitz, S.M., Tabuni, A., Kozel, T.R., MacGill, R.S., Ingalls, R.R., and Golenbock, D.T. (1997). Binding of *Cryptococcus neoformans* to heterologously expressed human complement receptors. *Infect. Immun.* 65: 931–935.
Lovchik, J.A. and Lipscomb, M.F. (1993). Role of C5 and neutrophils in the pulmonary intravascular clearance of circulating *Cryptococcus neoformans*. *J. Respir. Cell Mol. Biol.* 9: 617–627.
Lu, J., Thiel, S., Wiedemann, H., Timpl, R., and Reid, K.B.M. (1990). Binding of the pentamer/hexamer forms of mannan-binding protein to zymosan activates the proenzyme $C1r_2C1s_2$ complex, of the classical pathway of complement, without involvement of C1q. *J. Immunol.* 144: 2287–2294.
Lukasser-Vogl, E., Gruber, A., Lass-Florl, C., Eder, A., Hogasen, A.K., Morgan, B.P., Dierich, M.P., and Wurzner, R. (2000). Membrane attack complex formation on yeast as trigger of selective release of terminal complement proteins from human polymorphonuclear leukocytes. *FEMS Immunol. Med. Microbiol.* 28: 15–23.
Lyon, F.L., Hector, R.F., and Domer, J.E. (1986). Innate and acquired immune responses against

Candida albicans in congenic B10.D2 mice with deficiency of the C5 complement component. *J. Med. Vet. Mycol.* 24: 359–367.

MacGill, T.C., MacGill, R.S., Casadevall, A., and Kozel, T.R. (2000). Biological correlates of capsular (quellung) reactions of *Cryptococcus neoformans*. *J. Immunol.* 164: 4835–4842.

Macher, A.M., Bennett, J.E., Gadek, J.E., and Frank, M.M. (1978). Complement depletion in cryptococcal sepsis. *J. Immunol.* 120: 1686–1690.

Meri, T., Hartmann, A., Lenk, D., Eck, R., Wurzner, R., Hellwage, J., Meri, S., and Zipfel, P.F. (2002). The yeast *Candida albicans* binds complement regulators factor H and FHL-1. *Infect. Immun.* 70: 5185–5192.

Morelli, R. and Rosenberg, L.T. (1971). Role of complement during experimental *Candida* infection in mice. *Infect. Immun.* 3: 521–523.

Morrison, R.P. and Cutler, J.E. (1981). In vitro studies of the interaction of murine phagocytic cells with *Candida albicans*. *J. Reticuloendothel. Soc.* 29: 23–34.

Neth, O., Jack, D.L., Dodds, A.W., Holzel, H., Klein, N.J., and Turner, M.W. (2000). Mannose-binding lectin binds to a range of clinically relevant microorganisms and promotes complement deposition. *Infect. Immun.* 68: 688–693.

Ohta, M., Okada, M., Yamashina, I., and Kawasaki, T. (1990). The mechanism of carbohydrate-mediated complement activation by the serum mannan-binding protein. *J. Biol. Chem.* 265: 1980–1984.

Pfrommer, G.S.T., Dickens, S.M., Wilson, M.A., Young, B.J., and Kozel, T.R. (1993). Accelerated decay of C3b to iC3b when C3b is bound to the *Cryptococcus neoformans* capsule. *Infect. Immun.* 61: 4360–4366.

Pillemer, L. and Ecker, E.E. (1941). Anticomplementary factor in fresh yeast. *J. Biol. Chem.* 137: 139–142.

Pillemer, L., Blum, L., Lepow, I.H., Ross, O.A., Todd, E.W., and Wardlaw, A.C. (1954). Properdin system and immunity: Demonstration and isolation of new serum protein, properdin, and its role in immune phenomena. *Science* 120: 279–285.

Platts-Mills, T.A.E. and Ishizaka, K. (1974). Activation of the alternative pathway of human complement by rabbit cells. *J. Immunol.* 113: 348–357.

Ray, T.L. and Wuepper, K.D. (1976). Activation of the alternative (properdin) pathway of complement by *Candida albicans* and related species. *J. Invest. Dermatol.* 67: 700–703.

Rhie, G.E., Roehrl, M.H., Mourez, M., Collier, R.J., Mekalanos, J.J., and Wang, J.Y. (2003). A dually active anthrax vaccine that confers protection against both bacilli and toxins. *Proc. Natl. Acad. Sci. USA* 100: 10925–10930.

Rhodes, J.C. (1985). Contribution of complement component C5 to the pathogenesis of experimental murine cryptococcosis. *Sabouraudia* 23: 225–234.

Sahu, A., Kozel, T.R., and Pangburn, M.K. (1994). Specificity of the thioester-containing reactive site of human C3 and its significance to complement activation. *Biochem.* J. 302: 429–436.

Shapiro, S., Beenhouwer, D.O., Feldmesser, M., Taborda, C., Carroll, M.C., Casadevall, A., and Scharff, M.D. (2002). Immunoglobulin G monoclonal antibodies to *Cryptococcus neoformans* protect mice deficient in complement component C3. *Infect. Immun.* 70: 2598–2604.

Sturtevant, J. and Latgé, J.P. (1992). Participation of complement in the phagocytosis of the conidia of *Aspergillus fumigatus* by human polymorphonuclear cells. *J. Infect. Dis.* 166: 580–586.

Summerfield, J.A., Ryder, S., Sumiya, M., Thursz, M., Gorchein, A., Monteil, M.A., and Turner, M.W. (1995). Mannose binding protein gene mutations associated with unusual and severe infections in adults. *Lancet* 345: 886–889.

Tabona, P., Mellor, A., and Summerfield, J.A. (1995). Mannose binding protein is involved in the first-line host defense: Evidence from transgenic mice. *Immunology* 85: 153–159.

Thong, Y.H. and Ferrante, A. (1978). Alternative pathway of complement activation by *Candida albicans*. *Aust. N Z J. Med.* 8: 620–622.

Triebel, T., Grillhosl, B., Kacani, L., Lell, C.P., Fuchs, A., Speth, C., Lass-Florl, C., Steinmann, J., Dierich, M.P., and Wurzner, R. (2003). Importance of the terminal complement components for immune defence against *Candida*. *Int. J. Med. Microbiol.* 292: 527–536.

Van den Berg, C.W., Aerts, P.C., and van Dijk, H. (1991). In vivo anti-complementary activities of the cobra venom factors from *Naja naja* and *Naja haje*. *J. Immunol. Meth.* 136: 287–294.

von Dungern, E. (1900). Beitrage zur immunitatslehre. *Munchener Med. Wochenschr.* 47: 677–680.

Wilson, M.A. and Kozel, T.R. (1992). Contribution of antibody in normal human serum to early deposition of C3 onto encapsulated and nonencapsulated *Cryptococcus neoformans*. *Infect. Immun.* 60: 754–761.

Wilson, B.D. and Sohnle, P.G. (1988). Neutrophil accumulation and cutaneous responses in experimental cutaneous candidiasis of genetically complement-deficiency mice. *Clin. Immunol. Immunopathol.* 46: 284–293.

Young, B.J. and Kozel, T.R. (1993). Effects of strain variation, serotype and structural modification on the kinetics for activation and binding of C3 to *Cryptococcus neoformans*. *Infect. Immun.* 61: 2966–2972.

Zaragoza, O., Taborda, C.P., and Casadevall, A. (2004). The efficacy of complement-mediated phagocytosis of *Cryptococcus neoformans* is dependent on the location of C3 in the polysaccharide capsule and involves both direct and indirect C3-mediated interactions. *Eur. J. Immunol.* 33: 1957–1967.

Zhang, M.X. and Klein, B. (1997). Activation, binding, and processing of complement component 3 (C3) by *Blastomyces dermatitidis*. *Infect. Immun.* 65: 1849–1855.

Zhang, M.X. and Kozel, T.R. (1998). Mannan-specific immunoglobulin G antibodies in normal human serum accelerate binding of C3 to *Candida albicans* via the alternative complement pathway. *Infect. Immun.* 66: 4845–4850.

Zhang, M.X., Lupan, D.M., and Kozel, T.R. (1997). Mannan-specific IgG antibodies in normal human serum mediate classical pathway initiation of C3 binding to *Candida albicans*. *Infect. Immun.* 65: 3822–3827.

Zhang, M.X., Brandhorst, T.T., Kozel, T.R., and Klein, B.S. (2001). Role of glucan and surface protein BAD1 in complement activation by *Blastomyces dermatitidis* yeast. *Infect. Immun.* 69: 7559–7564.

19

Innate and Adaptive Immunity to Systemic *Candida albicans* Infection

Luigina Romani

1. Introduction

Candida albicans is associated with a wide spectrum of diseases in humans, including systemic forms of infection that may arise as localized primary diseases of deep organs or as hematogenously disseminated infection (Calderone, 2002). Candidal infections are a significant clinical problem for a variety of immunocompetent and immunocompromised patients (Calderone, 2002). *Candida* spp. now rank fourth on the list of microbes

Microbiology, Department of Experimental Medicine and Biochemical Science, University of Perugia, Perugia, Italy.

most frequently isolated from blood cultures (Jarvis, 1995) and mortality rates from systemic candidiasis can be as high as 50%. Not only are bloodstream infections with *C. albicans* and non-*C. albicans* spp. occurring more frequently, but the relative proportion of these infections due to non-*C. albicans* spp. is increasing, including species such as *C. glabrata*, *C. tropicalis*, *C. parapsilosis*, *C. krusei*, and *C. lusitaniae*. Common risk factors for bloodstream candidiasis include extremes of age (low-birth-weight infants and the elderly), immunosuppression, malignancy with leucopenia, major abdominal surgery, or trauma, as well as exposure to multiple antibacterial agents, central venous catheterization, prolonged length of stay in intensive care units, and parenteral nutrition (Jarvis, 1995).

Since early diagnosis of invasive infection is difficult, strategies for prevention would seem to be more attractive. Antifungal prophylaxis has been effective in reducing *Candida* infection in neutropenic patients with hematologic malignancies, however, there has been no proven benefit regarding the reduction in the overall mortality (Bohme et al., 1999). The beneficial effect of immunomodulators in clinical and preclinical models of the infection (Kullberg et al., 1994; Kullberg and Anaissie, 1998; Rodriguez-Adrian et al., 1998) suggests that maneuvers aimed at restoring the host defective antifungal immune responsiveness can be exploited in adjunctive antifungal therapies (Georgopapadakou and Walsh, 1996; Rodriguez-Adrian et al., 1998; Stevens et al., 1998; Stevens, 1998; Polonelli and Cassone, 1999). Therefore, understanding the components of this host response at a basic level is likely to lead to a better understanding of the pathogenesis of *C. albicans* infections and diseases in humans and result in optimization of preventive and therapeutic antifungal strategies. This chapter will focus on innate and adaptive immune reactivities to systemic *C. albicans* infection with particular attention given to innate immunity and its role in protection against infection, directing the adaptive immune response, and serving as an immunotherapeutic tool.

2. *Candida albicans:* A Unique Fungus

The complexity of interactions between *C. albicans* and its human host suggests that this fungus has numerous mechanisms to adapt to a diversity of host sites and also, in many cases, to occupy the host without causing overt disease. A crucial feature of this microorganism is its versatility that goes beyond its duality, as a pathogen as well as a commensal, to include the ability to survive and infect several anatomically distinct sites, each with its own specific set of environmental pressures (Calderone, 2002). *C. albicans* grows vegetatively in a variety of morphogenic forms, as it can exist as simple budding yeast or undergo morphogenesis and produce filaments in the form of pseudohyphae and/or hyphae. It is suggested that the mechanisms for rapid adaptation lie in the developmental programs of yeast-to-hypha transition and the high frequency of phenotypic switching (Nantel et al., 2002; Soll, 2002). Although morphological flexibility could be a key contributor to fungal virulence, neither molecular data unambiguously establish a role for fungal morphogenesis as a virulence factor for *Candida albicans*, nor can specific forms of *Candida* be regarded as absolutely indicative of saprophytism or infection at a given site. Mutant strains of *C. albicans* incapable of hyphal formation are, in general, avirulent in mouse models of disseminated candidiasis (Romani et al., 2003). However, decreased infectivity without changes in hyphal formation is also observed, and strains that are unable to grow in the yeast form were also less virulent (Romani et al., 2003). Therefore, defects other than the inability to form hyphae could be responsible for the reduced virulence of the mutant strains. In phenotypic switching, the white-to-opaque switch is a critical step in the mating process (Miller and Johnson, 2002), yet the inherent virulence of each phenotype is still controversial. Moreover, the fungus uses a common set of conserved pathways to regulate dimorphism, phenotypic switching, and virulence (Nantel et al., 2002) in addition to mating (Miller and Johnson, 2002) and metabolism (Lan et al., 2002). Therefore, as virulence genes are co-regulated with cell morphogenesis, the ability to switch from yeast to hyphal growth in response to various environmental signals is considered to be inherent to *Candida* virulence, but proof that links morphogenesis to virulence is still lacking and the issue remains controversial (Gow et al., 2002; Rooney and Klein, 2002; Romani et al., 2002).

The fact that commensals show infectivity only in patients with a variety of immunological defects indicates that a high degree of coexistence has evolved between *C. albicans* and its mammalian hosts which deviates into overt disease only under certain circumstances. The need for *C. albicans* is a stable host–parasite interaction that is achieved upon the implicit agreement that the elicited immune response be strong enough to allow host survival without pathogen elimination and to establish commensalism without excessive proinflammatory pathology. Therefore, the balance of proinflammatory and anti inflammatory signaling is a prerequisite for successful host–fungus interaction. In light of these considerations, although developments in fungal genomics may provide new insights into mechanisms of pathogenicity (Lorenz and Fink, 2001), the responsibility for virulence, regardless of the mode of its generation and maintenance, is shared by the host and the fungus at the pathogen–host interface. Studies with *C. albicans* have provided a paradigm that incorporates contributions from both the fungus and the host to explain the theme of the origin and maintenance of virulence for commensals (Romani et al., 2002). Through a high degree of flexibility, the model accommodates the concept of virulence as an important component of fungus fitness in vivo (that is, the reduction of host survival—that equals virulence—regarded as an unavoidable consequence of parasite adaptation and reproduction within the host) within the plasticity of the host immune system. Transition to the different fungal morphotypes is perceived by the host immune system in a morphotype-specific fashion (Gow et al., 2002; Rooney and Klein, 2002; Romani et al., 2002; Geiger et al., 2004). Dendritic cells (DCs) sense changes in the microorganism and determine the full range of host's immune relationships with *Candida*, from commensalism to infection. The exploitation of distinct recognition receptors on DCs is causally linked to fungal virulence (Romani et al., 2002, 2004). This may explain the interdependency of immunological reactivity and fungal infectivity, the relative importance of each single factor being dependent on the fungus and type of the infection.

3. Immunity to *C. albicans*

Host defense mechanisms against *C. albicans* are numerous and range from relatively primitive and constitutively expressed, nonspecific defenses to sophisticated adaptive mechanisms that are specifically induced during infection (Calderone, 2002). In the past decade, a dramatic shift has occurred in our mechanistic understanding of immunity to *C. albicans*. Precisely, the appreciation that activation of the innate immune system initiates, amplifies, and drives antigen-specific immune responses together with the identification of discrete cell types, specific receptors, and the signaling pathways involved in the activation of innate immunity has provided a multitude of new targets for exploitation by the developments of adjuvants for vaccines (Romani, 2003,

2004). Traditionally considered only as a first line of defense, the innate immunity has recently received considerable attention because this form of immunity effectively distinguishes self from nonself and activates the adaptive immune systems by provision of specific signals (Fearon and Locksley, 1996; Medzhitov and Janeway, 1997). Innate defense strategies are designed to detect broad and conserved patterns, which differ between pathogenic organisms and their multicellular hosts. This nonantigen-specific detection strategy is mediated by diverse and evolutionarily conserved families of pattern recognition receptors (PRRs) and Toll-like receptors (TLRs) that recognize and are triggered by evolutionarily conserved molecules essential to pathogen function (PAMPs, pathogen-associated molecular patterns) (Akira, 2003). By discriminating between different pathogens, and by contributing to discrimination between self and pathogens at the level of the adaptive T helper (Th) immunity, the innate immune system fulfills two important goals of the primary immune response: speed and specificity.

Candida spp. are detected and destroyed within hours by innate defense mechanisms (Cotter et al., 2000). For *C. albicans*, however, the state of commensalism with its vertebrate host is associated with the detection of underlying acquired immunity to the fungus, such as the occurrence of positive delayed-type hypersensitivity (DTH) reactivity and antigen-specific lymphoproliferation (Fidel and Sobel, 1994; Puccetti et al., 1995). The recognition of the fungus at sites of infection leads to the production of chemokines and cytokines that not only activate the innate cell population but also drive the adaptive immune response down different pathways of differentiation. Therefore, cytokines and other mediators play an essential role in the process and, indeed, may ultimately determine the type of effector response that is generated towards the fungus. As the different Th cell subsets are endowed with the ability to release a distinct panel of cytokines, capable of delivering activating and deactivating in feedback signals to effector phagocytes, the activation of an appropriate Th subset may be instrumental in the generation of a successful immune response to the fungus (Romani, 1999). To limit the pathologic consequences of an excessive inflammatory cell-mediated immune reactions, the immune system resorts to a number of protective mechanisms, including the reciprocal cross-regulatory effects of Th1- and Th2-type effector cytokines, such as interferon (IFN)-γ and interleukin (IL)-4, and the generation of regulatory T cells (Treg) (Montagnoli et al., 2002). Thus, despite a degree of redundancy of the anticandidal immune responses with respect to protection, innate and adaptive immune responses are intimately linked and controlled by sets of molecules and receptors that act to generate the most effective form of immunity for protection (Fig. 19.1).

As emphasized throughout this chapter, it has became apparent that understanding how immune responses are activated will enable the development of vaccine strategies that are effective at maintaining or eliciting acquired protective immunity to *C. albicans* in conditions of immunosuppression. The model has brought DCs to center stage as promising targets for intervention for immunotherapy and vaccine development (Steinman and Pope, 2002) and has shifted the emphasis from the "antigen" towards the "adjuvant" that best stimulates the appropriate type of response in immunosuppressed hosts.

4. The Innate Immune System

The constitutive innate mechanisms include the barrier functions of the body surfaces and mucosal epithelial of the respiratory, gastrointestinal, and genito-urinary tracts. *Candida* spp. possess a variety of complementary structures through which they adhere to cell surfaces and extracellular

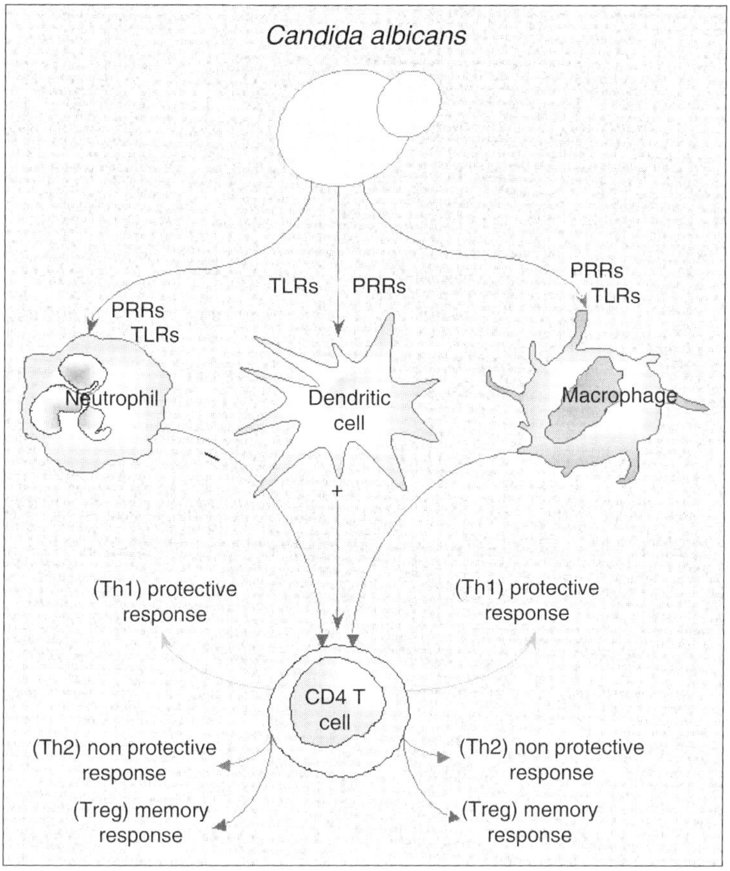

Figure 19.1. The immune response to *Candida albicans*, involving the "cross-talk" among many immune cells, including dendritic cells, macrophages, neutrophils, and CD4$^+$ T cells. Cells of the innate immune system discriminate between different forms of the fungus and produce sets of chemokines, cytokines, and costimulatory molecules through which signals to the adaptive T helper (Th) immune system. Protective and nonprotective Th cells release a distinct panel of cytokines, capable of delivering activating and inhibitory feedback signals to effector phagocytes. Together, the innate and adaptive immune systems contribute to the inflammatory response. Counter-regulatory T cells (Treg) may serve to dampen the excessive inflammatory reactions and to contribute to the development of memory antifungal immunity. (+) and (–) refer to positive and negative signals, respectively.

matrix (Calderone, 1994). When hematogenous dissemination to visceral organs is an important step in the pathogenesis of the infection, adherence and penetration to the endothelial lining of blood vessels to invade the deep tissues may occur (Sanchez et al., 2004) through a process that is actively induced by the fungus (Belanger et al., 2002). The susceptibility and outcome of invasive candidiasis also depends on serum level of iron, lipoproteins (Wanten et al., 2002), and may involve platelets (Romani, 2002).

The innate antifungal defense mechanisms against systemic *C. albicans* infection are built upon effector mechanisms mediated by cells, cellular receptors, and a number of humoral factors. The professional phagocytes consisting of polymorphonuclear leukocytes (PMNs, also known as neutrophils) play an essential role. The observation that invasive candidiasis occurs in concomitance with defects in neutrophil number and functions (Bodey et al., 1966), together with the detection of cells and mediators of the innate immune system with antifungal effector activities (Ashman, 1998), has led to one central dogma of resistance to candidiasis, i.e., that resistance to invasive candidiasis is mediated by the innate immune system. However, the antigen-independent recognition of the fungus by the innate immune system leads to the immediate mobilization of immune effector and regulatory mechanisms that provide the host with three crucial survival advantages: establishment of a first line of defense, which holds the pathogen in check during the maturation of the adaptive response; rapid initiation of the immune response (both innate and adaptive) and creation of the inflammatory and co-stimulatory context for antigen recognition; and steering of the adaptive response towards the cellular or humoral elements that are most appropriate for protection against the specific pathogen. Therefore, while the effectiveness of the innate system is undoubtedly acknowledged, it is now clear that optimal antifungal immune resistance results from the combined and interdependent effort of innate and adaptive immune mechanisms and that this can be achieved by targeting and manipulating cells and pathways of the innate immune system.

4.1. The Discrimination: The PAMP/TLR Recognition System

Toll was originally defined as a *Drosophila* gene important for ontogenesis and antimicrobial resistance. The sequence similarity of the cytoplasmic portion of *Drosophila* Toll and mammalian IL-1 receptor (IL-1R) intracellular domains suggested similarities in Toll and IL-1R signaling and illustrated the evolutionary conservation of both cell signaling systems (Hoffmann and Reichhart, 2002). A further piece of evidence comes from studies with *Galleria mellonella*, an insect capable of sensing the pathogenicity of *Candida* spp. in a manner similar to mammals (Cotter et al., 2000). TLRs are type I transmembrane proteins that are grouped into the same gene family based on their sequence similarity. Ten mammalian TLRs have been described so far, and TLR ligands include PAMPs and other ligands. Several putative endogenous TLR ligands, including members of the heat shock proteins (HSPs), have also been described. Evidence suggests that stimulation of TLRs by endogenous ligands could result in the maturation of DCs presenting host peptides and priming for autoimmunity (Millar et al., 2003). In contrast, the ability of PAMPs to induce costimulatory molecule expression on DCs suggests a permissive role of the PAMP/TLR system in the activation of T lymphocytes during antigen presentation. All TLRs activate a core set of stereotyped responses, including inflammation. However, individual TLRs can also induce specific programs in cells of the innate immune system that are tailored for a particular pathogen. TLRs and IL-1R share a similar signaling cascade, culminating in the activation of nuclear factor κB (NF-κB) and mitogen-activated protein kinases that activate the transcription of the inflammatory and adaptive immune responses. The common signal pathways utilized by IL-1R and TLRs involve the recruitment of the adapter protein MyD88 (*Drosophila* myeloid differentiation primary response gene 88) through the homophilic interaction of the TIR domain. MyD88, in turn, activates a series of IL-1R-associated kinases that are crucially involved in innate immunity, and signal is propagated via a specific member of the TNF receptor-associated factor family. However, in the case of TLR3- and TLR4-dependent lipopolysaccharide signaling, other proteins may also serve as adapter molecules with, or in place of, MyD88 (Yamamoto et al., 2003). It is recognized that the intricacies of how TLRs signal will ultimately provide an explanation for the molecular basis of how cells involved in innate immunity dictate the processes of host defense specific to the provoking pathogen (O'Neill et al., 2003). A number of cell wall components of *C. albicans* may act as PAMPs (Roeder et al., 2004) (Fig. 19.2). TLR2 signaling leads to the prevalent

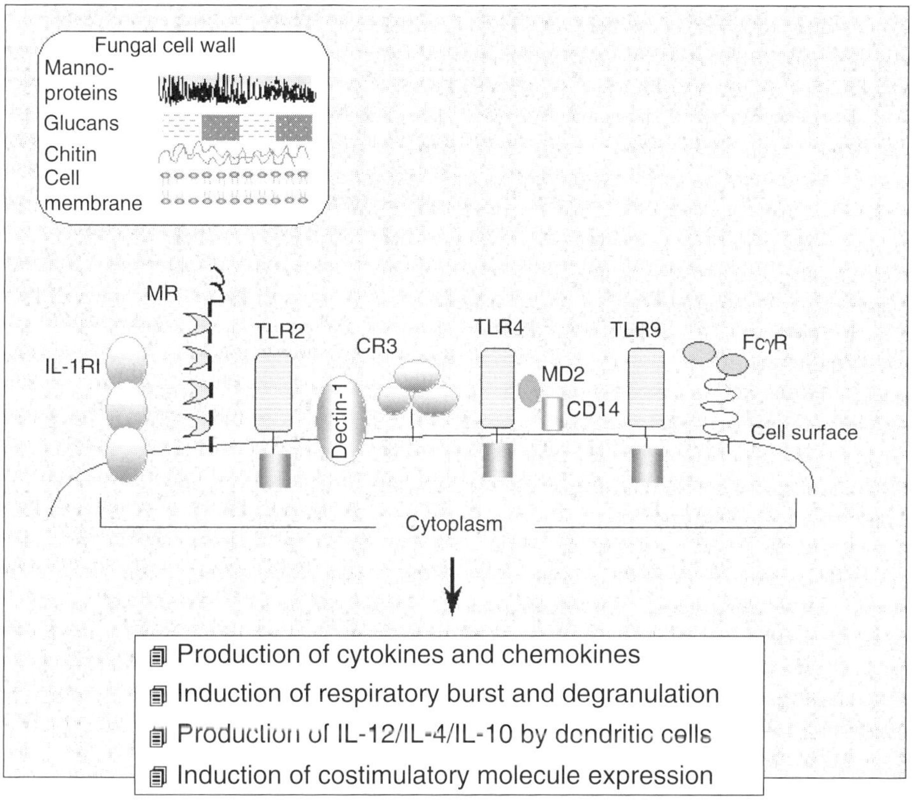

Figure 19.2. Pattern recognition receptors as activators of innate and adaptive immunity to fungi. Recognition of *Candida albicans* and fungal PAMPs, mainly associated with fungal cell wall (top left schematic icon) by Toll-like receptors (TLRs), mannose receptor (MR), complement receptor (CR3), and receptors for Fc (FcγR) leads to activation of specialized antifungal effector functions in neutrophils, such as respiratory burst and degranulation, and production of IL-12 p70 by dendritic cells (see text). As dendritic cells are equipped with pattern recognition receptors and TLRs, they are uniquely able at decoding the fungus-associated information and translating it in qualitatively different adaptive Th-immune responses. The engagement of distinct receptors by yeasts and hyphae translates into downstream signaling events, ultimately regulating costimulation, cytokine production, and development of Th and regulatory T cells. The functional plasticity of DCs at the pathogen–immune system interface may offer new interpretative clues to fungal virulence.

production of inflammatory (TNF-α and IL-1β) cytokines, although IL-10 is also produced occasionally (Netea et al., 2002b; Brown et al., 2003; Gantner et al., 2003; Jouault et al., 2003; Villamon et al., 2004). Signaling through TLR2 by zymosan occurs in collaboration with the β-glucan receptor Dectin-1 (Gantner et al., 2003), a finding that suggests the occurrence of collaborative recognition of distinct microbial components by different classes of innate immune receptors. TLR4 and CD14 also mediate the recognition of *C. albicans*-derived mannan (Tada et al., 2002). Although TNF-α and IL-1β production in response to *Candida* may also occur in a TLR4-independent manner, resistance to the systemic infection is decreased in TLR4-deficient mice along with the release of chemokines (Netea et al., 2002b). Therefore, TLR2 and TLR4 are both implicated in the elicitation of host defense to the fungus in the systemic compartment, a finding exemplifying the recruitment of different TLRs by one microbial species. The MyD88-dependent pathway is essential for the innate and acquired Th1-mediated resistance to the disseminated infection with the fungus. However, the contribution of individual TLRs may vary depending on fungal morphotypes. For instance, signaling by *C. albicans* essentially occurs through IL-1R, TLR2, and TLR4, each being implicated in different ways in the control of the disseminated infection with yeasts or hyphae (Bellocchio et al., 2004). Individual TLRs also activate specialized antifungal effector functions on neutrophils that correlate with susceptibility to the systemic infection. TLR expression on PMNs exposed to *C. albicans* is induced in a morphotype-specific manner. Although not affecting phagocytosis, TLRs affect specific antifungal programs of PMNs, such as respiratory burst and degranulation. TLR2 and TLR9 ligation by *Candida* yeasts preferentially activates the respiratory burst, while TLR4 engagement induces degranulation along with a more efficient fungal killing (Marr et al., 2003; Bellocchio et al., 2004). This finding is consistent with the ability of lipopolysaccharide (LPS) to restore anticandidal activity of PMNs from immunosuppressed mice (Yamamoto et al., 1993). As the quantity and specificity of delivery of toxic neutrophil products ultimately determine the relative efficiency of fungicidal activity versus inflammatory cytotoxicity to host cells, this implicates that TLRs may govern protection and immunopathology at the level of the innate immune response. The emerging picture calls for: (i) an essential requirement for the IL-1R1/MyD88-dependent pathway in the innate and Th1-mediated resistance to *C. albicans*; (ii) the occurrence of TLR signaling in a morphotype-specific manner, although the simultaneous engagement of multiple TLRs, as well as TLR cooperativity in vivo, make it difficult to gauge the relative contributions of individual fungal morphotypes in TLR activation and functioning, and (iii) the ability of individual TLRs to activate specialized antifungal effector functions in PMNs and DCs.

4.2. The Instructive Role: Chemokines and Cytokines

The instructive role of the innate immune system may be operative at the levels of expression of costimulatory molecules (Romani, 2003) and chemokine and cytokine production. Upon contact with *C. albicans*, cells of the innate immune system release a battery of chemokines (Herring and Huffnagle, 2001; Geiger et al., 2004) and cytokines that have profound effects on the functional activity of the innate response and on subsequent events. The local release of these effector molecules serve to regulate cell trafficking of various types of leukocytes, thus initiating the inflammatory response, to activate phagocytic cells to a microbicidal state and to direct Th cell development.

The inflammatory response to the fungus may serve to limit the infection but may also contribute to pathogenicity, as witnessed by the occurrence of severe fungal infection in patients with the immunorestitution disease (Cheng et al., 2000). These patients may experience intractable fungal infections despite the presence of innate and adaptive immune responses. Recovery from infection may not only depend on fungal growth restriction but also on resolution of inflammatory pathology. This imposes a new job to the immune system. In addition to efficient control of pathogens, tight regulatory mechanisms are required in order to balance protective immunity and immunopathology. In experimental systemic candidiasis, the course and outcome of the infection in different strains of mice correlate with fungal load but also with immunopathology (Ashman, 1998). To limit the pathologic consequences of excessive inflammatory cell-mediated immune reactions, the immune system resorts to a number of protective mechanisms, including the reciprocal cross-regulatory effects of Th1- and Th2-type effector cytokines, such as IFN-γ and IL-4, the generation of Treg and secretion of anti-inflammatory cytokines that are key for maintaining a healthy balance between protection and immunopathology. Thus, innate and adaptive immune responses are intimately linked and controlled by sets of molecules and receptors that act to generate the most effective form of immunity for protection against fungal pathogens (Romani, 2004).

One of the most important cytokines produced in the course of the infection is IL-10. IL-10 is readily produced by PMNs, macrophages, DCs, and Treg in response to the fungus and plays a crucial role in determining susceptibility to the infection in mice (Romani, 2003). High levels of IL-10 are also detected in patients with hepatosplenic candidiasis (Roilides et al., 1998). IL-10 acts as one major cytokine discriminating between virulent and less virulent forms of the fungus, impairs the antifungal effector functions of phagocytes, including secretion of inflammatory cytokines and IL-12, and the development of protective cell-mediated immunity (Romani, 2003). Circumstantial evidence suggests that IL-10 produced by cells of the innate immune system is responsible for prevention of an excessive activation of innate effector functions, whereas IL-10 secreted by Treg is mainly responsible for the establishment of commensalism (Romani, 2004). Similar to IL-10, transforming growth factor (TGF)-β is produced in invasive candidiasis (Letterio et al., 2001) and acts by inhibiting antifungal effector functions of phagocytes but also the excessive, Th1-dependent, inflammatory pathology (Montagnoli et al., 2002). Thus, like IL-10, TGF-β is a double-edged sword in the fight against the fungus. In addition to IL-10, IL-4 may act as one major discriminative factor of susceptibility and resistance in disseminated candidiasis (Romani, 1999). Ablation of IL-4 renders susceptible mice resistant to systemic candidiasis. IL-4 may both deactivate and activate phagocytes and DCs for certain specialized function. For instance, it may inhibit the antifungal effector activities of phagocytes yet may promote IL-12 production by DCs. Thus, the most important mechanism underlying the inhibitory activity of IL-4 in infection relies on its ability to promote Th2 reactivity, thus dampening protective Th1 responses. However, susceptibility to candidal infections may not always be associated with an overt production of IL-4. For instance, although an association between chronic disseminated candidiasis and genetic variants of IL-4 has been recently described (Choi et al., 2003), IL-4 or IL-5 is not always increased in patients with chronic mucocutaneous candidiasis (CMC), despite defective type 1 cytokine production (Lilic, 2002; Lilic et al., 2003).

Proinflammatory cytokines that are inhibited by IL-10 and are important to control the fungus are tumor necrosis factor (TNF)-α, IL-1β, IL-6, and IL-12, all of which are produced in response to the fungus (Romani,

2003). In addition to regulating the recruitment of inflammatory cells and triggering the respiratory burst, these cytokines are implicated, directly or indirectly, in the activation of protective Th1 responses to the fungus and in the occurrence of fungal-associated diseases (Romani, 2003). Blocking the biological activities of IL-18, IL-12, and IL-1β in patients may result in increased susceptibility to disseminated fungal infections (Netea et al., 2002a).

One of the more consistent dysregulation observed in response to the fungus is its ability to subvert the production of IL-12, which—as the main physiological inducer of IFN-γ and Th1 cell differentiation—is an essential cytokine for the development of acquired resistance to fungi (Romani, 2004). IL-12 production by PMNs, monocytes and, importantly DCs, occurs in a morphotype-dependent manner, probably through the exploitation of different recognition receptors and is inversely correlated with fungal virulence (Chiani et al., 2000; Liu et al., 2001). IL-18 may have a supporting role in the IL-12-dependent Th1 resistance to the systemic infection with the fungus (Mencacci et al., 2000; Stuyt et al., 2002, Netea et al., 2003).

IFN-γ is a key cytokine in the innate control of the infection in mice and humans (Romani, 2004). Defective IFN-γ production is associated with reduced resistance to candidiasis in humans (Lilic et al., 2003). A recent study suggests that deficient IFN-γ-receptor signaling may occur in neonatal macrophages (Marodi, 2002). It is produced by T and NK cells in response to both IL-12 and IL-18 released by cells of the innate immune system exposed to the fungus. IFN-γ, in turn, stimulates migration, phagocytosis, and oxidative killing of PMNs and favors the occurrence of Th1 reactivity. Experimental evidence indicates that IFN-γ may not work in a Th2 setting, a finding suggesting a degree of caution in evaluating patterns of IFN-γ production in human settings (Romani, 2002).

4.3. The Effector Activity

4.3.1. The Phagocytes

The antifungal effector functions of phagocytes include mechanisms of killing and growth inhibition of the fungus as well as pathways to oppose fungal infectivity, including effects on dimorphism and phenotypic switching (Romani, 2002; Mansour and Levitz, 2002). The restriction of fungal growth occurs by both oxygen-dependent and -independent mechanisms, the latter consisting of intracellular or extracellular release of effector molecules, defensins, neutrophil cationic peptides, and iron sequestration. Although phagocytes express intrinsic antifungal activity, in general, this activity could be increased by opsonins and T cell-derived cytokines, a finding implicating that the innate and adaptive immune systems do not work independently but are reciprocally regulated. Moreover, initiation of the oxidative metabolic burst and hydrogen peroxide production by neutrophils in response to opsonized or unopsonized forms of the fungus occurs through different modalities and involve different intracellular events (Romani, 2002; Mansour and Levitz, 2002). This means that if different events mediate phagocyte activation by opsonized and unopsonized fungal elements, candidacidal activity in vivo may vary under divergent conditions with specific localized sites of infection. As colony-stimulating factors, IFN-γ and TNF-α have disparate effect on the fungicidal activity of neutrophils. The candidacidal activity in vivo also reflects the local cytokine microenvironment (Romani, 2002; Mansour and Levitz, 2002). Enzymes such as the nicotinamide adenine dinucleotide phosphate (NADPH) oxidase and inducible nitric oxide (NO) synthase initiate the oxidative pathways known as respiratory burst. The respiratory burst produces toxic reactive oxygen intermediates and nitrogen oxidases the nature of which varies depending on the type of phagocytic cells. In retaliation, *Candida* has evolved strategies to selectively inhibit the respiratory burst (Hamilton and Holdon, 1999) or to adapt to oxidative stress (Chaunhan et al., 2003). The activation of NADPH-oxidase can be elicited by microbial products (such as LPS), by IFN-γ, IL-8, or by IgG-binding to FcR. The primary product of the reaction catalyzed by the NADPH-oxidase is superoxide (O_2^-), which can be converted to H_2O_2 by superoxide dismutase, to hydroxyl radicals (•OH) and hydroxyl anions (OH^-) by the iron-catalyzed Haber–Weiss reactions or, after dismutation to H_2O_2, to hypochlorous acid (HOCl) and chloramines either by myeloperoxidase-dependent or -independent mechanisms. Myeloperoxidase, a lysosomal hemoprotein found in azurophilic granules of neutrophils and monocytes, but not macrophages, is also a mediator in the oxygen-dependent killing. Not surprisingly, therefore, myeloperoxidase deficiency predisposes to pulmonary candidiasis, although it is unable to play a role in host defense in the absence of the NADPH oxidase (Aratani et al., 2002).

Additional toxic molecules produced by phagocytes are the reactive nitrogen intermediates. Different NO synthases convert the amino acid L-arginine and molecular oxygen to L-citrulline and NO (Bogdan et al., 2000). It is remarkable that the NO synthase of macrophages is stimulated by LPS and oppositely regulated by Th1 and Th2 cytokines (it is induced by IFN-γ and TNF-α and inhibited by IL-4, IL-10, IL-13, and TGF-β) (Raveh et al., 1998). Production but also inhibition of NO occurs in response to the fungus (Schroppel et al., 2001). The pleiotropic activity of NO, which may include a direct activity on fungal growth and on transition through different forms as well as a negative immunomodulatory activity, precludes a general conclusion on the significance of NO production in candidiasis, although a positive correlation has been found between NO production and inhibition of fungal growth (Jones-Carson et al., 1995).

PMNs are the most represented phagocyte population and generally the earliest to be recruited at sites of infection. Not surprisingly, therefore, quantitative (Bodey et al., 1966) or qualitative (Walsh et al., 1994) defects of PMNs are major predisposing factors to disseminated candidiasis. In general, their killing efficiency against *C. albicans* is relatively low, unless PMNs have been activated previously with activating cytokines. For instance, although phagocytosis and killing of blastospores by PMNs are superior to that of germ tubes and longer hyphae, only a fraction of engulfed *Candida* yeasts are digested (Marquis et al., 1991). Factors found to limit the intracellular killing of *C. albicans* by PMNs include, among others, the ability of some ingested cells to produce germ tube, a defective sealing of phagolysosomes, inhibition of PMN degranulation by fungal products, defective opsonization, and entry through a mannose-inhibitable receptor (Marquis, et al., 1991). However, the functions of PMNs may well go beyond microbicidal activity to include an immunoregulatory action on Th lymphocytes. Accumulating evidence indicates that cells of the myeloid lineage are capable of positive and negative regulation of T cell function (Bronte et al., 2003). Myeloid suppressor cells are responsible for the immunosuppression observed in pathologies as dissimilar as tumor growth, immunosuppression, overwhelming infections, graft vs. host disease, and pregnancy. A population of neutrophils suppressing Th1 cell activation is present in bone marrow-transplanted mice with systemic candidiasis (Mencacci et al., 2002), a finding suggesting that myeloid suppressor cells may prevent functional immunoreconstitution in transplantation. The reciprocal influence between PMNs and T lymphocytes further implies that the immune resistance to the fungus is a highly coordinate and unitary process, in the context of which the traditional dichotomy between neutropenia and T cell-specific defects may become inadequate. Further studies in mice have shown the ability of fungal cells to subvert neutrophil programs in a morphotype-dependent manner (Romani, 2002; Torosantucci et al., 2002; Mullick et al., 2004).

Macrophages may also play a role in the pathology of disseminated candidiasis (Vasquez-Torres and Balish, 1997). The extent to which these cells contribute to *Candida* pathogenicity is yet to be elucidated, although it is clear that they may favor survival and virulence of the fungus (Kapostza et al., 1999; Lorenz and Fink, 2001) also through altruistic suicidal apoptosis (Ibata-Ombetta et al., 2003).

4.3.2. The Receptors

Phagocytes bind and recognize opsonized and unopsonized *C. albicans* through a variety of receptors, including the receptors for different complement breakdown products (CR), Fc portion of immunoglobulins (FcR), mannosyl/fucosyl glycoconjugate ligands (MR), β-glucan (CR3 and Dectin-1), and TLRs (McKnight and Gordon, 2000). Both processes may occur in the absence of serum opsonins, but opsonins are required for optimal activation of the intracellular killing machinery. Each receptor on phagocytes not only mediates distinct downstream intracellular events related to clearance, but also participates in complex and disparate functions related to immunomodulation and activation of immunity, depending on cell types. The different receptors are called upon to serve early-warning systems and, not surprisingly, their ability to activate, in isolation, various effector functions is limited. Internalization via constitutively competent MR does not represent indeed an effective way of clearing of the fungus in the absence of opsonins. Unopsonized *C. albicans* yeasts can be internalized through the macrophage MR via a peroxisome proliferator activator receptor-gamma signaling (Coste et al., 2003), however, the highest killing activity is observed against opsonized yeasts. Actually, the enhancement of phagocytosis and killing of *C. albicans* by macrophages correlated with a decreased number of MR. The MR-mediated uptake of unopsonized *Candida* yeasts may lead to phagocyte abuse if not accompanied by the coordinate activation of the cell cytotoxic machinery (Marodi et al., 1993). Increased expression of the receptor with no induced cytotoxicity is induced upon exposure of macrophages to IL-4. In contrast, IFN-γ downregulates the expression of macrophage MR and nevertheless results in effective killing, presumably via increased coupling of the receptor to cytotoxic functions (Marodi et al., 1993). Thus, cooperation between Th1 and Th2 cytokines may be required for optimal stimulation of MR-mediated phagocytosis (Raveh et al., 1998). However, MR on DCs activates specific programs that are relevant for the development of antifungal immune responses (see below). CR3 (also known as CD11b/CD18) engagement is one most efficient uptake of opsonized and unopsonized *C. albicans* (Han et al., 2001) but it has the remarkable characteristic of a broad capacity for the recognition of diverse fungal ligands, such as iC3b, β-glucan, and zymosan. Stimulation of CR3-dependent phagocytosis or degranulation requires the simultaneous ligation of two distinct sites within CR3, one specific for iC3b and a second site specific for the fungal cell wall β-glucan. The multiplicity of binding sites and the existence of different activation states enables CR3 of disparate (both positive and negative) effector activities against the fungus (McKnight and Gordon, 2000). For instance, CR3-mediated phagocytosis of both serum-opsonized and unopsonized yeasts is the most efficient uptake by macrophages, a process inhibitable by cell wall components of the fungus. However, interaction with macrophage CR3 leads to suppression of the immune response to the microorganism. Thus, because signaling through CR3 may not lead to phagocyte activation without the concomitant engagement of FcR (van Spriel et al., 2001), the use of this receptor may contribute to the intracellular fungal parasitism. It is of interest, indeed, that *Candida* exploits entry through CR3 to survive inside DCs (Romani et al., 2002). In contrast, ligation of FcR, presumably FcγRI or FcαRI (van Spriel et al., 1999), is usually sufficient to trigger phagocytosis, a vigorous oxidative burst and generation of proinflammatory signals. Ultimately, recognition of antibody-opsonized particles represents a high-level threat. It is of interest that FcR-mediated phagocytosis may rescue the suppression of the respiratory burst, a finding explaining one possible mechanism through which T and B cells enhance the antifungal activity of effector phagocytes.

4.3.3. *The Soluble Mediators*

The complement system is a group of proteins, activated in cascade fashion to provide a rapid humoral defense against microorganisms. There are three pathways of complement activation. The classical pathway is triggered by the antibody (mainly IgG and IgM), and is thus part of the adaptive humoral immune response; the alternative pathway initiates directly on pathogen surfaces, does not depend on antibody, and is thus an important natural defense in non-immune host; the lectin pathway is activated by the binding of MBLs to mannans. Despite different activation mechanisms, all three lead to the three main effector functions of complement: opsonization of microbes, through deposition of C3b and its breakdown product iC3b on particles, recruitment of inflammatory cells, and direct killing of pathogens. The importance of the complement system in host resistance to *C. albicans* has been extensively described elsewhere (Kozel, 1998). *C. albicans* yeasts activate the complement cascade through both the classical and alternative pathways of initiation, eventually leading to deposition of C3 on the cell surface. Indeed, C3 deposition is greatly accelerated through activation of the classical pathway by naturally occurring anti-mannan IgG antibody (Kozel et al., 2004). This finding, while suggesting that the different pathways normally operate together, also points to the important role of antibodies directed against the cell surface to serve as an amplification of C3b deposition and opsonization once either the classical or lectin pathway has been activated (Kozel, 1998; Kozel et al., 2004). The presence of complement receptors on most pathogenic *Candida* spp. suggests a role in pathogenesis. Indeed, complement receptors act as fungal adhesions play a role in iron acquisition by the fungus, and C3b deposition on fungal surfaces signals the ultimate destruction of the pathogen by phagocytic cells. This occurs by the specific recognition of bound complement components by CRs on phagocytes (Calderone, 1994). By targeting specific CRs on phagocytic cells, the complement system may not only fulfill the requirement of a first-line defense against the fungus, but also will contribute to the innate control of the subsequent adaptive immunity.

4.4. Dendritic Cells as an Interface between Host and *C. albicans*

Since their original discovery in 1973, DCs have assumed center stage as the key initiatior of adaptive immunity (Steinman and Pope, 2002). As DCs are equipped with several PRRs and TLRs, they are the main connectors of the innate and adaptive immune systems. DCs are bone marrow-derived cells of both lymphoid and myeloid stem cell origins that populate all lymphoid organs as well as nearly all nonlymphoid tissues and organs. DCs are uniquely adept at decoding the fungus-associated information and translating it in qualitatively different adaptive Th-cell immune responses (Fè d'Ostiani et al., 2000; Claudia et al., 2002; Buentke and Scheynius, 2003; Romani et al., 2004; Bozza et al., 2004). PRRs and TLRs determine the functional plasticity of DCs in response to *C. albicans* and contribute to the discriminative recognition of the different fungal morphotypes. *Candida* proved to be a useful pathogen model to dissect events occurring at the fungus–DC interface (Fè d'Ostiani et al., 2000; Huang et al., 2001; Newman and Holly, 2001; Romagnoli et al., 2003; Romani et al., 2004; Torosantucci et al., 2004). A unique feature of DCs is represented by their ability to internalize different fungal morphotypes. For instance, DCs internalize both *Candida* yeasts and hyphae. Phagocytosis occurs through distinct morphologies and involves different recognition receptors. Recognition and internalization of yeasts occurs predominantly by coiling phagocytosis, through the engagement of MR of different sugar specificity, DC-SIGN (Cambi et al., 2003) and, partly, CR3. In contrast, entry of hyphae occurs by a more conventional, zipper-type phagocytosis, and involves the cooperative action of FcγR and CR3 (Romani et al., 2002). Phagocytosis of either fungal form does not require TLR2, TLR4, TLR9, or MyD88 (Bellocchio et al., 2004).

The engagement of distinct receptors by yeasts and hyphae translates into downstream signaling events, ultimately regulating cytokine production and costimulation, an event greatly influenced by fungal opsonins (Romani et al., 2002, 2004). Entry through MR results in the production of proinflammatory cytokines, including IL-12, upregulation of costimulatory molecules and histocompatibility class II antigens, and activation of protective Th1-cell responses. These events are suppressed upon entry through CR3. In contrast, co-ligation of CR3 with FcγR, as in the phagocytosis of hyphae or opsonized yeasts, results in the production of IL-4 and/or IL-10, upregulation of costimulatory molecules and histocompatibility class II antigens, and activation of Th2/Treg cells (Montagnoli et al., 2003). A recent in vivo study confirmed that hyphal formation by *C. albicans* induces Th2 or IL-10-dominant host responses in tissues (Spellberg et al., 2003). Signaling through the MyD88 pathway is essentially required for IL-12 production by DCs in response to *Candida* yeasts with the implication of distinct TLRs, such as IL-1RI; however, TLR2, but not MyD88, signaling is required for IL-10 production (Bellocchio et al., 2004).

Opsonins and antibodies greatly modify receptor exploitation on DCs by the different fungal morphotypes and qualitatively affect DC activation. MBL opsonization, for instance, increases the uptake of yeasts through CR3 and prevents DC activation and production of IL-12. It is of interest that collectins appear to favor phagocytosis of the fungus without implicating the production of cytokine messengers to the immune system, an activity compatible with a primitive mechanism of host defense and in line with their ability to downregulate the inflammatory response to fungi. Antibodies also may subvert the portal of entry of yeasts and hyphae (Montagnoli et al., 2003; Romani et al., 2004). Thus, by subverting the morphotype-specific program of activation of DCs, opsonins may qualitatively affect DC functioning and Th selection in vivo, ultimately impacting on fungal virulence. Likewise, the different ability of antibodies to opsonize fungi for DC recognition could contribute to the determination of protective and nonprotective activity of antibodies in fungal infections. A remarkable and important feature of Peyer's patches DCs is the production of IL-10 in response to *Candida*, an event occurring by signaling through CR3 and requiring the presence of opsonizing antibodies (Montagnoli et al., 2002). These IL-10-producing DCs activate $CD4^+CD25^+$ Treg cells that negatively affect antifungal Th1 reactivity (see below). It is conceivable that tissue-dependent factors and opsonins modulate receptor usage by DCs at different body sites, and may contribute to the functional plasticity of DCs at the pathogen–immune system interface.

This scenario may offer new interpretative clues to fungal virulence. In fact, the qualitative development of the Th response to the fungus may not primarily depend on the nature of the fungal form being phagocytosed and presented. Rather, the nature of the cell response is strongly affected by the type of cell signaling initiated by the ligand–receptor interaction in DCs. The paradigm would predict that dimorphism per se can neither be considered as the single most important factor in determining commensalism versus infection, nor can specific forms of the fungus be regarded as absolutely indicative of saprophytism or infection at a given site. The selective exploitation of receptor-mediated entry into DCs could explain the full range of host's immune relationships with the fungus, including saprophytism and infection. Usage of CR3, and the consequent attenuation of IL-12 production, might favor commensalism of the fungus at human mucosal surfaces, including gut and vagina, where a condition of immune tolerance is desirable to the host. Averting cellular activation through the interaction with CR3 may ultimately represent an important evasive strategy for fungi, a condition common to different pathogens (McKnight and Gordon, 2000). Interestingly, the entry of heat-inactivated fungi may occur through different pathways, as inactivated *Candida* yeasts were internalized mainly through CR3 (Claudia et al., 2002), a finding that may have important implications in terms of vaccination strategies against fungi.

Lastly, as both fungal morphotypes, but particularly hyphae, activate gut DCs for the local induction of Treg, and because the morphogenesis of *C. albicans* is activated in vivo by a wide range of signals (Brown, 2002), it appears that the discriminative response towards Treg is of potential teleological meaning. It could indeed allow for fungal persistence in the absence of pathological consequences of an exaggerated immunity and possible autoimmunity, which represents the very essence of fungal commensalism. Therefore, in addition to the induction of phase-specific products enhancing fungal survival within the host, transition to the hyphal phase of the fungus could implicate the induction of immunoregulatory events that will benefit the host.

Studies in vivo confirm that DCs sample the fungus at mucosal surfaces and initiate disparate Th responses to the different fungal morphotypes (Montagnoli et al., 2003). Furthermore, they suggest the utility of DCs for fungal vaccines (Table 19.1). The adoptive transfer of DCs pulsed with *Candida* yeasts or transfected with fungal RNA restores protective antifungal immunity in a murine model of allogeneic bone marrow transplantation (Bacci et al., 2002). We have demonstrated that an imbalanced production of Th1 and Th2 cytokines was responsible for the susceptibility to candidiasis in our model. However, readdressing the balance between Th1 and Th2 subsets, as by treatment with Th2 cytokine antagonists, accelerated the recovery of Th1-mediated antifungal resistance (Mencacci et al., 2001).

Table 19.1. Dendritic Cells Vaccination against *Candida albicans*

DC pulsed with	Th priming	Resistance to infection	References
Candida yeasts	Th1	Increased	Fè d'Ostiani et al; 2000
Yeast RNA	Th1+Treg	Increased	Bacci et al; 2002
Candida hyphae	Th2	Decreased	Fè d'Ostiani et al; 2000
Hyphal RNA	Th2	Decreased	Bacci et al; 2002

The recovery of functional Th1 cells producing IFN-γ was also accelerated by the infusion of fungus-pulsed or RNA-transfected DCs, a finding suggesting that DCs may contribute to the educational program of T cells in transplantation (Bacci et al., 2002).

5. Adaptive Immunity

5.1. Th1, Th2, and Treg Cells

The dichotomous Th-cell model has proven to be a useful construct that sheds light on the general principle that diverse effector functions are required for eradication of different fungal infections (Romani, 1999). Although, perhaps, through the limitations of a continued popularity and a "Procrustean" usage under many different circumstances (Gor et al., 2003), this paradigm has greatly contributed to our current understanding of the host response to the fungus from a regulatory perspective, and has been most helpful in accommodating the clinical findings in a conceptual framework amenable to strategies of immunointerventions. There is extensive plasticity in the T cell response to the fungus. The heterogeneity of the $CD4^+$ and $CD8^+$ T cell repertoire may account for the multiplicity and redundancy of effector mechanisms through which T lymphocytes participate in the control of the infection. The flexible program of T lymphocytes also implicates the production of a number of mediators, including cytokines. Due to their action on circulating leukocytes, the cytokines produced by fungus-specific T cells are instrumental in mobilizing and activating antifungal effectors, thus providing prompt and effective control of infectivity once the fungus has established itself in tissues or spread to internal organs. Therefore, host resistance to *Candida* is dependent on the induction of cellular immunity, driven by IL-12 and mediated by Th1 lymphocytes, cytokines, and a number of effector phagocytes. Experimental data have demonstrated the deleterious effects of IL-12 or IFN-γ ablation on the course and outcome of the disseminated infection (Romani, 1999). Through the production of the signature cytokine IFN-γ and help for opsonizing antibodies, the activation of Th1 cells is instrumental in the optimal activation of phagocytes at sites of infection. That acquired immunity to *C. albicans* correlates with the expression of local or peripheral Th1 reactivity has also been confirmed by studies in adult healthy humans (Fidel and Sobel, 1994; Puccetti et al., 1995). Underlying acquired immunity to the fungus, such as the expression of a positive DTH, is demonstrable in adult immunocompetent individuals, and is presumed to prevent mucosal colonization from progression to symptomatic infection (Fidel and Sobel, 1994; Puccetti et al., 1995). Not surprisingly, DTH to *Candida* antigens is a standard in in vivo assays for T cell-mediated immunity in humans. DTH reactivity is usually detectable in more than 80% of the normal adult population (Calderone, 2002) and human lymphocytes show strong proliferative responses after stimulation with *Candida* antigens and produce a number of different cytokines (La Sala et al., 1996, La Valle et al., 2000). The expression of this cutaneous reactivity is often defective in neonates, in immunocompromised individuals as well as in patients with recurrent or persistent infection with the fungus, or immunopathology associated with it (Fidel and Sobel, 1994; Puccetti et al., 1995). In contrast, ablation of IL-4 increases resistance and enhances immunity in experimental models of infections (Romani, 2003). IL-4 may both deactivate and activate phagocytes and DCs for certain specialized functions; for instance, it may inhibit the antifungal effector activities of phagocytes, yet may promote IL-12 production by DCs. Thus, the most important mechanism underlying the inhibitory activity of IL-4 in candidal infections relies on its ability to act as the most potent proximal signal for commitment to Th2 reactivity that dampens protective Th1 responses and favors fungal allergy. In atopic subjects, the suppressed DTH response to the fungus is associated with elevated levels of antifungal IgE, IgA, and IgG (Puccetti et al., 1995).

However, susceptibility to infection may not always be associated with an overt production of IL-4. For instance, although an association between chronic disseminated candidiasis and genetic variants of IL-4 has been recently described (Choi et al., 2003), IL-4 or IL-5 is not always increased in patients with CMC, despite a defective type 1 cytokine production (Lilic, 2002). More often, the defective type 1 cytokine production in CMC occurs concomitantly with the increase of IL-10 (Lilic et al., 2003). A number of clinical observations suggest an inverse relationship between IFN-γ and IL-10 production in patients with fungal infections. High levels of IL-10, negatively affecting IFN-γ production, are detected in chronic disseminated candidal diseases (Lilic, 2002; Roilides et al., 1998). Fungal polysaccharides are known to negatively modulate cell-mediated immunity through the production of IL-10, a finding suggesting that IL-10 production may be a consequence of infection. It has long been presumed that the ability of *C. albicans* to persist in host tissues might involve primarily the immunosuppressive property of cell wall glycoproteins. Mannan and oligosaccharide fragments thereof could be potent inhibitors of cell-mediated immunity and appear to reproduce the immune deficiency of patients with CMC (Ashman, 1998). As already mentioned, tolerance to *Candida* can be achieved through the induction of Treg cells capable of fine-tuning antifungal Th reactivity (Montagnoli et al., 2002). Different types of Treg have been defined that are implicated in the control of organ-specific autoimmunity, transplantation tolerance, and inflammatory responses evoked by enteric organisms (Read and Powrie, 2001). In candidiasis, although protective immunity is mediated by antigen-specific Th1 cells, paradoxically, some Th2 cytokines are required for the maintenance of the antifungal immune resistance (Romani, 1999). Therefore, in addition to the Th1/Th2 balance, other mechanisms seem to be involved in the regulation of Th1 immunity to the fungus. $CD4^{+}CD25^{+}$ T cells negatively regulating antifungal Th1 reactivity was observed in mice with gastrointestinal candidiasis (Montagnoli et al., 2002). Activation of Treg required DCs expressing costimulatory molecules and producing IL-10, the last activity being strictly dependent on local levels of opsonizing antibodies (Montagnoli et al., 2003). Administration of IL-10-producing, *Candida*-pulsed DCs or $CD4^{+}CD25^{+}$ Treg prevented sterilization of the fungus from the gastrointestinal tract and allowed fungal persistence and the occurrence of memory immunity. Therefore, after over a decade of eclipse, suppressor T cells have regained a reputation as key controllers of antifungal immunity.

CMC, although encompassing a variety of clinical entities, has been associated with autoimmune polyendocrinopathy–candidiasis–ectodermal dystrophy, a condition in which the mutated gene has been shown to be involved in the ontogeny of $CD25^{+}$ Treg cells (Liston et al., 2003) In CMC, both anergy and active lymphoproliferation and variable DTH reactivity to the fungus are observed. Similarly, both the recovery of the fungus from the gastrointestinal tract and the detection of underlying Th1 reactivity, such as DTH and lymphoproliferation, may fluctuate in healthy subjects (Calderone, 2002). It is tempting to speculate that specific, yet unknown, tissue-dependent factors may modulate receptor usage by DCs at different body sites, thus shaping the local immune antifungal reactivity. In CMC, the pattern of cytokine production and T cell activation would be consistent with the hypothesis that an inherent alteration in receptor-mediated signaling in response to fungal polysaccharide (Lilic, 2002) may predispose patients to a dysfunctional induction of Treg, negatively affecting the capacity of the Th1-dependent clearance of the fungus, without inducing nonprotective Th2 cells. The engagement of distinct TLRs on DCs and the ensuing production of IL-6 are crucial events mediating the inhibition of Treg-cell functionality (Pasare and Medzhitov, 2003). This is in agreement with the failure of IL-6-deficient mice to activate antifungal Th1 responses concomitantly with a heightened IL-10 production (Romani et al., 1996).

5.2. Antibodies

Although the elevated serum levels of polyclonally activated and specific antibodies frequently observed in mice and humans with progressive infection suggest that the levels of circulating antibodies may not correlate with protection, the existence of protective and nonprotective monoclonal antibodies to *C. albicans* (Casadevall et al., 2002; Bromuro et al., 2002) have greatly helped clarify the controversial issue on the role of antibodies in the systemic infection. It is now clear that differences in the composition and proportion of protective and nonprotective antibodies produced in infection may underlie the variable results obtained with polyclonal sera in experimental systemic infections as well as the lack of correlation of the presence of specific antibody with protection (Bromuro et al., 2002). However, the presence of antibodies to a 47-kDa breakdown product of HSP90 is associated with recovery from *C. albicans* infections and protection against disseminated disease in patients with AIDS (Matthews and Burnie, 2001). Sera from patients who have recovered from disseminated candidiasis confer protection upon passive transfer into infected mice. Antibodies to HSP90 also synergize with antifungal chemotherapy (Matthews and Burnie, 2001). Additional evidence points to the existence of protective antibody. First, both polyclonal sera and IgM monoclonal antibodies to a mannan adhesin fraction are able to passively transfer protection against disseminated and vaginal candidiasis in mice (Cutler et al., 2002). A crude extract of the phosphomannan complex encapsulated into a liposome and given to intact or immunocompromised mice elicits protection, clearly attributable to agglutinating antibodies. The sharing of the same isotype, specificity, and agglutinating function is not sufficient to confer protective value to monoclonal antibodies. Second, antibodies specific for the idiotype of antibodies reactive with yeast killer toxin (anti-idiotypic antibodies) are lethal to strains of *C. albicans* expressing the receptor for toxin (Magliani et al., 1997, 2001). Anti-idiotypic antibody, single chain of it or synthetic killer anti-idiotypic antibody fragment, displays broad fungicidal activity and have therapeutic efficacy in experimental infections (Magliani et al., 1997; Polonelli et al., 2003; Wellington et al., 2003). Third, antibodies may have an influence over Th1/Th2 cytokine balance and induction of Treg (Montagnoli et al., 2003). Finally, indirect evidence for the protective role of antibodies come from the observation that *C. albicans* has evolved strategies to evade antibody immunity, such as the production of proteases which may degrade immunoglobulins and antigenic variation (Romani, 2002). All together, these results indicate that humoral immunity, either independently or through augmentation of complement activity or protective cell mediated immunity, may contribute to host resistance to *C. albicans*.

Research in the field is now in progress as a pursuit to identify those antibodies that are protective, the peptide mimetics that specifically elicit them, and putative candidate vaccines eliciting the protective humoral immunity (Magliani et al., 2001).

6. Conclusions and Future Vision

The past decade has witnessed the rising of a wide range of new approaches to elucidate events occurring at the host–fungus interface. Recognition of the importance of activation of the innate immune system to the eventual induction of antigen-specific immunity has kindled enthusiasm to identify cytokines and ligands for these receptors as potential new-generation immunomodulators to be used for therapy and immunotherapy or as adjuvants for fungal vaccines. A variety of cytokines and growth factors proved to be beneficial in experimental systemic candidiasis (Kullberg et al., 1994; Georgopapadakou and Walsh, 1996; Kullberg and Anaissie, 1998; Rodriguez-Adrian et al., 1998; Poynton et al., 1998). However, establishing the clinical utility of cytokines as therapy for fungal infections in patients has been difficult. The basic strategies pursued include the increase of number, function, and mobility of phagocytic effector cells, as it is now accepted that cytokines, effector cells (Stevens, 1998), and antifungals work synergistically to oppose the fungal growth. Recently, however, the Th1/Th2 balance itself was found to be the target of immunotherapy as well (Poynton, 1997; Polonelli and Cassone, 1999; Stevens et al., 1998; Roilides et al., 2002). The therapeutic efficacy of antifungals in experimental candidiasis is significantly increased by the concomitant inhibition of Th2 cytokines, such as IL-4 and IL-10, more than the addition of Th1 cytokines, such as IL-12 (Cenci et al., 1997; Mencacci et al., 2000). Interestingly, the efficacy of combination therapy with the antifungals and selected cytokines appears to be largely dependent on the host immune reactivity. Thus, the efficacy of the combined treatment with amphotericin B and IL-4 antagonists was superior in neutropenic, as compared to nonneutropenic mice. In contrast, the efficacy of combined treatment with fluconazole and IL-12 was superior in nonneutropenic, as compared to neutropenic mice. It is clear that the dynamics of the interaction of the fungus with cells of the innate immune system may greatly contribute to fungal survival and virulence in the systemic compartment and may condition the efficacy of and responsiveness to antifungal therapy.

Acknowledgments

I thank Lara Bellocchio for editorial assistance. This study was supported by the National Research Project on AIDS, contract 50F.30.

References

Akira, S. (2003). Mammalian Toll-like receptors. *Curr. Opin. Immunol.* 15: 5–11.

Aratani, Y., Kura, F., Watanabe, H., Akagawa, H., Takano, Y., Suzuki, K., Dinauer, M.C., Maeda, N., and Koyama, H. (2002). Relative contribution of myeloperoxidase and NADPH-oxidase to the early host defense against pulmonary infections with *Candida albicans* and *Aspergillus fumigatus*. *Med. Mycol.* 40: 557–563.

Ashman, R.B. (1998). *Candida albicans*: Pathogenesis, immunity and host defence. *Res. Immunol.* 149: 281–288.

Bacci, A., Montagnoli, C., Perruccio, K., Bozza, S., Gaziano, R., Pitzurra, L., Velardi, A., d'Ostiani, C.F., Cutler, J.E., and Romani, L. (2002). Dendritic cells pulsed with fungal RNA induce protective immunity to *Candida albicans* in hematopoietic transplantation. *J. Immunol.* 168: 2904–2913.

Belanger, P.H., Johnston, D.A., Fratti, R.A., Zhang, M., and Filler, S.G. (2002). Endocytosis of *Candida albicans* by vascular endothelial cells is associated with tyrosine phosphorylation of specific host cell proteins. *Cell. Microbiol.* 4: 805–812.

Bellocchio, S. Montagnoli, C., Bozza, S., Gaziano, R., Rossi, G., Mambula, S.S., Vecchi, A., Mantovani, A., Levitz, S.M., and Romani, L. (2004). The contribution of the Toll-like receptor superfamily to innate and adaptive immunity to fungal pathogens in vivo. *J. Immunol.* 172: 3059–3069.

Bodey, G. P., Buckley, M., Sathe, Y. S., and Freireich, E. J. (1966). Quantitative relationships between circulating leukocytes and infection in patients with acute leukemia. *Ann. Intern. Med.* 64: 328–340.

Bogdan, C., Rollinghoff, M., and Diefenbach, A. (2000). Reactive oxygen and reactive nitrogen intermediates in innate and specific immunity. *Curr. Opin. Immunol.* 12: 64–76.

Bohme, A., Karthaus, M., and Hoelzer, D. (1999). Antifungal prophylaxis in neutropenic patients with hematologic malignancies: Is there a real benefit? *Chemotherapy* 45: 224–232.

Bozza, S., Montagnoli, C., Gaziano, R., Rossi, G., Nkwanyuo, G., Bellocchio, S., and Romani, L. (2003). Dendritic cell-based vaccination against opportunistic fungi. *Vaccine* 22: 857–864.

Bromuro, C., Torosantucci, A., Chiani, P., Conti, S., Polonelli, L., and Cassone, A. (2002). Interplay between protective and inhibitory antibodies dictates the outcome of experimentally disseminated candidiasis in recipients of a *Candida albicans* vaccine. *Infect. Immun.* 70: 5462–5470.

Bronte, V., Serafini, P., Mazzoni, A., Segal, D. M., and Zanovello, P. (2003). L-Arginine metabolism in myeloid cells controls T-lymphocyte functions. *Trends Immunol.* 24: 302–306.

Brown, A.J. (2002). Expression of growth form-specific factors during morphogenesis in *Candida albicans*. In R.A. Calderone (ed.), *Candida and Candidiasis*. ASM Press, Washington, DC, pp. 87–106.

Brown, G.D., Herre, B., William, D.L., Willment, J.A., Marshall, A.S., and Gordon, S. (2003). Dectin-1 mediates the biological effects of β-glucans. *J. Exp. Med.* 197: 1119–1124.

Buentke, E. and Scheynius, A. (2003). Dendritic cells and fungi. *APMIS* 111: 789–796.

Calderone, R.A. (eds.) *Candida and Candidiasis*. ASM Press, Washington, DC, 2002.

Calderone, R. (1994). Molecular pathogenesis of fungal infections. *Trends Microbiol.* 2: 461–463.

Cambi, A., Gijzen, K., de Vries, J.M., Torensma, R., Joosten, B., Adema, G.J., Netea, M.G., Kullberg, B.J., Romani, L., and Figdor, C.G. (2003). The C-type lectin DC-SIGN (CD209) is an antigen-uptake receptor for *Candida albicans* on dendritic cells. *Eur. J. Immunol.* 33: 532–538.

Casadevall, A., Feldmesser, M., and Pirofski, L. -A. (2002). Induced humoral immunity and vaccination against major human fungal pathogens. *Curr. Opin. Microbiol.* 5: 386–391.

Cenci, E., Mencacci, A., Del Sero, G., Bistoni, F., and Romani L. (1997). Induction of protective Th1 responses to *Candida albicans* by antifungal therapy alone or in combination with an interleukin-4 antagonist. *J. Infect. Dis.* 176: 217–226.

Chauhan, N., Inglis, D., Roman, E., Pla, J., Li, D., Calera, J.A., and Calderone, R. (2003). *Candida albicans* response regulator gene SSK1 regulates a subset of genes whose functions are associated with cell wall biosynthesis and adaptation to oxidative stress. *Eukaryot. Cell.* 2: 1018–1024.

Cheng, V.C., Yuen, K.Y., Chan, W.M., Wuong, S.S., Ma, E.S., and Chan, R.M. (2000). Immunorestitution disease involving the innate and adaptive response. *Clin. Infect. Dis.* 30: 882–892.

Chiani, P., Bromuro, C., and Torosantucci, A. (2000). Defective induction of interleukin-12 in human monocytes by germ-tube forms of *Candida albicans*. *Infect. Immun.* 68: 5628–5634.

Choi, E.H., Foster, C.B., Taylor, J.G., Erichsen, H.C., Chen, R.A., Walsh, T.J., Anttila, V.J., Ruutu, T., Palotie, A., and Chanock, S.J. (2003). Association between chronic disseminated candidiasis in adult acute leukemia and common IL4 promoter haplotypes. *J. Infect. Dis.* 187: 1153–1156.

Claudia, M., Bacci, A., Silvia, B., Gaziano, R., Spreca, A., and Romani, L. (2002). The interaction of fungi with dendritic cells: Implications for T_H immunity and vaccination. *Curr. Mol. Med.* 2: 507–524.

Cotter, G., Doyle, S., and Kavanagh, K. (2000). Development of an insect model for the in vivo pathogenicity testing of yeasts. *FEMS Immunol. Med. Microbiol.* 27: 163–169.

Coste, A., Duboourdeau, M., Linas, M.D., Cassaing, S., Lepert, J.C., Balard, P., Chalmeton, S., Bernard, J., Orfila, C., Seguela, J.P., and Pipy, B. (2003). PPARgamma promotes mannose receptor gene expression in murine macrophages and contributes to the induction of this receptor by IL-13. *Immunity* 19: 329–339.

Cutler, J.E., Granger, B.L., and Han, Y. (2002). Immunoprotection against Candidiasis. In R.A. Calderone (ed.), *Candida and Candidiasis*. ASM press, Washington DC: , pp. 243–256.

Fearon, D.T. and Locksley, R.M. (1996). The instructive role of innate immunity in the acquired immune response. *Science* 272: 50–53.

Fè d'Ostiani, C., Del Sero, G., Bacci, A., Montagnoli, C., Spreca, A., Mencacci, A.,

Ricciardi-Castagnoli, P., and Romani, L. (2000). Dendritic cells discriminate between yeasts and hyphae of the fungus *Candida albicans*. Implications for initiation of T helper cell immunity in vitro and in vivo. *J. Exp. Med.* 191: 1661–1674.

Fidel, P. L., Jr. and Sobel, J. D. (1994). The role of cell-mediated immunity in candidiasis. *Trends Microbiol.* 6: 202–206.

Gantner, B.N., Simmons, R.M., Canavera, S.J., Akira, S., and Underhill, D.M. (2003). Collaborative induction of inflammatory responses by Dectin-1 and Toll-like receptor 2. *J. Exp. Med.* 197: 1107–1117.

Geiger, J., Wessels, D., Lockhart, S.R., and Soll, D.R. (2004). Release of a potent polymorphonuclear leukocyte chemoattractant is regulated by white-opaque switching in *Candida albicans. Infect. Immun.* 72: 667–677.

Georgopapadakou, N.H. and Walsh, T.J. (1996). Antifungal agents: Chemotherapeutic targets and immunologic strategies. *Antimicrob. Agents Chemother.* 40: 279–291.

Gor, D.O., Rose, N.R., and Greenspan, N.S. (2003). T_H1–T_H2: A procustean paradigm. *Nat. Immunol.* 4: 503–505.

Gow, N.A., Brown, A.J., and Odds, F.C. (2002). Fungal morphogenesis and host invasion. *Curr. Opin. Microbiol.* 5: 366–371.

Hamilton, A.J. and Holdon, M.D. Antioxidant systems in the pathogenic fungi of man and their role in virulence. *Med. Mycol.* 37: 375–389.

Han, Y., Kozel, T.R., Zhang, M.X., MacGill, R.S., and Carroll, M.C. (2001). Complement is essential for protection by an IgM and IgG3 monoclonal antibody against experimental, hematogenously disseminated candidiasis. *J. Immunol.* 167: 1550–1557

Herring, A.C. and Huffnagle, G.B. (2001). Innate immunity to fungi. In S.H.E. Kaufmann, A. Sher, and R. Ahmed (eds), *Immunology of Infectious Diseases*. ASM Press, Washington, DC, pp. 127–137.

Hoffmann, J.A. and Reichhart, J.M. (2002). *Drosophila* innate immunity: An evolutionary perspective. *Nat. Immunol.* 3: 121–126.

Huang, Q., Liu, D., Majewski, P., Schulte, L.C., Korn, J.M., Young, R.A., Lander, E.S., and Hacohen, N. (2001). The plasticity of dendritic cell responses to pathogens and their components. *Science* 294: 870–875.

Ibata-Ombetta, S., Idziorek, T., Trinel, P.A., Poulain, D., and Jouault, T. (2003). *Candida albicans* phospholipomannan promotes survival of phagocytosed yeasts through modulation of bad phosphorylation and macrophage apoptosis. *J. Biol. Chem.* 278: 13086–13093.

Jarvis, W.R. (1995). Epidemiology of nosocomial fungal infections, with emphasis on *Candida* species. *Clin. Infect. Dis.* 20: 1526–1530.

Jones-Carson, J., Vazquez-Torres, A., van der Heyde, H.C., Warner, T., Wagner, R.D., and Balish, E. (1995). Gamma delta T cell-induced nitric oxide production enhances resistance to mucosal candidiasis. *Nat. Med.* 1: 552–557.

Jouault, T., Ibata-Ombetta, S., Takeuchi, O., Trinel, P.A., Sacchetti, P., Lefebvre, P., Akira, S., and Poulain, D. (2003). *Candida albicans* phospholipomannan is sensed through Toll-like receptors. *J. Infect. Dis.* 188: 165–172.

Kaposzta, R., Marodi, L., Hollinshead, M., Gordon, S., and da Silva R.P. (1999). Rapid recruitment of late endosomes and lysosomes in mouse macrophages ingesting *Candida albicans. J. Cell Sci.* 112: 3237–3248.

Kozel, T.R. (1998). Complement activation by pathogenic fungi. *Res. Immunol.* 149: 309–320.

Kozel, T.R., MacGill, R.S., Percival, A., and Zhou, Q. (2004). Biological activities of naturally occurring antibodies reactive with *Candida albicans* mannan. *Infect. Immun.* 72: 209–218.

Kullberg, B., Vogels, M.T.E., and van der Meer, J.W.M. (1994). Immunomodulators in bacterial and fungal infections. A review of their therapeutic potential. *Clin. Immunother.* 1: 43–55.

Kullberg, B.J. and Anaissie, E.J. (1998). Cytokines as therapy for opportunistic fungal infections. *Res. Immunol.* 149: 478–488.

Lan, C.Y., Newport, G., Murillo, L.A., Jones, T., Scherer, S., Davis, R.W., and Agabian, N. (2002). Metabolic specialization associated with phenotypic switching in *Candida albicans. Proc. Natl. Acad. Sci. USA* 99: 14907–14912.

La Sala, A., Urbani, F., Torosantucci, A., Cassone, A., and Ausiello, C. (1996). Mannoproteins from *Candida albicans* elicit a Th1-type-1 cytokine profile in human *Candida* specific long-term T cell cultures. *J. Biol. Regul. Homeost. Agents* 10: 8–12.

La Valle, R., Sandini, S., Gomez, M.J., Mondello, F., Romagnoli, G., Nisini, R., and Cassone, A. (2000). Generation of a recombinant 65-kilodalton mannoprotein, a major antigen target of cell-mediated immune response to *Candida albicans. Infect. Immun.* 68: 6777–6784.

Letterio, J.J., Lehrnbecher, T., Pollack, G., Walsh, T.J., and Chanock, S.J. (2001). Invasive candidiasis stimulates hepatocyte and monocyte production of active transforming growth factor beta. *Infect. Immun.* 69: 5115–5120.

Lilic, D. (2002). New perspectives on the immunology of chronic mucocutaneous candidiasis. *Curr. Opin. Infect. Dis.* 15: 143–147.

Lilic, D., Gravenor, I., Robson, N., Lammas, D.A., Drysdale, P., Calvert, J.E., Cant, A.J., and Abinum, M. (2003). Deregulated production of protective cytokines in response to *Candida albicans* infection in patients with chronic mucocutaneous candidiasis. *Infect. Immun.* 71: 5690–5699.

Liston, A., Lesage, S., Wilson, J., Peltonen, L., and Goodnow, C. C. (2003). Air regulates negative selection of organ-specific T cells. *Nat. Immunol.* 4: 350–435.

Liu, L., Kang, K., Takahara, M., Cooper, K.D., and Ghannoum, M.A. (2001). Hyphae and yeasts of *Candida albicans* differentially regulate interleukin-12 production by human blood monocytes: Inhibitory role of *C. albicans* germination. *Infect. Immun.* 69: 4695–4697.

Lorenz, M.C. and Fink, G.R. (2001). The glyoxylate cycle is required for fungal virulence. *Nature* 412: 83–86.

Magliani, W., Conti, S., de Bernardis, F., Gerloni, M., Bertolotti, D., Mozzoni, P., Cassone, A., and Polonelli, L. (1997). Therapeutic potential of antiidiotypic single chain antibodies with yeast killer toxin activity. *Nat. Biotechnol.* 15: 155–158.

Magliani, W., Conti, S., Arseni, S., Frazzi, R., Salati, A., and Polonelli, L. (2001). Killer anti-idiotypes in the control of fungal infections. *Curr. Opin. Investig. Drugs* 2: 477–479.

Mansour, M.K. and Levitz, S.M. (2002). Interactions of fungi with phagocytes. *Curr. Opin. Microbiol.* 5: 359–365.

Marodi, L. (2002). Deficient interferon-gamma receptor-mediated signalling in neonatal macrophages. *Acta Paediatr. Suppl.* 91: 117–119.

Marodi, L., Schreiber, S., Anderson, D.C., MacDermott, R.P., Korchak, H.M., and Johnston, R.B. Jr. (1993). Enhancement of macrophage candidacidal activity by interferon-gamma. Increased phagocytosis, killing, and calcium signal mediated by a decreased number of mannose receptors. *J. Clin. Invest.* 91: 2596–2601.

Marquis, G., Garzon, S., Montplaisir, S., Strykowski, H., and Benhamou, N. (1991). Histochemical and immunochemical study of the fate of *Candida albicans* inside human neutrophil phagolysosomes. *J. Leukoc. Biol.* 50: 587–599.

Marr, K.A., Balajee, S.A., Hawn, T.R., Ozinsky, A., Pham, U., Akira, S., Aderem, A., and Liles, W.C. (2003). Differential role of MyD88 in macrophage-mediated responses to opportunistic fungal pathogens. *Infect. Immun.* 71: 5280–5286.

Matthews, R. and Burnie, J. (2001). Antifungal antibodies: A new approach to the treatment of systemic candidiasis. *Curr. Opin. Investig. Drugs* 2: 472–476.

McKnight, A. and Gordon, S. (2000). Forum in Immunology: Innate recognition systems. *Microbes Infect.* 2: 239–336.

Medzhitov, R. and Janeway, C.A. Jr. (1997). Innate immunity: The virtues of a nonclonal system of recognition. *Cell* 91: 295–298.

Mencacci, A., Bacci, A., Cenci, E., Montagnoli, C., Fiorucci, S., Casagrande, A., Flavell, R.A., Bistoni, F., and Romani, L. (2000). Interleukin-18 restores detective Th1 immunity to *Candida albicans* in caspase 1-deficient mice. *Infect. Immun.* 68: 5126–5131.

Mencacci, A., Cenci, E., Bacci, A., Bistoni, F., and Romani, L. (2000). Host immune reactivity determines the efficacy of combination immunotherapy and antifungal chemotherapy in candidiasis. *J. Infect. Dis.* 181: 686–694.

Mencacci, A., Perruccio, K., Bacci, A., Cenci, E., Benedetti, R., Martelli, M. F., Bistoni, F., Coffman, R., Velardi, A., and Romani, L. (2001). Defective antifungal T-helper 1 (TH1) immunity a murine model of allogeneic T-cell-depleted bone marrow transplantation and its restoration by treatment with TH2 cytokine antagonists. Blood 97: 1483–1490.

Mencacci, A., Montagnoli, C., Bacci, A., Cenci, E., Pitzurra, L., Spreca, A., Kopf, M., Sharpe, A.H., and Romani, L. (2002). $CD80^{+}Gr\text{-}1^{+}$ myeloid cells inhibit development of antifungal TH1 immunity in mice with candidiasis. *J. Immunol.* 169: 3180–3190.

Millar, D.G., Garza, K.M., Odermatt, B., Elford, A.R., Ono, N., Li, Z., and Ohashi, P.S. (2003). HPS70 promotes antigen-presenting cell function and converts T-cell tolerance to autoimmunity in vivo. *Nat. Med.* 9: 1469–1476.

Miller, M.G. and Johnson, A.D. (2002). White-opaque switching in *Candida albicans* is controlled by mating-type locus homeodomain proteins and allows efficient mating. *Cell* 110: 293–302.

Montagnoli, C., Bacci, A., Bozza, S., Gaziano, R., Mosci, P., Sharpe, H.A., and Romani, L. (2002). B7/CD28-dependent $CD4^+CD25^+$ regulatory T cells are essential components of the memory protective immunity to *Candida albicans*. *J. Immunol.* 169: 6298–6308.

Montagnoli, C., Bozza, S., Bacci, A., Gaziano, R., Mosci, P., Morschhauser, J., Pitzurra, L., Kopf, M., Cutler, J., and Romani, L. (2003). A role for antibodies in the generation of memory antifungal immunity. *Eur. J. Immunol.* 33: 1193–1204.

Mullick, A., Elias, M., Harakidas, P., Marcil, A., Whiteway, M., Ge, B., Hudson, T.J., Caron, A.W., Bouget, L., Picard, S., Jovcevski, O., Massie, B., and Thomas, D.Y. (2004). Gene expression in HL60 granulocytoid and human polymorphonuclear leukocytes exposed to *Candida albicans*. *Infect. Immun.* 72: 414–429.

Nantel, A., Dignard, D., Bachewich, C., Harcus, D., Marcil, A., Bouin, A.P., Sensen, C.W., Hogues, H., van het Hoog, M., Gordon, P., et al. (2002). Transcription profiling of *Candida albicans* cells undergoing the yeast-to-hyphal transition. *Mol. Biol. Cell.* 13: 3452–3465.

Newman, S.L. and Holly, A. (2001). *Candida albicans* is phagocytosed, killed, and processed for antigen presentation by human dendritic cells. *Infect. Immun.* 69: 6813–6822.

O'Neill, L.A., Fitzgerald, K.A., and Bowie, A.G. (2003). The Toll-IL-1 receptor adaptor family grows to five members. *Trends Immunol.* 24: 286–290.

Netea, M.G., Stuyt, R. J., Kim, S.H., Van der Meer, J.W., Kullberg, B.J., and Dinarello, C.A. (2002a). The role of endogenous interleukin (IL)-18, IL-12, IL-1β, and tumor necrosis factor-α in the production of interferon-γ induced by *Candida albicans* in human whole-blood cultures. *J. Infect. Dis.* 185: 963–970.

Netea, M.G., Van Der Graaf, C.A., Vonk, A.G., Verschueren, I, Van Der Meer, J.W., and Kullberg, B.J. (2002b). The role of Toll-like receptor (TLR) 2 and TLR4 in the host defense against disseminated candidiasis. *J. Infect. Dis.* 185: 1483–1489.

Netea, M.G., vonk, A.G., van den Hoven, M., Verschueren, I., Joosten, L.A., van Krieken, J.H., van den Berg., Van deer Meer, J.W., and Kullberg, B.J. (2003). Differential role of IL-18 and IL-12 in the host defense against disseminated *Candida albicans* infection. *Eur. J. Immunol.* 33: 3409–3417.

Pasare, C. and Medzhitov, R. (2003). Toll pathway-dependent blockade of $CD4^+CD25^+$ T cell-mediated suppression by dendritic cells. *Science* 299: 1033–1036.

Polonelli, L., Magliani, W., Conti, S., Bracci, L., Lozzi, L., Neri, P., Adriani, D., De Bernardis, F., and Cassone, A. (2003). Therapeutic activity of an engineered synthetic killer antiidiotypic antibody fragment against experimental mucosal and systemic candidiasis. *Infect. Immun.* 71: 6205–6212.

Poynton, H.C. (1997). Immune modulation by cytokines in the treatment of opportunistic infections. *Curr. Opin. Infect. Dis.* 10: 275–280.

Poynton, C.H., Barnes, R.A., and Rees, J. (1998). Interferon γ and granulocyte-macrophage colony-stimulating factor for the treatment of hepatosplenic candidosis in patients with acute leukemia. *Clin. Inf. Dis.* 26: 239–240.

Puccetti, P., Romani, L., and Bistoni, F. (1995). A T_H1-T_H2-like switch in candidiasis: New perspectives for therapy. *Trends Microbiol.* 3: 237–240.

Raveh, D., Kruskal, B.A., Farland, J., and Ezekowitz, R.A. (1998). Th1 and Th2 cytokines cooperate to stimulate mannose-receptor-mediated phagocytosis. *J. Leukoc. Biol.* 64: 108–113.

Read, S. and Powrie, F. (2001). $CD4^+$ regulatory T cells. *Curr. Opin. Immunol.* 13: 644–649.

Rodriguez-Adrian, L.J., Grazziutti, M.L., Rex, H.J., and Anaissie, E.J. (1998). The potential role of cytokine for fungal infections in patients with cancer: Is recovery from neutropenia all that is needed? *Clin. Infect. Dis.* 26: 1270–1278.

Roeder, A., Kirscning, C.J., Rupec, R.A., Schaller, M., and Korting, H.C. (2004). Toll-like receptors and innate antifungal responses. *Trends Microbiol.* 12: 44–49.

Roilides, E., Sein, T., Schaufele, R., Chanock, S.J., and Walsh, T.J. (1998). Increased serum concentrations of interleukin-10 in patients with hepatosplenic candidiasis. *J. Infect. Dis.* 178: 589–592.

Roilides, E., Lamaignere, C.G., and Farmaki, E. (2002). Cytokines in immunodeficient patients with invasive fungal infections: An emerging therapy. *Int. J. Infect. Dis.* 6: 154–163.

Romagnoli, G., Nisini, R., Chiani, P., Mariotti, S., Teloni, R., Cassone, A., and Torosantucci, A.

(2004). The interaction of human dendritic cells with yeasts and germ-tube forms of *Candida albicans* leads to efficient fungal processing, dendritic cell maturation, and acquisition of a Th1 response-promoting function. *J. Leukoc. Biol.* 75: 117–126.

Romani, L. (2004). Immunity to fungal infections. *Nat. Rev. Immunol.* 4: 11–23.

Romani, L. (2002). Innate immunity against fungal pathogens. In R.A. Calderone and L.R. Cihlar (eds), *Fungal Pathogenesis. Principles and Clinical Applications*. Marcel Dekker, New York, pp. 401–432.

Romani, L. (2003). Cytokines in the innate and adaptive immunity to *Candida albicans*. In M. Kotb and T. Calandra (eds), *Cytokines and Chemokines in Infectious Diseases Handbook*. Humana Press, Totowa, NJ, pp. 227–241.

Romani, L. (1999). Immunity to *Candida albicans:* Th1, Th2 cells and beyond. *Curr. Opin. Microbiol.* 2: 363–367.

Romani, L., Montagnoli, C., Bozza, S., Perruccio, K., Spreca, A., Allavena, P., Verbeek, S., Calderone, R.A., Bistoni, F., and Puccetti, P. (2004). The exploitation of distinct recognition receptors in dendritic cells determines the full range of host's immune relationships with *Candida albicans. Int. Immunol.* 16: 149–161.

Romani, L., Bistoni, F., and Puccetti, P. (2003). Adaptation of *Candida albicans* to the host environment: The role of morphogenesis in virulence and survival in mammalian hosts. *Curr. Opin. Microbiol.* 6: 338–343.

Romani, L., Bistoni, F., and Puccetti, P. (2002). Fungi, dendritic cells and receptors: A host perspective of fungal virulence. *Trends Microbiol.* 10: 508–514.

Romani, L., Mencacci, A., Cenci, E., Spaccapelo, R., Toniatti, C., Puccetti, P., Bistoni, F., and Poli, V. (1996). Impaired neutrophil response and $CD4^+$ T helper cell 1 development in interleukin 6-deficient mice infected with *Candida albicans. J. Exp. Med.* 183: 1345–1355.

Rooney, P.J. and Klein, B.S. (2002). Linking fungal morphogenesis with virulence. *Cell. Microbiol.* 4: 127–137.

Sanchez, A.A., Johnston D.A., Myers, C., Edwards, J.E. Jr., Mitchell, A.P., and Miller, S.G. (2004). Relationship between *Candida albicans* virulence during experimental hematogenously disseminated infection and endothelial cell damage in vitro. *Infect. Immun.* 72: 598–601.

Schroppel, K., Kryk, M., Herrmann, M., Leberer, E., Rollinghoff, M., and Bogdan, C. (2001). Suppression of type 2 NO-synthase activity in macrophages by *Candida albicans. Int. Med. Microbiol.* 290: 659–668.

Soll, D.R. (2002). *Candida* commensalism and virulence: The evolution of phenotypic plasticity. *Acta Trop.* 81: 101–110.

Spellberg, B., Johnston, D., Phan, Q.T., Edwards, J.E., French, S.W., Ibrahim, A.S., and Filler, S.G. (2003). Parenchymal organ, and not splenic, immunity correlates with host survival during disseminated candidiasis. *Infect. Immun.* 71: 5756–5764.

Steinman, R.M. and Pope, M. (2002). Exploiting dendritic cells to improve vaccine efficacy. *J. Clin. Invest.* 109: 1519–1526.

Stevens, D.A. (1998). Combination immunotherapy and antifungal chemotherapy. *Clin. Infect. Dis.* 26: 1266–1269.

Stevens, D.A., Walsh, T.J., Bistoni, F., Cenci, E., Clemons, K.V., Del Sero, G., Fè d'Ostiani, C., Kullberg, B.J., Mencacci, A., Roilides, E., and Romani, L. (1998). Cytokines and mycoses. *Med. Mycol.* 36(S1): 174–182.

Stuyt, R.J., Netea, M.G., Verschueren, I., Fantuzzi, G., Dinarello, C.A., Van Der Meer, J.W., and Kullberg, B.J. (2002). Role of interleukin-18 in host defense against disseminated *Candida albicans* infection. *Infect. Immun.* 70: 3284–3286.

Tada, H., Nemoto, E., Shimauchi, H., Watanabe, T., Mikami, T., Matsumoto, T., Ohno, N., Tamura, H., Shibata, K., Akashi, S., Miyake, K., Sugawara, S., and Takada, H. (2002). *Saccharomyces cerevisiae*- and *Candida albicans*-derived mannan induced production of tumor necrosis factor alpha by human monocytes in a CD14- and Toll-like receptor 4-dependent manner. *Microbiol. Immunol.* 46: 503–512.

Torosantucci, A., Chiani, P., De Bernardis, F., Cassone, A., Calera, J.A., and Calderone, R. (2002). Deletion of the two-component histidine kinase gene (CHK1) *Candida albicans* contributes to enhanced growth inhibition and killing by human neutrophils in vitro. *Infect. Immun.* 70: 985–987.

Torosantucci, A., Romagnoli, G., Chiani, P., Stringaro, A., Crateri, P., Mariotti, S., Teloni, R., Arancia, G., Cassone, A., and Nisini, R. (2004). *Candida albicans* yeast and germ tube forms interfere differently with human monocyte differentiation into dendritic cells: A novel dimorphism-dependent mechanism to escape the host's immune response. *Infect. Immun.* 72: 833–843.

van Spriel, A.B., van den Herik-Oudijk, I.E., van Sorge, N.M., Vile, H.A., van Strijp, J.A., and van de Winkel, J.G. (1999). Effective phagocytosis and killing of *Candida albicans* via targeting FcgammaRI (CD64) or FcalphaRI (CD89) on neutrophils. *J. Infect. Dis.* 179: 661–669.

van Spriel, A.B., Leuse, J.H.W., van Egmond, M., Dijkman, H.B.P.M., Assmann, K.J.M., Mayadas, T.N., and van de Winkel, J.G. (2001). Mac-1 (CD11b/Cd18) is essential for Fc receptor-mediated neutrophil cytotoxicity and immunologic synapse formation. *Blood* 97: 2478–2486.

Vasquez-Torres, A. and Balish, E. (1997). Macrophages in resistance to candidiasis. *Microbiol. Mol. Rev.* 61: 170–192.

Villamon, E., Gozalbo, D., Roig, P., O'Connor, J.E., Fradelizi, D., and Gil, M.L. (2004). Toll-like receptor-2 is essential in murine defenses against *Candida albicans* infections. *Microbes Infect.* 6: 1–7.

Walsh, T.J., Hiemenz, J., and Pizzo, P.A. (1994). Evolving risk factors for invasive fungal infections-all neutropenic patients are not the same. *Clin. Infect. Dis.* 18: 793–798.

Wanten, G.J., Netea, M.G., Naber, T.H., Curfs, J.H., Jacobs, L.E., Verver-Jansen, T.J., and Kullberg, B.J. (2002). Parenteral administration of medium- but not long-chain lipid emulsions may increase the risk for infections by *Candida albicans. Infect. Immun.* 70: 6471–6474.

Wellington, M., Bliss, J.M., and Haidaris, C.G. (2003). Enhanced phagocytosis of *Candida* species mediated by opsonization with a recombinant human antibody single-chain variable fragment. *Infect. Immun.* 71: 7228–7231.

Yamamoto, M., et al. (2003). Role of adaptor TRIF in the MyD88-independent Toll-like receptor signaling pathway. *Science* 301: 640–643.

Yamamoto, Y., Specter, S., and Friedman, H. (1993). Lipopolysaccharide restores anti-*Candida albicans* growth inhibition activity of polymorphonuclear neutrophils from retrovirus-immunosuppressed mice. *Infect. Immun.* 61: 2216–2219.

20

Interactions of Fungi with Endothelial Cells

Scott G. Filler[1,2] and Donald C. Sheppard[1,3]

1. Introduction

In the past, endothelial cells were thought to be passive cells whose only function was to keep the various blood components inside the vascular tree. However, it is now clear that endothelial cells play an important role in maintaining homeostasis and regulating the host inflammatory response. For example, endothelial cells govern vascular tone and permeability, and regulate the activity of the coagulation cascade.

[1] Los Angeles Biomedical Research Institute at Harbor-UCLA Medical Center, Torrance, CA 90502, USA.
[2] David Geffen School of Medicine, Los Angeles, CA 90024, USA.
[3] *Current address:* McGill University, Department of Microbiology and Immunology, Montreal, Quebec, Canada.

In addition, they can influence the inflammatory response by secreting pro-inflammatory cytokines and prostaglandins, and expressing leukocyte adhesion molecules and platelet-activating factor. Endothelial cells can even express MHC class II molecules and act as antigen-presenting cells. Thus, the endothelial cell response to fungal infection has the potential to significantly influence the outcome of infection.

Fungi that cause invasive infections can interact with either the luminal or abluminal surface of vascular endothelial cells. Organisms that disseminated hematogenously must cross the endothelial cell lining of the vasculature to invade the deep tissues. These blood-borne organisms therefore interact with the luminal surface of the endothelial cells. Fungi that are known to disseminate hematogenously include the *Candida* species, *Cryptococcus neoformans*, and *Aspergillus* species. Other fungi that disseminate hematogenously relatively infrequently include *Coccidioides immitis*, *Histoplasma capsulatum*, *Blastomyces dermatiditis*, and *Sporothrix schenckii*. A second type of endothelial cell interaction occurs during angioinvasion. In this process, fungi elements growing at a focus of infection extend to and invade blood vessels by passing from the external surface into the vascular lumen. Thus, these organisms interact first with the abluminal surface of endothelial cells. Once the organisms gain access to the vascular lumen, they can disseminate hematogenously. Angioinvasion is limited to a few molds, such as *Aspergillus* species and members of the *Mucorales* family.

2. *Candida* Species

The species of *Candida* that are the most common cause of hematogenously disseminated candidiasis are *Candida albicans*, *Candida glabrata*, *Candida parapsilosis*, *Candida tropicalis*, and *Candida krusei* (Hajjeh et al., 2004). Of these species, only the interactions of *C. albicans* with vascular endothelial cells have been studied in detail. In fact, more is known about the interactions of endothelial cells with this organism than is known about the endothelial cell interactions of any other fungus.

2.1. Adherence

The first step in fungal invasion across the endothelial cell lining of the vasculature is likely adherence to the luminal surface of endothelial cells. The first experiments to investigate candidal adherence to endothelial cells were reported by Klotz et al. (1983). They studied the adherence of *Candida* sp. to the endothelial cell lining of porcine blood vessels *ex vivo* and found that *C. albicans* adheres to endothelial cells most avidly, whereas *C. tropicalis*, *C. glabrata*, *C. parapsilosis*, and *C. krusei* are less adherent. This relative hierarchy of adherence has been confirmed by other investigators using human umbilical vein endothelial cell grown in tissue culture (Rotrosen et al., 1985). Furthermore, the finding that *C. albicans* is most adherent to endothelial cells suggests that adherence is a significant virulence factor, because *C. albicans* is most common species of *Candida* to be isolated from the blood.

The *C. albicans* proteins encoded by the *ALS* gene family are the only adhesins that are known to mediate binding to vascular endothelial cells in vitro and have been characterized at the molecular level. Hoyer and colleagues discovered this gene family, which has at least eight members (Hoyer et al., 1995, 1998a,b; Hoyer and Hecht, 2000). Subsequently, other investigators have determined that Als1p, Als3p, and Als5p mediate adherence to endothelial cells in vitro (Fu et al., 1998, 2002; Sheppard et al., 2004b). The substrate-binding regions of Als1p and Als5 p have been localized to the N-terminal region of these proteins (Loza et al., 2004; Sheppard et al., 2004b). Interestingly, this region is characterized by antiparallel β sheets, indicating that the Als proteins are members of the immunoglobulin superfamily (Hoyer and Hecht, 2001; Sheppard et al., 2004b). In vitro, Als1p, Als3p, and Als5p mediate binding to multiple substrates in addition to endothelial cells, including fibronectin, laminin, collagen, and an oral epithelial cell line (Gaur and Klotz, 1997; Fu et al., 1998; Gauret al., 1999; Klotz et al., 2004; Sheppard et al., 2004b).

Other, less well-characterized adhesins also mediate the adherence of *C. albicans* to endothelial cells. *C. albicans* yeast and germ tubes express one or more molecules on their surface that are antigenically and functionally similar to human $\alpha_V\beta_3$ and $\alpha_V\beta_5$ integrins, which bind to vitronectin (Spreghini et al., 1999; Santoni et al., 2001). Antibodies to these integrins can block the binding of *C. albicans* to vitronectin and an endothelial cell line in vitro. Endothelial cell adherence can also be blocked with RGD peptides (containing the amino acid sequence arginine–glycine–aspartic acid), suggesting that the *C. albicans* integrin-like molecules bind to similar substrate motifs as do human integrins. Klotz et al. (2001) screened a *C. albicans* cDNA library that was expressed in *S. cerevisiae* for clones that were recognized by a polyclonal antiserum to the human fibronectin receptor (the $\alpha_5\beta_1$ integrin). They discovered that the *S. cerevisiae* clones recognized by this antiserum expressed *C. albicans* alcohol dehydrogenase. These clones were also recognized by antiserum against the human $\alpha_V\beta_3$ integrin. Thus, it is possible that alcohol dehydrogenase may function as an integrin-like adhesin for endothelial cells. However, it was not reported whether clones of *S. cerevisiae* that expressed *C. albicans* alcohol dehydrogenase had increased adherence to endothelial cells. Also, the endothelial cell adherence of *C. albicans* strains that lack alcohol dehydrogenase has not been described.

C. albicans also expresses on its surface a molecule that is recognized by antibodies against $\alpha_M\beta_2$ (also called CR3 or CDllb/CD18). Both the human $\alpha_M\beta_2$ and the candidal $\alpha_M\beta_2$-like molecule bind the complement fragment iC3b (Alaei et al., 1993; Edwards et al., 1986; Gilmoreet al., 1988). Antibodies against this receptor block the adherence of *C. albicans* to human dermal microvascular endothelial cells in vitro and improve the survival of mice with experimental hematogenously disseminated candidiasis (Lee et al., 1997). The identity of the candidal $\alpha_M\beta_2$-like adhesin is controversial. Gale et al. (1996) reported that this molecule was encoded by *INT1*. There is limited expression of Int1p on the surface of *C. albicans* cells and an *int1/int1* null mutant has reduced adherence to epithelial cells (Gale et al., 1998). However, it has subsequently been determined that Int1p has significant structural and functional homology to Bud4p in *S. cerevisiae*, which is involved in septin ring localization and formation. Thus, it is likely that one or more proteins other than Int1p constitute the $\alpha_M\beta_2$-like molecule in *C. albicans*.

In mammalian cells, binding of an integrin to its ligand activates signal transduction pathways that result in cell-specific responses such as changes in cell motility and induction of gene expression. Focal adhesion kinase (FAK) is a cytoskeletal-associated signaling protein in mammalian cells that is tyrosine-phosphorylated in response to integrin binding. Phosphorylated FAK in turn phosphorylates other proteins and thereby activates the mitogen-activated protein kinase pathway. Santoni et al. (2002) reported that *C. albicans* possesses a protein that is recognized by anti-FAK antibodies and is tyrosine phosphorylated when the organism adheres to either an endothelial cell line or vitronectin. Furthermore, treatment of *C. albicans* with broad-spectrum tyrosine kinase inhibitors blocks the phosphorylation of this FAK-like protein and reduces *C. albicans* adherence to host substrates. These results suggest that adherence of *C. albicans* to endothelial cells may induce a specific set of responses in the organism. These responses are currently unknown, but could include upregulation of adhesins, stimulation of thigmotropism, or induction of hyphal formation.

The exact identity of the *C. albicans* FAK-like protein remains to be determined, as there are no obvious FAK orthologs in the *C. albicans* genome.

Virtually all of the investigations of the mechanisms by which *C. albicans* adheres to endothelial cells have been performed under static conditions. However, Glee et al. (2001) studied the adherence of *C. albicans* blastospores to endothelial cells grown in capillary tubes under conditions that simulated physiologic shear. They found that hydrophobic proteins on the fungal cell surface mediated adherence to endothelial cells under shear conditions. One of these proteins may be Csh1p (Singleton et al., 2001; Singleton and Hazen, 2004).

It was also discovered that *C. albicans* adherence to endothelial cells under shear conditions was increased when the endothelial cells were stimulated with tumor necrosis factor α (TNF-α) (Glee et al., 2001). These results suggest that *C. albicans* binds to molecules on the endothelial cell surface that are upregulated when the endothelial cells are stimulated. One such molecule is intercellular adhesion molecule 1 (ICAM-1), which is a known a ligand for the $\alpha_M\beta_2$ integrin. It has been reported that antibodies against ICAM-1 block adherence of *C. albicans* to rat pulmonary artery endothelial cells in vitro, and prolong survival in rats with candidemia (Yokomura et al., 2001). Although these results suggest that *C. albicans* adherence to ICAM-1 is an important virulence factor, experiments with mice that are genetically deficient in ICAM-1 do not support this conclusion. ICAM-1 knockout mice have aberrant leukocyte recruitment, higher organ fungal burden, and greater mortality during candidemia (Davis et al., 1996). One possible explanation for these disparate results is that ICAM-1 may be more important for leukocyte recruitment during candidemia in mice than it is in rats. In support of this hypothesis, we have found that ICAM-1 is expressed by leukocytes at foci of disseminated candidiasis in mice (Cannom et al., 2002).

It virtually certain that *C. albicans* also binds to molecules other than ICAM-1 on the endothelial cells surface. These additional ligands have not yet been characterized.

2.2. Invasion

Blood-borne fungi must penetrate through the endothelial cell lining of the vasculature to invade from the lumen of the blood vessels into the deep tissues. There are at least three possible mechanisms by which blood-borne organisms can escape from the vasculature. First, they can pass through the endothelial cell monolayer, either by directly or via a paracellular pathway. Second, they can be phagocytized by circulating leukocytes and be carried across the endothelial cell monolayer within the leukocytes. This mechanism would be unlikely to occur in profoundly leukopenic patients. Third, they could penetrate through gaps in the endothelial cell monolayer that could form as a result of trauma or cytotoxic chemotherapy. During their early studies of the interactions of *C. albicans* with porcine blood vessels *ex vivo*, Klotz et al. (1983) observed that live blastospores could directly traverse the endothelial cell lining. However, an extremely high inoculum of *C. albicans* was used in these experiments. Subsequently, Rotrosen et al. (1985) examined the interactions of *C. albicans* hyphae with human umbilical vein endothelial cells by transmission electron microscopy. They observed that endothelial cells responded to contact with *C. albicans* hyphae by producing pseudopods that surrounded the hyphae and pulled them into the cells. Similar findings have been observed with cultured human brain microvascular endothelial cells (Jong et al., 2001). These results suggest that *C. albicans* invades endothelial cells in vitro by inducing its own uptake.

The mechanisms by which *C. albicans* induces its own uptake have been studied in some detail. Endocytosis is induced maximally by true hyphae (Filler et al., 1995; Phan et al., 2000). Mutants of *C. albicans* that grow as either blastospores or pseudohyphae on human umbilical vein endothelial cells are endocytosed poorly compared to their wild-type parent strain that forms true hyphae on these cells. However, it has been reported that blastospores are endocytosed by porcine aortic endothelial cells (Klotz et al., 1983), and that a mixture of blastospores and pseudohyphae are endocytosed by human brain microvascular endothelial cells (Jong et al., 2001). Unfortunately, the endocytic capacity of endothelial cells from different vascular beds has not been compared directly. Nevertheless, it is possible that some types of endothelial cells may be able to endocytose nonhyphal forms of *C. albicans* relatively efficiently.

The endocytosis of *C. albicans* is passive on the part of the organism because killed hyphae are endocytosed as avidly as are live hyphae (Phan et al., 2000). Recently, we have discovered that *S. cerevisiae* expressing *C. albicans* Als3p are endocytosed by endothelial cells, suggesting that Als3p functions as an endothelial cell invasin-like protein (Sheppard et al., 2004b). Als3p is expressed most strongly on true hyphae (Hoyer et al., 1998), providing an explanation as to why hyphae are endocytosed more efficiently than other forms of *C. albicans*.

Jong et al. (2003) have reported that *C. albicans* enolase binds plasminogen and plasmin, and that *C. albicans* cells that are coated with plasmin have an increased ability to transcytose across human brain microvascular endothelial cells. However, other investigators used a proteomics approach to identify *C. albicans* surface proteins that bound plasminogen. The eight candidal surface proteins that were found to bind plasminogen did not include enolase. It was also discovered that *C. albicans* cells coated with plasmin did not have increased ability to invade and injure human umbilical vein endothelial cells (Crowe et al., 2003). Therefore, it is possible that plasmin acts as a bridging molecule that induces the endocytosis of *C. albicans* by microvascular brain endothelial cells, but not human umbilical vein endothelial cells.

Experiments with cytochalasin D, which disrupts microfilaments, indicate that intact endothelial cell microfilaments are required for the endocytosis of *C. albicans* hyphae. Additional studies with fluorescently labeled phalloidin, which binds to filamentous actin, demonstrate that during the process of endocytosis, endothelial cell microfilaments surround the portion of the organism that is being internalized. These microfilaments disappear after endocytosis is complete (Filler et al., 1995).

Intact endothelial cell microtubules are also necessary for the endocytosis of *C. albicans*, because agents such as taxol and colchicines that disrupt microtubules inhibit endocytosis of the organism. However, contact with the organism does not induce visible changes in endothelial cells microtubule organization, unlike it does with microfilaments (Filler et al., 1995).

There is substantial evidence that the endothelial cell endocytosis of *C. albicans* is governed by the tyrosine phosphorylation of endothelial cell proteins in vitro. Using indirect immunofluorescence with an anti-phosphotyrosine monoclonal antibody we observed that tyrosine-phosphorylated endothelial cell proteins surround organisms that are being endocytosed. Immunoblotting experiments with the antiphosphotyrosine antibody demonstrate that endocytosis of wild-type *C. albicans* is accompanied by the tyrosine phosphorylation of two endothelial cell proteins with molecular masses of 80 and 82 kDa. The phosphorylation of these proteins is closely associated with the endocytosis of *C. albicans* because these proteins are phosphorylated in response to the endocytosis of both live and killed hyphae, but they are not phosphorylated in endothelial cells infected with a poorly endocytosed strain of *C. albicans*. Furthermore, the broad-spectrum tyrosine kinase inhibitors genistein and tyrphostin 47 block the phosphorylation of the two endothelial cell proteins and significantly reduce endocytosis of *C. albicans* hyphae (Filler et al., 1995). Collectively, these results indicate that *C. albicans* induces its own endocytosis by stimulating the tyrosine phosphorylation of two endothelial cell proteins. The identity of these proteins is currently unknown.

2.3. Endothelial Cell Stimulation

Edwards and colleagues infected endothelial cells with *C. albicans* and then added human neutrophils to the infected monolayer. The interactions among the three different cell types were monitored by videomicroscopy. They observed that the neutrophils were recruited to the foci of infection, where they phagocytized and eventually killed the hyphae. During this process, the endothelial cells were protected from injury, indicating that the neutrophils were activated sufficiently to kill the organisms, but not so much as to injure the endothelial cells (Edwards et al., 1987). These results suggested that there is an exchange of signals between the endothelial cells and neutrophils during their combined response to *C. albicans*.

Subsequently, the response of endothelial cells to *C. albicans* invasion has been investigated, with a focus on responses that have the potential to influence leukocyte function during candidal infection. Endothelial cells respond to *C. albicans* infection in vitro by secreting prostacyclin (Filler et al., 1991, 1994), interleukin-6 (IL-6), IL-8, and monocyte chemoattractant protein 1 (MCP-1) (Filleret al., 1996). In addition, *C. albicans* stimulates endothelial cells to express the leukocyte adhesion molecules, E-selectin, ICAM-1, and vascular cell adherence molecule 1 (VCAM-1) (Filler et al., 1996). It is likely that the production of these pro-inflammatory mediators in vivo contributes to the recruitment of leukocytes to foci of candidal infection.

We have also investigated the mechanisms by which *C. albicans* stimulates a pro-inflammatory response by endothelial cells. Stimulation of endothelial cell IL-8 secretion and leukocyte adhesion molecule expression requires the endocytosis of viable *C. albicans* (Filler et al., 1996). Analysis of *C. albicans* mutants that lack different components of the signal transduction pathways that regulate the yeast-to-hyphal transition have yielded insights into the candidal factors that are required to stimulate endothelial cells. Both a *cph1/cph1* null mutant and an *efg1/efg1* null mutant stimulate endothelial cells to express E-selectin and ICAM-1, whereas an *efg1/efg1 cph1/cph1* double mutant does not. The failure of the double mutant to stimulate endothelial cells is not due to its inability to form hyphae or invade endothelial cells because the *efg1/efg1* null mutant also does not form hyphae on endothelial cells and is endocytosed poorly (Phan et al., 2000). Therefore, some candidal factor under control of Efg1p and Cph1p is required for *C. albicans* to stimulate expression of E-selectin and ICAM-1. The identity of this factor remains to be determined.

Interestingly, different pro-inflammatory endothelial cell responses to *C. albicans* are induced by distinct mechanisms in vitro. We have found that *C. albicans* induces endothelial cells to synthesize TNF-α, which in turn stimulates the infected endothelial cells to secrete IL-8 and express E-selectin. Endothelial cell VCAM-1 expression is induced by a similar autocrine mechanism that involves the combination of TNF-α, IL-1α, and IL-1β, all of which are synthesized by the infected endothelial cells. All three of these cytokines remain predominantly cell-associated. In contrast, induction of ICAM-1 expression is independent of TNF-α, IL-1α, and IL-1β (Orozco et al., 2000). Whether other species of *Candida* are able to induce endothelial cells to synthesize pro-inflammatory mediators via similar mechanisms is currently unknown.

2.4. Endothelial Cell Injury

When human umbilical vein endothelial cells are infected with *C. albicans* in vitro, significant endothelial cell injury is detectable within 2 to 4 h (Edwards et al., 1987; Filler et al., 1991, 1995; Crowe et al., 2003). In contrast, *C. tropicalis* and *C. glabrata* do not cause detectable endothelial cell injury, even after 6 h of incubation (Filler et al., 1991). Two lines of evidence suggest that *C. albicans* cells must be endocytosed by endothelial cells to cause injury. First, treating endothelial cells with cytochalasin D, interferon-γ, or iron chelators blocks endocytosis of *C. albicans* and protects the cells from *C. albicans*-induced injury (Filler et al., 1995; Fratti et al., 1996, 1998). Second, mutants of *C. albicans* that are endocytosed poorly by endothelial cells have reduced capacity to induce endothelial cell injury (Phan et al., 2000).

Surprisingly, although human brain microvascular endothelial cells endocytose *C. albicans* cells, they do not appear to be injured by this organism (Jong et al., 2001). However, the investigations of the interactions of *C. albicans* with brain microvascular endothelial cells were performed under conditions in which the organisms grew only as blastospores and pseudohyphae. These forms of *C. albicans* also cause minimal injury to human umbilical vein endothelial cells (Phan et al., 2000). Therefore, it is not clear whether human brain microvascular endothelial cells are truly more resistant to injury by *C. albicans* than are human umbilical vein endothelial cells.

Endothelial cell injury also requires fungal viability, as killed *C. albicans* cells are endocytosed by human umbilical vein endothelial cells but do not cause injury (Filler et al., 1995). One explanation for these results is that viable *C. albicans* cells must synthesize factors that injure the endothelial cells. *C. albicans* is known to produce a variety of lytic enzymes including secreted aspartyl proteinases (Saps) and phospholipases (Magee et al., 1993; Monod et al., 1994; Hoover et al., 1998; Sugiyama et al., 1999). Most of these enzymes have greatest activity at a low pH, which is likely present within the endothelial cell endocytic vacuole. Consistent with the hypothesis that enzymes secreted by *C. albicans* are responsible for endothelial cell injury, Ibrahim et al. (1998) found that a *sap2/sap2* null mutant had a modest reduction in its capacity to injure endothelial cells.

Other multiple mutants of *C. albicans* have been identified that have reduced capacity to injure endothelial cells (Davis et al., 2000; Phan et al., 2000; Bensen et al., 2002; Blankenship et al., 2003; Sanchez et al., 2004). Many of these mutants have defects in signal transduction pathways that govern hyphal formation (Cla4p, Efg1p, Cph1p, Tec1p) and regulate the pH response (Mds3p, Phr1p, Rim101p). Some of these pathways also govern the secretion of lytic enzymes (Lane et al., 2001; Felk et al., 2002). However, a strain that lacks Czf1p, which forms only short hyphae on the endothelial cells, causes a similar amount of endothelial cell injury as does the wild-type parent strain. Therefore, not all hyphal regulatory pathways govern endothelial cell injury by *C. albicans*. Another strain that has reduced capacity to injure endothelial cells is a *pmt1/pmt1* null mutant, which is defective in *O*-mannosylation of multiple proteins (Timpel et al., 1998). This strain is likely defective in causing endothelial cell injury because the reduced mannosylation of surface proteins prevents the organism from adhering to and invading endothelial cells.

The collective data suggest that induction of endothelial cell injury requires three steps: (1) adherence of *C. albicans* to the endothelial cell, (2) endothelial cell endocytosis of the organism, and (3) secretion of lytic enzymes by *C. albicans*. Therefore, a *C. albicans* mutant that has a defect in any one of these steps is likely to have reduced capacity to cause endothelial cell injury. The ability to injure endothelial cells, and perhaps other host cells, is likely an important virulence factor of *C. albicans*. In support of this hypothesis, we have found that most *C. albicans* mutants that are defective in their capacity to cause endothelial cell injury in vitro also have attenuated virulence in the mouse model of hematogenously disseminated candidiasis (Sanchez et al., 2004). Thus, the interactions of *C. albicans* with endothelial cells in vitro can serve as a model for some aspects of the host–pathogen interaction.

3. *Cryptococcus neoformans*

During the pathogenesis of cryptococcal meningitis, the organisms are inhaled into the alveoli, from which they invade the pulmonary parenchyma and enter the bloodstream. How *Cryptococcus neoformans* traverses from the abluminal to luminal surface of the vasculature and gains access to the bloodstream is currently unknown, but it is possible that the organisms are transported into the vascular lumen inside of leukocytes. This process is distinct from the angioinvasion that occurs during infection with filamentous fungi because there is no evidence that *C. neoformans* grows directly across the blood vessel wall and into the vascular lumen.

3.1. Adherence and Invasion

Once *C. neoformans* cells have entered the bloodstream, they have a predilection for causing infection in the central nervous system. One potential explanation for this tropism is that blood-borne *C. neoformans* cells are specifically able to adhere to and invade the endothelial cell lining of the cerebral vasculature. Chen et al. (2003) reported that both encapsulated and unencapsulated strains of *C. neoformans* adhered to and transcytosed brain microvascular endothelial cells in vitro. Adherent organisms induced ruffling of the endothelial cell plasma membrane, rearrangement of endothelial cell microfilaments, and loss of tight junctions between the endothelial cells. There were also changes in the morphology of the endothelial cell nuclei and mitochondria, which suggested that the endothelial cells were injured by the organisms. Olszewski et al. (2004) demonstrated that production of urease by *C. neoformans* was required for the organism to pass through intact endothelium from the blood to the brain and other tissues. Ibrahim et al. (1995) investigated the interactions of encapsulated and unencapsulated strains of *C. neoformans* with human umbilical vein endothelial cells in vitro. They found that encapsulated strains, which are likely the pathogenic form of the organism, had reduced adherence to and invasion of these endothelial cells. They also caused almost no endothelial cell injury. In contrast, an acapsular strain of *C. neoformans* avidly adhered to and invaded the human umbilical vein cells, and induced significant injury. Although there are significant methodological differences between the studies of the in vitro interactions of *C. neoformans* with brain microvascular and human umbilical vein endothelial cells, it is possible that the organism interacts with these two endothelial cell types differently.

It is known that endothelial cells from different vascular beds express different surface antigens (Ghitescu and Robert, 2002). Also, Prasadarao et al. (1999) found that the K-1 strain of *Escherichia coli*, which causes neonatal meningitis, invades brain microvascular endothelial cells in vitro by binding to a 95-kDa glycoprotein. *E. coli* is unable to invade aortic or human umbilical vein endothelial cells because these cells do not express the glycoprotein receptor for this organism. It is therefore reasonable to hypothesize that the endothelial cells lining the central nervous system vasculature similarly express a surface protein that acts as a receptor for *C. neoformans*. To date, such a receptor has not been identified.

Chrétien et al. (2002) studied the pathogenesis of cerebral cryptococcosis in mice that were inoculated intravenously. They found that the majority of circulating organisms were contained within peripheral blood mononuclear cells. These investigators also used transmission electron microscopy to examine the brains of mice that developed cryptococcal meningitis. They observed that some organisms in the leptomeningeal capillaries appeared to have been internalized by endothelial cells. Interestingly, the organisms that were contained within either endothelial cells or monocyte/macrophages had small capsules, whereas organisms that were free in the tissues had large capsules. Thus, it is possible that during cryptococcal meningitis, organisms with a small capsule initiate hematogenous dissemination and cerebral vascular invasion. The organisms then form large capsules once they are within the brain tissue.

3.2. Endothelial Cell Stimulation

In addition to being targets of cryptococcal adherence and invasion, endothelial cells have the potential to influence the host response to *C. neoformans*. Roseff and Levitz (1993) found that neutrophils and monocytes caused greater growth inhibition of *C. neoformans* when the organisms were in contact with human umbilical vein endothelial cells than when they were on bare plastic. Neutrophil inhibition of *C. neoformans* was enhanced even further when the endothelial cells were prestimulated with IL-1β. The ability of endothelial cells to augment the anti-cryptococcal activity of neutrophils was due in part to enhanced neutrophil survival, as well as an increase in the number of neutrophils that surrounded individual organisms. Although the salutary effects of the endothelial cells on neutrophil function appeared to require direct contact between the endothelial cells and neutrophils, these effects could not be reversed by the addition of neutralizing antibodies directed against E-selectin or ICAM-1. Thus, the mechanism by which endothelial cells enhance the anti-cryptococcal activity of neutrophils remains unclear.

C. neoformans can influence the interactions between leukocytes and endothelial cells. Glucuronoxylomannan (GXM) is a major component of the cryptococcal capsule that circulates in high concentrations in patients with cryptococcosis. Exposure to GXM induces the shedding of L-selectin from the surface of neutrophils and T lymphocytes in vitro (Dong and Murphy, 1996; Dong et al., 1999). In addition, pretreatment of either neutrophils or endothelial cells with GXM reduces neutrophil adherence to endothelial cells in vitro. This reduction in neutrophil adherence is due to reduced binding to E-selectin and ICAM-1 on the endothelial cell surface (Ellerbroek et al., 2002). Finally, it has been found that GXM inhibits the secretion of chemokines by endothelial cells that are stimulated with TNF-α in vitro (Mozaffarian et al., 2000). Collectively, these results suggest that the inhibitory effects of GXM on leukocyte–endothelial cell interactions may contribute to the poor recruitment of leukocytes to foci of cryptococcal infection.

4. *Aspergillus fumigatus*

Aspergillus fumigatus and a handful of other molds, such as the etiologic agents of mucormycosis, are characterized by the unique pathologic finding of prominent angioinvasion. Unlike infections with *C. albicans* or *C. neoformans*, infection with these molds begins as a focal infection, most commonly an invasive pneumonitis. Hyphae within these lesions then grow by extension and invade neighboring blood vessels from the abluminal surface (Denning, 2000; Marret al., 2002). There are two major consequences of this angioinvasion. First, it results in pulmonary hemorrhage and vascular thrombosis at the site of the initial infection. Thrombosis of the pulmonary vasculature leads to tissue infarction, which permits fungi at the center of these infarcted regions to grow unchecked, as there is poor delivery of leukocytes as well as antifungal agents to these areas. Second, angioinvasion is the mechanism by which hyphal fragments disseminate via the bloodstream to other organs, a process that is associated with a dismal prognosis. During both angioinvasion and dissemination to deep organs, the fungi must interact with the endothelial cell lining of the blood vessels to gain entry to and exit from the bloodstream. A schematic illustration of these processes is depicted in Fig. 20.1.

4.1. Interactions with the Abluminal Surface of Endothelial Cells during Angioinvasion

Surprisingly little is known about the mechanisms by which angioinvasion occurs, and all studies of the interactions of *Aspergillus* and endothelial cells have focused on *Aspergillus fumigatus*. Murine models of invasive pulmonary aspergillosis are characterized by prominent invasion of the blood vessels, and can therefore give some insight into the nature of this unique biological process (Sheppard et al., 2004a).

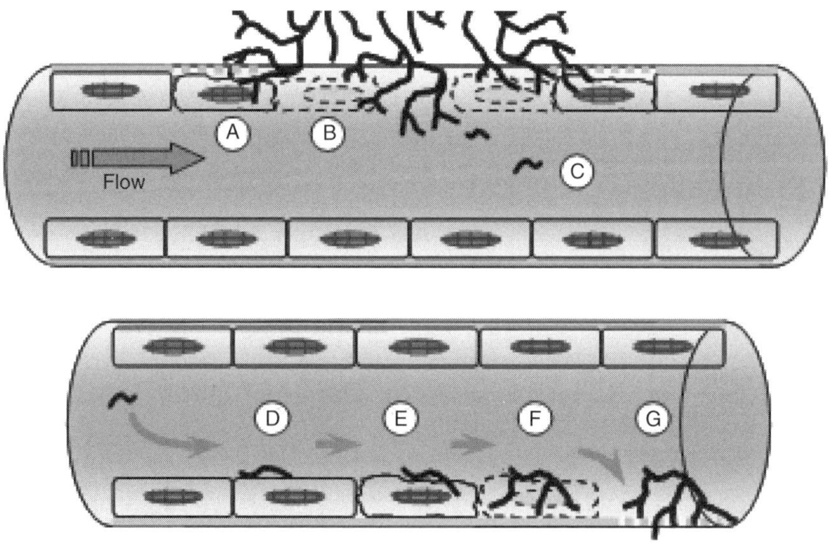

Figure 20.1. Model of angioinvasion and dissemination by *A. fumigatus*. These processes occur via the following steps: (A) abluminal endothelial cell invasion, (B) endothelial cell injury from the abluminal surface, (C) hematogenous dissemination of hyphal fragments, (D) hyphal adherence to the luminal endothelial cell surface, (E) luminal endothelial cell invasion, (F) endothelial cell injury from the luminal surface, and (G) extravascular invasion of deep organs. Steps (A)–(C) occur in the pulmonary blood vessels while steps (D)–(G) occur in the systemic blood vessels.

Histopathologic studies of animals infected with *A. fumigatus* clearly demonstrate prominent abluminal vascular invasion by hyphae (Fig. 20.2A). This invasion is associated with destruction of the endothelial cell lining of these blood vessels, and the development of intravascular thrombosis at the site of invasion. Thrombosis is likely the cause of the tissue infarction and hemorrhage seen on gross pathologic examination. As the mice recover from leukopenia, neutrophil margination within the infected blood vessel can be seen (Fig. 20.2B), indicating that the endothelial cells within the vessel are stimulated to express leukocyte adhesion molecules. Interestingly, this neutrophil margination occurs in locations close to, but not necessarily in direct contact with the actual site of angioinvasion, suggesting that soluble factors may induce this endothelial cell response.

The mechanisms by which *A. fumigatus* hyphae invade the abluminal surface of endothelial cells and the response of endothelial cells to abluminal invasion are completely unknown. While interactions of hyphae with the luminal surface of endothelial cells have been investigated (discussed below; Paris et al., 1997; Taramelli et al., 1996; Lopes-Bezerra and Filler, 2003), very little is known about the interactions of hyphae with the abluminal surface of endothelial cells.

It is known that endothelial cells are polarized. For example, some cell membrane proteins such as the glucose transporter are highly enriched on the abluminal and lateral surfaces of endothelial cells, whereas other proteins such as mast-cell growth factor are present mainly on the luminal surface (Weiss et al., 1995; Virgintino et al., 2000). Further, endothelial cells respond differently to the same stimulus depending on whether it is applied to the luminal or abluminal surface. For instance, endothelial cells exhibit a greater increase in permeability when TNF-α is applied to their luminal surface compared to their abluminal surface (Mark and Miller, 1999). Thus it is likely that the abluminal interactions of hyphae with endothelial cells are different from their luminal interactions.

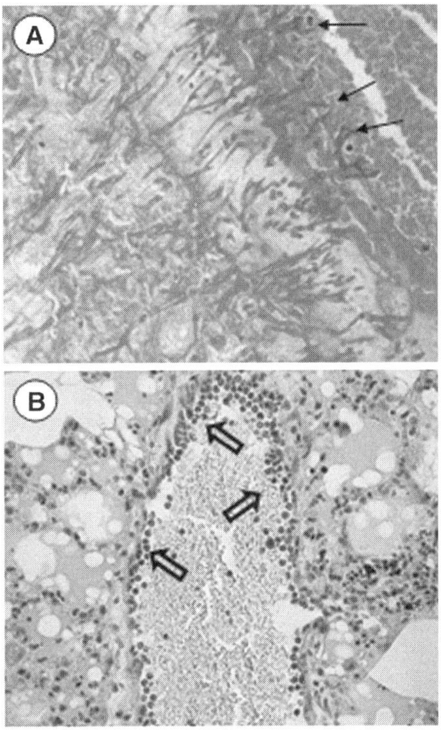

Figure 20.2. Histopathology of invasive pulmonary aspergillosis. Periodic-acid Schiff (PAS) stained thin sections from lungs of mice infected with *A. fumigatus* for 7 and 10 days respectively. (A) Abluminal angioinvasion by hyphae. Note that endothelial cells are absent at the site of the invading hyphae (arrows). (B) Neutrophil margination (open arrows) occurs in the vicinity of *A. fumigatus* lesions. Note that neutrophils have attached to the vessel wall in large numbers, suggesting that these endothelial cells are activated to express leukocyte adhesion molecules.

4.2. Adherence to the Luminal Surface of Endothelial Cells

Once *A. fumigatus* hyphae enter the lumen of the blood vessels, hyphal fragments break off and disseminate throughout the bloodstream to gain access to distal sites of infection such as brain, liver, and spleen. In order for this deep organ infection to develop, the blood-borne hyphal fragments must adhere to the luminal surface of the endothelial cells that line the vasculature of the target organs before invading into the deep tissues. While *A. fumigatus* conidia have been reported to adhere to a type II pneumocyte cell line (DeHart et al., 1997) and pulmonary alveolar macrophages (Kan and Bennett, 1988), surprisingly little is known about the adherence of hyphae to vascular endothelial cells. We recently discovered that hyphae are at least eightfold more adherent to endothelial cells than are conidia in vitro (Chiang et al., 2004), and that hyphae, but not conidia, bind to specific endothelial cell membrane proteins.

It is also possible that during dissemination, blood-borne hyphal fragments adhere to subendothelial extracellular matrix constituents. Indeed, conidia have been shown to adhere to laminin, collagen, fibronectin, and fibrinogen in vitro (Kan and Bennett, 1988; Bromley and Donaldson, 1996; Gil et al., 1996; Penalver et al., 1996; Bouchara et al., 1997; DeHart et al., 1997; Wasylnka and Moore, 2000). Cross-blocking of adherence can be achieved between some of these matrix proteins, suggesting that conidia likely express receptors that are capable of binding multiple substrates (Gil et al., 1996). In contrast, we have found that hyphae adhere avidly to fibronectin and laminin, but only poorly to Type I collagen. Thus, the ligands mediating hyphal adherence are likely different from those mediating adherence of conidia, although the relative contribution of subendothelial cell matrix proteins to the adherence of blood-borne hyphal fragments is unknown.

4.3. Invasion through the Luminal Endothelial Cell Surface

After blood-borne *A. fumigatus* hyphae adhere to endothelial cells, they must penetrate through the luminal surface of these cells to escape from the blood vessel and invade the deep tissues. Both *A. fumigatus* conidia and hyphae are able to invade the luminal surface of human umbilical vein endothelial cells in vitro (Paris et al., 1997; Wasylnka and Moore, 2002; Lopes-Bezerra and Filler, 2004). However, given that only hyphae and not conidia are seen in foci of invasive aspergillosis, the physiological relevance of conidial–endothelial cell interactions is uncertain. The invasion of the luminal surface of endothelial cells by *A. fumigatus* hyphae in vitro is relatively rapid, occurring after 45 min of infection. Addition of cytochalasin D, a microfilament inhibitor, causes an 80% reduction in their uptake, indicating that hyphae are actively endocytosed by endothelial cells. This hypothesis is also consistent with the results of microfilament staining, which demonstrates that endocytosis of hyphae is accompanied by the polymerization of endothelial cell actin around the organisms, which disappears after endocytosis is complete (Lopes-Bezerra and Filler, 2004).

4.4. Endothelial Cell Injury during Luminal Infection

A. fumigatus hyphae induce endothelial cell injury when they are added to the luminal surface of these cells (Lopes-Bezerra and Filler, 2004). Viable hyphae cause significant endothelial cell injury after 8 h of infection. Surprisingly, killed *A. fumigatus* hyphae induce the same degree of injury as do live hyphae, suggesting that injury is induced by a pre-formed component of the fungal cell. This finding is markedly different from what we have observed with *C. albicans*, which must be viable to induce any endothelial cell injury (Filler et al., 1995). Endothelial cell injury by *A. fumigatus* hyphae was reduced by 89% when cytochalasin D was added to the medium, and completely abrogated when tissue culture inserts were interposed between the endothelial cells and the hyphae (Lopes-Bezerra and Filler, 2004). These results indicate that *A. fumigatus* must be endocytosed to cause endothelial cell injury.

4.5. Endothelial Cell Stimulation

The presence of thrombosis and dramatic neutrophil margination at sites of infection with *A. fumigatus* suggests that endothelial cells are activated to express procoagulant factors as well as leukocyte adhesion molecules. Indeed, hyphae added to the luminal surface of endothelial cells in vitro induce the expression of tissue factor activity by these cells (Lopes-Bezerra and Filler, 2004). Additionally, we have recently found that, under similar conditions, hyphae strongly induce the surface expression of E-selectin, weakly induce expression of VCAM-1, but do not induce expression of intracellular adhesion molecule 1 (ICAM-1). In contrast, conidia do not induce the expression of any of the leukocyte adhesion molecules or tissue factor activity. The response of endothelial cells to *A. fumigatus* hyphae is significantly different from their response to *C. albicans*, which induces the expression of all three leukocyte adhesion molecules, but not tissue factor (Orozco et al., 2000; Lopes-Bezerra and Filler, 2004). The expression of E-selectin and VCAM-1 by endothelial cells infected with *A. fumigatus* hyphae on their luminal surface likely assists the recruitment of leukocytes to foci of hematogenous infection. Also, the increased tissue factor activity of the infected endothelial cells may contribute to the intravascular thrombosis that is characteristic of disseminated aspergillosis.

5. Other Fungi

There is one report of the ability of *S. schenckii* to adhere to and invade human umbilical vein endothelial cells in vitro (Figueiredo et al., 2004). This organism rapidly adheres to endothelial cells. It invades endothelial cells by inducing its own endocyotsis, which is largely complete within 90 min of infections. *S. schenckii* likely binds to an inducible molecule on the endothelial cell surface because the number of organisms that are cell-associated (adherent plus endocytosed) with the endothelial cells is increased when the endothelial cells are stimulated with IL-1β. Interestingly, internalized *S. schenckii* cells do not induce detectable endothelial cell injury even after 24 h of infection. This result suggests the possibility that *S. schenckii* may be able to persist in endothelial cells in vivo.

Other fungi that can cause a hematogenously disseminated infection include *C. immitis*, *H. capsulatum*, and *B. dermatitidis*. All of these organisms likely initiate foci of pneumonitis and then spread via the bloodstream to other organs. During the process of dissemination, they must interact with endothelial cells. However, the interactions of these fungi with endothelial cells have not yet been reported.

References

Alaei, S., Larcher, C., Ebenbichler, C., Prodinger, W.M., Janatova, J., and Dierich, M.P. (1993). Isolation and biochemical characterization of the iC3b receptor of *Candida albicans*. *Infect. Immun.* 61: 1395–1399.

Bensen, E.S., Filler, S.G., and Berman, J. (2002). A forkhead transcription factor is important for true hyphal as well as yeast morphogenesis in *Candida albicans*. *Eukaryot. Cell* 1: 787–798.

Blankenship, J.R., Wormley, F.L., Boyce, M.K., Schell, W.A., Filler, S.G., Perfect, J.R., and Heitman, J. (2003). Calcineurin is essential for *Candida albicans* survival in serum and virulence. *Eukaryot. Cell* 2: 422–430.

Bouchara, J.P., Sanchez, M., Chevailler, A., Marot-Leblond, A., Lissitzky, J.C., Tronchin, G., and Chabasse, D. (1997). Sialic acid-dependent recognition of laminin and fibrinogen by *Aspergillus fumigatus* conidia. *Infect. Immun.* 65: 2717–2724.

Bromley, I.M. and Donaldson, K. (1996). Binding of *Aspergillus fumigatus* spores to lung epithelial cells and basement membrane proteins: Relevance to the asthmatic lung. *Thorax* 51: 1203–1209.

Cannom, R.R.M., French, S.W., Johnston, D., Edwards, J.E. Jr., and Filler, S.G. (2002). *Candida albicans* stimulates local expression of leukocyte adhesion molecules and cytokines in vivo. *J. Infect. Dis.* 186: 389–396.

Chen, S.H., Stins, M.F., Huang, S.H., Chen, Y.H., Kwon-Chung, K.J., Chang, Y., Kim, K.S., Suzuki, K., and Jong, A.Y. (2003). *Cryptococcus neoformans* induces alterations in the cytoskeleton of human brain microvascular endothelial cells. *J. Med. Microbiol.* 52: 961–970.

Chiang, L.Y., Sheppard, D.C., Edwards, J.E. Jr., and Filler, S.G. (2004, Abstract F-102). *Aspergillus fumigatus* adherence to and stimulation of endothelial cells in vitro. Paper presented at the 104th General Meeting of the American Society for Microbiology, New Orleans, LA.

Chretien, F., Lortholary, O., Kansau, I., Neuville, S., Gray, F., and Dromer, F. (2002). Pathogenesis of cerebral *Cryptococcus neoformans* infection after fungemia. *J. Infect. Dis.* 186: 522–530.

Crowe, J.D., Sievwright, I.K., Auld, G.C., Moore, N.R., Gow, N.A.R., and Booth, N.A. (2003). *Candida albicans* binds human plasminogen: Identification of eight plasminogen-binding proteins. *Mol. Microbiol.* 47: 1637–1651.

Davis, S.L., Hawkins, E.P., Mason, E.O. Jr., Smith, C.W., and Kaplan, S.L. (1996). Host defenses against disseminated candidiasis are impaired in intercellular adhesion molecule 1-deficient mice. *J. Infect. Dis.* 174: 435–439.

Davis, D., Edwards, J.E. Jr., Mitchell, A.P., and Ibrahim, A.S. (2000). *Candida albicans RIM101* pH response pathway is required for host–pathogen interactions. *Infect. Immun.* 68: 5953–5959.

DeHart, D.J., Agwu, D.E., Julian, N.C., and Washburn, R.G. (1997). Binding and germination of *Aspergillus fumigatus* conidia on cultured A549 pneumocytes. *J. Infect. Dis.* 175: 146–150.

Denning, D.W. (2000). *Aspergillus* species. In G.L. Mandell, J.E. Bennett, and R. Dolin (eds), *Mandell, Douglas, and Bennett's Principles and Practice of Infectious Diseases*, 5th edn. Churchill Livingstone, Philadelphia, pp. 2674–2684.

Dong, Z.M. and Murphy, J.W. (1996). Cryptococcal polysaccharides induce L-selectin shedding and tumor necrosis factor receptor loss from the surface of human neutrophils. *J. Clin. Invest.* 97: 689–698.

Dong, Z.M., Jackson, L., and Murphy, J.W. (1999). Mechanisms for induction of L-selectin loss from T lymphocytes by a cryptococcal polysaccharide, glucuronoxylomannan. *Infect. Immun.* 67: 220–229.

Edwards, J.E. Jr., Gaither, T.A., O'Shea, J.J., Rotrosen, D., Lawley, T.J., Wright, S.A., Frank, M.M., and Green, I. (1986). Expression of specific binding sites on *Candida* with functional and antigenic characteristics of human complement receptors. *J. Immunol.* 137: 3577–3583.

Edwards, J.E. Jr., Rotrosen, D., Fontaine, J.W., Haudenschild, C.C., and Diamond, R.D. (1987). Neutrophil-mediated protection of cultured human vascular endothelial cells from damage by growing *Candida albicans* hyphae. *Blood* 69: 1450–1457.

Ellerbroek, P.M., Hoepelman, A.I., Wolbers, F., Zwaginga, J.J., and Coenjaerts, F.E. (2002). Cryptococcal glucuronoxylomannan inhibits adhesion of neutrophils to stimulated endothelium in vitro by affecting both neutrophils and endothelial cells. *Infect. Immun.* 70: 4762–4771.

Felk, A., Kretschmar, M., Albrecht, A., Schaller, M., Beinhauer, S., Nichterlein, T., Sanglard, D., Korting, H.C., Schafer, W., and Hube, B. (2002). *Candida albicans* hyphal formation and the expression of the Efg1-regulated proteinases Sap4 to Sap6 are required for the invasion of parenchymal organs. *Infect. Immun.* 70: 3689–3700.

Figueiredo, C.C., De Lima, O.C., De Carvalho, L., Lopes-Bezerra, L.M., and Morandi, V. (2004). The in vitro interaction of *Sporothrix schenckii* with human endothelial cells is modulated by cytokines and involves endothelial surface molecules. *Microb. Pathog.* 36: 177–188.

Filler, S.G., Ibe, B.O., Luckett, P.M., Raj, J.U., and Edwards, J.E. Jr. (1991). *Candida albicans* stimulates endothelial cell eicosanoid production. *J. Infect. Dis.* 164: 928–935.

Filler, S.G., Ibe, B.O., Ibrahim, A.S., Ghannoum, M.A., Raj, J.U., and Edwards, J.E. Jr. (1994). Mechanisms by which *Candida albicans* induces endothelial cell prostaglandin synthesis. *Infect. Immun.* 62: 1064–1069.

Filler, S.G., Swerdloff, J.N., Hobbs, C., and Luckett, P.M. (1995). Penetration and damage of endothelial cells by *Candida albicans*. *Infect. Immun.* 63: 976–983.

Filler, S.G., Pfunder, A.S., Spellberg, B.J., Spellberg, J.P., and Edwards, J.E. Jr. (1996). *Candida albicans* stimulates cytokine production and leukocyte adhesion molecule expression by endothelial cells. *Infect. Immun.* 64: 2609–2617.

Fratti, R.A., Ghannoum, M.A., Edwards, J.E. Jr., and Filler, S.G. (1996). Gamma interferon protects endothelial cells from damage by *Candida albicans* by inhibiting endothelial cell phagocytosis. *Infect. Immun.* 64: 4714–4718.

Fratti, R.A., Belanger, P.H., Ghannoum, M.A., Edwards, J.E. Jr., and Filler, S.G. (1998). Endothelial cell injury caused by *Candida albicans* is dependent on iron. *Infect. Immun.* 66: 191–196.

Fu, Y., Rieg, G., Fonzi, W.A., Belanger, P.H., Edwards, J.E. Jr., and Filler, S.G. (1998). Expression of the *Candida albicans* gene *ALS1* in *Saccharomyces cerevisiae* induces adherence to endothelial and epithelial cells. *Infect. Immun.* 66: 1783–1786.

Fu, Y., Ibrahim, A.S., Sheppard, D.C., Chen, Y.C., French, S.W., Cutler, J.E., Filler, S.G., and Edwards, J.E. (2002). *Candida albicans* Als1p: An adhesin that is a downstream effector of the *EFG1* filamentation pathway. *Mol. Microbiol.* 44: 61–72.

Gale, C., Finkel, D., Tao, N., Meinke, M., McClellan, M., Olson, J., Kendrick, K., and Hostetter, M. (1996). Cloning and expression of a gene encoding an integrin-like protein in *Candida albicans*. *Proc. Natl. Acad. Sci. USA* 93: 357–361.

Gale, C.A., Bendel, C.M., McClellan, M., Hauser, M., Becker, J.M., Berman, J., and Hostetter, M.K. (1998). Linkage of adhesion, filamentous growth, and virulence in *Candida albicans* to a single gene, *INT1*. *Science* 279: 1355–1358.

Gaur, N.K. and Klotz, S.A. (1997). Expression, cloning, and characterization of a *Candida albicans* gene, *ALA1*, that confers adherence properties upon *Saccharomyces cerevisiae* for extracellular matrix proteins. *Infect. Immun.* 65: 5289–5294.

Gaur, N.K., Klotz, S.A., and Henderson, R.L. (1999). Overexpression of the *Candida albicans* *ALA1* gene in *Saccharomyces cerevisiae* results in aggregation following attachment of yeast cells to extracellular matrix proteins, adherence properties similar to those of *Candida albicans*. *Infect. Immun.* 67: 6040–6047.

Ghitescu, L. and Robert, M. (2002). Diversity in unity: The biochemical composition of the endothelial cell surface varies between the vascular beds. *Microsc. Res. Tech.* 57: 381–389.

Gil, M.L., Penalver, M.C., Lopez-Ribot, J.L., O'Connor, J.E., and Martinez, J.P. (1996). Binding of extracellular matrix proteins to *Aspergillus fumigatus* conidia. *Infect. Immun.* 64: 5239–5247.

Gilmore, B.J., Retsinas, E.M., Lorenz, J.S., and Hostetter, M.K. (1988). An iC3b receptor on *Candida albicans*: Structure, function, and correlates for pathogenicity. *J. Infect. Dis.* 157: 38–46.

Glee, P.M., Cutler, J.E., Benson, E.E., Bargatze, R.F., and Hazen, K.C. (2001). Inhibition of hydrophobic protein-mediated *Candida albicans* attachment to endothelial cells during physiologic shear flow. *Infect. Immun.* 69: 2815–2820.

Hajjeh, R.A., Sofair, A.N., Harrison, L.H., Lyon, G.M., Arthington-Skaggs, B.A., Mirza, S.A., Phelan, M., Morgan, J., Lee-Yang, W., Ciblak, M.A., Benjamin, L.E., Sanza, L.T., Huie, S., Yeo, S.F., Brandt, M.E., and Warnock, D.W. (2004). Incidence of bloodstream infections due to *Candida* species and in vitro susceptibilities of isolates collected from 1998 to 2000 in a population-based active surveillance program. *J. Clin. Microbiol.* 42: 1519–1527.

Hoover, C.I., Jantapour, M.J., Newport, G., Agabian, N., and Fisher, S.J. (1998). Cloning and regulated expression of the *Candida albicans phospholipase B* (*PLB1*) gene. *FEMS Microbiol. Lett.* 167: 163–169.

Hoyer, L.L. and Hecht, J.E. (2000). The *ALS6* and *ALS7* genes of *Candida albicans*. *Yeast* 16: 847–855.

Hoyer, L.L. and Hecht, J.E. (2001). The *ALS5* gene of *Candida albicans* and analysis of the Als5p N-terminal domain. *Yeast* 18: 49–60.

Hoyer, L.L., Scherer, S., Shatzman, A.R., and Livi, G.P. (1995). *Candida albicans ALS1*: Domains related to a *Saccharomyces cerevisiae* sexual agglutinin separated by a repeating motif. *Mol. Microbiol.* 15: 39–54.

Hoyer, L.L., Payne, T.L., Bell, M., Myers, A.M., and Scherer, S. (1998a). *Candida albicans ALS3* and insights into the nature of the *ALS* gene family. *Curr. Genet.* 33: 451–459.

Hoyer, L.L., Payne, T.L., and Hecht, J.E. (1998b). Identification of *Candida albicans ALS2* and *ALS4* and localization of als proteins to the fungal cell surface. *J. Bacteriol.* 180: 5334–5343.

Ibrahim, A.S., Filler, S.G., Alcouloumre, M.S., Kozel, T.R., Edwards, J.E. Jr., and Ghannoum, M.A. (1995). Adherence to and damage of endothelial cells by *Cryptococcus neoformans* in vitro: Role of the capsule. *Infect. Immun.* 63: 4368–4374.

Ibrahim, A.S., Filler, S.G., Sanglard, D., Edwards, J.E. Jr., and Hube, B. (1998). Secreted aspartyl proteinases and interactions of *Candida albicans* with human endothelial cells. *Infect. Immun.* 66: 3003–3005.

Jong, A.Y., Stins, M.F., Huang, S.H., Chen, S.H., and Kim, K.S. (2001). Traversal of *Candida albicans* across human blood-brain barrier in vitro. *Infect. Immun.* 69: 4536–4544.

Jong, A.Y., Chen, S.H.M., Stins, M.F., Kim, K.S., Tuan, T.-L., and Huang, S.-H. (2003). Binding of *Candida albicans* enolase to plasmin(ogen) results in enhanced invasion of human brain microvascular endothelial cells. *J. Med. Microbiol.* 52: 615–622.

Kan, V.L. and Bennett, J.E. (1988). Lectin-like attachment sites on murine pulmonary alveolar macrophages bind *Aspergillus fumigatus* conidia. *J. Infect. Dis.* 158: 407–414.

Klotz, S.A., Drutz, D.J., Harrison, J.L., and Huppert, M. (1983). Adherence and penetration of vascular endothelium by *Candida* yeasts. *Infect. Immun.* 42: 374–384.

Klotz, S.A., Pendrak, M.L., and Hein, R.C. (2001). Antibodies to alpha5beta1 and alpha(v)beta3 integrins react with *Candida albicans* alcohol dehydrogenase. *Microbiology* 147: 3159–3164.

Klotz, S.A., Gaur, N.K., Lake, D.F., Chan, V., Rauceo, J., and Lipke, P.N. (2004). Degenerate peptide recognition by *Candida albicans* adhesins Als5p and Als1p. *Infect. Immun.* 72: 2029–2034.

Lane, S., Birse, C., Zhou, S., Matson, R., and Liu, H. (2001). DNA array studies demonstrate convergent regulation of virulence factors by Cph1, Cph2, and Efg1 in *Candida albicans. J. Biol. Chem.* 276: 48988–48996.

Lee, K.H., Yoon, M.S., and Chun, W.H. (1997). The effects of monoclonal antibodies against iC3b receptors in mice with experimentally induced disseminated candidiasis. *Immunology* 92: 104–110.

Lopes-Bezerra, L.M. and Filler, S.G. (2004). Interactions of *Aspergillus fumigatus* with endothelial cells: Internalization, injury, and stimulation of tissue factor activity. *Blood.* 103: 2143–2149.

Loza, L., Fu, Y., Ibrahim, A.S., Sheppard, D.C., Filler, S.G., and Edwards, J.E. Jr. (2004). Functional analysis of the *Candida albicans ALS1* gene product. *Yeast* 21: 473–482.

Magee, B.B., Hube, B., Wright, R.J., Sullivan, P.J., and Magee, P.T. (1993). The genes encoding the secreted aspartyl proteinases of *Candida albicans* constitute a family with at least three members. *Infect. Immun.* 61: 3240–3243.

Mark, K.S. and Miller, D.W. (1999). Increased permeability of primary cultured brain microvessel endothelial cell monolayers following TNF-alpha exposure. *Life Sci.* 64: 1941–1953.

Marr, K.A., Patterson, T., and Denning, D. (2002). Aspergillosis. Pathogenesis, clinical manifestations, and therapy. *Infect. Dis. Clin. North Am.* 16: 875–894.

Monod, M., Togni, G., Hube, B., and Sanglard, D. (1994). Multiplicity of genes encoding secreted aspartic proteinases in *Candida* species. *Mol. Microbiol.* 13: 357–368.

Mozaffarian, N., Casadevall, A., and Berman, J.W. (2000). Inhibition of human endothelial cell chemokine production by the opportunistic fungal pathogen *Cryptococcus neoformans. J. Immunol.* 165: 1541–1547.

Olszewski, M.A., Noverr, M.C., Chen, G.H., Toews, G.B., Cox, G.M., Perfect, J.R., and Huffnagle, G.B. (2004). Urease expression by *Cryptococcus neoformans* promotes microvascular sequestration, thereby enhancing central nervous system invasion. *Am. J. Pathol.* 164: 1761–1771.

Orozco, A.S., Zhou, X., and Filler, S.G. (2000). Mechanisms of the pro-inflammatory response of endothelial cells to *Candida albicans* infection. *Infect. Immun.* 68: 1134–1141.

Paris, S., Boisvieux-Ulrich, E., Crestani, B., Houcine, O., Taramelli, D., Lombardi, L., and Latge, J.P. (1997). Internalization of *Aspergillus fumigatus* conidia by epithelial and endothelial cells. *Infect. Immun.* 65: 1510–1514.

Penalver, M.C., O'Connor, J.E., Martinez, J.P., and Gil, M.L. (1996). Binding of human fibronectin to *Aspergillus fumigatus* conidia. *Infect. Immun.* 64: 1146–1153.

Phan, Q.T., Belanger, P.H., and Filler, S.G. (2000). Role of hyphal formation in interactions of *Candida albicans* with endothelial cells. *Infect. Immun.* 68: 3485–3490.

Prasadarao, N.V., Wass, C.A., Huang, S.H., and Kim, K.S. (1999). Identification and characterization of a novel Ibe10 binding protein that contributes to *Escherichia coli* invasion of brain microvascular endothelial cells. *Infect. Immun.* 67: 1131–1138.

Roseff, S.A. and Levitz, S.M. (1993). Effect of endothelial cells on phagocyte-mediated anticryptococcal activity. *Infect. Immun.* 61: 3818–3824.

Rotrosen, D., Edwards, J.E. Jr., Gibson, T.R., Moore, J.C., Cohen, A.H., and Green, I. (1985). Adherence of *Candida* to cultured vascular endothelial cells: Mechanisms of attachment and endothelial cell penetration. *J. Infect. Dis.* 152: 1264–1274.

Sanchez, A.A., Johnston, D.A., Myers, C., Edwards, J.E. Jr., Mitchell, A.P., and Filler, S.G. (2004). Relationship between *Candida albicans* virulence during experimental hematogenously disseminated Infection and endothelial cell damage in vitro. *Infect. Immun.* 72: 598–601.

Santoni, G., Spreghini, E., Lucciarini, R., Amantini, C., and Piccoli, M. (2001). Involvement of alpha(v)beta3 integrin-like receptor and glycosaminoglycans in *Candida albicans* germ tube adhesion to vitronectin and to a human endothelial cell line. *Microb. Pathog.* 31: 159–172.

Santoni, G., Lucciarini, R., Amantini, C., Jacobelli, J., Spreghini, E., Ballarini, P., Piccoli, M., and Gismondi, A. (2002). *Candida albicans* expresses a focal adhesion kinase-like protein that undergoes increased tyrosine phosphorylation upon yeast cell adhesion to vitronectin and the EA.hy 926 human endothelial cell line. *Infect. Immun.* 70: 3804–3815.

Sheppard, D.C., Rieg, G., Chiang, L.Y., Filler, S.G., Edwards, J.E. Jr., and Ibrahim, A.S. (2004a). Novel inhalational murine model of invasive pulmonary aspergillosis. *Antimicrob. Agents Chemother.* 48: 1908–1911.

Sheppard, D.C., Yeaman, M.R., Welch, W.H., Phan, Q.T., Fu, Y., Ibrahim, A.S., Filler, S.G., Zhang, M., Waring, A.J., and Edwards, J.E. Jr. (2004b). Functional and structural diversity in the Als protein family of *Candida albicans*. *J. Biol. Chem.* (in press).

Singleton, D.R. and Hazen, K.C. (2004). Differential surface localization and temperature-dependent expression of the *Candida albicans* CSH1 protein. *Microbiology* 150: 285–292.

Singleton, D.R., Masuoka, J., and Hazen, K.C. (2001). Cloning and analysis of a *Candida albicans* gene that affects cell surface hydrophobicity. *J. Bacteriol.* 183: 3582–3588.

Spreghini, E., Gismondi, A., Piccoli, M., and Santoni, G. (1999). Evidence for alphavbeta3 and alphavbeta5 integrin-like vitronectin (VN) receptors in *Candida albicans* and their involvement in yeast cell adhesion to VN. *J. Infect. Dis.* 180: 156–166.

Sugiyama, Y., Nakashima, S., Mirbod, F., Kanoh, H., Kitajima, Y., Ghannoum, M.A., and Nozawa, Y. (1999). Molecular cloning of a second phospholipase B gene, *caPLB2* from *Candida albicans*. *Med. Mycol.* 37: 61–67.

Taramelli, D., Sala, G., Malabarba, M.G., Malacarne, F., Saresella, M., Ferrante, P., Frigerio, S., and Lombardi, L. (1996). *Aspergillus fumigatus* conidia adhere and activate human endothelial cells. *Mikol. Lek.* 3: 75–81.

Timpel, C., Strahl-Bolsinger, S., Ziegelbauer, K., and Ernst, J.F. (1998). Multiple functions of Pmt1p-mediated protein *O*-mannosylation in the fungal pathogen *Candida albicans*. *J. Biol. Chem.* 273: 20837–20846.

Virgintino, D., Robertson, D., Benagiano, V., Errede, M., Bertossi, M., Ambrosi, G., and Roncali, L. (2000). Immunogold cytochemistry of the blood–brain barrier glucose transporter GLUT1 and endogenous albumin in the developing human brain. *Brain Res. Dev. Brain Res.* 123: 95–101.

Wasylnka, J.A. and Moore, M.M. (2000). Adhesion of *Aspergillus* species to extracellular matrix proteins: Evidence for involvement of negatively charged carbohydrates on the conidial surface. *Infect. Immun.* 68: 3377–3384.

Wasylnka, J.A. and Moore, M.M. (2002). Uptake of *Aspergillus fumigatus* conidia by phagocytic and nonphagocytic cells in vitro: Quantitation using strains expressing green fluorescent protein. *Infect. Immun.* 70: 3156–3163.

Weiss, R.R., Whitaker-Menezes, D., Longley, J., Bender, J., and Murphy, G.F. (1995). Human dermal endothelial cells express membrane-associated mast cell growth factor. *J. Invest. Dermatol.* 104: 101–106.

Yokomura, I., Iwasaki, Y., Nagata, K., Nakanishi, M., Natsuhara, A., Harada, H., Kubota, Y., Ueda, M., Inaba, T., and Nakagawa, M. (2001). Role of intercellular adhesion molecule 1 in acute lung injury induced by candidemia. *Exp. Lung Res.* 27: 417–431.

21

Immunology of Cutaneous Candidiasis

Srividya Srinivasan, David K. Wagner, and Peter G. Sohnle

Division of Infectious Diseases, Department of Medicine, Medical College of Wisconsin, Milwaukee, WI.
Infectious Diseases Section, Consultant Care Division, VA Medical Center, Milwaukee, WI.

1. Introduction

This chapter will review the major mechanisms involved in the defense against cutaneous candidiasis. In the latter condition the epidermis of the skin is infected by *Candida albicans* and occasionally certain non-*C. albicans* species, with chronic mucocutaneous candidiasis representing a subgroup of syndromes with particularly chronic and recalcitrant cutaneous, nail and mucosal *Candida* infections. Local and systemic defenses against *Candida* and cutaneous candidiasis will be reviewed with an emphasis on innate immunity and the immunological predispositions that have been described in chronic mucocutaneous candidiasis. In particular, this discussion will cover the elements of the cutaneous immune system, the mechanisms of immunologic deficits in chronic mucocutaneous candidiasis, and the role of cytokines in the defense against cutaneous *Candida* infections. Implications for possible reversal of the immunologic abnormalities as an adjunct to the use of antifungal drugs for the treatment of chronic mucocutaneous candidiasis will also be addressed.

2. Characteristics of Cutaneous Candidiasis

Cutaneous candidiasis is an infection of the skin that is generally caused by the fungus *C. albicans* and which can be either acute or chronic in nature. Cases are sometimes seen of cutaneous candidiasis caused by other *Candida* species, including *C. parapsilosis* or *C. tropicalis*, but these are rare. Recently, *C. glabrata* has developed increased importance as a cause of human disease and currently ranks second or third as the agent of superficial (cutaneous or mucosal) or deep candidiasis (Fidel et al., 1999). *C. albicans* is part of the normal flora of the gastrointestinal (GI) tract rather than that of the skin, although it can be found on the skin occasionally. This organism can grow as either yeast cells or filamentous forms, with mixtures of the two phases often seen in the cutaneous infections. The virulence of *C. albicans* has been attributed variously to its ability to grow at particular temperatures, its ability to produce filamentous forms, its adherence capabilities, and the activity of its different enzymes.

Acute cutaneous candidiasis may present as intertrigo with production of intense erythema, edema, creamy exudate, and satellite pustules within folds of the skin. Other infections may be more chronic, as in the feet where there can be a thick white layer of infected stratum corneum overlaying the epidermis of the interdigital spaces. *Candida* paronychia is marked by infections of the periungual skin and the nail itself, resulting in the typical swelling and redness of this type of *Candida* infection.

In some cases superficial *C. albicans* infections may be particularly severe and recalcitrant to treatment, producing the uncommon disorder known as chronic mucocutaneous candidiasis. This condition consists of persistent and recurrent infections of the mucous membranes, skin and nails, along with a variety of other manifestations. The superficial infections last for years in the affected patients unless they are properly treated; however, deep *Candida* infections are very rare in this situation (Kauffman et al., 1981). Oral thrush and *Candida* vaginitis are fairly common in patients with chronic mucocutaneous candidiasis. There is often infection of the esophagus, although further extension into the viscera is unusual. The typical skin lesions are generally red, raised, and hyperkeratotic, but usually are not painful. Epidermal neutrophilic microabscesses, which are common in acute cutaneous candidiasis, are rare in the lesions of chronic mucocutaneous candidiasis. Nail involvement can be severe in this condition, producing marked thickening, distortion, and fragmentation of the nails, with chronic swelling of the distal phalanx. The oral thrush and vaginitis in chronic mucocutaneous candidiasis closely resemble the acute mucous membrane infections in other patients, except that they are more chronic in nature. The oral lesions are generally tender and painful.

There are a number of other disorders that are associated with the syndrome of chronic mucocutaneous candidiasis (Kirkpatrick and Sohnle, 1981; Filler and Edwards, 1993). Especially prominent are certain types of endocrine dysfunction, such as hypoadrenalism, hypoparathyroidism, hypothyroidism, ovarian insufficiency, pernicious anemia, and diabetes mellitus. The combination of chronic superficial candidiasis and endocrine hypofunction has been termed the "*Candida* endocrinopathy" syndrome. More recently the term autoimmune polyendocrinopathy-candidiasis-ectodermal dystrophy (APECED) has been used to describe this syndrome (Bjorses et al., 2000). A particular gene, AIRE (for autoimmune regulator), appears to be responsible for this syndrome in both humans and mice (Rosatelli et al., 1998; Mittaz et al., 1999). The product of the AIRE gene is predicted as a proline-rich polypeptide with two zinc-finger motifs and a putative nuclear targeting signal, suggesting involvement in the regulation of transcription; this protein is expressed in the thymus, as well as the pancreas and adrenal cortex, and may be involved in the molecular pathogenesis of APECED and other types of autoimmunity (Bjorses et al., 1998).

Sometimes found in patients with chronic mucocutaneous candidiasis are alopecia totalis, vitiligo, malabsorption, chronic hepatitis, dysplasia of the dental enamel, congenital thymic dysplasia, thymomas, and other infections. Amongst the latter, chronic dermatophytosis, recurrent bacterial infections, and occasional opportunistic infections such as cryptococcosis, histoplasmosis, and *Pneumocystis carinii* pneumonia are the most common (Kirkpatrick et al., 1971; Filler and Edwards, 1993; Eppinger et al., 1999). In these patients dermatophytosis may cause extensive skin lesions that may be misidentified as cutaneous candidiasis and then perhaps not be treated optimally (Chappler et al., 1978). Chronic mucocutaneous candidiasis no doubt represents a group of syndromes, in addition to APECED, with a variety of predisposing or secondary abnormalities in host defense function. Therefore it may be difficult to describe an immunologic pattern that includes all patients. The most common deficiency appears to be one of cell-mediated immune responses against *Candida* antigens, as discussed below, although abnormalities in chemotaxis or phagocytic cell function have also been reported; other host defense mechanisms, such as humoral immunity and the complement system, are generally normal in these patients, with some exceptions.

Although the superficial infections of chronic mucocutaneous candidiasis are generally not life threatening, they can be very disfiguring. Before the azole antifungal agents became available, the treatment of this condition was quite difficult. Whereas amphotericin B produced prompt clearance of the cutaneous lesions, relapses usually occurred, presumably because of the underlying immunodeficiency state. At present, long-term treatment with azole antifungal drugs can produce good results in chronic mucocutaneous candidiasis, although occasional failures have occurred due to the development of resistant strains of *C. albicans.* Also, endocrine dysfunction, including life-threatening adrenal crises, can develop after presentation of the candidiasis, so these patients need to be followed for this possibility. Patients who present with chronic mucocutaneous candidiasis should also be evaluated for the presence of infection with the human immunodeficiency virus (HIV), and if presenting as adults, for the possibility of thymoma.

3. Cutaneous Defenses

3.1. Predisposing Factors to Cutaneous Candidiasis

A variety of local and systemic factors predispose to superficial fungal infections. Cutaneous candidiasis most frequently occurs when there are warm, moist conditions such as in skin folds, under the diapers of newborns, and also in tropical climates or during the summer months. Otherwise, treatment with corticosteroids, cytotoxic agents, broad-spectrum antibiotics, and oral contraceptives all predispose to various forms of candidiasis. Diabetes mellitus and infection with HIV are both strongly associated with superficial candidiasis, although disseminated candidiasis is unusual in these conditions. In diabetes mellitus a variety of disturbances in immune and phagocytic cell functions may be involved in the increased susceptibility to infection, and particularly with *C. albicans* there may be increased adherence to diabetic cells (Geerlings and Hoepelman, 1999). Deficiency of the neutrophil enzyme myeloperoxidase may be associated with cutaneous candidiasis, presumably because of diminished ability to produce fungicidal oxidants (Nguyen and Katner, 1997). In fact, addition of recombinant human myeloperoxidase enhances the ability of activated macrophages to kill *C. albicans* in vitro (Marodi et al., 1998). Genetic predisposition may be important in chronic mucocutaneous candidiasis in that approximately 25% of these patients have relatives with this disease (Herrod, 1990). The hyper IgE syndrome is another condition in which cutaneous candidiasis as well as recurrent staphylococcal abscesses are common; this syndrome has complicated effects on the host defense system, possibly mediated in part by IgE antibodies against *Candida* or staphylococcal antigens (Chappler et al., 1978; de la Torre Morin et al., 1997).

3.2. Nonimmunologic Cutaneous Defenses—Innate Immunity

The skin, like the mucosa, is generally colonized by large numbers of microorganisms and therefore must represent an initial barrier to the entry of these potential pathogens to the deeper tissues. A variety of mechanisms are available for this purpose. Some of these appear to be merely mechanical, whereas others are more complicated and have some capacity to react. The skin structure itself would suggest a physical barrier, although more recent studies have suggested that it represents more complicated mechanisms of host defense. Similarly, evidence is mounting for an intricate sensing mechanism to allow the inflammatory cells to differentiate between substances released from pathogens and those from the host. The entire system of nonimmunologic cutaneous defenses allows for immediacy of its effect and multiple overlapping mechanisms.

3.2.1. Structure of the Skin

The physical and chemical structure of the skin represents a form of defense against fungal pathogens. In keratinized epithelia the stratum corneum has a structure of protein-enriched corneocytes embedded in a continuous, lipid-enriched, intercellular matrix in the "bricks and mortar" model (Elias, 1983; Elias and Feingold, 1999; Schurer and Elias, 1991). As the keratinocytes make their transition to corneocytes, they lose 45% to 86% of their dry weight and form into a flattened shape that helps to provide mechanical protection at the skin surface (Haake and Holbrook, 1999). This makeup lends tensile strength to the skin and also may protect it from invasion by microorganisms. In addition, the skin surface is relatively inhospitable to fungal growth because of exposure to ultraviolet light, low moisture conditions, and competition from the normal bacterial flora of this site. Therefore, this surface acts as a barrier to the entry of fungi. The stratum corneum is made up of keratin, which most microorganisms cannot use for nutrition. In fact, high molecular mass (>60 kDa) keratins stabilized by intermolecular disulfide bonds, account for up to 80% of the mass of the corneocytes (Haake and Holbrook, 1999). However, *C. albicans* produces proteases (keratinases) that hydrolyze this substance and facilitate the growth of these organisms in the stratum corneum itself (Negi et al., 1984). These enzymes are secreted aspartyl proteases, and in one study of *C. parapsilosis* were found in higher concentrations in skin versus blood isolates (De Bernardis et al., 1999). The very superficial site of infection in the stratum corneum may protect the infecting organisms from direct contact with at least some of the effector cells of the immune system. Although neutrophils and small numbers of lymphocytes may enter the epidermis, the major infiltrates of cell-mediated immune responses are generally confined to the dermis.

3.2.2. Keratinization and Epidermal Proliferation

The process by which the stratum corneum is continually renewed through keratinization of the epidermal cells may also present a form of defense against organisms infecting this site. The anatomy of the normal skin is shown in Fig. 21.1. Basal epidermal cells produce continued growth of the epidermis as they undergo repeated cell divisions that move the resulting daughter cells (keratinocytes) outward, toward the surface. As they mature these cells lose their nuclei and become flattened

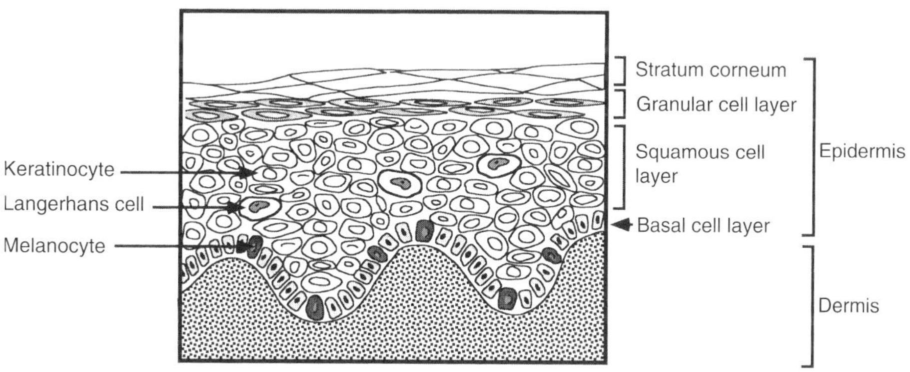

Figure 21.1. Anatomy of the normal skin.

to form the keratinized cells. This process results in shedding of the stratum corneum, which also may remove infecting fungal microorganisms residing there. Keratinocytes in the periphery of a similar kind of superficial fungal infection, annular dermatophytosis, have been found to divide at an increased rate (Berk et al., 1976). Inflammation, including that produced by cell-mediated immune reactions, appears to enhance epidermal proliferation so that rates of transit of epidermal cells towards the stratum corneum are increased (Lepper and Anger, 1976). Epidermal proliferation in experimental cutaneous candidiasis appears to be enhanced by cell-mediated immune responses to fungal antigens in the infected skin and may play a role in the defense against cutaneous candidiasis (Sohnle and Kirkpatrick, 1978). As will be discussed below, it is possible that increased proliferation and/or differentiation of keratinocytes may promote increased expression of certain antimicrobial proteins.

3.2.3. Antifungal Substances

3.2.3.1. Lipids Lipids of adult hair contain saturated fatty acids that are fungistatic against *Microsporum audouini,* formerly a common cause of hair and scalp infections (Rothman et al., 1947). In particular, various types of sphingosines, particularly sphinganine, sphingosine, and dimethylsphingosine, have been found to be active against certain dermatophytes and *C. albicans* (Bibel et al., 1993). This type of antimicrobial activity is calcium-dependent (Bibel et al., 1992). Whereas the sebum of adults may not be significantly more fungistatic than that from children on a weight per weight basis, older individuals appear to produce quantitatively more of this material than do children (Kligman and Ginsberg, 1950). Epidermal lipids, in addition to those from sebum, also have antimicrobial activity, which is related to free fatty acids, polar lipids, and glycosphingolipids (Miller et al., 1988).

3.2.3.2. Metal-Binding Proteins Unsaturated transferrin is present in serum and can prevent the growth of *Candida* (Esterly et al., 1967); presence of this substance in the dermis may confine the organisms to the epidermis and in inflamed skin it might also make its way into the epidermis. It has been shown that the serum of infected animals, but not that of uninfected animals, is inhibitory of *Candida* growth in vitro through an iron-dependent mechanism; therefore, increase in levels of this protein as an acute phase reactant may also contribute to host defense in the skin (Radke et al., 1994). Also, the siderophore iron transport system of *C. albicans* appears necessary for epithelial invasion, suggesting that the ability to acquire iron from host tissues may be important in superficial *Candida* infections (Heymann et al., 2002).

Calprotectin is a calcium- and zinc-binding protein of neutrophils and keratinocytes that has potent, broad-spectrum antimicrobial activity based on its ability to bind zinc (Sohnle, 1997). Production of this substance is markedly upregulated in differentiating keratinocytes (Madsen et al., 1992; Siegenthaler et al., 1997). This process could be a mechanism by which epidermal proliferation produces an environment in the epidermis that is inhospitable to fungal growth because available zinc is lacking at that site.

3.2.3.3. Other Antimicrobial Substances Human β-defensin 2 (HBD2), is a small cationic, cysteine-rich peptide expressed in skin keratinocytes and airway epithelium; this substance is produced following stimulation of keratinocytes by contact with bacteria or cytokines, has microbicidal activity against *Candida* and bacteria, and is inhibited by sodium chloride (Liu et al., 1998; Schroder and Harder, 1999). In human epidermal cell cultures, monocyte-derived cells acting through interleukin 1 (IL-1) greatly amplify the induction of HBD2 (Liu et al., 2003). A variety of other antimicrobial substances are expressed by human epidermal cells, including peptide LL-37 (a cathelicidin), granzyme B, adrenomedullin, and antileukoprotease (Berthou et al., 1997; Frohm et al., 1997; Martinez et al., 1997; Wiedow et al., 1998). Note that the expression of LL-37 has been shown to be upregulated in inflammatory skin disorders (Frohm et al., 1997). Melanins have also been postulated to be important in cutaneous host defense (Mackintosh, 2001) and certain other fungicidal proteins have also been isolated from normal epidermis and could play some role in the defense against cutaneous fungal infections (Kashima et al., 1989).

3.2.4. Phagocytic Cells and the Inflammatory Response

3.2.4.1. Mechanisms of the Innate Immune System The innate immune system represents a first line of defense against invading pathogens and does not require a preliminary exposure to microbial antigens to generate an effective response. This system is largely mediated by leukocytes such as macrophages and neutrophils, which phagocytose and kill pathogens while also eliciting an inflammatory response. Within the macrophages the pathogen is killed in the phagosome and microbial components are presented to T lymphocytes to activate the adaptive immune system. A critical part of this process is the ability of the macrophage to discriminate between itself and a large number of potential pathogens using a restricted number of germ-line encoded receptors (reviewed in Aderem, 2001; Cook et al., 2003). These receptors recognize conserved motifs on pathogens that are not found in higher eukaryotes; such motifs are called pathogen-associated molecular patterns (PAMPs) and include mannans in the yeast cell wall, formylated peptides, lipopolysaccharides (LPS), peptidoglycans, and teichoic acids. There are different pattern recognition receptors for mediating phagocytosis and for activating the proinflammatory pathways (Aderem, 1999).

The role of the innate immune system is especially prominent in those surfaces contacting the external environment, such as the skin, digestive and genitourinary tracts, and airways (reviewed in Hackett, 2003). The innate defenses are based on phagocytic cells as discussed above, but in addition are mediated also by certain others that are permanently located within tissues or are recruited to the site as needed. These include the Langerhans cells of the skin, tissue dendritic cells, macrophages, tissue-associated lymphocytes, and certain epithelial cells themselves. Interactions and functions of the particular skin cell types are described more fully in the section on the cutaneous immune system below. In many cases there is a close relationship between innate and adaptive immune processes in the skin.

Critical to the rapid innate immune responses are the expression of the receptors against PAMPs, primarily the family of Toll-like receptors (TLRs, reviewed in Aderem, 1999; Ong et al., 2002; Cook et al., 2003). To date ten different TLRs have been described in mammals, with the molecular ligands for most not having been identified yet. Different PAMPs are recognized by distinct combinations of TLRs, suggesting that the TLRs can establish a combinatorial repertoire to discriminate among the large number of PAMPs found in nature. Once the TLR recognizes a PAMP it elicits a cell-signaling cascade that initiates defensive responses directed at eliminating the pathogen. Each of the TLRs can signal through the adaptor molecule MyD88 and lead to activation of nuclear factor kappa beta. MyD88 signaling has been shown to mediate phagocytosis and killing of *C. albicans*, but not *Aspergillus fumigatus* (Marr et al., 2003). In *C. albicans* it is a unique glycolipid, called phospholipomannan, which stimulates TLRs; both TLR2 (Joualt et al., 2003) and TLR4 (Tada et al., 2002) have been found to be involved in the signaling responses of mononuclear cells to this organism. Dendritic antigen-presenting cells function as a link between innate and adaptive immunity and are therefore important in the recognition of pathogens; dendritic cells express different patterns of TLRs and are strongly activated by fungal products to produce costimulatory molecules and cytokines that in turn lead to different T lymphocyte responses (Buentke and Scheynius, 2003).

3.2.4.2. Chemotactic Mechanisms Although cutaneous candidiasis is generally limited to the most superficial layers of the skin, these infections can be highly inflammatory even in patients with evidence for various kinds of immune dysfunction. One can observe in the infected skin a variety of gross changes including scaling, pustules, and erythema. Evidence of epidermal proliferation may also be seen in the chronic infections as hyperkeratosis and parakeratosis. Microscopically, the lesions are characterized by an accumulation of neutrophils in the infected skin of acute infections, or a mononuclear cell infiltrate in the dermis of the more chronic ones. The acute inflammatory responses may be manifested as epidermal microabscesses in which the *Candida* yeast cells or filamentous forms can be seen with appropriate special stains.

A variety of mechanisms have been described by which inflammatory cells are attracted into the sites of cutaneous fungal infections, including cutaneous candidiasis. *C. albicans* has been shown to activate complement through the alternative pathway (Ray and Wuepper, 1976). Animals deficient in C5 clear experimental cutaneous *C. albicans* infections more slowly than do normal animals, but the C5-deficient animals do appear to accumulate neutrophils in the skin normally and develop normal epidermal proliferative responses (Wilson and Sohnle, 1988). A collagenous serum lectin, called mannose-binding lectin, binds strongly to a variety of microorganisms, including *Candida* species, and promotes C4 deposition in a concentration-dependent manner (Neth et al., 2000); this mechanism may be of importance in innate immunity and may represent a type of first-line defense against these organisms. A patient has been described with deficiency of mannan-binding lectin-associated serine protease 2, which helps to generate the C3 convertase after the mannan-binding lectin binds to microorganisms; this patient had recurrent pneumococcal infections and a chronic inflammatory state, but apparently not superficial fungal infections (Stengaard-Pedersen et al., 2003). Whereas the complement system may represent an important nonspecific skin defense mechanism, it also may be responsible for producing symptoms of superficial fungal infections at that site through production of proinflammatory products (Tagami, 1992).

C. albicans also produces low molecular weight chemotactic factors analogous to the ones made by growing bacteria (Cutler, 1977). These factors may be of two different types, including one that seems to act through the formyl peptide receptor of neutrophils, and another that is not inhibited by an antagonist to this receptor and appears to attract macrophages through a different mechanism (Edens et al., 1999). Finally, as discussed more fully below, keratinocytes themselves, when properly stimulated, can generate chemotactic cytokines that could also be responsible for some of the inflammation in the lesions of cutaneous fungal infections. Other elements of the cutaneous immune system may also be involved in generating an inflammatory response in the infected skin of cutaneous candidiasis.

3.2.4.3. Antifungal Mechanisms of Phagocytic Cells Neutrophils and monocytes/macrophages appear to be important in the defense against fungi, including those involved in the cutaneous mycoses. Neutrophils can directly attack pathogens using a variety of microbicidal processes (reviewed in Nauseef and Clark, 2000). Some of these processes depend upon microbicidal oxidants, including superoxide, hydrogen peroxide, hypochlorous acid, and monochloramine (Grisham et al., 1983; Test et al., 1984). Alternatively, the neutrophil killing mechanisms may involve nonoxidative granule microbicidal substances, such as the defensins (Ganz et al., 1985), bactericidal/permeability-increasing protein (Weiss et al., 1978), lactoferrin (Arnold et al., 1980), lysozyme (Collins and Pappagianis, 1974), azuricidin (Campanelli et al., 1990), and cathelicidin (Zanetti et al., 1996). Most of these substances have been studied primarily for their ability to kill the organisms, although lactoferrin may have both microbistatic and microbicidal effects (Arnold et al., 1981). In studies of neutrophil-mediated damage to *C. albicans* hyphae, confocal microscopy and quantification of cell wall glycoprotein release reveal that both oxidative and nonoxidative mechanisms are required for maximal effects on the target fungal cells (Christin et al., 1997). Macrophages have an additional antimicrobial mechanism whereby they can use production of nitric oxide to inhibit growth of ingested fungal pathogens, such as *Cryptococcus neoformans* (Alspaugh and Granger, 1991). This mechanism might potentially be active against the organisms causing superficial fungal infections also.

Neutrophils also appear to have significant growth inhibitory activity in addition to their microbicidal processes. These cells contain large amounts of a calcium- and zinc-binding protein, called calprotectin, which is also produced by keratinocytes, as discussed above. Neutrophil-derived calprotectin has potent microbistatic activity against *C. albicans* and other fungi (Steinbakk et al., 1990; Sohnle et al., 1991). This protein is released into inflammatory exudates as neutrophils die at sites of infection (Sohnle et al., 1991) and could supplement other host defenses in the infected skin by controlling growth of *C. albicans* or other fungi there.

3.3. The Cutaneous Immune System—Adaptive Immunity

3.3.1. *Potential Role in Cutaneous Candidiasis*

Since cutaneous fungal infections are more frequent and more severe in patients with immunologic defects, immune responses to fungal antigens would seem to play an important role in the host defense against these infections. Immunologic host defense mechanisms in normal hosts seem to be effective even when the infections are limited to superficial locations such as the stratum corneum. A number of studies suggest that the epidermis of the skin acts as a unique immunologic organ in addition to its role as a passive barrier against entry of infecting organisms. In 1983, a hypothesis regarding the skin-associated lymphoid tissue (SALT) concept was advanced wherein the skin acted as an immune surveillance unit (Streilein, 1983). A variety of cell types are believed to have involvement in this cutaneous immune system and will be reviewed below. The mechanisms employed are complex, involving a network of fixed or mobile cells interacting either by trafficking of the cells themselves from one site to another or by the production of cytokines that influence the function of other cells. The innate immune system probably is involved in initiating or amplifying these responses. Such skin-initiated immune responses act against a broad-spectrum of foreign antigens and PAMPs and it is likely that they are also active against *C. albicans* when it is involved in infections of the stratum corneum. Therefore, this system is probably responsible for initiating immune responses that work to eliminate the infecting organisms in the immune host. In addition, such responses may also produce some of the inflammation that results in much of the symptomatology of these infections. The cutaneous immune system has been reviewed in detail (Ring and Thewes, 1999; Stingl et al., 1999) and will be summarized briefly here.

3.3.2. Cells with Immunologic Potential in the Skin

3.3.2.1. Epidermal Langerhans Cells Langerhans cells develop as dendritic cells from bone marrow stem cells and home into selected tissues. At least five distinct subsets of dendritic cells have been recognized, including Langerhans cells in epithelial tissues, dendritic cells in peripheral blood or lymph, interdigitating dendritic cells in T cell-dependent areas of lymphoid tissues, follicular dendritic cells in B cell-dependent areas, and dermal dendritic cells (Bergstresser et al., 1992). Epidermal Langerhans cells make up approximately 2% to 5% of the total epidermal cell population, and vary in density depending upon anatomic location. These cells express a variety of antigenic markers on their surface (Stingl, 1993) and function to present antigens in an immunologically relevant fashion to both naive and sensitized T lymphocytes.

3.3.2.2. Dermal Dendritic Cells The dermis contains a population of antigen-presenting cells that constitute one of the five subsets described above. These cells have dendritic processes, are motile, and express a variety of markers, including high levels of class II major histocompatibility complex (MHC) antigen as well as certain proteins involved in adherence of one cell type to another. These cells also act as antigen-presenting cells and probably are important in the initiation of immunologic responses in the skin, particularly those involving antigens in the dermis.

3.3.2.3. Epidermal T Lymphocytes Although the lymphoid infiltrates characteristic of cutaneous cell-mediated immune responses are generally confined to the dermis of the skin, there are small numbers of T lymphocytes that are present within the epidermis (Bos et al., 1990). T lymphocyte antigen receptors are of two types, with most being of the $\alpha\beta$ heterodimer phenotype and a small population expressing the $\gamma\delta$ heterodimer. In the papillary dermis up to 80% of T lymphocytes are $\alpha\beta$-positive and approximately 7% are $\gamma\delta$-positive. In contrast, only 60% of the T lymphocytes in the epidermis are $\alpha\beta$-positive, with 18% to 29% being $\gamma\delta$-positive. Sensitized T lymphocytes can occur in the epidermis, either through antigenic stimulation of resting T lymphocytes at this site or attraction of already sensitized T lymphocytes by chemotactic cytokines, possibly including members of the IL-8 family produced by keratinocytes.

3.3.2.4. Keratinocytes Keratinocytes not only have an important structural role in forming a physical barrier to foreign antigens and microorganisms, but are also important functionally in mediating cutaneous immune reactions. These cells are by far the most numerous in the epidermis, although other cells types including melanocytes and Langerhans cells are also found there (see Fig. 21.1). The interfollicular epidermis is divided into a series of proliferating units, known as epidermal proliferative units (Potten, 1974). Within an epidermal proliferative unit there are slow and fast cycling basal keratinocytes, which are distinct populations that could possibly have different functions. Other neighboring cells, Langerhans cells, and cells in the dermis appear to have a regulatory effect on keratinocytes and may lead to cellular diversity within the basal layer. Keratinocytes secrete a number of soluble factors that are capable of upregulating and downregulating immune responses. The IL-7 that they produce has been shown to serve as a growth factor for epidermal T lymphocytes in mice (Matsue et al., 1993).

3.3.2.5. Microvascular Endothelial Cells Microvascular endothelial cells are located near the microenvironment where the important cutaneous immunologic reactions occur. Endothelial cells are known to be active participants in a variety of functions, including wound healing, angiogenesis, production of clotting factors, and maintenance of vascular tone. Their role in epidermal immunologic events is not entirely clear, although there is increasing evidence for their participation in this area. Like the keratinocytes, microvascular endothelial cells secrete a number of soluble factors capable of inducing inflammation and recruiting leukocytes, and express a variety of adhesion molecules.

3.3.3. Initiation and Expression of Cutaneous Immune Responses

According to the SALT concept, the skin contains an immune surveillance system consisting of antigen-presenting Langerhans cells, cytokine-producing keratinocytes, epidermotropic T lymphocytes, and draining peripheral lymph nodes. Much work has been done since that time to confirm and expand this concept. In the working hypothesis proposed for mechanisms and pathways involved in these cutaneous immune responses (Stingl, 1993; Ring and Thewes, 1999), foreign antigens entering the epidermis are first ingested and processed by Langerhans cells so that the antigenic fragment is complexed to MHC-encoded antigens. Concomitantly, there is antigen-induced enhancement of cytokine production by keratinocytes, leading to activation of the Langerhans cells. Within a short time, the antigen-processing Langerhans cells leave the epidermis, enter the dermal lymphatics, and migrate as veiled cells to the draining lymph nodes. Here they present the antigen–MHC complex on their surface to the proper receptors on resting T lymphocytes and elicit an antigen-specific response in these cells. Through a second signal (IL-1) produced by the Langerhans cells there is T lymphocyte stimulation and subsequent clonal expansion. The resulting T lymphocyte blasts then migrate back to the dermis and epidermis by homing to cytokine-activated microvascular endothelial cells in this area. Once in this location the T lymphocytes can be further stimulated by other antigen-presenting cells to undergo continued clonal expansion and generation of effector cells that can help to eliminate the pathogenic microorganisms. Other aspects of this immune surveillance mechanism are continuing to be elucidated and include other possible functions for the dermal dendritic cells, keratinocytes, and epidermal T lymphocytes. Each of these cell types may have other less well-defined roles in the above-described immune pathway, or they may play a more or less prominent role against a particular type of infection or other antigenic insult to the skin. The exact role of each cell type in producing immune responses against the organisms causing cutaneous mycoses have not yet been defined, although it is very likely that the immune surveillance mechanism described above is heavily involved in the defense against cutaneous candidiasis.

4. Immunology of Cutaneous Candidiasis

4.1. Immune Responses to *Candida* Antigens

Inoculation into the skin of viable *C. albicans* yeast cells in mice has been shown to elicit cell-mediated immune responses to various antigens of this organism (Moser et al., 1980). Experimental cutaneous candidiasis also sensitizes the infected animals so that a second infection is cleared more rapidly than is the initial one in both guinea pigs (Sohnle et al., 1976) and mice (Wilson and Sohnle, 1986). Clearance of the organisms in these experimental infections appears to be mediated at least in part by a vigorous epidermal proliferative response associated with cell-mediated immune responses to the antigens of the organisms (Sohnle et al., 1976; Sohnle and Kirkpatrick, 1978). On the other hand a certain degree of epidermal proliferation occurs in the infected skin of immunosuppressed mice, suggesting that other factors are also involved (Sohnle and Hahn, 1989).

Depending on environmental conditions, *C. albicans* can grow in either yeast or filamentous forms, with the latter being postulated to be more invasive. Therefore, it is possible that phase-specific immune responses could develop to antigens that are different between the two phases. Indeed, specific antigens have been found on the surface of cultured hyphal forms that are not present on yeast cells (Sundstrom and Kenny, 1984). In addition, it has been shown that antibodies in sera from some patients with candidiasis react only with germinating *C. albicans*, whereas those from normal individuals react preferentially with yeast cells (Ho et al., 1979).

Antibody against *C. albicans* is often found in high titers in human patients with chronic mucocutaneous candidiasis (Kirkpatrick et al., 1971; Axelsen et al., 1974; Mobacken et al., 1977). Whereas an occasional patient with this condition lacks anti-*Candida* antibodies in either serum (Chipps et al., 1979; Herrod, 1990) or saliva (Lehner et al., 1972), most seem to have intact humoral immunity to *C. albicans*. Also, the patients who have been reported to have abnormal antibody production appear to be indistinguishable from other patients with chronic mucocutaneous candidiasis, so the significance of these abnormalities is uncertain. More specific tests of B cell function may show abnormalities in patients with this condition in that Schick tests have been reported to be abnormal in some patients (Cahill et al., 1974) and in vitro antibody production to *Candida* mannan by cells from patients with active *Candida* infection was found to be deficient in another study (Durandy et al., 1987). Patients with the hyper IgE syndrome often have chronic superficial *C. albicans* infections along with elevated levels of IgE antibodies to this organism (Berger et al., 1980; Schmitt and Ballet, 1983). A syndrome of chronic mucocutaneous candidiasis has been described in which the patients have selective antibody deficiencies, particularly of IgG2, IgG4, and/or IgA (Kalfa et al., 2003).

Most noninfected humans have evidence of cell-mediated immunity (CMI) to *C. albicans*, as demonstrated by skin testing (Ferguson et al., 1977; Sohnle et al., 1983), in vitro lymphocyte stimulation (Bice et al., 1974; Gettner and Mackenzie, 1981), and lymphokine production (Bice et al., 1974; Sohnle et al., 1983). On the other hand patients with chronic mucocutaneous candidiasis often demonstrate significant immunologic defects in cell-mediated immune responses to *C. albicans* antigens, as discussed below. Even so, the pattern of immunologic abnormalities does not correlate very well with other manifestations of chronic mucocutaneous candidiasis. Also, since some uninfected relatives of patients with this condition also have diminished responsiveness to *Candida* antigens (Rothschild et al., 1976), this abnormality cannot entirely explain why the patients are susceptible to the fungal infections.

4.2. Mechanisms of Immunologic Defects in Cutaneous Candidiasis

4.2.1. Deficient CMI to Candida Antigens

In patients with chronic mucocutaneous candidiasis the most common immunologic abnormalities found are defects in CMI (Kirkpatrick et al., 1971; Kirkpatrick and Sohnle, 1981; Herrod, 1990; Filler and Edwards, 1993). Although most of the patients have normal numbers of T lymphocytes, they often do not manifest delayed hypersensitivity responses to *Candida* extracts when skin tested. Obviously lack of exposure to the antigens cannot explain the negative skin tests since the patients are chronically infected with the organism. In vitro correlates of delayed hypersensitivity responses, including lymphocyte transformation and lymphokine production, are also abnormal in many of these patients. These deficient responses fall into the general patterns of anergy to all antigens tested, unresponsiveness to *Candida* antigens only, and normal responses to all antigens, including those from *Candida*. For example, in one study, 10 out of 26 patients appeared to have normal CMI to *Candida* antigens (Valdimarsson et al., 1973). However, other patients appear to have significant abnormalities in lymphocyte function, with some having complete anergy to a battery of recall antigens and negative in vitro lymphocyte proliferation responses to mitogens and all antigens (Kirkpatrick and Sohnle, 1981).

The abnormalities in either cutaneous delayed hypersensitivity responses or in vitro lymphocyte function do not appear to relate directly to the clinical manifestations of the mucocutaneous *Candida* infections (Filler and Edwards, 1993). For example, subgroups of chronic mucocutaneous candidiasis patients, such as those with APECED or thymoma, do not all have the same patterns of reactivity in skin testing or in vitro lymphocyte assays, and some in each group may have apparently normal responses to *Candida* antigens in all the standard assays. Normal persons, without evidence of chronic superficial *Candida* infections, do not all react to *Candida* antigens in these assays, either; however, in this case it is possible that lack of exposure may account for negative tests in some people. In any event, it seems likely that the predisposition to chronic *Candida* infections in some patients with chronic mucocutaneous candidiasis and normal immunologic responsiveness may be due to factors other than deficient CMI; on the other hand, it may be that our immunologic assays are too crude to pick up subtle defects in CMI that do predispose the patients to these infections. In other cases it is possible that some nonimmunologic factor like antibiotic usage could initiate superficial *Candida* infections that suppress CMI secondarily and lead to more chronic infections; possible mechanisms involved in this type of suppression are discussed below.

Certain patients have been found to have specific cellular defects that might explain their susceptibility to superficial *Candida* infections. A group of 11 related chronic mucocutaneous candidiasis patients from Sicily were shown to be deficient in intercellular adhesion molecule 1 (ICAM-1 or CD54), a member of the immunoglobulin superfamily with a central role in cellular immune responses (Zuccarello et al., 2002). Other patients with chronic mucocutaneous candidiasis have been found to have impaired natural killer cell activity as well as increased *Candida* antigen-induced apoptosis of their lymphocytes (De Moraes-Vasconcelos et al., 2001).

4.2.2. Serum Inhibitors

Serum inhibitors appear to account for some of the immunologic defects in patients with chronic mucocutaneous candidiasis (Valdimarsson et al., 1973; Twomey et al., 1975; Kirkpatrick and Windhorst, 1979; Burford-Mason et al., 1987), and sometimes these defects disappear after antifungal therapy (Kirkpatrick and Smith, 1974; Twomey et al., 1975; Drouhet and Dupont, 1980). Parenteral administration of viable *C. albicans* yeast cells or extracts of this organism to experimental animals can result in suppression of CMI (Rogers and Balish, 1978; Rivas and Rogers, 1983; Carrow and Domer, 1985). Carbohydrate antigens from *C. albicans*, primarily mannans, have been shown to persist in the serum of patients with chronic mucocutaneous candidiasis and suppress lymphocyte proliferation responses of cells from control subjects (Fischer et al., 1987). Defective handling of mannan by monocytes from patients with chronic mucocutaneous candidiasis has been postulated as the reason why this substance accumulates in the serum of these patients (Fischer et al., 1982). Mannan-derived oligosaccharides from *C. albicans* can inhibit in vitro lymphocyte proliferation induced by *Candida* antigens (Podzorski et al., 1990). Therefore, catabolism of mannan in vivo may generate immunoinhibitory oligosaccharides that cause the defects in CMI in some patients with chronic mucocutaneous candidiasis. However, other patients with this syndrome probably have immunologic abnormalities due to other mechanisms, and still others have no demonstrable immunologic abnormalities at all and may be susceptible to chronic superficial *C. albicans* infections for other reasons.

4.2.3. Imbalance of Th1 versus Th2 Responses

T lymphocyte subpopulations include the CD4 helper cells that secrete cytokines and the CD8 cells that are mainly cytotoxic killer cells. There are two major types of CD4 cells, including type 1 (Th1) helper cells that secrete IL-2 and interferon gamma (IFN-γ) and type 2 (Th2) cells that secrete IL-4, 5, 6, and 10, but not IL-2 or IFN-γ (Delves and Riott, 2000). Cytokine production influences the type of immune response needed to protect against particular types of infectious agents and may also normally reduce allergic or autoimmune responses. In particular, the production of cytokines by Th1 cells facilitates CMI, including the activation of macrophages and T cell-mediated cytotoxicity; alternatively, Th2 cells help the B lymphocytes to produce antibodies. Th1 and Th2 cells may inhibit each other; for example, secretion of IFN-γ by Th1 cells inhibits Th2 cells, and secretion of IL-10 by Th2 cells reciprocally inhibits Th1 cells (Mosmann and Sad, 1996). Since the activity of Th1 cells promotes protective cell-mediated immune responses, overactivity by Th2 cells might work to inhibit these responses and predispose the host to certain types of infection.

Studies in mice have demonstrated that resistance to *C. albicans* infections results from the development of Th1 cell responses, which generate cytokines that activate macrophages and neutrophils and increase their candidacidal abilities (Romani, 1999). Alternatively, IL-4, a Th2 cytokine, has been shown to inhibit uptake and killing of *C. albicans* cells by human mononuclear phagocytes (Roilides et al., 1997). Therefore, coordination of Th1 and Th2 responses is required for efficient host defense against this organism. Lymphocytes from patients with chronic mucocutaneous candidiasis have been found to show impaired in vitro secretion of IL-2 (a Th1 cytokine), but increased secretion of IL-6 (a Th2 cytokine) in response to stimulation by *Candida* antigens (Lilic et al., 1996). Another study demonstrated markedly decreased *Candida*-specific production of IL-12 in these patients, but increased production of IL-6 and IL-10 (Lilic et al., 2003). Therefore, *Candida* antigens appear to trigger predominantly a Th2 response in chronic mucocutaneous candidiasis patients, perhaps leading to their increased susceptibility to this type of infection.

4.3. Role of Cytokines in Cutaneous Candidiasis

Cytokines appear to enhance the ability of phagocytic cells to damage or kill *C. albicans* cells. Three types of colony-stimulating factors, including granulocyte colony-stimulating factor (G-CSF), macrophage colony-stimulating factor (M-CSF), and granulocyte-macrophage colony-stimulating factor (GM-CSF), as well as IL-2, IFN-γ, and tumor necrosis factor alpha TNF-α), have been shown in vitro to enhance the fungicidal activity of phagocytic cells against *Candida* species (reviewed in Rodriguez-Adrian et al., 1998). GM-CSF also appears to work in concert with neutrophil myeloperoxidase to augment killing of *C. albicans* by macrophages (Marodi et al., 1998). Neutrophils from human volunteers given G-CSF were found in one study to more effectively damage the pseudohyphae of *C. albicans* (Gavira et al., 1999). Other cytokines, including IL-12 and IL-15, may also act to enhance neutrophil killing of *Candida* (Rodriguez-Adrian et al., 1998; Vazquez et al., 1998). Alternatively, IL-4 and IL-10 characterize the Th2 response and appear to decrease the antifungal activity of macrophages against *C. albicans* (Cenci et al., 1993). Since neutrophils can enter the stratum corneum and contact the infecting organisms in cutaneous candidiasis, it is likely that modulation of the fungicidal mechanisms of these cells by various cytokines, in either a positive or negative manner, could significantly affect the ability of the host to clear this type of infection.

5. Therapeutic Implications

Standard therapy of chronic mucocutaneous candidiasis involves long treatment courses (6–9 months) with oral azole antifungals such as ketoconazole or fluconazole. For other forms of cutaneous candidiasis, therapy can be attempted with topical preparations of azoles, amphotericin B or nystatin, or cyclopirox. These therapies are generally effective, although relapses can occur particularly in chronic mucocutaneous candidiasis when the treatment is stopped or if a resistant organism is encountered. Therefore, in chronic mucocutaneous candidiasis maintenance therapy is usually required after the initial antifungal treatment has cleared the cutaneous and mucosal lesions. In some patients, the defects in CMI may resolve after antifungal therapy; this improvement may be due to disappearance of circulating inhibitory serum factors related to mannan products from the organism itself, as discussed above.

Early attempts at immunological treatment used transplants of whole thymic tissue, lymphocytes, or bone marrow, or leukocyte-derived factors such as transfer factor or thymosin (Kirkpatrick and Smith, 1974; Filler and Edwards, 1993). In some cases immunologic reconstitution was achieved, but generally these therapies were difficult and only marginally effective. The development and approval of various cytokines for use in humans has provided a possible new therapy for difficult mucocutaneous *Candida* infections. To date, there are only limited data on the use of cytokines as adjuvant therapy for fungal infections in general. However, in experimental animals in vivo synergy between antifungal drugs and various cytokines has been convincingly demonstrated (reviewed in Stevens, 1998). Formal clinical trials will be required to determine if administration of cytokines can significantly enhance the treatment of fungal infections, perhaps including relapsing forms of chronic mucocutaneous candidiasis.

6. Summary

Cutaneous candidiasis represents infections of the epidermis, primarily the stratum corneum of the skin, with *C. albicans* and occasionally certain non-*C. albicans* species. The condition known as chronic mucocutaneous candidiasis consists of a variety of syndromes with varying degrees of immune dysfunction and resulting chronic infections of the skin, nails, and mucous membranes with *Candida* organisms. The various forms of cutaneous candidiasis have a number of predispositions, such as warmth, moisture, and occlusion at the local site, various kinds of natural or iatrogenic immunosuppression, and perhaps some degree of inherited susceptibility. The immune system, particularly CMI, appears to be important in the defense against this type of infection. In the skin the mechanisms involved in generating immunologic reactions are particularly complex, with epidermal Langerhans cells, other dendritic cells, lymphocytes, microvascular endothelial cells, and the keratinocytes themselves all playing important roles. Studies of cutaneous candidiasis have elucidated a number of immunologic defects, which in some cases may be preexistent and in others may be secondary to the infection itself. Different mechanisms may cause immunologic dysfunction in individual patients and lead to the development of chronic infections. Although an inability to develop protective immune responses appears to be involved in the chronicity of certain cutaneous *Candida* infections, treatment at the present time depends primarily on antifungal medications; therapeutic modalities aimed at reversing the underlying immunologic defects remain experimental.

References

Aderem, A.A. (1999). Mechanisms of phagocytosis in macrophages. *Annu. Rev. Biochem.* 17: 593–623.

Aderem, A.A. (2001). Role of toll-like receptors in inflammatory response in macrophages. *Crit. Care Med.* 29: S16–S18.

Alspaugh, J.A. and Granger, D.L. (1991). Inhibition of *Cryptococcus neoformans* replication by nitrogen oxides supports the role of these molecules as effectors of macrophage-mediated cytostasis. *Infect. Immun.* 59: 2291–2296.

Arnold, R.R., Brewer, M., and Gauthier, J.J. (1980). Bactericidal activity of human lactoferrin: Sensitivity of a variety of microorganisms. *Infect. Immun.* 23: 893–898.

Arnold, R.R., Russell, J.E., Champion, W.J., and Gauthier, J.J. (1981). Bactericidal activity of human lactoferrin—influence of physical conditions and metabolic state of the target microorganism. *Infect. Immun.* 32: 655–660.

Axelsen, N.H., Kirkpatrick, C.H., and Buckley, R.H. (1974). Precipitins to *Candida albicans* in chronic mucocutaneous candidiasis studied by crossed immunoelectrophoresis with intermediate gels. *Clin. Exp. Immunol.* 17: 385–394.

Berger, M., Kirkpatrick C.H., Goldsmith P.K., and Gallin, J.I. (1980). IgE antibodies to *Staphylococcus aureus* and *Candida albicans* in patients with the syndrome of hyperimmunoglobulin E and recurrent infections. *J. Immunol.* 125: 2437–2443.

Bergstresser, P.R., Cruz, P.D. Jr., Niederkorn, J.Y., and Takashima, A. (1992). Third international workshop on Langerhans cells: Discussion overview. *J. Invest. Dermatol.* 99: 1S–4S.

Berk, S.H., Penneys, N.S., and Weinstein, G.D. (1976). Epidermal activity in annular dermatophytosis. *Arch. Dermatol.* 112: 485–488.

Berthou, C., Michel, L., Soulie, A., Jean-Louis, F., Flageul, B., Dubertret, L., Sigaux, F., Zhang, Y., and Sasportes, M. (1997). Acquisition of granzyme B and Fas ligand proteins by human keratinocyte contributes to epidermal cell defense. *J. Immunol.* 159: 5293–5300.

Bibel, D.J., Aly, R., and Shinefield, H.R. (1992). Antimicrobial activity of sphingosines. *J. Invest. Dermatol.* 98: 269–273.

Bibel, D.J., Aly, R., Shah, S., and Shinefield, H.R. (1993). Sphingosines: Antimicrobial barriers of the skin. *Acta Derm. Venereol. (Stockh.)* 73: 407–411.

Bice, D.E., Lopez, M., Rothschild, H., and Salvaggio, J. (1974). Comparison of *Candida* delayed hypersensitivity skin test size with lymphocyte transformation, migration inhibitory factor production and antibody titer. *Int. Arch. Allergy Appl. Immunol.* 47: 54–62.

Bjorses, P., Aaltonen, J., Horelli-Kuitunen, N., Yaspo, M.L., and Peltonen, L. (1998). Gene defect behind APECED: A new clue to autoimmunity. *Hum. Mol. Genet.* 7: 1547–1553.

Bjorses, P., Halonen, M., Palvimo, J.J., Kolmer, M., Aaltonen, J., Ellonen, P., Perheentupa, J., Ulmanen, I., and Peltonen, L. (2000). Mutations in the AIRE gene: Effects on subcellular location and transactivation function of the autoimmune polyendocrinopathy-candidiasis-ectodermal dystrophy protein. *Am. J. Human Gen.* 66: 378–392.

Bos, J.D., Teunissen, M.B.M., Cairo, I., Krieg, S.R., Kapsenberg, M.L., Das, P.K., and Borst, J. (1990). T-cell receptor $\gamma\delta$ bearing cells in normal human skin. *J. Invest. Dermatol.* 94: 37–42.

Buentke, E. and Scheynius, A. (2003). Dendritic cells and fungi. *Acta Pathol. Microbiol. Immunol. Scand.* 111: 789–796.

Burford-Mason, A.P., Matthews, R.C., and Williams, J.R.B. (1987). Transient abrogation of immunosuppression in a patient with chronic mucocutaneous candidiasis following vaccination with *Candida albicans*. *J. Infect.* 14: 147–157.

Cahill, L.T., Ainbender, E., and Glade, P.R. (1974). Chronic mucocutaneous candidiasis: T cell deficiency associated with B cell dysfunction in man. *Cell. Immunol.* 14: 215–225.

Campanelli, D., Detmers, P.A., Nathan, C.F., and Gabay, J.E. (1990). Azuricidin and a homologous serine protease from neutrophils. Differential antimicrobial and proteolytic properties. *J. Clin. Invest.* 85: 904–915.

Carrow, E.W. and Domer, J.E. (1985). Immunoregulation in experimental murine candidiasis: Specific suppression induced by *Candida albicans* cell wall glycoprotein. *Infect. Immun.* 49: 172–181.

Cenci, E., Romani, L., Mencacci, A., Spaccapelo, R., Schiaftella, E., Pucetti, P., and Bistoni, F. (1993). Interleukin-4 and IL-10 inhibit nitric oxide-dependent macrophage killing of *Candida albicans*. *Eur. J. Immunol.* 23: 1034–1038.

Chappler, R.R., Maibach, H.I., Conant, M.K.A., and Aly, R. (1978). Mucocutaneous candidiasis or mucocutaneous microbiosis? *J. Am. Med. Assoc.* 239: 428–429.

Chipps, B.E., Saulsbury, F.T., Hsu, S.H., Hughes, W.T., and Winkelstein, J.A. (1979). Non-*Candida* infections in children with chronic mucocutaneous candidiasis. *Johns Hopkins Med.* J. 144: 175–179.

Christin, L., Wysong, D.R., Meshulam, T., Wang, S., and Diamond, R.D. (1997). Mechanisms and target sites of damage in killing of *Candida albicans hyphae* by human polymorphonuclear neutrophils. *J. Infect. Dis.* 176: 1567–1578.

Collins, M.S. and Pappagianis, D. (1974). Inhibition by lysozyme of growth of the spherule phase of *Coccioides immitis* in vitro. *Infect. Immun.* 10: 616–623.

Cook, D.N., Hollingsworth, J.W.II, and Schwartz, D.A. (2003). Toll-like receptors and the genetics of innate immunity. *Curr. Opin. Allergy Clin. Immunol.* 3: 523–529.

Cutler, J.E. (1977). Chemotactic factor produced by *Candida albicans*. *Infect. Immun.* 18: 568–573.

De Bernardis, F., Mondello, F., San Millan, R., Ponton, J., and Cassone, A. (1999). Biotyping and virulence properties of skin isolates of *Candida parapsilosis*. *J. Clin. Microbiol.* 37: 3481–3486.

de la Torre Morin, F., Garcia Robaina, J.C., Bonnet Moreno, C., and Fonta, G.L. (1997). Hyper IgE syndrome. Presentation of three cases. *Allergy Immunopathol.* 25: 30–35.

De Moraes-Vasconcelos, D., Morii, N., Romano, C.C., Igueoka, R.Y., and da S. Duarte, A.J. (2001). Characterization of the cellular immune function of patients with chronic mucocutaneous candidiasis. *Clin. Exp. Immunol.* 123: 247–253.

Delves, P.J. and Riott, I.M. (2000). The immune system. *N. Engl. J. Med.* 343: 108–117.

Drouhet, E. and Dupont, B. (1980). Chronic mucocutaneous candidiasis and other superficial and systemic mycoses successfully treated with ketoconazole. *Rev. Infect. Dis.* 2: 606–619.

Durandy, A, Fischer, A., Le Deist, F., Drouhet, E., and Griscelli, C. (1987). Mannan-specific and mannan-induced T-cell suppressive activity in patients with chronic mucocutaneous candidiasis. *J. Clin. Immunol.* 7: 400–409.

Edens, H.A., Parkos, C.A., Liang, T.W., Jesaitis, A.J., Cutler, J.E., and Miettinen, H.M. (1999). Non-serum-dependent chemotactic factors produced by *Candida albicans* stimulate chemotaxis by binding to the formyl peptide receptor on neutrophils and to an unknown receptor on macrophages. *Infect. Immun.* 67: 1063–1071.

Elias, P.M. (1983). Epidermal lipids, barrier function, and desquamation. *J. Invest. Dermatol.* 80: 44s–49s.

Elias, P.M. and Feingold, K.R. (1999). Skin as an organ of protection. In I.M. Freedberg, A.Z. Eisen, K. Wolff, K.F. Austen, L.A. Goldsmith, S.I. Katz, and T.B. Fitzpatrick (eds), *Dermatology in General Medicine*, 5th edn. McGraw-Hill, New York, pp 164–174.

Eppinger, T.M., Aronson, J.E., Fonacier, L.S., and Cunningham-Rundles, C. (1999). *Pneumocystis carinii* pneumonia in a 15 year old with chronic mucocutaneous candidiasis. *Scand. J. Infect. Dis.* 31: 203–206.

Esterly, N.B., Brammer, S.R., and Crounse, R.G. (1967). The relationship of transferrin and iron to serum inhibition of *Candida albicans*. *J. Invest. Dermatol.* 49: 437–442.

Ferguson, A.C., Kershnar, H.E., Collin, W.K., and Stiehm, E.R. (1977). Correlation of cutaneous hypersensitivity with lymphocyte response to *Candida albicans. Am. J. Clin. Pathol.* 68: 499–504.

Fidel, P.L. Jr., Vazquez, J.A., and Sobel, J.D. (1999). *Candida glabrata:* Review of epidemiology, pathogenesis, and clinical disease with comparison to *C. albicans. Clin. Microbiol. Rev.* 12: 80–96.

Filler, S.G. and Edwards, J.E. Jr. (1993). Chronic mucocutaneous candidiasis. In J.W. Murphy, H. Friedman, and M. Bendinelli (eds), *Fungal Infections and Immune Responses.* Plenum Press, New York, pp. 117–133.

Fischer, A.J., Pichat, L., Audinot, M., and Griscelli, C. (1982). Defective handling of mannan by monocytes in patients with chronic mucocutaneous candidiasis resulting in a specific cellular unresponsiveness. *Clin. Exp. Immunol.* 47: 653–660.

Fischer, A.J., Ballet, J.J., and Griscelli, C. (1987). Specific inhibition of the in vitro *Candida*-induced lymphocyte proliferation by polysaccharide antigens present in the serum of patients with chronic mucocutaneous candidiasis. *J. Clin. Invest.* 62: 1005–1013.

Frohm, M., Agerberth, B., Ahangari, G., Stahle-Backdahl, M., Liden, S., Wigzell, H., and Gudmundsson, G.H. (1997). The expression of the gene coding for the antibacterial peptide LL-37 is induced in human keratinocytes during inflammatory disorders. *J. Biol. Chem.* 272: 15258–15263.

Ganz, T., Selsted, M.E., Szklarek, D., Harwig, S.S.L., Dahler, K., Bainton, D.F., and Lehrer, R.I. (1985). Defensins: Natural peptide antibiotics of human neutrophils. *J. Clin. Invest.* 76: 1427–1435.

Gavira, J.M., van Burik, J.A., Dale, D.C., Root, R.K., and Liles, W.C. (1999). Modulation of neutrophil-mediated activity against the pseudohyphal form of *Candida albicans* by granulocyte colony-stimulating factor (G-CSF) administered in vivo. *J. Infect. Dis.* 179: 1301–1304.

Geerlings, S.E. and Hoepelman, A.I. (1999). Immune dysfunction in patients with diabetes mellitus. *FEMS Immunol. Med. Microbiol.* 26: 259–265.

Gettner, S.M.M. and Mackenzie, D.W.R. (1981). Responses of human peripheral lymphocytes to soluble and insoluble antigens of *Candida albicans. J. Med. Microbiol.* 14: 333–340.

Grisham, M.B., Jefferson, M.M., Melton, D.F., and Thomas, E.L. (1983). Chlorination of exogenous amines by isolated neutrophils. Ammonia dependent bactericidal, cytotoxic, and cytolytic activities of the chloramines. *J. Biol. Chem.* 258: 10404–10413.

Haake, A.R. and Holbrook, K. (1999). The structure and development of the skin. In I.M. Freedberg, A.Z. Eisen, K. Wolff, K.F. Austen, L.A. Goldsmith, S.I. Katz, and T.B. Fitzpatrick (eds), *Dermatology in General Medicine*, 5th edn. McGraw-Hill, New York, pp 70–97.

Hackett, C.J. (2003). Innate immune activation as a broad-spectrum biodefense strategy—perspectives and research challenges. *J. Allergy Clin. Immunol.* 112: 686–694.

Herrod, H.G. (1990). Chronic mucocutaneous candidiasis in childhood and complications of non-*Candida* infection—a report of the pediatric immunodeficiency study group. *J. Pediatr.* 116: 377–382.

Heymann, P., Gerads, M., Schaller, M., Dromer, F., Winkelmann, G., and Ernst, J.F. (2002). The siderophore iron transporter of *Candida albicans* (Sit1P/Arn1P) mediates uptake of ferrichrome-type siderophores and is required for epithelial invasion. *Infect. Immun.* 70: 5246–5255.

Ho, Y., Ng, M., and Huang, C.T. (1979). Antibodies to germinating and yeast cells of *Candida albicans* in human and rabbit sera. *J. Clin. Pathol.* 32: 399–405.

Jouault, T., Ibaya-Ombetto, S., Takeuchi, O., Trinel, P.A., Sacchetti, P., Lefebvre, P., Akira, S., and Poulain, D. (2003). *Candida albicans* phosphomannan is sensed through toll-like receptors. *J. Infect. Dis.* 188: 165–172.

Kalfa, V.C., Roberts R.L., and Steihm, E.R. (2003). The syndrome of chronic mucocutaneous candidiasis with selective antibody deficiency. *Ann. Allergy Asthma Immunol.* 90: 259–264.

Kashima, M., Takahashi, H., Shimozuma, M., Epstein, W.L., and Fukuyama, K. (1989). Candidacidal activities of proteins partially purified from rat epidermis. *Infect. Immun.* 57: 186–190.

Kauffman, C.A., Shea, M.J., and Frame, P.R. (1981). Invasive fungal infections in patients with chronic mucocutaneous candidiasis. *Arch. Intern. Med.* 141: 1076–1078.

Kirkpatrick, C.H. and Smith, T.K. (1974). Chronic mucocutaneous candidiasis: Immunologic and antibiotic therapy. *Ann. Intern. Med.* 80: 310–320.

Kirkpatrick, C.H. and Sohnle, P.G. (1981). Chronic mucocutaneous candidiasis. In B. Safai and R.A. Good (eds), *Immunodermatology*. Plenum Press, New York, pp. 495–514.

Kirkpatrick, C.H. and Windhorst, D.B. (1979). Mucocutaneous candidiasis and thymoma. *Am. J. Med.* 66: 939–945.

Kirkpatrick, C.H., Rich, R.R., and Bennett, J.E. (1971). Chronic mucocutaneous: Model building in cellular immunity. *Ann. Intern. Med.* 74: 955–978.

Kligman, A.M. and Ginsberg, D. (1950). Immunity of the adult scalp to infection with *Microsporum audouini*. *J. Invest. Dermatol.* 14: 345–356.

Lehner, T.J., Wilton, M.A., and Ivanyi, L. (1972). Immunodeficiencies in chronic mucocutaneous candidiasis. *Immunology* 22: 775–787.

Lepper, A.W.D. and Anger, H.S. (1976). Experimental bovine *Trichophyton verrucosum* infection. Comparison of the rate of epidermal cell proliferation and keratinization in non-infected and reinoculated cattle. *Res. Vet. Sci.* 20: 117–121.

Lilic, D., Cant, A.J., Abinum, M., Calvert, J.E., and Spickett, G.P. (1996). Chronic mucocutaneous candidiasis. I. Altered antigen-stimulated IL-2, IL-4, IL-6 and interferon-gamma (IFN-gamma) production. *Clin. Exp. Immunol.* 105: 205–212.

Lilic, D., Gravenor, I., Robson, N., Lammas, D.A., Drysdale, P., Calvert, J.E., Cant, A.J., and Abinun, M. (2003). Deregulated production of protective cytokines in response to *Candida albicans* infection in patients with chronic mucocutaneous candidiasis. *Infect. Immun.* 71: 5690–5699.

Liu, L., Wang, L., Jia, H.P., Zhao, C., Heng, H.H.Q., Schutte, B.C., McCray, P.B. Jr., and Ganz, T. (1998). Structure and mapping of the human β-defensin HBD-2 gene and its expression at sites of inflammation. *Gene* 222: 237–244.

Liu, L., Roberts, A.A., and Ganz, T. (2003). By IL-1 signaling, monocytic-derived cells dramatically enhance the epidermal antimicrobial response to lipopolysaccharide. *J. Immunol.* 170: 575–580.

Mackintosh, J.A. (2001). The antimicrobial properties of melanocytes, melanosomes, and melanin, and the evolution of black skin. *J. Theor. Biol.* 211: 101–113.

Madsen, P., Rasmussen, H.H., Leffers, H., Honore, B., and Celis, J.E. (1992). Molecular cloning and expression of a novel keratinocyte protein (psoriasis-associated fatty acid-binding protein) that is highly upregulated in psoriatic skin and that shares similarity to fatty acid-binding proteins. *J. Invest. Dermatol.* 99: 299–305.

Marodi, L., Tournay, C., Kaposzta, R., Johnston, R.B. Jr., and Moguilevsky, N. (1998). Augmentation of human macrophage candidacidal capacity by recombinant human myeloperoxidase and granulocyte-macrophage colony-stimulating factor. *Infect. Immun.* 66: 2750–2754.

Marr, K.A., Balajee, S.A., Hawn, T.R., Ozinsky, A., Phom, U., Akira, S., Aderem, A., and Liles, W.C. (2003). Differential roles of MyD88 in macrophage-mediated responses to opportunistic fungal pathogens. *Infect. Immun.* 71: 5280–5286.

Martinez, A., Elsasser, T.H., Muro-Cacho, C., Moody, T.W., Miller, M.J., Macri, C.J., and Cuttitta, F. (1997). Expression of adrenomedullin and its receptor in normal and malignant human skin: A potential pluripotent role in the integument. *Endocrinology* 138: 5597–5604.

Matsue, H., Bergstresser, P.R., and Takashima, A. (1993). Keratinocyte-derived IL-7 serves as a growth factor for dendritic epidermal T cells in mice. *J. Immunol.* 151: 6012–6019.

Miller, S.J., Aly, R., Shinefield, H.R., and Elias, P.M. (1988). In vitro and in vivo antistaphylococcal activity of human stratum corneum lipids. *Arch. Dermatol.* 124: 209–215.

Mittaz, L., Rossier, C., Heino, M., Peterson, P., Krohn, K.J., Gos, A., Morris, M.A., Judoh, J., Shimizu, N., Antonarakis, S.E., and Scott, H.S. (1999). Isolation and characterization of the mouse AIRE gene. *Biochem. Biophys. Res. Comm.* 255: 483–490.

Mobacken, H., Lindholm, L., and Olling, S. (1977). Deficient neutrophil function in a patient with chronic mucocutaneous candidiasis, thymoma and myasthenia gravis. *Acta Derm. Venereol.* 57: 335–339.

Moser, S.A., Domer, J.E., and Mather, F.J. (1980). Experimental murine candidiasis: Cell-mediated immunity after cutaneous challenge. *Infect. Immun.* 27: 140–149.

Mosmann, T.R. and Sad, S. (1996). The expanding universe of T cell subsets: Th1, Th2 and more. *Immunol. Today* 17: 138–146.

Nauseef, W.M. and Clark, R.A. (2000). Granulocytic phagocytes. In G.L. Mandel, J.E. Bennett, and R. Dolin (eds), *Principles and Practice of Infectious Diseases*. Churchill Livingstone, Philadelphia, pp. 89–112.

Negi, M., Tsuboi, R., Matsui, T., and Ogawa, H. (1984). Isolation and characterization of proteinase from *Candida albicans*—substrate specificity. *J. Invest. Dermatol.* 83: 32–36.

Neth, O., Jack, D.L., Dodds, A.W., Holzel, H., Klein, N.J., and Turner, M.W. (2000). Mannose-binding lectin binds to a range of clinically relevant microorganisms and promotes complement deposition. *Infect. Immun.* 68: 688–693.

Nguyen, C. and Katner, H.P. (1997). Myeloperoxidase deficiency manifesting as pustular candidal dermatitis. *Clin. Infect. Dis.* 24: 258–260.

Ong, P.Y., Ohtake, T., Brandt, C., Strickland, I., Boguniewicz, M., Ganz, T., Gallo, R.L., and Leung, D.Y.M. (2002). Endogenous antimicrobial peptides and skin infections in atopic dermatitis. *N. Engl. J. Med.* 347: 1151–1160.

Podzorski, R.P., Gray, G.R., and Nelson, R.D. (1990). Different effects of native *Candida albicans* mannan and mannan-derived oligosaccharides on antigen-stimulated lymphoproliferation in vitro. *J. Immunol.* 144: 707–716.

Potten, C.S. (1974). The epidermal proliferative unit—the possible role of the central basal cell. *Cell Tissue Kinet.* 7: 77–88.

Radke, L.L., Hahn, B.L., Wagner, D.K., and Sohnle, P.G. (1994). Comparison of metal-binding antimicrobial activities in serum and abscess fluid supernatants. *J. Med. Veter. Mycol.* 32: 295–301.

Ray, T.L. and Wuepper, K.D. (1976). Activation of the alternative (properdin) pathway of complement by *Candida albicans* and related species. *J. Invest. Dermatol.* 67: 700–703.

Ring, J. and Thewes, M. (1999). The clinical expression of allergy in the skin. *Allergy* 54: 192–197.

Rivas, V. and Rogers, T.J. (1983). Studies on the cellular nature of *Candida albicans*—induced suppression. *J. Immunol.* 130: 376–379.

Rodriguez-Adrian, L.J., Grazziutti, M.L., Rex, J.H., and Anaissie, E.J. (1998). The potential role of cytokine therapy for fungal infections in patients with cancer—is recovery from neutropenia all that is needed? *Clin. Infect. Dis.* 26: 1270–1278.

Rogers, T.J. and Balish, E. (1978). Suppression of lymphocyte blastogenesis by *Candida albicans*. *Clin. Immunol. Immunopathol.* 10: 298–305.

Roilides, E., Kadiltsoglou, I., Dimitriadou, A., Hatzistilianou, M., Manitsa, A., Karpouzas, J., Pizzo, P.A., and Walsh, T.J. (1997). Interleukin 4 suppresses antifungal activity of human mononuclear phagocytes against *Candida albicans* in association with decreased uptake of blastoconidia. *FEMS Immunol. Med. Microbiol.* 19: 169–180.

Romani, L. (1999). Immunity to *Candida albicans:* Th1, Th2 cells and beyond. *Curr. Opin. Microbiol.* 2: 363–367.

Rosatelli, M.C., Meloni, A., Meloni, A., Devoto, M., Cao, A., Scott, H.S., Peterson, P., Heino, M., Krohn, K.J., Nagamine, K., Kodoh, J., Shimizu, N., and Antonarakis, S.E. (1998). A common mutation in Sardinian autoimmune polyendocrinopathy-candidiasis-ectodermal dystrophy patients. *Hum. Genet.* 103: 428–434.

Rothman, S., Smiljanic, A., Shapiro, A.L., and Weitkamp, A.W. (1947). The spontaneous cure of tinea capitis in puberty. *J. Invest. Dermatol.* 8: 81–98.

Rothschild, H., Wilson, M., Lopez, M., Salvaggio, J., and Bice, D. (1976). An immunological investigation of a family with chronic mucocutaneous candidiasis. *Int. Arch. Allergy Appl. Immunol.* 52: 291–296.

Schmitt, C. and Ballet, J.J. (1983). Serum IgE and IgG antibodies to tetanus toxoid and candidin in immunodeficient children with the hyper-IgE syndrome. *J. Clin. Immunol.* 3: 178–183.

Schroder, J.M. and Harder, J. (1999). Human beta-defensin 2. *Int. J. Biochem. Cell Biol.* 31: 645–651.

Schurer, N.Y. and Elias, P.M. (1991). The biochemistry and function of stratum corneum lipids. *Adv. Lipid Res.* 24: 27–56.

Siegenthaler, G., Roulin, K., Chatellard-Gruaz, D., Hotz, R., Saurat, J.H., Hellman, U., and Hagens, G. (1997). A heterocomplex formed by the calcium-binding proteins MRP 8 (S100A8) and MRP 14 (S100A9) binds unsaturated fatty acids with high affinity. *J. Biol. Chem.* 272: 9371–9377.

Sohnle, P.G. (1997). Antimicrobial defence through competition for zinc. *Rev. Med. Microbiol.* 8: 217–234.

Sohnle, P.G. and Hahn, B.L. (1989). Epidermal proliferation and the neutrophilic infiltrates of experimental cutaneous candidiasis in mice. *Arch. Dermatol. Res.* 281: 279–283.

Sohnle, P.G. and Kirkpatrick, C.H. (1978). Epidermal proliferation in the defense against cutaneous candidiasis. *J. Invest. Dermatol.* 70: 130–133.

Sohnle, P.G., Frank, M.M., and Kirkpatrick, C.H. (1976). Mechanisms involved in elimination of organisms from experimental cutaneous *Candida albicans* infection in guinea pigs. *J. Immunol.* 117: 523–530.

Sohnle, P.G., Collins-Lech, C., and Huhta, K.E. (1983). Kinetics of lymphokine production by lymphocytes from elderly humans. *Gerontology* 29: 169–175.

Sohnle, P.G., Collins-Lech, C., and Wiessner, J.H. (1991). The zinc-reversible antimicrobial activity of neutrophil lysates and abscess fluid supernatants. *J. Infect. Dis.* 164: 137–142.

Steinbakk, M., Naess-Andresen, C.F., Lingass, E., Dale, I., Brandtzaeg, P., and Fagerhol, M.K. (1990). Antimicrobial actions of calcium binding leucocyte L1 protein, calprotectin. *Lancet* 336: 763–765.

Stengaard-Pedersen, K., Thiel, S., Gadjeva, M., Moller-Kristensen, M., Sorensen, R., Jensen, L.T., Sjoholm, A.G., Fugger, L., and Jensenius, J.C. (2003). Inherited deficiency of mannan-binding lectin-associated serine protease 2. *N. Engl. J. Med.* 349: 554–560.

Stevens, D.A. (1998). Combination immunotherapy and antifungal chemotherapy. *Clin. Infect. Dis.* 26: 1266–1269.

Stingl, G. (1993). This skin: Initiation and target site of immune responses. *Recent Results Cancer Res.* 128: 45–57.

Stingl, G., Maurer, D., Hauser, C., and Wolff, K. (1999). The epidermis–an immunologic microenvironment. In I.M. Freedberg, A.Z. Eisen, K. Wolff, K.F. Austen, L.A. Goldsmith, S.I. Katz, and T.B. Fitzpatrick (eds), *Dermatology in General Medicine*, 5th edn. McGraw-Hill, New York, pp. 343–370.

Streilein, J.W. (1983). Skin-associated lymphoid tissues (SALT)—origins and functions. *J. Invest. Dermatol.* 80: 12S–16S.

Sundstrom, P.M. and Kenny, G.E. (1984). Characterization of antigens specific to the surface of germ tubes of *Candida albicans* by immunofluorescence. *Infect. Immun.* 43: 850–855.

Tada, H., Nemoto, E., Shimauchi, H., Watanabe, T., Mikami, T., Matsumato, T., Ohno, N., Tamura, H., Shibata, K., Akashi, S., Miyake, K., Sugawara, S., and Takada, H. (2002). *Saccharomyces cerevisae*- and *Candida albicans*-derived mannan induced production of tumor necrosis factor alpha by human monocytes in a CD14- and toll-like receptor 4-dependent manner. *Microbiol. Immunol.* 46: 503–512.

Tagami, H. (1992). The role of complement-derived mediators in inflammatory skin diseases. *Arch. Dermatol. Res.* 284(Suppl. 1): S2–S9.

Test, S.T., Lampert, M.B., Ossanna, P.J., Thoene, J.G., and Weiss, S.J. (1984). Generation of nitrogen-chlorine oxidants by human phagocytes. *J. Clin. Invest.* 74: 1341–1349.

Twomey, J.T., Waddel, C.C., Krantz, S., O'Reilly, R., L'Esperance, P., and Good, R.A. (1975). Chronic mucocutaneous candidiasis with macrophage dysfunction, a plasma inhibitor and coexistent aplastic anemia. *J. Lab. Clin. Med.* 85: 968–977.

Valdimarsson, H., Higgs, J.M., Wells, R.S., Yamamura, M., Hobbs, J.R., and Holt, P.J.L. (1973). Immune abnormalities associated with chronic mucocutaneous. *Cell Immunol.* 6: 348–361.

Vazquez, N., Walsh, T.J., Friedman, D., Chanock, S.J., and Lyman, C.A. (1998). Interleukin-15 augments superoxide production and microbicidal activity of human monocytes against *Candida albicans. Infect. Immun.* 66: 145–150.

Weiss, J., Elsbach, P., Olsson, I., and Odeberg, H. (1978). Purification and characterization of a potent bactericidal and membrane active protein from the granules of human polymorphonuclear leukocytes. *J. Biol. Chem.* 253: 2664–2672.

Wiedow, O., Harder, J., Bartels, J., Streit, V., and Christophers, E. (1998). Antileukoprotease in human skin: An antibiotic peptide constitutively produced by keratinocytes. *Biochem. Biophys. Res. Commun.* 248: 904–909.

Wilson, B.D. and Sohnle, P.G. (1986). Participation of neutrophils and cell-mediated immunity in the defense against experimental cutaneous candidiasis in mice. *Am. J. Pathol.* 123: 241–249.

Wilson, B.D. and Sohnle, P.G. (1988). Neutrophil accumulation and cutaneous responses in experimental cutaneous candidiasis of genetically complement-deficient mice. *Clin. Immunol. Immunopathol.* 46: 284–293.

Zanetti, M., Gennaro, R., and Romeo, D. (1996). Cathelicidins: A novel protein family with a common proregion and a variable C-terminal antimicrobial domain. *FEBS Lett.* 374: 1–5.

Zuccarello, D., Salpietro, D.C., Gangemi, S., Toscano, V., Merlino, M.V., Briuglia, S., Bisignano, G., Mangino, M., Mingarelli, R., and Dallapiccola, B. (2002). Familial chronic nail candidiasis with ICAM-1 deficiency—a new form of chronic mucocutaneous candidiasis. *J. Med. Genet.* 39: 671–675.

22

Immune Surveillance against Dermatophyte Infection

Tetsuya Koga

Department of Dermatology, Fukuoka Red Cross Hospital, Japan.

1. Immune Surveillance against Microorganisms in the Skin

The skin is the largest and most visible of all organs. The major function of the skin is a barrier between the outer world and the body. The skin is exposed to variable microorganisms, therefore the immune system has developed a special subsystem in the skin to eliminate them.

The innate immunity and acquired immunity (the recruitment of memory T cells that have clonally expanded in response to microorganism's antigens encountered at the skin) are both required for cutaneous immune surveillance against microorganisms at the skin. The local factors are instrumental in directing acquired immunity into the set of action. An example is the complex interplay between proinflammatory cytokines and chemokines produced in the skin after invasion of microorganisms.

2. Innate Immunity in the Skin

2.1. Proinflammatory Cytokines and Chemokines

Epidermal keratinocytes not only have an important structural role in forming a physical barrier to microorganisms but also are important functionally in mediating cutaneous immune reactions. Keratinocytes, which are the major cellular constituent of the epidermis, can produce IL-1α, TNF-α, and IL-8 in response to microorganisms. After binding to their receptors, these proinflammatory cytokines activate several cellular signaling pathways, including the NF-κB pathway and induce the translocation of NF-κB to the nucleus and the transcription of genes that play an important part in cutaneous inflammation (Barnes and Karin, 1997). These genes regulated by NF-κB include those for E-selectin, chemokines, cytokines, defensins, and cell adhesion molecules.

2.2. Antimicrobial Peptides

The antimicrobial peptides participate in the innate immune response by providing a rapid first-line defense against infection. The antimicrobial peptides directly kill a broad spectrum of microorganisms, including bacteria, fungi, and certain viruses. In addition, these peptides act as signaling molecules that activate host cell processes involved in immune defense and repair (Gallo et al., 2002). The innate immune system of human skin contains antimicrobial peptides known as cathelicidins and beta-defensins (Harder et al., 1997; Ong et al., 2002). In normal skin these peptides are negligible, but they accumulate in skin affected by inflammatory diseases. A deficiency in the expression of antimicrobial peptides may account for the susceptibility to skin infection (Milner and Ortega, 1999). The skin reacts rapidly by increased production of antimicrobial peptides from the keratinocytes and deposition of antimicrobial peptides from degranulation of recruited neutrophils. The chemotactic activity of antimicrobial peptides might further amplify this process by stimulating additional neutrophils recruitment.

2.3. Toll-like Receptors (TLRs)

TLRs, a family of innate immune cell surface receptors, also signal through NF-κB (Medzhitov et al., 1997; Hoffmann et al., 1999). TLRs recognize conserved molecules derived from microorganisms. TLR2 recognizes various ligands expressed by gram-positive bacteria, while TLR3, TLR4, and TLR5 are specific for double-stranded RNA, gram-negative lipopolysaccharides, and bacterial flagellin, respectively. Although their extracellular ligands are different, TLRs use multiple intracellular molecular elements in common with primary cytokine receptors. Many TLRs have been described in keratinocytes. Epidermal keratinocytes in normal skin constitutively express TLR1, TLR2, and TLR5, while TLR3 and TLR4 are, in most cases, barely detectable (Baker et al., 2003). Human keratinocytes are capable of expressing functional TLR2 (Kawai et al., 2002) and TLR4 (Song et al., 2002). Thus, TLRs seems to be involved in the antimicrobial responses of epidermal keratinocytes.

3. Acquired Immunity in the Skin

3.1. Dendritic Cells

Skin contains large numbers of dendritic cells in the epidermis and the dermis (Banchereau and Steinman, 1998). Epidermal Langerhans cells make up approximately 2% to 5% of the total epidermal cell population and have a dendritic shape and contain rod-shaped organelles called Birbeck granules. Macromolecules derived from microorganisms are internalized by dendritic cells and after enzymatic processing in the endosomes of these cells, the antigens are bound to antigen-presenting molecules, and the resulting complex is expressed on the cell surface for presentation to T cells (Porcelli et al., 1998). These dendritic cells migrate through afferent lymphatics and collect in lymph node, where they come into contact with naive T cells.

3.2. Cutaneous Lymphocyte Antigen (CLA)-Positive T Cells

Once naive T cells have been activated by an antigen, they proliferate and express activation molecules, undergoing the transition to memory T cells. There is a subgroup of memory T cells (CLA-positive T cells) with the ability to circulate preferentially to the skin. These CLA-positive T cells are generated in lymph nodes draining skin and are recruited back to the skin during inflammation. CLA is an adhesion molecule that mediates the initial tethering of T cells to the endothelium in cutaneous vessels (Fuhlbrigge et al., 1997). E-selectin is the endothelial ligand for CLA, and the interactions between CLA and E-selectin are required as the initial step in the extravasation of T cells from the blood into the skin CLA (Picker et al., 1991).

CLA-positive T cells represent 10% to 15% of all circulating T cells in peripheral blood, and their T cell antigen-receptor specificities are heterogeneous. CLA-positive T cells may be positive for either CD4 or CD8, and once activated, they may produce either Th1 cytokines (IFN-γ, IL-2) or Th2 cytokines (IL-4, 5, 10, and 13). This heterogeneity of phenotype and function may be important for a successful and flexible host response to microorganisms encountered in the skin.

3.3. Recruitment of CLA-Positive T Cells to the Skin

NF-κB transcriptional activation induces cutaneous inflammation, favoring the recruitment of CLA-positive T cells to the skin through E-selectin, chemokines, and cell adhesion molecules. Thus, cutaneous inflammation preferentially recruits CLA-positive T cells that have been activated by skin-related antigens. This mechanism of immune surveillance mediated by CLA-positive T cells is based on the principle that antigens encountered previously in the skin may be responsible for the new insult into the skin (Robert and Kupper, 1999). Extravasation of CLA-positive T cells from the blood into the skin does not require antigen recognition by T cells.

3.4. Activation of Antigen-Specific, CLA-Positive T Cells in the Skin

For CLA-positive T cells to perform effector functions in the skin, however, they must recognize antigen through their antigen receptors. They then become activated, producing effector molecules, including Th1 or Th2 cytokines. Therefore, only CLA-positive T cells that encounter the antigen for which their antigen receptor is specific will be activated in the skin, resulting in clinically apparent T cell-mediated immune response.

4. Immune Surveillance against Dermatophyte Infection

4.1. Overview

Infections with dermatophytes are generally confined to the keratinized stratum corneum and the cutaneous appendages like the hair and nails. The stratum corneum is made up of keratin. The dermatophytes produce keratinases, which hydrolyze this substance and facilitate the growth of these organisms in the stratum corneum (Takiuchi et al., 1982). Thus, the dermatophyte infections are limited to superficial locations of the skin. This superficial site of infection may protect the infecting dermatophytes from direct contact with some of the effector cells of the immune system. Since dermatophyte infections are more frequent and more severe in immunodeficient patients, immune responses to dermatophyte antigens would seem to play an important role in the host defense against dermatophyte infections. However, it appears that this immunity is not complete and is probably less than that found in animals (Grappel et al., 1974). A delayed-type hypersensitivity (DTH) response to a dermatophyte antigen is one of the host defense mechanisms. Furthermore, the pathogenesis in dermatophytosis may depend on a number of factors, such as immunogenicity and invasiveness of the infecting organism, the site of infection, and the patient's immune response. The early literature on the immunology against dermatophyte infection is reviewed by Wagner and Sohnle (1995), Weitzman and Summerbell (1995), and Calderon (1989). Although various components of the host–dermatophyte relationship have been explored, the mechanisms of innate immunity involved in the prevention and control of dermatophytosis has not yet been investigated in detail.

4.2. Nonspecific Cutaneous Defenses

4.2.1 Structure, Keratinization, and Epidermal Proliferation

The physical and chemical structure of the skin represents a form of defense against dermatophytes. The skin surface acts as a barrier to the entry of dermatophytes. The stratum corneum is continually renewed through keratinization of the epidermal cells. This process results in continuous shedding of the stratum corneum, which also may remove infecting dermatophytes residing there. Epidermal proliferation is also important in the defense against superficial dermatophytosis (Berk et al., 1976). Inflammation, including that produced by T cell-mediated immune reactions, appears to enhance epidermal proliferation.

4.2.2. Accumulation of Neutrophils in the Epidermis

One can sometimes observe pustules in the infected skin of acute dermatophyte infections. Microscopically, the lesions are characterized by an accumulation of neutrophils in the epidermis (epidermal microabscesses). The mechanism by which neutrophils are attracted to the sites of dermatophyte infection has already been partially clarified. Both *Trichophyton rubrum* and *T. mentagrophytes* have been shown to be capable of activating complement by the alternative pathway, which thus produces chemotactic activity for neutrophils (Swan et al., 1983; Davies and Zaini, 1984). *T. mentagrophytes* produce low molecular weight chemotactic factors by themselves (Tagami et al., 1982). In response to stimulation with dermatophyte antigens, keratinocytes can generate chemotactic cytokine (IL-8) that could also be responsible for an accumulation of neutrophils in the lesions of dermatophyte infection (Koga et al., 1996). The neutrophils adhere to opsonized and unopsonized hyphae to inhibit growth of the dermatophyte and perhaps damage or kill it (Dahl, 1994). The neutrophil oxidative mechanisms are capable of killing *Trichophyton* sp. in vitro (Calderon and Hay, 1987). Thus, an accumulation of neutrophils could have a role in the defense against dermatophyte infections.

4.2.3. Antifungal Substances

Not much is known about the substances, which can eliminate the dermatophytes or prevent invasion into the deeper viable tissue. Unsaturated transferrin (King et al., 1975) and α2-macroglobulin keratinase inhibitor (Yu et al., 1972) are thought to be active against dermatophyte invasion.

4.3. Specific Immune Response

Even though dermatophyte infections are very superficial in location, they appear to sensitize the host to the antigens of dermatophyte. Both humoral immunity and cell-mediated immunity (CMI) respond against dermatophyte infection. The T cell-mediated DTH response to dermatophyte antigens may play a central role in both pathogenesis of the typical skin lesions and an acquired, relative resistance that affords partial immunity to the host. The development of CMI, which is correlated with DTH, is usually associated with clinical cure and ridding the stratum corneum of the offending dermatophyte (Jones, 1993). In contrast, the lack of CMI prevents an effective response and predisposes the host to chronic or recurrent dermatophyte infections (Jones, 1986). However, the exact form of effector T cell immunity and the cellular and molecular mechanisms, which eliminate dermatophytes from the skin, are poorly understood. Recently several studies about cytokines have been demonstrated.

4.3.1. Dermatophyte Antigens

The dermatophytes, like other fungi, have a very complicated antigenic makeup. There are two major classes of dermatophyte antigens: glycopeptides and keratinases. The protein portion of the glycopeptides preferentially stimulates CMI, whereas the polysaccharide portion of the glycopeptides preferentially stimulates humoral immunity (Dahl, 1993). Keratinase elicits strong DTH responses, and antibodies that inhibit the proteolytic activity produce this enzyme (Grappel and Blank, 1972). Dermatophytes have many antigenic determinants in common with each other as well as with unrelated fungi (Grappel et al., 1974). Extracts of various dermatophyte species contain a mixture of antigens that are either species-specific or broadly cross-reactive with those of other dermatophytes or those of other fungi. Infection with *Microsporum canis* can induce antibody titers and DTH reaction to itself as well as cross-reacting antibody titers to *T. equinum* and *T. mentagrophytes* and DTH reactions to *T. mentagrophytes*, suggesting establishment of a broad-based immunity following infection with a single dermatophyte (Pier et al., 1995). Studies of dermatophyte antigens by monoclonal antibodies would help to identify specific antigens.

4.3.2. CMI

CMI (T cell-mediated DTH) is the major immunologic defense in clearing dermatophyte infections. Experimental animal models have been used to study the role of CMI during dermatophytosis and the results are summarized by Calderon (1989). Athymic rats that lack T cell-mediated immunity could not clear *T. mentagrophytes* infections compared with genetically matched euthymic control rats (Green et al., 1983). Furthermore, in experimentally infected mice, immunity to dermatophyte infection can be achieved by adoptive transfer of lymphoid cells, but not by serum, of infected donors (Calderon, 1989). The resolution of the disease in both naturally and experimentally infected humans and animals correlates with the development of DTH response, whereas persistence of infection is frequently accompanied by poor in vitro lymphocyte transformation response. absence of DTH response, and enhanced proliferation of the skin in the DTH reaction. DTH reaction is mediated by Th1 cells and macrophages, and enhanced proliferation of the skin in response to this DTH reaction may be one of the final mechanisms that remove the dermatophytes from the skin by epidermal desquamation (Dahl, 1993). The Th1 response, which is characterized by interferon gamma (IFN-γ) release, is thought to be involved in the host defense against dermatophytes and to reflect cutaneous manifestations in dermatophytosis.

4.3.2.1. Th1 Response Several in vitro systems were previously studied to assess CMI in dermatophyte-infected hosts, e.g., lymphocyte transformation (Helander, 1978) and leukocyte migration inhibition (Hay and Brostoff, 1977). Recently, cytokine production is used in vitro assay of T cell immunity (Koga et al., 1993a). One of the key functional parameters determining the immune response to dermatophyte antigen is the nature of cytokines produced by T cells. Th1 cytokines are involved in the elicitation of the DTH response, and IFN-γ is regarded as a major factor in the effector phase of the DTH reaction (Fong and Mosmann, 1989). In recent studies, the production of IFN-γ has been investigated on the DTH response in dermatophytosis. Peripheral blood mononuclear cells from patients with acute dermatophytosis produce a high level of IFN-γ in response to dermatophyte antigen (Koga et al., 1993b, 1995). The presence of IFN-γ mRNA in skin lesions of dermatophytosis has been detected by using reverse transcription-polymerase chain reaction (RT-PCR) (Miyata et al., 1996; Ohta et al., 1998). Immunohistochemically, IFN-γ-positive cells have been detected in situ at the protein level in the upper dermis of the skin lesions (Koga et al., 2001a). These findings suggested that the skin lesion of dermatophytosis is associated with a Th1 response.

Dermatophyte infections can be acute and inflammatory or chronic and noninflammatory. In response to dermatophyte antigen in vitro, IFN-γ was produced in peripheral lymphocytes obtained from patients with acute inflammatory dermatophytosis (Koga et al., 1993b). In contrast, markedly lower levels of IFN-γ production were found in chronically infected patients (Koga et al., 1995). Thus, in vitro T lymphocyte hyposensitivity to dermatophyte antigen was shown by measuring the release of the Th1 cytokine. Patients with chronic dermatophyte infection may suffer from an immune imbalance, which has characteristics of a Th2-type response (Leibovici et al., 1995; Sato and Tagami, 2003).

In normal healthy persons with no clinical evidence of dermatophytosis, IFN-γ production in response to dermatophyte antigen is divided into two groups: high responder and low responder, with high responders being correlated with a clinical history of previous tinea pedis (Koga et al., 2001b). This finding suggests that a history of cured tinea pedis may confer long-lasting T cell recall response, whereas persons with no such history may be immunologically naive or low responders to dermatophyte antigens.

4.3.2.2. Langerhans Cells The inflammatory dermal infiltrates of dermatophytosis mainly consist of CD4-positive T cells and CD8-positive T cells, complemented by

CD68-positive macrophages and CD1a-positive Langerhans cells (Brasch and Sterry, 1992; Brasch et al., 1993; Koga et al., 2001a). Considerable amount of CD1a-positive Langerhans cells are present in the upper dermis and epidermis of the dermatophyte lesions (Emtestam et al., 1985; Johansson et al., 1986), supporting the notion of an antigen-presenting situation. Langerhans cells have been shown to be capable of inducing a T cell response to trichophytin in dermatophytosis in vitro (Braathen and Kaaman, 1983). Langerhans cells are responsible for the uptake and processing of antigens in the lesional Th1 response in dermatophyte infection.

4.3.2.3. Humoral Immunity The host develops a variety of antibodies to dermatophyte infection. Antibodies has been demonstrated in human dermatophytosis, using a variety of techniques such as ELISA. However, humoral immunity apparently does not play a role to eliminate the infection since the highest level of antibodies is found in patients with chronic dermatophyte infection (Dahl, 1987). A frequent pattern seen in chronic patients is the presence of high immediate hypersensitivity and low or waning DTH to dermatophyte antigens (Hunziker and Brun, 1980; Jones, 1993). Immediate hypersensitivity (anti-*Trichophyton* IgE-mediated) may interfere with the development of a protective DTH response. However, many patients with chronic dermatophytosis neither are atopic nor manifest immediate hypersensitivity to dermatophyte antigens, indicating that other factors must also be involved in producing susceptibility to this type of infection.

4.4. Dermatophyte-Induced Suppression of Immune Response

Certain dermatophytes, like *T. rubrum*, produce substances that diminish the immune response. Mannan, a glycoprotein component of the fungal cell wall, may suppress the inflammatory response especially in atopic or other persons susceptible to the mannan-induced suppression of cellular immune response (Dahl, 1993). Incubation of purified *T. rubrum* mannan with peripheral blood mononuclear cells suppressed lymphoblast formation and inhibited the lymphocyte proliferation response to mitogens and a variety of antigenic stimuli (Blake et al., 1991b). *T. rubrum* mannan inhibits keratinocyte proliferation, thus slowing epidermal turnover (Cabrera et al., 1991) and interferes with accessory cell functions of the monocyte (Grando et al. 1992). The increased amount and potency of *T. rubrum* mannan compared with that of *M. canis* may explain why *T. rubrum* elicits less inflammation and causes a more chronic infection than *M. canis* (Blake et al., 1991a). Some of the primary chronic trichophytosis appears to be associated with defective phagocytosis of peripheral blood leukocytes and this defect is probably caused by the fungus itself (Gregurek-Novak et al., 1993).

References

Baker, B.S., Ovigne, J.M., Powles, A.V., Corcoran, S., and Fry, L. (2003). Normal keratinocytes express toll-like receptors (TLRs) 1, 2 and 5: Modulation of TLR expression in chronic plaque psoriasis. *Br. J. Dermatol.* 148: 670–679.

Banchereau, J. and Steinman, R.M. (1998). Dendritic cells and the control of immunity. *Nature* 392: 245–252.

Barnes, P.J. and Karin, M. (1997). Nuclear factor-κB—a pivotal transcription factor in chronic inflammatory diseases. *N. Engl. J. Med.* 336: 1066–1071.

Berk, S.H., Penneys, N.S., and Weinstein, G.D. (1976). Epidermal activity in annular dermatophytosis. *Arch. Dermatol.* 112: 485–488.

Blake, J.S., Cabrera, R.M., Dahl, M.V., Herron, M.J., and Nelson, R.D. (1991a). Comparison of the immunoinhibitory properties of cell wall mannan glycoproteins from *Trichophyton rubrum* and *Microsporum canis*. *J. Invest. Dermatol.* 96: 601.

Blake, J.S., Dahl, M.V., Herron, M.J., and Nelson, R.D. (1991b). An immunoinhibitory cell wall glycoprotein (mannan) from *Trichophyton rubrum*. *J. Invest. Dermatol.* 96: 657–661.

Braathen, L.R. and Kaaman, T. (1983). Human epidermal Langerhans cells induce cellular immune response to trichophytin in dermatophytosis. *Br. J. Dermatol.* 109: 295–300.

Brasch, J. and Sterry, W. (1992). Immunophenotypical characterization of inflammatory cellular infiltrates in tinea. *Acta Derm. Venereol. (Stockh.)* 72: 345–347.

Brasch, J., Martens, H., and Sterry, W. (1993). Langerhans cell accumulation in chronic tinea pedis and pityriasis versicolor. *Clin. Exp. Dermatol.* 18: 329–332.

Cabrera, R.M., Blake, J.S., Dahl, M.V., Herron, M.J., and Nelson, R.D. (1991). Inhibition of keratinocyte proliferation by a mannan glycoprotein isolated from *Trichophyton rubrum*. *J. Invest. Dermatol.* 96: 616.

Calderon, R.A. (1989). Immunoregulation of dermatophytosis. *Crit. Rev. Microbiol.* 16: 338–368.

Calderon, R.A. and Hay, R.J. (1987). Fungicidal activity of human neutrophils and monocytes on dermatophytic fungi, *Trichophyton quinckeanum* and *Trichophyton rubrum*. *Immunology* 61: 289–295.

Dahl, M.V. (1987). Immunological resistance to dermatophyte infections. *Adv. Dermatol.* 2: 305–320.

Dahl, M.V. (1993). Suppression of immunity and inflammation by products produced by dermatophytes. *J. Am. Acad. Dermatol.* 28: S19–S23.

Dahl, M.V. (1994). Dermatophytosis and the immune response. *J. Am. Acad. Dermatol.* 31: S34–S41.

Davies, R.R. and Zaini, F. (1984). *Trichophyton rubrum* and the chemotaxis of polymorphonuclear leucocytes. *Sabouraudia* 22: 65–71.

Emtestam, L., Kaaman, T., Hovmark, A., and Asbrink, E. (1985). An immunohistochemical staining of epidermal Langerhans cells in tinea cruris. *Acta Derm. Venereol. (Stockh.)* 65: 240–243.

Fong, T.A.T. and Mosmann, T.R. (1989). The role of IFN-γ in delayed type hypersensitivity mediated by Th1 clones. *J. Immunol.* 143: 2887–2893.

Fuhlbrigge, R.C., Kieffer, J.D., Armerding, D., and Kupper, T.S. (1997). Cutaneous lymphocyte antigen is a specialized form of PSGL-1 expressed on skin-homing T cells. *Nature* 389: 978–981.

Gallo, R.L., Murakami, M., Ohtake, T., and Zaiou, M. (2002). Biology and clinical relevance of naturally occurring antimicrobial peptides. *J. Allergy Clin. Immunol.* 110: 823–831.

Grando, S.A., Hostager, B.S., Herron, M.J., Dahl, M.V., and Nelson, R.D. (1992). Binding of *Trichophyton rubrum* mannan to human monocytes *in vitro*. *J. Invest. Dermatol.* 98: 876–880.

Grappel, S.F. and Blank, F. (1972). Role of keratinases in dermatophytosis. I. Immune responses of guinea pigs infected with *Trichophyton mentagrophytes* and guinea pigs immunized with keratinases. *Dermatologica* 145: 245–255.

Grappel, S.F., Bishop, C.T., and Blank, F. (1974). Immunology of dermatophytes and dermatophytosis. *Bacteriol. Rev.* 38: 222–250.

Gregurek-Novak, T., Rabatic, S., and Silobrcic, V. (1993). Defective phagocytosis in chronic trichophytosis. *J. Med. Vet. Mycol.* 31: 115–120.

Green, F., Weber, J.K., and Balish, E. (1983). The thymus dependency of acquired resistance to *Trichophyton mentagrophytes* dermatophytosis in rats. *J. Invest. Dermatol.* 81: 31–38.

Harder, J., Bartels, J., Christophers, E., and Schroder, J.M. (1997). A peptide antibiotic from human skin. *Nature* 387: 861.

Hay, R.J. and Brostoff, J. (1977). Immune responses in patients with chronic *Trichophyton rubrum* infection. *Clin. Exp. Dermatol.* 2: 373–380.

Helander, I. (1978). The lymphocyte transformation test in dermatophytosis. *Mykosen* 21: 71–80.

Hoffmann, J.A., Kafatos, F.C., Janeway, C.A., and Ezekowitz, R.A. (1999). Phylogenetic perspectives in innate immunity. *Science* 284: 1313–1318.

Hunziker, N. and Brun, R. (1980). Lack of delayed reaction in presence of cell-mediated immunity in trichophytin hypersensitivity. *Arch. Dermatol.* 116: 1266–1268.

Johansson, S., Scheynius, A., and Faergemann, J. (1986). Fungal infections inducing HLA-DR but not HLA-DQ transplantation antigens on keratinocytes. *Acta Derm. Venereol. (Stockh.)* 66: 277–280.

Jones, H.E. (1986). Cell mediated immunity in the immunopathogenesis of dermatophytosis. *Acta Derm. Venereol. Suppl.* 121: 73–83.

Jones, H.E. (1993). Immune response and host resistance to human dermatophyte infection. *J. Am. Acad. Dermatol.* 28: S12–S18.

Kawai, K., Shimura, H., Minagawa, M., Ito, A., Tomiyama, K., and Ito, M. (2002). Expression of functional toll-like receptor 2 on human epidermal keratinocytes. *J. Dermatol. Sci.* 30: 185–194.

King, R.D., Khan, H.A., Foye, J.C., Greenberg, J.H., and Jones, H.E. (1975). Transferrin, iron, and dermatophytes. I. Serum dermatophyte inhibitory component definitively identified as unsaturated transferrin. *J. Clin. Med.* 86: 204–212.

Koga, T., Ishizaki, H., Matsumoto, T., and Hori, Y. (1993a). Cytokine production of peripheral blood mononuclear cells in a dermatophytosis patient in response to stimulation with trichophytin. *J. Dermatol.* 20: 441–443.

Koga, T., Ishizaki, H., Matsumoto, T., and Hori, Y. (1993b). In vitro release of interferon-γ by peripheral blood mononuclear cells of patients with dermatophytosis in response to stimulation with trichophytin. *Br. J. Dermatol.* 128: 703–704.

Koga, T., Ishizaki, H., Matsumoto, T., and Hori, Y. (1995). Decreased release of interferon-γ by peripheral blood mononuclear cells of patients with chronic dermatophytosis in response to stimulation with trichophytin. *Acta Derm. Venereol. (Stockh.)* 75: 81–82.

Koga, T., Ishizaki, H., Matsumoto, T., and Toshitani, S. (1996). Enhanced release of interleukin-8 from human epidermal keratinocytes in response to stimulation with trichophytin in vitro. *Acta Derm. Venereol. (Stockh.)* 76: 399–400.

Koga, T., Duan, H., Urabe, K., and Furue, M. (2001a). Immunohistochemical detection of interferon-γ-producing cells in dermatophytosis. *Eur. J. Dermatol.* 11: 105–107.

Koga, T., Shimizu, A., and Nakayama, J. (2001b). Interferon-γ production in peripheral lymphocytes of patients with tinea pedis: Comparison of patients with and without *Tinea unguium. Med. Mycol.* 39: 87–90.

Leibovici, V., Evron, R., Axelrod, O., Westerman, M., Shalit, M., Barak, V., and Frankenburg, S. (1995). Imbalance of immune responses in patients with chronic and widespread fungal skin infection. *Clin. Exp. Dermatol.* 20: 390–394.

Medzhitov, R., Preston-Hurlburt, P., and Janeway, C.A. Jr. (1997). A human homologue of the Drosophila Toll protein signals activation of adaptive immunity. *Nature* 388: 394–397.

Milner, S.M. and Ortega, M.R. (1999). Reduced antimicrobial peptide expression in human burn wounds. *Burns* 25: 411–413.

Miyata, T., Fujimura, T., Masuzawa, M., Katsuoka, K., and Nishiyama, S. (1996). Local expression of IFN-γ mRNA in skin lesion of patients with dermatophytosis. *J. Dermatol. Sci.* 13: 167–171.

Ohta, Y., Saitoh, N., Tanuma, H., Fujimura, T., and Katsuoka, K. (1998). Local cytokine expression in steroid-modified tinea faciei. *J. Dermatol.* 25: 362–366.

Ong, P.Y., Ohtake, T., Brandt, C., Strickland, I., Boguniewicz, M., Ganz, T., Gallo, R.L., and Leung, D.Y. (2002). Endogenous antimicrobial peptides and skin infections in atopic dermatitis. *N. Engl. J. Med.* 347: 1151–1160.

Picker, L.J., Kishimoto, T.K., Smith, C.W., Warnock, R.A., and Butcher, E.C. (1991). ELAM-1 is an adhesion molecule for skin-homing T cells. *Nature* 349: 796–799.

Pier, A.C., Hodges, A.B, Lauze, J.M., and Raisbeck, M. (1995). Experimental immunity to *Microsporum canis* and cross reactions with other dermatophytes of veterinary importance. *J. Med. Vet. Mycol.* 33: 93–97.

Porcelli, S.A., Segelke, B.W., Sugita, M., Wilson, I.A., and Brenner, M.B. (1998). The CD1 family of lipid antigen-presenting molecules. *Immunol. Today* 19: 362–368.

Robert, C. and Kupper, T.S. (1999). Inflammatory skin diseases, T cells, and immune surveillance. *Allergy/Immunology* 341: 1817–1828.

Sato, N. and Tagami, H. (2003). Severe measles in a young female patient with chronic, generalized *Trichophyton rubrum* infection showing type 2 helper T cell-dominant immunologic reactivity. *J. Am. Acad. Dermatol.* 48: S43–S46.

Song, P.I., Park, Y.M., Abraham, T., Harten, B., Zivony, A., Neparidze, N., Armstrong, C.A., and Ansel, J.C. (2002). Human keratinocytes express functional CD14 and toll-like receptor 4. *J. Invest. Dermatol.* 119: 424–432.

Swan, J.W., Dahl, M.A., Coppo, P.A., and Hammerschmidt, D.E. (1983). Complement activation by *Trichophyton rubrum. J. Invest. Dermatol.* 80: 156–158.

Tagami, H., Natsume, N., Aoshima, T., Inoue, F., Suehisa, S., and Yamada, M. (1982). Analysis of transepidermal leucocyte chemotaxis in experimental dermatophytosis in guinea pigs. *Arch. Dermatol. Res.* 273: 205–217.

Takiuchi, I., Higuchi, D., Sei, Y., and Koga, M. (1982). Isolation of an extracellular proteinase (keratinase) from *Microsporum canis. Sabouraudia* 20: 281–288.

Wagner, D.K. and Sohnle, P.G. (1995). Cutaneous defenses against dermatophytes and yeasts. *Clin. Microbiol. Rev.* 8: 317–335.
Weitzman, I. and Summerbell, R.C. (1995). The dermatophytes. *Clin. Microbiol. Rev.* 8: 240–259.
Yu, R.J., Grappel, S.F., and Blank, F. (1972). Inhibition of keratinases by α2-macroglobulin. *Experientia* 28: 886.

23

Immune Surveillance against *Sporothrix schenckii* Infection

Takeshi Uenotsuchi[1], Tetsuo Matsuda[1], Masutaka Furue[1], and Tetsuya Koga[2]

1. Introduction

Sporotrichosis is a granulomatous, cutaneous, or subcutaneous mycotic infection with a subacute or chronic course. It is caused by *Sporothrix schenckii*, a dimorphic fungus, which exists as conidia and yeast cells. The fungus generally enters the body at sites of trauma, where it becomes implanted. The size of the initial fungal inoculum, the immune state of the host, the virulence of the fungus, the depth of traumatic inoculation, and thermal tolerance are all thought to play a part in the development of sporotrichosis.

The disease sporotrichosis occurs in different clinical forms, depending on the patient's immune condition. The main clinical manifestation is on the skin, where it presents as two major clinical types (lymphocutaneous and fixed-cutaneous); these two forms are commonly observed in patients

[1] Department of Dermatology, Graduate School of Medical Sciences, Kyushu University, Fukuoka, Japan.
[2] Department of Dermatology, Fukuoka Red Cross Hospital, Fukuoka, Japan.

with good immunological response. Disseminated cutaneous sporotrichosis is rarely reported. Hematogenous spread is thought to underlie cutaneous dissemination (Morris-Jones, 2002). Immunosuppression caused by conditions such as alcoholism, diabetes, chronic obstructive pulmonary disease, malignancies, transplantation, corticosteroid therapy, and human immunodeficiency virus (HIV) infection increases the probability of disseminated, hematogenous, pulmonary, and visceral sporotrichosis (Bonifaz et al., 2001; Carvalho et al., 2002).

The immunological mechanisms involved in the prevention, control, and eradication of sporotrichosis are not fully understood. However, it is believed to involve nonspecific and specific immune defense systems, both of which are discussed below.

2. Nonspecific Cutaneous Defenses

The mechanisms of innate immunity involved in the prevention and control of sporotrichosis have not been investigated in detail as yet. Phagocytosis is considered to provide an important barrier to the course of sporotrichosis (Cunningham et al., 1979; Ramos-Zepeda and González-Mendoza, 1986). In addition, it has been reported that both neutrophils and monocytes can readily kill *S. schenckii* and that this killing can be blocked by adding inhibitors of oxidative metabolism (Rex and Bennett, 1990).

2.1. Neutrophils

Sporotrichosis presents as a nonspecific, chronic, and granulomatous inflammation with a necrotic or pyogenic center, consisting mainly of lymphocytes, epithelioid cells, multinucleated giant cells, dendritic cells, and neutrophils. In man, the fungal cells within the sporotrichosis lesions are frequently phagocytosed by neutrophils (Hiruma et al., 1992). Thus, the lesions are characterized by an infiltration of neutrophils in the granuloma. A study using mouse models showed that a lack of killing activity by neutrophils in immunocompromised nude mice contributed more to the impaired defense of these animals than the lack of macrophage activation by T cells, suggesting a possible role of neutrophils in host defense (Lei et al., 1993).

2.2. Monocytes and Macrophages

Activated macrophages, including those produced by T cell-mediated immune reactions, appears to play an important role in the resistance to *S. schenckii* in mice. Pretreatment of mice with OK-432 (Picibanil), a macrophage-activating agent, enhanced resistance to *S. schenckii* infection, while pretreatment with carrageenan, a macrophage inhibitor, impaired their resistance (Shiraishi et al., 1992). The same authors reported that, in vitro, *S. schenckii* was intracellularly killed by peritoneal macrophages from OK-432-treated mice. Nitric oxide is a key cytotoxic mediator involved in the macrophage defense against *S. schenckii*. The differential susceptibility of two types of conidia to the cytotoxic effect of macrophages seems to depend not only on a differential phagocytosis but also on their differential resistance to the effects of nitric oxide (Fernandes et al., 2000).

3. Specific Immune Response

Both humoral and cellular-specific immune response mechanisms are involved in combating a *S. schenckii* infection. Cell-mediated immunity (CMI), via T cell-mediated delayed-type hypersensitivity (DTH) to *S. schenckii* antigen, is the major immunologic defense mechanism used to deal with this infection. Of particular interest and importance in the host's defense against *S. schenckii*, as we discuss below, is granuloma formation, which is thought to be a result of a Th1 cell-dependent inflammatory response.

3.1. CMI

There are several indications of the involvement of cell-mediated immune response against infection with *S. schenckii*. The results of delayed hypersensitivity skin and lymphocyte transformation tests with *S. schenckii* antigen showed a depression in cellular immune response. This is correlated with the severity of the disease, and implied a greater involvement of the host (Carlos et al., 1992). In a murine model, it was confirmed that both CD4-positive T cells and macrophages were required for the development of cellular immunity against *S. schenckii* antigen (Tachibana et al., 1999). CD4-positive Th 1 cells, which produce the cytokines interleukin-2 (IL-2) and interferon gamma (IFN-γ), are chiefly responsible for DTH responses. The granuloma formation in sporotrichosis is coupled with a Th1 response, which provides a strong defense.

3.1.1. Th1 Response

Recent studies have investigated the effect of the DTH response in sporotrichosis on the pattern of cytokine production. Peripheral blood mononuclear cells from a patient with lymphocutaneous sporotrichosis produced a high level of IFN-γ in response to stimulation with sporotrichin (Koga et al., 1996). Using a mouse model, Tachibana et al. (1999) demonstrated that protection in vivo could be transferred to naive congenitally athymic nude mice using lymph node cells taken from immune mice. The same authors reported that, in vitro, inhibition of fungal growth was observed when both immune lymph node cells and macrophages were combined. Both the protection in vivo and the growth inhibition in vitro were reduced after depletion of CD4-positive T cells. Immune lymph node cells expressed IFN-γ mRNA after stimulation with heat-killed *S. schenckii* (Tachibana et al., 1999). Taken together these results suggest that acquired immunity against *S. schenckii* is expressed mainly by macrophages activated by Th1 cells.

Granuloma formation is a critical event in the immune response and an essential component of a host's normal defense. Immunohistochemical procedures have shown that IFN-γ-positive cells can be detected in the periphery of the granulomatous lesions of sporotrichosis, and that CD4-positive T cells are the dominant phenotype (Koga et al., 2002). Using reverse transcription polymerase chain reaction (RT-PCR) techniques, IFN-γ mRNA has been detected in the skin lesions of sporotrichosis (Fujimura et al., 1996). These findings indicate that granuloma formation in sporotrichosis is associated with a Th1 response in the skin lesions. This Th1 response, which is characterized by IFN-γ release, would result in activation of macrophages that would kill intracellular *S. schenckii*. Interestingly in another study, stimulation of murine macrophages with IFN-γ induced nitric oxide production and inhibited the growth of *S. schenckii* (Fernandes et al., 2000).

3.1.2. Dendritic Cells

Dendritic cells are considered to be the most potent of the antigen-presenting cells, and CD83 is expressed at a high level in immunocompetent, activated, and mature dendritic cells. A small but significant subpopulation of CD83-positive dendritic cells have been identified in the granulation tissue of sporotrichosis (Koga et al., 2001). This indicates that activated and mature dendritic cells may play a role in the immune response to sporotrichosis.

3.1.3. *Epithelioid Cells and Multinucleated Giant Cells*

Epithelioid cells (which are derived from activated macrophages) and multinucleated cells (which are fused epithelioid cells) are typical of granulomatous hypersensitivity. The majority of the epithelioid cells and multinucleated giant cells within sporotrichosis granulomas are CD68-positive cells (Koga et al., 2002). Inducible nitric oxide synthetase (iNOS) is expressed by activated macrophages and results in the production of nitric oxide (MacMicking et al., 1997). The expression of iNOS was not detected in the epithelioid cells and multinucleated giant cells within the granulomas of patients with sporotrichosis (Koga et al., 2002).

3.2. Humoral Immunity

Precipitating antibodies against *S. schenckii* antigens have been found in the sera of patients with sporotrichosis (de Alborno et al., 1984). The serologic response to *S. schenckii* has been investigated in patients with sporotrichosis using solid-phase enzyme-linked immunosorbent assays and Western immunoblot techniques (Scott and Muchmore, 1989). The authors of this study proposed that the purification of specific antigen fractions could provide the basis of a sensitive and specific serodiagnostic test to indicate the presence and activity of extracutaneous sporotrichosis. However, it would appear that humoral immunity does not play a pivotal role in eliminating the infection since immune serum does not enhance resistance against *S. schenckii* infection (Tachibana et al., 1999).

4. Differential Susceptibility of *S. schenckii* to Host Defenses

Melanin has been implicated in the pathogenesis of several important human fungal pathogens. *S. schenckii* produces melanin or melanin-like compounds (Morris-Jones et al., 2003). Melanins have properties that enable them to bind metals and function as a physiological redox buffer (thereby possibly acting as a sink for harmful unpaired electrons), provide structural rigidity to cell walls, and store water and ions, thus helping to prevent desiccation. The mechanism by which they interfere in the phagocytosis of a microorganism by macrophages has not been fully understood. However, surface charge effects are likely to play an important role because melanins are charged polymers and phagocytosis is inversely correlated with cell charge. Melanization appears to protect *S. schenckii* against phagocytosis and subsequent killing by human monocytes and macrophages (Langfelder et al., 2002).

It is interesting to look at the role of cell wall compounds in the immune response to sporotrichosis. The effect of cell wall compounds and exoantigen, obtained from *S. schenckii*, on macrophage–fungus interaction has recently been analyzed. The *S. schenckii* conidia cultured for 4 to 7 days were more virulent than the *S. schenckii* conidia cultured for 10 to 12 days. The differences in the virulence of these two types of conidia, which were from a single strain of *S. schenckii*, correlated with the ratio of their cell wall sugars (rhamnose:mannose) (Fernandes et al., 1999), and the differences in the virulence could be ascribed to a differential susceptibility to nitric oxide produced by activated macrophages (Fernandes et al., 2000). Another in vitro study has shown that the lipid compound of the cell wall plays an important role in the pathogenesis of sporotrichosis. It was found that this component of the cell wall could inhibit the phagocytic process and induce a high level of release of nitric oxide and tumor necrosis factor alpha (TNF-α) in macrophage cultures (Carlos et al., 2003).

Adhesion is the first step involved in the infection of pathogens in the host. Adherence of *S. schenckii* to host tissues such as endothelial cells and extracellular matrix proteins is regarded as prerequisite for systemic sporotrichosis. The two morphological forms of *S. schenckii*, yeast cells and conidia, can bind to fibronectin, laminin, and type II collagen. It has been demonstrated that the binding capacities differ between the two forms. The cell surface glycoconjugates of *S. schenckii* participated in the binding to human fibronectin via carbohydrate or peptide moieties (Lima et al., 1999; 2001).

References

Bonifaz, A., Peniche, A., Mercadillo, P., and Saul, A. (2001). Successful treatment of AIDS-related disseminated cutaneous sporotrichosis with itraconazole. *AIDS Patient Care STDS* 15: 603–606.

Carlos, I.Z., Sgarbi, D.B., Angluster, J., Alviano, C.S., and Silva, C.L. (1992). Detection of cellular immunity with the soluble antigen of the fungus *Sporothrix schenckii* in the systemic form of the disease. *Mycopathologia* 117: 139–144.

Carlos, I.Z., Sgarbi, D.B.G., Santos, G.C., and Placeres, M.C.P. (2003). *Sporothrix schenckii* lipid inhibits macrophage phagocytosis: Involvement of nitric oxide and tumor necrosis factor-α. *Scand. J. Immunol.* 57: 214–220.

Carvalho, M.T.M., de Castro, A.M., Baby, C., Werner, B., Neto, J.F., and Queiroz-Telles, F. (2002). Disseminated cutaneous sporotrichosis in a patient with AIDS: Report of a case. *Rev. Soc. Bras. Med. Trop.* 35: 655–659.

Cunningham, K.M., Blumer, G.S., and Rhoades, E.R. (1979). Phagocytosis: An intracellular fate of *Sporothrix schenckii*. *J. Infect. Dis.* 140: 815–817.

de Alborno, M.B., Villamueva, E., and de Torres, E.D. (1984). Application of immunoprecipitation techniques to the diagnosis of sporotrichosis. *Mycopathologia* 85: 177–183.

Fernandes, K.S., Mathews, H.L., and Lopes Bezerra, L.M. (1999). Differences in virulence of *Sporothrix schenckii* conidia related to culture conditions and cell-wall components. *J. Med. Microbiol.* 48: 195–203.

Fernandes, K.S., Coelho, A.L., Lopes Bezerra, L.M., and Barja-Fidalgo, C. (2000). Virulence of *Sporothrix schenckii* conidia and yeast cells, and their susceptibility to nitric oxide. *Immunology* 101: 563–569.

Fujimura, T., Asai, T., Muguruma, K., Masuzawa, M., and Katsuoka, K. (1996). Local expression of migration inhibitory factor and Th1 type cytokine mRNA in sporotrichosis lesions. *Acta Derm. Venereol.* (*Stockh.*) 76: 321–322.

Hiruma, M., Kawada, A., Noda, T., Yamazaki, M., and Ishibashi, A. (1992). Tissue response in sporotrichosis: Light and electron microscopy studies. *Mycoses* 35: 35–41.

Koga, T., Matsuda, T., Ota, K., Ishizaki, H., Matsumoto, T., and Hori, Y. (1996). Cytokine production of peripheral blood mononuclear cells in a patient with sporotrichosis in response to stimulation with sporotrichin. *Acta Derm. Venereol.* (*Stockh.*) 74: 328.

Koga, T., Duan, H., Urabe, K., and Furue, M. (2001). Immunohistochemical localization of activated and mature $CD83^+$ dendritic cells in granulomas of sporotrichosis. *Eur. J. Dermatol.* 11: 527–529.

Koga, T., Duan, H., and Furue, M. (2002). Immunohistochemical detection of interferon-γ-producing cells in granuloma formation of sporotrichosis. *Med. Mycol.* 40: 111–114.

Langfelder, K., Streibel, M., Jahn, B., Haase, G., and Brakhage, A.A. (2002). Biosynthesis of fungal melanins and their importance for human pathogenic fungi. *Fungal Genet. Biol.* 38: 143–158.

Lei, P.C., Yoshiike, T., Yaguchi, H., and Ogawa, H. (1993). Histopathological studies of *Sporothrix schenckii*-inoculated mice. Possible functions of polymorphonuclear leukocytes in normal and immunocompromised (congenitally athymic nude) mice. *Mycopathologia* 122: 89–93.

Lima, O.C., Figueiredo, C.C., Pereria, B.A., Coelho, M.G., Morandi, V., and Lopez-Bezerra, L.M. (1999). Adhesion of the human pathogen *Sporothrix schenckii* to several extracellular matrix proteins. *Braz. J. Med. Biol. Res.* 32: 651–657.

Lima, O.C., Figueiredo, C.C., Previato, J.O., Mendonca-Previato, L., Morandi, V., and Lopez-Bezerra, L.M. (2001). Involvement of fungal cell wall components in adhesion of *Sporothrix schenckii* to human fibronectin. *Infect. Immun.* 69: 6974–6980.

MacMicking, J., Xie, Q., and Nathan, C. (1997). Nitric oxide and macrophage function. *Annu. Rev. Immunol.* 15: 323–350.

Morris-Jones, R. (2002). Sporotrichosis. *Clin. Exp. Dermatol.* 27: 427–431.

Morris-Jones, R., Youngchim, S., Gomez, B.L., Aisen, P., Hay, R.J., Nosanchuk, J.D., Casadevall, A., and Hamilton, A.J. (2003). Synthesis of melanin-like pigments by *Sporothrix schenckii* in vitro and during mammalian infection. *Infect. Immun.* 71: 4026–4033.

Ramos-Zepeda, R. and González-Mendoza, A. (1986). Metabolic activity of phagocytes in experimental sporotrichosis. *Mycopathologia* 93: 109–112.

Rex, J.H. and Bennett, J.E. (1990). Administration of potassium iodide to normal volunteers does not increase killing of *Sporothrix schenckii* by their neutrophils or monocytes. *J. Med. Vet. Mycol.* 28: 185–189.

Scott, E.N. and Muchmore, H.G. (1989). Immunoblot analysis of antibody responses to *Sporothrix schenckii. J. Clin. Microbiol.* 27: 300–304.

Shiraishi, A., Nakagaki, K., and Arai, T. (1992). Role of cell-mediated immunity in the resistance to experimental sporotrichosis in mice. *Mycopathologia* 120: 15–21.

Tachibana, T., Matsuyama, T., and Mitsuyama, M. (1999). Involvement of $CD4^+$ T cells and macrophages in acquired protection against infection with *Sporothrix schenckii* in mice. *Med. Mycol.* 37: 397–404.

24

Innate and Acquired Immunity in *Cryptococcus neoformans* Infections of the Central Nervous System

Kent L. Buchanan

Program in Molecular Pathogenesis and Immunity, Department of Microbiology and Immunology, Tulane University Health Sciences Center, New Orleans, LA 70112.

1. Introduction

Cryptococcosis is a life-threatening disease that develops following the inhalation and dissemination of the encapsulated fungal pathogen, *Cryptococcus neoformans*. In most individuals with normal resistance mechanisms, following inhalation of cryptococcal yeast cells or basidiospores, the cryptococci remain localized in the lungs and are eventually cleared from the host. However, in individuals with deficiencies in cell-mediated immunity, such as acquired immunodeficiency syndrome (AIDS) patients, the organisms frequently disseminate to extrapulmonary sites via the bloodstream. *C. neoformans* has a predilection for the central nervous system (CNS); thus, mortality due to *C. neoformans* is most frequently associated with meningitis or meningoencephalitis. Much has been learned about how *C. neoformans* causes disease and how the host fights off the yeast in the lung; however, less is known about immune responses in the CNS against this pathogen.

In this chapter, the epidemiology, pathology, innate host response, and acquired immune reactivity to *C. neoformans* as they relate to infections of the CNS will be discussed. Much of the information described herein was obtained from experimental animal models, thus an attempt was made to correlate the experimental data with the clinical picture of human cryptococcosis.

2. Epidemiology

2.1. Environmental Sources and Acquisition of *C. neoformans*

C. neoformans strains currently are classified into three variants based on genetic differences and into four predominant serotypes due to differences in capsular polysaccharide structure (Casadevall and Perfect, 1998; Franzot et al., 1999; Perfect and Casadevall, 2002). *C. neoformans* var. *neoformans* (serotype D) and *C. neoformans* var. *grubii* (serotype A) strains are typically found in the environment in dust, debris, or soil associated with avian excreta, whereas *C. neoformans* var. *gattii* (serotypes B and C) isolates have been found mostly associated with eucalyptus trees in tropical and subtropical areas (Kwon-Chung and Bennett, 1984; Ellis and Pfeiffer, 1990, 1992). Although definitive evidence is lacking, cryptococcosis is thought to be acquired by inhalation of yeast cells or basidiospores followed by dissemination from the initial pulmonary infection. However, direct invasion of the CNS from the nasal passage should not be ruled out as a possible route of infection (Gomes et al., 1997).

For a pulmonary route to be the portal of entry, the infectious propagule would need to be sufficiently small (<5 μm) to be deposited in the alveolar spaces (Kwon-Chung, 1992; Buchanan and Murphy, 1998). *C. neoformans* basidiospores typically range in size from 1.8 to 3 μm in diameter (Kwon-Chung, 1992); thus, these spores are small enough for direct deposition in the alveoli. Cryptococcal yeast cells isolated from soil or pigeon excreta are typically desiccated and mostly nonencapsulated (Ishaq et al., 1968; Farhi et al., 1970; Neilson et al., 1977), in contrast to the appearance of clinical specimens in which the yeast cells are usually 4–6 μm in size and are surrounded by a prominent polysaccharide capsule that ranges from 1 μm to >30 μm in diameter (Levitz, 1991). Desiccated and nonencapsulated yeast cells <1 μm in size have been isolated from aerosolized soil (Neilson et al., 1977) and pigeon droppings (Powell et al., 1972; Ruiz and Bulmer, 1981; Ruiz et al., 1981). These desiccated yeast cells are not only viable but also virulent, and their size is compatible with alveolar deposition following inhalation (Neilson et al., 1977; Ruiz et al., 1981). Regardless of the nature of the infectious particle, it is generally thought that once the infectious propagule is deposited in the lung, it becomes rehydrated or transforms into the yeast stage. The resulting yeast cells then produce the thick polysaccharide capsule that is evident in clinical specimens. At this point the primary pulmonary infection may be asymptomatic, or could elicit mild pneumonia-like symptoms. In most individuals with normal resistance, inhaled cryptococci remain localized in the lungs and are eventually eliminated by innate and/or acquired immune responses.

Until recently, the general belief was that disease caused by *C. neoformans*, especially in immunocompromised individuals, was due to recent exposure to the ubiquitous organisms. Serological evidence indicates that most humans are exposed to the organism even early in life (Chen et al., 1999; Goldman et al., 2001). Growing evidence suggests that *C. neoformans* may lay dormant in a host for several years and reemerge or reactivate to cause disease once the hosts' immune system is compromised (Dromer et al.,1992, 1996; Garcia-Hermoso et al.,1999; Goldman et al., 2000). For instance, Dromer et al. (1992) propose that the first reported case in France of cryptococcosis attributed to *C. neoformans* var. *gattii* was not acquired in France, but instead was due to a much earlier exposure to the organism in Cambodia or Zaire. Using genetic typing, Garcia-Hermosa et al (1999) analyzed 103 *C. neoformans* isolates obtained from 29 cryptococcosis patients as part of a study in France. Seventeen of the patients were born in Europe, whereas nine patients had been born in Africa and had lived in France a median time of 110 months prior to diagnosis, with no recent return trips to Africa reported (Garcia-Hermoso et al., 1999). Based on genetic analyses of the isolates obtained from these patients, these investigators reported a statistically significant clustering of isolate subtypes from African-born patients compared to the isolates obtained from patients born in Europe (Garcia-Hermoso et al., 1999). The results suggest that the patients originating from African countries had acquired *C. neoformans* before immigrating to France, and further, that reactivation of a subclinical or dormant infection was likely involved in these cryptococcosis cases.

Goldman et al. (2000) developed a rat model to study latent cryptococcal infections. In these studies, rats were infected in the lungs and the pulmonary infection was resolved by a host response that was previously characterized as granulomatous in nature (Goldman et al., 1994, 1996b). Although the host restricted dissemination of the organisms from the lung in this model, the yeast apparently survived inside macrophages and epithelioid cells and reemerged later to cause disease when the immune system was suppressed by glucocorticoids (Goldman et al., 2000). In addition, there is evidence that *C. neoformans* can take sanctuary in the prostate of immunocompromised individuals during antifungal treatment (Staib et al., 1990; Ndimbie et al., 1994; Yip et al., 1998). For this reason, especially in AIDS patients, lifelong antifungal drug therapy is often prescribed for cryptococcosis (Powderly, 1992; Spitzer et al., 1993). Additional epidemiological and experimental studies are needed to determine the role of dormancy and reactivation in disease caused by *C. neoformans*.

2.2. Predisposing Conditions

C. neoformans, especially var. *gattii*, can cause disease in apparently normal individuals (Speed and Dunt, 1995; Chen et al., 2000). However, in most cases of cryptococcosis, an underlying deficiency in immunity predisposes an individual for acquisition of disease or reactivation of a dormant infection. Individuals with depressed immune function due to malignancy or lymphoproliferative disease (Collins et al., 1951; Lewis and Rabinovich, 1972), corticosteroid therapy (Collins et al., 1972; Diamond and

Bennett, 1974), organ transplantation (Gallis et al., 1975; John et al., 1994; Gupta et al., 2004), HIV infection or AIDS (Kovacs et al., 1985; Bottone and Wormser, 1986; Eng et al., 1986; Mackenzie, 1989; Clark et al., 1990), non-HIV causes of T lymphocytopenia (Duncan et al., 1993; Dev et al., 1994), hypogammaglobulinemia (Gupta et al., 1987), or hyper IgM syndrome (Tabone et al., 1994), are more susceptible to progressive cryptococcosis and in these individuals the organisms frequently disseminate to extrapulmonary sites via the bloodstream. It is unclear at this time whether gender, race, or ethnic differences contribute to risk of infection with *C. neoformans*. However, there is a marked disparity in the numbers of pediatric cases of cryptococcosis compared to adults (Speed and Kaldor, 1997). Considering that greater than 75% of children older than 2 years of age in a New York City study were seropositive for anticryptococcal antibody, which suggests previous exposure to *C. neoformans* by the children (Goldman et al., 2001), then the disparity in pediatric cryptococcosis cases is not likely due to lack of exposure in the pediatric population.

3. Pathogenesis

C. neoformans has been described as a neurotropic fungus with a predilection for the central nervous system. Although numerous reasons for the neurotropism have been suggested, it has still not been established why this organism behaves as it does in the host. Because immunocompetent hosts can contain cryptococcal infections, it has been proposed that *C. neoformans* may colonize in the CNS because the CNS is somewhat immunoprivileged and infectious agents like *C. neoformans* may be able to evade the immune system by hiding out in the CNS. Another long-held theory is that *C. neoformans* utilizes catecholamine-like molecules that are abundant in the CNS to make and deposit melanin in the cryptococcal cell wall. Melanin could provide protection from nitrogen- and oxygen-derived oxidants, antimycotic drugs, and even inhibit phagocytosis by macrophages or macrophage-like cells of the CNS (Wang and Casadevall, 1994a,b; Wang et al., 1995; Hamilton and Holdom, 1999; Hamilton and Gomez, 2002). In support of this theory, melanin has been detected in the cell walls of cryptococcal yeast cells in animal models (Nosanchuk et al., 1999; Rosas et al., 2000) and in human cryptococcal meningoencephalitis tissue sections (Nosanchuk et al., 2000). However, it should be kept in mind that melanin production, as well as the production of other virulence factors, such as the polysaccharide capsule, are probably accidental virulence attributes in the human host. These virulence factors likely did not evolve in the fungus to aid in causing disease in man, but to help in survival in nature.

3.1. Dissemination of Cryptococcosis

Besides the CNS, other tissues, such as the skin and prostate, can be infected with *C. neoformans* following dissemination from the lungs. In general, the different varieties of *C. neoformans* cause somewhat different manifestations of cryptococcosis. As mentioned above, *C. neoformans* var. *gattii* more frequently causes disease in apparently immunocompetent individuals compared to varieties *neoformans* and *grubii* (Chen et al., 2000). In these cases, the organisms are often found associated with granulomas that can become quite large in the brain parenchyma during cryptococcal meningoencephalitis (Chen et al., 2000). In addition, *C. neoformans* var. *neoformans* isolates tend to be more dermatotropic than var. *grubii* strains, most likely due to an increased sensitivity of var. *neoformans* to heat as compared to var. *grubii* organisms (Martinez et al., 2001).

Although the lungs are likely the primary site of infection, diagnosis of cryptococcosis often is not made until neurological symptoms arise as a result of dissemination of the organisms into the CNS. At this time, little is known about the mechanisms for dissemination from the lungs and into the CNS. Considering the barriers to infection of the CNS (see Section 3.2 below), invasion of CNS tissues likely supplies some selective advantage to invading microorganisms.

3.2. Physical Barriers to Infection of the CNS

Under normal circumstances, entry of cells, pathogenic microorganisms, and even small molecules into the CNS is restricted by a tight blood–brain barrier (BBB). This BBB prevents blood constituents from getting into the brain parenchyma and into the cerebrospinal fluid (CSF) and, depending on the site in the CNS, the barrier is maintained by either endothelial cells or epithelial cells. The barrier between the bloodstream and the brain parenchyma is composed of microvessel endothelial cells with tight junctions that are, in part, dependent on pericytes, the basement membrane, and the perivascular glia limitans, which consists of astrocytes and microglial cells (Janzer and Raff, 1987; Janzer, 1993; Tuomanen, 1996; Ring and Tuomanen, 1997). Astrocytes, in particular, appear to be important in maintenance of the integrity of the BBB by virtue of contact with the endothelial cells of the blood vessels via foot processes and/or the production of soluble factors that stimulate the endothelial cells to form tight junctions (Ring and Tuomanen, 1997). Pathogens crossing into the CNS through the endothelial BBB of the microvessels would be found initially in the perivascular areas of the brain parenchyma, with possible dissemination into the CSF and meningeal spaces occurring later.

The second area of restricted access to the CNS is at the blood–CSF interface in the choroid plexus. The endothelial cell junctions of the blood vessels in the choroid plexus are leaky, thus blood–CSF restriction is maintained by tight junction formation of polarized epithelial cells (Tuomanen, 1996; Ring and Tuomanen, 1997). Entry of a pathogen at the choroid plexus would result in access to the ventricles and quick spread through the CSF. CSF is normally sterile and devoid of host defense components, such as leukocytes and complement components, making it an attractive sanctuary for invading organisms. However, CSF is also poor in nutrients needed for the growth of some microorganisms, which may impede the spread or dissemination of pathogenic organisms throughout the CSF.

3.3. Mechanisms of Entry Across the BBB

Three main routes have been proposed for entry of pathogenic organisms into the CNS (Tuomanen, 1996). Transcellular migration involves uptake by endothelial cells of BBB microvessels or epithelial cells of the choroid plexus followed by emigration through the cells and into the brain parenchyma (Tuomanen, 1996). In this case, the pathogen may help facilitate its own uptake by encoding surface molecules that aid in binding to receptors on the endothelium or epithelium or in altering vesicular transport of the host cell. Several bacteria and the fungal pathogen, *Candida albicans*, have been reported to cross the BBB by this mechanism (Tuomanen, 1996; Jong et al., 2001). Pathogens may also migrate between the endothelial cells or the epithelial cells of the BBB by disrupting tight junction formation. Lastly, pathogens may migrate through the BBB by hitching a ride on or within leukocytes, such as monocytes or possibly T lymphocytes, using a process termed the "Trojan Horse" mechanism (Tuomanen, 1996). Few studies have been conducted to determine the mechanism of *C. neoformans* entry into the CNS. Historically, the general assumption was that *C. neoformans* would first initiate meningeal infection with subsequent movement into the brain parenchyma via the Virchow–Robin spaces connected to the subarachnoid space, however, it has also been postulated that once in the blood, *C. neoformans* crosses the endothelial cells comprising the BBB and initiates CNS infection in the brain parenchyma.

Both in vitro and in vivo approaches have been used to identify the mechanisms involved in *C. neoformans* dissemination into the CNS. Using a mouse model of meningoencephalitis following intravenous infection with viable yeast cells, Chretien et al. (2002) observed cryptococci inside monocytes and macrophages associated with the leptomeningeal capillaries and leptomeningeal space, respectively, as well as, inside endothelial cells. The association of cryptococci with monocytes and endothelial cells in the leptomeningeal capillaries suggested to these authors that *C. neoformans* crossed into the CNS at the level of the endothelial BBB and that likely both monocytes and endothelial cells played a role in the traversal of the BBB (Chretien et al., 2002).

Chen et al. (2003) developed an in vitro BBB composed of SV40-transformed human brain microvascular endothelial cells (HBMEC) to examine binding of cryptococci to the endothelial cells and potential emigration of the yeast cells across the in vitro barrier. Binding of *C. neoformans* to the in vitro BBB was associated with morphological changes in the HBMEC, suggestive of actin cytoskeletal reorganization (Chen et al., 2003). However, these investigators did not observe cryptococci inside the endothelial cells of the in vitro BBB suggesting that *C. neoformans* was not crossing the in vitro BBB by a transcellular route (Chen et al., 2003).

More recently, Olszewski et al. (2004) observed that intravenous as well as intratracheal infection with the virulent *C. neoformans* var. *grubii* strain H99 resulted in colonization of the brain parenchyma in close proximity to blood vessels occluded by cryptococcal cells. The lack of observable yeast cells in the subarachnoid space, leptomeninges, and the CSF of the ventricles contributed to the conclusion that the organisms were entering the CNS by direct transfer across the endothelial BBB (Olszewski et al., 2004). The direct transcytosis of *C. neoformans* across the endothelial BBB was corroborated by Chang et al. (2004) using *C. neoformans* var. *neoformans*. These investigators used both an in vivo mouse intravenous infection model coupled with an in vitro BBB composed of non-transformed HBMEC to investigate the mechanism of *C. neoformans* transcytosis across the BBB. In this study, shortly after adding cryptococci to HBMEC monolayers, the HBMEC form microvilli-like projections that eventually engulf the yeast cells (Fig. 24.1) (Chang et al., 2004). Furthermore, cryptococci traversing the HBMEC barrier were observed inside vacuoles and not in between cells as would be expected if a paracellular route of migration was involved. Finally, in vivo the cryptococci were seen in the brain parenchyma early after intravenous infection and only later in infection were the meninges involved; invading yeast cells were not observed in the choroid plexus even late in infection (Chang et al., 2004). Based on their results, the authors concluded that the endothelial BBB in the microvessels and not the choroid plexus epithelial barrier is the site of entry of *C. neoformans* into the CNS and the mechanism of emigration involves a transcellular route (Chang et al., 2004).

Lastly, a phospholipase mutant of *C. neoformans* reportedly was unable to infect the CNS of mice following intravenous inoculation unless the mutant was provided to the mice engulfed inside a mononuclear phagocyte (Santangelo et al., 2004). Presumably, the mutant yeast gained access into the CNS by virtue of riding along with the monocyte

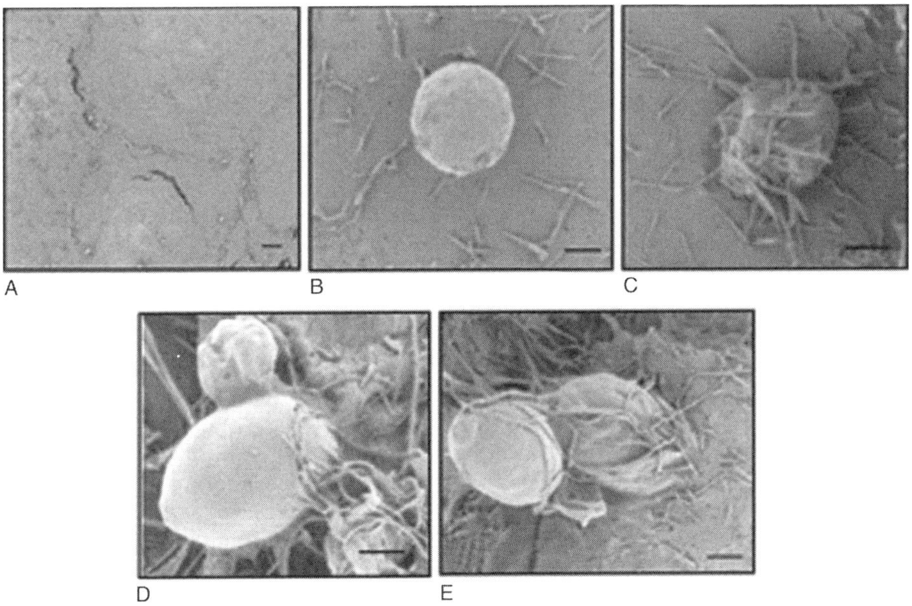

Figure 24.1. Adherence of *C. neoformans* to human brain microvessel endothelial cells (HBMEC). Primary HBMEC cells were grown to confluency on collagen coated glass cover slips. *C. neoformans* strain B-3501 (Serotype D) was added for the indicated time, followed by washing with culture medium, fixing and preparation for scanning electron microscopy (SEM). Confluent growth of these same cells in transwell inserts resulted in the development of an in vitro BBB with tight junctions (Chang et al., 2004). A. Surface of the HBMEC at 0 time point (control). B. Extensive microvilli-like projections observed 15 min after addition of B-3501 cells to HBMEC monolayer. C. Microvilli-like projections are covering yeast cells at 30 min. D and E. Penetration of yeast cells into HBMEC (Scale bar = 4 μm). The figure, courtesy of Dr. June Kwon-Chung (NIH), originally appeared in reference (Chang et al., 2004) and is reproduced here with permission.

following intravenous injection (Santangelo et al., 2004), the so-called "Trojan Horse" mechanism of CNS entry by pathogens. It is clear that additional studies are required to identify precisely how *C. neoformans* enters the CNS and determine if all *C. neoformans* variants or serotypes use the same mechanisms and/or receptor–ligand interactions to cross the BBB.

3.4. Pathology of Cryptococcal CNS Infections

Historically, inflammatory disease due to cryptococcal infection of the CNS has been termed cryptococcal meningitis. In fact, the brain parenchyma is usually involved during cryptococcal disease of the CNS, leading to the more appropriate term meningoencephalitis to describe most of the cryptococcal disease of the CNS. Tissue responses to invading cryptococci in the CNS range from no apparent inflammatory response to granulomatous inflammation, although granuloma formation is typically less frequent in the brain compared to the lung. In the case of little or no inflammatory responses described by Freeman (1931), lesions or cysts composed of encapsulated *C. neoformans* yeast cells can form gelatinous masses that have the appearance of "soapsuds."

Granulomatous responses typically involve T lymphocytes, macrophages, and multinucleated giant cells forming granulomas with yeast cells in the interior and usually intracellular. Neutrophils may be associated with the granulomas as well. These granulomas, termed cryptococcomas, usually keep the yeast cells walled off and, at least in immunocompetent hosts, retard the growth of the organisms (Schwartz, 1988). If the yeast continues to replicate inside, the cryptococcomas can become quite large and are readily visible by radiology (Sabetta and Andriole, 1985).

The variability in human responses to *C. neoformans* is aptly illustrated by a study of 27 autopsy cases of cryptococcal meningoencephalitis that included 13 AIDS patients (Lee et al., 1996). Analysis of inflammatory infiltrates revealed that 13 of 14 non-AIDS patients had prominent lymphocytic infiltration and 12 of the 14 non-AIDS patients exhibited granulomatous inflammation (Lee et al., 1996). T lymphocytes and macrophages were abundant in the granulomatous lesions of non-AIDS patients along with prominent multinucleated giant cell formation and the involvement of epithelioid macrophages. Neutrophils were frequently observed in the granulomas as well (Lee et al., 1996). In contrast, no granulomatous inflammatory response was evident in the brain tissue of AIDS patients with cryptococcal meningoencephalitis and when some inflammation was observed, neutrophils were not evident and nonepithelioid macrophages were the principal inflammatory cell present (Lee et al., 1996). In six of the 13 AIDS patients, T lymphocytes were observed, but the lymphocytes were not associated with macrophages or cryptococcal lesions. Lastly, these investigators observed a significant involvement of microglial cells in association with the yeast cells in both AIDS and non-AIDS patients suggesting that microglial cells may play an important role in resistance (Lee et al., 1996).

Similar variability in tissue reactivity has been reported in animal models of cryptococcal meningoencephalitis. For example, Dobrick et al. (1995) infected mice intravenously and observed tissue responses in the CNS compared to the liver over time. Two weeks after infection in the brain parenchyma, collections of *C. neoformans* were observed that formed what these authors described as pseudocysts that were surrounded by both $CD4^+$ T cells and $CD8^+$ T cells (Dobrick et al., 1995). Subsequently, monocytes and neutrophils infiltrated the pseudocysts, but by 4 weeks postinfection most lesions were scars devoid of viable yeasts (Dobrick et al., 1995). Inflammatory lesions of the meninges were composed primarily of monocytes and $CD4^+$ T cells. Although granulomatous-type reactions were also observed in the liver, inflammatory responses were markedly delayed in the CNS compared to the liver (Dobrick et al., 1995).

Using outbred (OF1) mice, Chretien et al. (2002) showed that fungemia following intravenous injection could elicit similar CNS infection and tissue reactivity as observed in AIDS patients. Limited inflammation was observed in the brain tissue from AIDS patients and outbred mice, and except for the relative lack of $CD4^+$ T cells in AIDS patients, the inflammatory infiltrates consisted of $CD4^+$ and $CD8^+$ T cells but only rarely B cells surrounding cysts composed of numerous yeast cells (Chretien et al., 2002). Later in infection and lesion development in the brain parenchyma, activated microglial cells were observed along with increased numbers of astrocytes in both human cases and in the mice. Mice that recovered from the infection exhibited granulomatous-like scars with few yeasts that were very similar in appearance to a human case with resolved cryptococcal meningoencephalitis (Chretien et al., 2002). Although mice are inherently susceptible to cryptococcosis, especially CNS infections, these results suggest that mouse models of cryptococcal meningoencephalitis can be good systems for studying the pathogenesis of cryptococcosis.

In contrast to mice, rats appear to be similar to humans when it comes to resistance to cryptococcosis. Goldman et al. (1996a) infected rats intracisternally to induce cryptococcal meningitis with limited brain parenchyma involvement. In this model, the cryptococci disseminate from the CNS to extracerebral sites whereby a granulomatous reaction apparently contains the infection (Goldman et al., 1996a). A similar granulomatous response restricts growth of the yeast in the meninges, however, as was observed by Dobrick et al. (1995), the response in the CNS was delayed in comparison to extracerebral tissues (Goldman et al., 1996a).

Lastly, Huffnagle and coworkers used gene knockout mice to identify chemokines and chemokine receptors involved in pathogenesis and host defense of cryptococcosis (Huffnagle and McNeil, 1999; Huffnagle et al., 1999). Mice genetically deficient in macrophage inflammatory protein-1α (MIP-1α, CCL3) had significantly more cryptococci in the brain compared to wild-type mice following intratracheal infection (Huffnagle and McNeil, 1999). Increased brain fungal burden was associated with milder inflammatory responses due to decreased leukocyte recruitment into brains of MIP-1α knockout mice compared to wild-type mice (Huffnagle and McNeil, 1999). Likewise, 8 weeks after intratracheal infection, mice defective in CCR5, the receptor for MIP-1α, as well as other chemokines, had decreased survival, significantly higher brain fungal burden, increased meningeal and parenchymal swelling, and decreased inflammatory reactions in the CNS compared to wild-type mice suggesting that CCR5 was involved in optimal leukocyte recruitment in response to *C. neoformans* infection of the CNS (Huffnagle et al., 1999).

In summary, the type of pathological reaction to *C. neoformans* infection of the CNS depends largely on the immune status and capabilities of the host. Loss of T lymphocytes or inhibition of cell-mediated immunity leads to less granulomatous-type responses, increased cryptococcal growth with more lesions and larger numbers of cryptococci per lesion, increased involvement of the brain parenchyma, and ultimately a poorer prognosis.

4. Host Defense and Immune Responses

4.1. Innate Mechanisms of Resistance

For *C. neoformans* to establish an infection in the CNS, the organism has to withstand a formidable onslaught of defense mechanisms in the lung and bloodstream, as well as successfully navigate through a restricted barrier maintained by endothelial and epithelial cells of the BBB. The plethora of cells, soluble factors, and killing mechanisms of the innate host defense system that participate in restricting the growth of or killing *C. neoformans* in extracerebral tissues are described in great detail elsewhere (Casadevall and Perfect, 1998) and include defensins, surfactant proteins and collectins, complement, neutrophils, natural killer cells, macrophages, eosinophils, mast cells, and toxic by-products of these cells such as nitric oxide and H_2O_2. Those innate host defense mechanisms that have been shown experimentally to play a role in host resistance in the CNS against *C. neoformans* are discussed below.

4.1.1. *Complement Deposition on the Cryptococcal Cell Surface*

The importance of complement in host defense against *C. neoformans* in the lung and other extracerebral tissues has been known for some time (Kozel, 1996).

However, in vivo analyses indicate that *C. neoformans* yeast cells in the CNS do not have complement component C3 on the surface (Truelsen et al., 1992). In vitro assays using effector cells of CNS origin to kill or restrict the growth of *C. neoformans* often rely on complement provided by serum for optimal growth inhibition (see Table 24.1 and Section 4.1.1 below on in vitro studies with CNS effector cells). Presumably, complement is serving as an opsonin in these in vitro assays, but it is possible that the CNS effector cells are further activated by complement deposited on the cryptococci.

Much of the complement components found in the blood are produced in the liver, however, the BBB restricts access of complement components into the CNS and the CSF is normally devoid of significant quantities of complement components. Thus, if complement is present in the CNS and is deposited on *C. neoformans* while in the CNS, then the complement components are likely produced by cells locally during an innate or acquired immune response. In fact, human astrocytes can produce all necessary components of the complement cascade and production of complement by astrocytes is increased by exposure to IFN-γ (Gasque et al., 1995, 2000; van Beek et al., 2003). To define the precise role of complement in host defense against *C. neoformans* in the CNS, experiments that allow specific depletion or neutralization of complement components in the CNS during infection will need to be devised.

4.1.2. Antimicrobial Molecules

Nitric oxide has been implicated in host defense against many infectious agents in animal models (MacMicking et al., 1997), including *C. neoformans* (Alspaugh and Granger, 1991; Lee et al., 1994; Lovchik et al., 1995; Blasi et al., 1995b; Hoag et al., 1997; Gross et al., 1999; Kawakami et al., 1999a; Rossi et al., 1999). Nitric oxide is produced by an enzymatic reaction catalyzed by nitric oxide synthase (NOS). Three NOS isoforms are present in mammals; however, only inducible NOS (iNOS) made primarily by macrophages appears to play a significant role in host defense (MacMicking et al., 1997). The role of iNOS in host defense in humans has been controversial; however, there is clear evidence that cytokine-activated human macrophages can produce functional iNOS (Lee and Brosnan, 1996; Chao et al., 1997; Persichini et al., 1997; Binion et al., 1998; Taylor and Geller, 2000). Thus, effector cell expression of iNOS and production of nitric oxide following cytokine stimulation likely contributes to acquired host defense against *C. neoformans*. In fact, iNOS expression has been detected in human granulomas caused by *C. neoformans* (Facchetti et al., 1999). The contribution of nitric oxide in in vitro growth inhibition of *C. neoformans* by CNS effector cells is described below and in Table 24.1.

Because of the tight BBB, in vivo neutralization to determine the effects of nitric oxide and other soluble mediators in the CNS has been difficult. Barluzzi et al. (1997) reported that intracerebral injection of *Candida albicans* induced regional activation of CNS effector cells, leading to increased inflammatory reactions upon subsequent infection with *C. neoformans*. Inflammatory reactions were associated with increased expression of IL-1β and TNF-α, and to a lesser extent IFN-γ and iNOS (Barluzzi et al., 1997). Treatment of *Candida*-activated mice with the iNOS inhibitor, aminoguanidine, during *C. neoformans* CNS infection partially abrogated the protective effects, suggesting that nitric oxide produced by iNOS was important in host defense against *C. neoformans* in this model (Barluzzi et al., 1997).

C. neoformans may be able to neutralize the effects of nitric oxide itself (Trajkovic et al., 2000). *C. neoformans* produces two enzymes involved in detoxifying the effects of nitric oxide production (de Jesus-Berrios et al., 2003). Flavohemoglobin denitrosylase (FHB1) reportedly consumes nitric oxide, and *S*-nitrosoglutathione (GSNO) reductase

Table 24.1. In Vitro Anticryptococcal Activity of CNS Effector Cells

Species	Cell type	Opsonin	Stimulation	Activity	Ref.
Rabbit	CSF macrophage	Rabbit serum, rabbit anticryptococcal antibody	Intracisternal infection with *C. neoformans*	No fungicidal or fungistatic activity noted	Perfect et al. (1988)
Mouse	BV-2 microglial cell line (immortalized with retrovirus) (Blasi et al., 1990)	Mouse serum or none	No additional stimuli	Growth inhibition significantly higher with opsonized yeast	Blasi et al. (1992, 1993); Bocchini et al. (1992)
Human	Primary astrocytes	None	IL-1β + IFN-γ	Growth inhibition dependent on NO	Lee et al. (1994)
Human	Primary fetal microglial cells	Mouse-human chimeric anticapsule antibody	No additional stimuli	Antibody opsonization increased phagocytosis	Zebedee et al. (1994)
Rat	C6 glioma cell line	None	None	Adherence inhibited by certain carbohydrates	Merkel and Scofield (1993, 1994)
Mouse	BV-2 microglial cell line (Blasi et al., 1990)	Mouse serum or none	IFN-γ + LPS or IFN-γ	Growth inhibition dependent on NO; melanized yeast are more resistant	Blasi et al. (1995b), Mucci et al. (2003)
Human	Primary fetal microglial cells	Anticapsule antibody (specific for GXM)	No additional stimuli except addition of iNOS and ROI inhibitors	Growth inhibition significantly increased by opsonization but not dependent on NO or ROI	Lee et al. (1995a)

Continues

Table 24.1. (continued)

Species	Cell type	Opsonin	Stimulation	Activity	Ref.
Mouse	BV-2 microglial cell line (Blasi et al., 1990)	Anti-GXM antibody	Chloroquine	Chloroquine enhances growth inhibition by BV-2 microglial cell line	Mazolla et al. (1997)
Swine	Primary microglial cells	None	Morphine	Morphine-inhibited phagocytosis	Sowa et al. (1997)
Swine	Primary microglial cells	None	None	Blockade of CD14 decreases phagocytosis by swine microglial cells	Lipovsky et al. (1997)
Human	Primary fetal microglial cells	Human serum	None	Morphine enhanced phagocytosis of opsonized cryptococci	Lipovsky et al. (1998a)
Human	Primary fetal microglial cells	Human serum or none	IFN-γ, GM-CSF, or IFN-γ + GM-CSF	Microglial cells inhibited the growth of opsonized yeast, but cytokine treatment did not affect anticryptococcal activity	Lipovsky et al. (1998b)
Mouse	BV-2 microglial cell line (Blasi et al., 1990)	Mouse serum	IFN-γ or co-culture with immune CD4+ or CD8+ T cells	IFN-γ and immune CD4+ T cells augment anticryptococcal activity of BV-2 cells	Aguirre et al. (2004)

Abbreviations: CSF, cerebrospinal fluid; NO, nitric oxide; LPS, lipopolysaccharide; GXM, glucuronoxylomannan; iNOS, inducible nitric oxide synthetase; ROI, reactive oxygen intermediates.

metabolizes GSNO (de Jesus-Berrios et al., 2003). Mutants of FHB1 and GSNO reductase are less virulent in vivo except in iNOS knockout mice (de Jesus-Berrios et al., 2003). Furthermore, an FHB1 mutant was susceptible to killing by activated macrophages in vitro, unless iNOS activity was inhibited (de Jesus-Berrios et al., 2003). The importance of FHB1 in resistance of *C. neoformans* to nitric oxide was confirmed in a study in which random mutagenesis resulted in two mutants with increased sensitivity to nitric oxide stress (Idnurm et al., 2004). Both of the mutations were due to insertion into the FHB1 gene, indicating that FHB1 is needed for optimal resistance to nitric oxide (Idnurm et al., 2004).

Additional molecules may be present in the CSF or brain parenchyma that have anticryptococcal properties. For instance, the iron sequestering molecule, transferrin, has been isolated from human CSF and reportedly inhibits the growth of *C. neoformans* in vitro (Ahluwalia et al., 2001). In addition, expression of the collectin family member, long pentraxin (PTX3), is upregulated in the CNS in response to *C. neoformans* (Polentarutti et al., 2000), and may play a role in activation of innate immune mechanisms in the CNS. Production of antimicrobial substances in the CNS is likely tightly regulated to prevent unnecessary accumulation of toxic metabolites or substances that could damage the nervous tissue. Future studies on innate mechanisms of immunity against CNS pathogens should take into account the detrimental effects of the immune response on the CNS tissue in addition to the protective effects in inhibiting the growth of the organism.

4.1.3. In Vitro Studies of Anticryptococcal Activity of CNS Effector Cells

In vitro assays to investigate the mechanisms of killing of *C. neoformans* by mammalian effector cells, such as macrophages and neutrophils, have been performed for many years, however, it is only recently that effector cells obtained from the CNS have been examined for activity in vitro. A listing of in vitro studies examining the activity of CNS effector cells is shown in Table 24.1. Perfect et al. (1988) used a rabbit model of cryptococcal meningitis to elicit macrophages to the CSF. Infection of rabbits intracisternally resulted in the accumulation of macrophage-like cells in the CSF (Perfect et al., 1988). Using the production of H_2O_2 and tumoricidal activity as a readout for activation, these investigators found that the elicited CSF macrophages were activated as a result of the infection; however, the CSF macrophages were unable to limit the growth of *C. neoformans* in vitro even if the yeast cells were opsonized with rabbit serum or rabbit anticryptococcal antibody (Perfect et al., 1988).

Much of the in vitro work done with rodent models or cells has involved the use of immortalized cell lines. Blasi et al. (1990) developed the BV-2 microglial cell line by transforming mouse microglial cells with a recombinant retrovirus expressing v-raf and v-myc. The first study using the BV-2 microglial cell line showed that the cells could inhibit the growth of *C. neoformans* in vitro, especially if the yeast cells were opsonized with fresh mouse serum (Bocchini et al., 1992). Further studies demonstrated that BV-2 cell anticryptococcal activity against serum-opsonized cryptococci was significantly enhanced by stimulation with IFN-γ and LPS and was dependent on the production of nitric oxide (Blasi et al., 1995b). BV-2 cells were also active in vitro against antibody-opsonized cryptococcal cells and treatment with chloroquine, a weak base that accumulates in acidic vacuoles, enhanced the in vitro anticryptococcal activity (Mazzolla et al., 1997). Consequently, intracerebral injection of chloroquine enhanced resistance of mice to intracerebral infection with *C. neoformans* by an as yet defined manner (Mazzolla et al., 1997). More recently, Aguirre et al. (2004)

reported that co-culture of BV-2 cells with $CD4^+$ T cells from mice previously vaccinated against *C. neoformans* augmented the activity of the microglial cells. Finally, adherence of *C. neoformans* to the rat C6 glioma cell line was inhibited by exogenous *N*-acetyl-D-glucosamine, sucrose, and inositol, suggesting that these glial cells bind to sugar moieties on the cryptococci (Merkel and Scofield, 1993, 1994).

In contrast to the studies with mouse BV-2 microglial cell line, primary human microglial cells appear to act differently in in vitro assays for growth inhibition of *C. neoformans*. For example, in vitro growth inhibition of *C. neoformans* by human fetal microglial cells was dependent on opsonization with anticapsular antibody, but was neither dependent on nitric oxide nor on the production of reactive oxygen intermediates, such as H_2O_2, O_2^-, hydroxyl radicals (OH), and singlet oxygen ($^1O_2$) (Lee et al., 1995a). Furthermore, treatment of human fetal microglial cells with the cytokines IFNγ and/or GM-CSF did not increase the anticryptococcal activity against opsonized or unopsonized yeast (Lipovsky et al., 1998b). Lee et al. (1995b) provided evidence that cryptococci can survive inside human microglial cells and can, in fact, replicate. The discrepancy between the activity of human and rodent microglial cells may be due to differences in the source of cells (fetal in the case of human) and/or the treatment of the cells, such as immortalization of BV-2 cells with recombinant retrovirus.

In contrast to the lack of cytokine activation of human microglial cells, cytokine treatment of human fetal astrocytes results in significantly enhanced in vitro growth inhibition of *C. neoformans* (Brosnan et al., 1994; Lee et al., 1994). The in vitro growth inhibition of *C. neoformans* by human astrocytes was dependent on the synthesis of nitric oxide, and nitric oxide production was increased by treatment with IL-1β plus IFNγ, IL-1β plus TNF-α, or IFN-γ alone (Brosnan et al., 1994; Lee et al., 1994).

Taken together, the in vitro growth inhibition studies indicate that care should be taken when comparing data from in vitro rodent models to innate host defense in human cryptococcosis. Although the rodent models and cell systems have proven to be valuable in understanding *C. neoformans* pathogenesis in the CNS and how the host might fight off this yeast, clearly differences in the mammalian systems should be taken into account when analyzing the data.

4.1.4. Nonspecific Activation of Innate Mechanisms in the CNS

Studies have demonstrated that nonspecific activation of CNS effector cells or macrophages recruited from the periphery can aid in inhibiting the growth of *C. neoformans* (Blasi et al., 1993, 1995a; Aguirre et al., 1996; Barluzzi et al., 1997; Mazzolla et al., 1997). Aguirre et al. (1996) infected mice with a sublethal dose of the neurotropic parasite, *Toxoplasma gondii*. By 6 weeks, infection with *T. gondii* induced an inflammatory reaction in the brains that inhibited the colonization of *C. neoformans* in the CNS but not in the lung. In a similar study, an inflammatory response was induced in the CNS 7 days after intracerebral injection of a weakly virulent isolate of *Candida albicans* (Barluzzi et al., 1997). Mice infected with *Candida* yeast cells survived significantly longer and exhibited reduced CNS colonization with *C. neoformans* compared to control mice (Barluzzi et al., 1997). The inflammatory response that protected against *C. neoformans* was associated with increased transcript levels of IL-1β and TNF-α and to a lesser extent IFN-γ and iNOS (Barluzzi et al., 1997).

Intracerebral administration of heat-killed *C. neoformans* also induces an inflammatory state in the CNS (Blasi et al., 1992, 1994, 1995a). In fact, within 24 h of intracerebral injection of heat-killed cryptococci an inflammatory response develops that (a) delays colonization following intravenous infection with viable *C. neoformans* and (b) increases survival of mice infected intracerebrally with viable *C. neoformans* (Blasi et al., 1995a). Analysis of cytokine gene expression revealed that IL-1β and IL-6 transcript levels were significantly higher in brains of mice that received heat-killed cryptococci compared to controls (Blasi et al., 1995a). Intracerebral injection of IL-1β or IL-6 inhibited growth of cryptococci in the brain and increased survival of intracerebrally infected mice (Blasi et al., 1995a).

Mazzolla et al. (1997) reported that chloroquine enhances the anticryptococcal activity of the mouse BV-2 microglial cell line in vitro. These investigators also observed that intracerebral injection of chloroquine increases survival and reduces brain fungal burden of intracerebrally infected mice (Mazzolla et al., 1997). Although the enhanced anticryptococcal activity of chloroquine-treated mice was likely due to effects of chloroquine on the acidic phagosomes of effector cells in the CNS, increased transcript levels of IL-1β and IL-6 were also observed suggesting that enhanced anticryptococcal activity was in part due to cytokine activation of effector cells (Mazzolla et al., 1997).

In summary, the evidence to date indicates that inflammatory processes in the CNS can restrict the growth of *C. neoformans*. Other infectious agents or local administration of cytokines or drugs can induce anticryptococcal inflammatory responses in the CNS. Whether these "nonspecific" responses, in conjunction with viable or killed cryptococci, will eventually lead to long-lasting immunity in the CNS against *C. neoformans* is yet to be determined. It is likely, however, that acquired resistance mechanisms work by augmenting the innate resistance components to more effectively limit the growth of *C. neoformans* in the CNS.

4.2. Acquired Immunity in Cryptococcosis

Acquired or adaptive immunity is composed of two limbs that cooperate with each other and with natural effector cells, such as macrophages, to limit the growth of or clear pathogenic organisms from the host. These two arms of acquired immunity are humoral immunity and cell-mediated immunity. Antibodies produced by B cells and plasma cells mediate humoral immunity, which can be transferred by immune antisera. In contrast, cell-mediated immunity is elicited by T lymphocytes and the cytokines and chemokines that they produce and sensitized T cells must be adoptively transferred to confer cell-mediated immunity to a naïve host. Antibodies contribute greatly to opsonization of pathogenic organisms and, thus, cooperate with phagocytic cells and complement components for enhanced phagocytosis of invading pathogens. Likewise, T cells are important in helping B cells make more specific antibodies and activating effector cells to more readily phagocytize and/or kill cryptococcal yeast cells. Each of these arms of acquired immunity has been shown to play a role in host defense in the CNS and will be discussed separately in the section below.

4.2.1. Humoral Immunity

Passive transfer of monoclonal antibodies specific for cryptococcal glucuronoxylomannan (GXM), the major component of the polysaccharide capsule, has been found to confer protection in a mouse model (Mukherjee et al., 1992). Multiple routes of infection and antibody administration have been investigated, and all provide some level of protection as measured by survival of the mice (Mukherjee et al., 1993). Further investigation revealed that both protective and nonprotective antibodies can be produced, and this distinction is based at least partially on the isotype of the antibody (Mukherjee et al., 1995; Yuan et al., 1995, 1998). Significantly, T cell function is needed for protection mediated by passive transfer of protective antibody and both Th1- and Th2-type cytokines are required for antibody efficacy (Beenhouwer et al., 2001). Yuan et al. (1997) reported that protection following anticryptococcal antibody transfer was not observed in mice deficient in $CD4^+$ T cells or mice incapable of producing IFNγ. Vecchiarelli et al. (2002) suggested a mechanism for the cooperative cellular response to passive antibody transfer involving the IL-12 receptor β2 subunit (IL-12Rβ2). IL-12 is involved in the development of cell-mediated immunity, specifically in the induction of Th1 cells. IL-12 signals through the IL-12 receptor; and the β2 subunit of the receptor can be used as a marker of Th1 cells. Vecchiarelli et al. (2002) demonstrated that stimulation of leukocytes with unencapsulated cryptococci induced the expression of IL-12Rβ2 on T cells; however, when the yeasts were encapsulated with GXM, a lower percentage of T cells became $IL\text{-}12R\beta2^+$. Administration of specific anti-GXM antibody, but not irrelevant antibody, reversed this downregulation. These observations and others led to the conclusion that GXM inhibits effective phagocytosis and antigen presentation, thus preventing the induction of Th1 cells; however, specific antibody allows for appropriate antigen presentation and induction of Th1 cells that can produce IFN-γ and mediate protective cell-mediated immune responses.

4.2.2. Cell-Mediated Immunity

There is abundant clinical and experimental evidence that clearly demonstrates the importance of cell-mediated immunity in host resistance to cryptococcosis (Gentry et al., 1977; Kaplan et al., 1977; Cauley and Murphy, 1979; Heenan and Dawkins, 1981; Borton and Wintroub, 1984; Kovacs et al., 1985; Gal et al., 1986, 1987; Edson et al., 1987; Salkowski et al., 1987). Much of the in vivo work on host resistance to *C. neoformans* has focused on the lung, where the infection begins (Mody et al., 1990, 1993, 1994; Hill and Harmsen, 1991; Huffnagle et al., 1991a,b, 1994, 1995, 1996, 1997, 2000; Lovchik and Lipscomb, 1993; Hoag et al., 1995, 1997; Lovchik et al., 1995; Huffnagle, 1996). Anticryptococcal resistance in the lung is associated with T helper 1 (Th1) cells and the cytokines they produce, such as IFN-γ (Huffnagle et al., 1994; Kawakami et al., 1995, 1996a, 1999b, 2001). In addition, TNFα is required for induction of host resistance in cryptococcosis (Huffnagle et al., 1996; Bauman et al., 2003), and IL-12 augments protection (Kawakami et al., 1996b, 1999a,b, 2000; Hoag et al., 1997; Qureshi et al., 1999). Clearance of *C. neoformans* has also been associated with production of IL-4 and IL-10 in lung homogenates and increased transcription of IL-2, IFN-γ, lymphotoxin (LT), IL-4, IL-6, IL-10, IL-12p40, IL-18, transforming growth factor-beta (TGF-β), and IL-1β in the lungs (Huffnagle et al., 1994; Hoag et al., 1995; Kawakami et al., 1995, 1997, 2000; Lovchik et al., 1995). In addition, the chemokine, monocyte chemotactic protein-1 (MCP-1, CCL2) has been reported to play a role in cellular infiltration into *C. neoformans*-infected lungs (Huffnagle et al., 1995). MIP-1α, another chemokine, is important in cellular infiltration into an anticryptococcal CMI reaction site and in protection (Doyle and Murphy, 1997; Huffnagle et al., 1997; Olszewski et al., 2000, 2001) as is the CC chemokine TCA-3 (CCL1) (Doyle and Murphy, 1999). The protective anticryptococcal response induced by pulmonary infection with *C. neoformans* is complex and involves a large number of cells and soluble factors interacting to produce optimal protection.

4.3. Acquired Host Defense against *C. neoformans* in the CNS

In contrast to the lung, less is known about the mechanisms of resistance to *C. neoformans* in the CNS. Because the CNS has a restrictive

BBB and unique effector cells (microglial cells and astrocytes) (Fabry et al., 1994), it is possible that resistance mechanisms in the CNS may be different from the lung. However, these unique features of the CNS can also make it more difficult to study. For example, to analyze the role of a cytokine in host defense, many investigators simply add an antibody specific for that cytokine to a model system and observe the effects of neutralization of the cytokine on the ensuing response. In the case of the CNS, the restrictive BBB will inhibit the movement of an antibody or other reagent from the blood into the CNS unless the BBB has been perturbed in some manner. Thus, it may be necessary to bypass the BBB and administer reagents directly into the CNS via intracerebral or intracisternal injection in order to examine the role of a specific soluble mediator in the anticryptococcal response in the CNS.

4.3.1. Role of B Cells and Antibodies in CNS Defense

Mice deficient in B cells were examined for their ability to control the growth of *C. neoformans* in lungs and brains following intravenous infection (Aguirre and Johnson, 1997). No difference in brain fungal burden was observed in B cell-deficient compared to wild-type control mice during the primary response to infection (Aguirre and Johnson, 1997). To induce a protective immune response, mice were vaccinated by sublethal intratracheal infection that resolved within 6 weeks. Mice vaccinated in this way can contain CNS infection with *C. neoformans* following intravenous infection more readily than unvaccinated mice (Hill and Aguirre, 1994; Aguirre et al.,1995). As observed in the primary response to *C. neoformans* infection, no difference in brain or lung fungal burden was observed in vaccinated B cell-deficient mice compared to vaccinated B cell-sufficient mice (Aguirre and Johnson, 1997). These investigators further reported that adoptive transfer of immune leukocytes from B cell-sufficient mice into SCID mice enhanced resistance to intravenous infection whereas infusion of immune leukocytes from B cell-deficient mice did not (Aguirre and Johnson, 1997). However, their analyses were performed 11 days after infection when CD4 T cell numbers were three times lower in SCID mice infused with B cell-deficient immune leukocytes compared to SCID mice infused with B cell-sufficient immune leukocytes. B cells reportedly are important in maintaining CD4 T cell integrity (Liu et al., 1995), thus, B cells may not be directly involved in host resistance in this model. In fact, a specific B cell need not be present at the site of infection so long as sufficient antibody is produced by the B cell to travel through the body fluids to the site of infection.

Specific anticryptococcal antibody has been detected in the CSF of cryptococcosis patients (Porter et al., 1977) and in experimental models of cryptococcal meningitis (Hobbs et al., 1990). The general lack of B cells in CNS suggests that the antibody is made elsewhere and migrates into the CSF, however, evidence is lacking on the source of anticryptococcal antibody in the CSF. Traversal of antibody across the BBB is evident in a study in which a monoclonal antibody specific for cryptococcal GXM was injected intraperitoneally into mice infected intracerebrally with *C. neoformans* (Mukherjee et al., 1993). The antibody treatment significantly lengthened the lifespan of the intracerebrally infected mice, as well as reduced the brain fungal burden, suggesting that the antibody crossed the BBB and participated in host resistance directly in the CNS (Mukherjee et al., 1993).

The role of specific anticryptococcal antibody in host defense in the CNS likely involves a significant role in opsonization for more efficient phagocytosis by effector cells in the CNS (see Table 24.1 and Section 4.1.3 on in vitro studies of anticryptococcal activity of CNS effector cells). In addition, antibody may also play an important role in clearing capsular polysaccharide from the tissue (Vecchiarelli and Casadevall, 1998).

4.3.2. Role of T Lymphocytes in CNS Defense

Blasi et al. (1994) used intracerebral injection of heat-killed *C. neoformans* yeast cells to induce a protective response in mice. The protective response generated, as determined by reduced cryptococcal colony-forming units (CFU) in the brain following intracerebral challenge with viable *C. neoformans*, was characterized by a vigorous inflammatory response in the brain and development of delayed-type hypersensitivity (DTH) responsiveness to heat-killed yeast cells (Blasi et al., 1994). Similar treatment of nude mice, which are T cell-deficient, did not induce any of these characteristics suggesting that T cell involvement was necessary for the protection (Blasi et al., 1994).

Hill and Aguirre (1994) induced a protective response by infecting mice intratracheally with a sublethal dose of viable *C. neoformans*. Ten weeks later, these immune mice had significantly fewer yeast cells in the brain following intravenous infection compared to nonimmune mice (Hill and Aguirre, 1994). Depletion of $CD4^+$ cells, but not $CD8^+$ cells, ablated the protective response (Hill and Aguirre, 1994). In addition, adoptive transfer of CD4-intact immune leukocytes to SCID mice significantly limited seeding of the brain with *C. neoformans* and/or enhanced clearance of the organisms from the brains of the SCID mice following infection with viable cryptococci, but adoptive transfer of CD4-depleted immune populations did not (Hill and Aguirre, 1994). Although it appears that $CD4^+$ T lymphocytes are important in limiting the numbers of cryptococci present in the brain in this study (Hill and Aguirre, 1994), it is possible that the $CD4^+$ T cells are not directly involved in clearance of the infection from the CNS but instead the $CD4^+$ T cells aid in limiting the growth of the organism in extracerebral tissues, leading to decreased cryptococci seeding the brain.

To examine direct anticryptococcal activity in the CNS, Buchanan and Doyle (2000) used a nonreplicating cryptococcal antigen (CneF) to induce protective immunity followed by intracerebral infection to deposit *C. neoformans* directly into the brain. Using this model, it was shown that $CD4^+$ T cells, $CD8^+$ T cells, macrophages, and even neutrophils infiltrate into *C. neoformans*-infected brains of immune mice, and the ensuing immune response limits the growth of *C. neoformans* in the CNS (Buchanan and Doyle, 2000). $CD4^+$ T lymphocytes, but not $CD8^+$ T lymphocytes, were required for both optimal recruitment and accumulation of leukocytes in *C. neoformans*-infected brains and for growth inhibition of *C. neoformans* in the CNS (Buchanan and Doyle, 2000). Thus, $CD4^+$ T cells appear to be major players in protective anticryptococcal responses in the brain.

Barluzzi et al. (2000) induced protective immunity in the CNS by injecting mice with a strain of *C. neoformans* that was avirulent due to the inability to produce melanin. Mice given the nonmelanogenic strain intracerebrally developed a regional immune response capable of reducing brain fungal burden and extending survival of mice subsequently infected with a virulent melanin-producing strain (Barluzzi et al., 2000). The immune response was associated with the induction of a cell-mediated immune response as measured by delayed-type hypersensitivity response to *C. neoformans* and with increased expression of IL-12, TNF-α, IL-1β, IFN-γ, and iNOS transcripts in CNS tissue as measured by RT-PCR (Barluzzi et al., 2000). In addition, significantly higher levels of IL-12, TNF-α, and IL-1β were detected in brain homogenates by specific enzyme-linked immunosorbent assay (ELISA) (Barluzzi et al., 2000).

Recently, Uicker et al. (2005) reported that subcutaneous immunization with the cryptococcal antigen, CneF, emulsified in complete Freund's adjuvant (CFA) induces an immune response that significantly prolongs the life of mice infected intracerebrally with viable *C. neoformans* (Fig. 24.2). In this study, the immune response was apparently sterilizing as surviving mice had no culturable *C. neoformans* in brains, spleen, or lungs (Uicker et al., 2005). The protective response was associated with significant increases in transcripts of the chemokines, MCP-1, RANTES (CCL5), IP-10 (CXCL10), and MIP-2 (CXCL8), the chemokine receptors CCR1, CCR2, and CCR5, and the cytokines, TNF-α, IFN-γ, IL-1β, and IL-1ra (Uicker et al., 2005). Significant increases in TNF-α and IFN-γ were detected in brain homogenates of immune mice infected with *C. neoformans* compared to nonimmune mice (Uicker et al., 2005). Lastly, immunohistochemical analyses revealed that IFN-γ was produced in the vicinity of mononuclear infiltrates containing $CD4^+$ T cells in brains of immune mice but not in nonimmune mice (Uicker et al., 2005). The authors conclude from their results that a Th1-type cell-mediated immune response was elicited in the CNS of *C. neoformans*-infected immune mice and this response limited the growth of *C. neoformans* in the CNS (Uicker et al., 2005).

4.3.3. Mechanisms of Acquired Resistance in the CNS

Host defense in the brain can be provided by activated T cells and monocytes entering the brain via the BBB or by endogenous glial cells (astrocytes and microglial cells) acting as effector cells or antigen-presenting cells to stimulate T cells or other immunologically

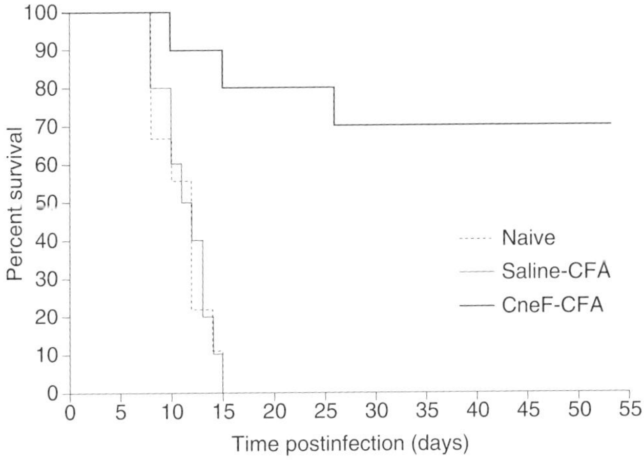

Figure 24.2. Immunization with cryptococcal antigen extends survival of mice infected intracerebrally with *C. neoformans*. Groups of 10 mice were either untreated, injected subcutaneously with saline emulsified in complete Freund's adjuvant (CFA), or were immunized with cryptococcal culture filtrate antigen (CneF) emulsified in CFA (CneF-CFA) 6 days before intracerebral infection with 200 CFU of *C. neoformans*. Survival of infected animals was monitored daily up to day 57 postinfection when the experiment was terminated. The figure originally appeared in reference (Uicker et al., 2004) and is reproduced here with permission.

competent cells (Shrikant and Benveniste, 1996). Many of the studies reporting a protective immune response in the CNS against *C. neoformans* have also described an association with at least the expression of IL-1β and, in some cases, IL-6, TNF-α, and IFN-γ. Other studies describe additional cytokines and chemokines as part of the overall immune response. It is clear that IFN-γ plays an important role in extracerebral clearance of *C. neoformans* and likely plays a role in the CNS as well. For instance, microglial cells stimulated with IFN-γ become more phagocytic and express higher levels of Class II MHC and B7-1 (CD80) molecules that are important for antigen presentation to T cells (Shrikant and Benveniste, 1996). In vitro studies have shown that human fetal astrocytes (Lee et al., 1995a) or a transformed mouse microglial cell line (Blasi et al., 1995b) can inhibit the growth of *C. neoformans* more readily if the cells are activated with IFNγ. In both reports, cryptococcal growth inhibition was due to enhanced production of nitric oxide following activation of the astrocyte or microglial cell by IFN-γ. In light of the fact that IFN-γ is produced during an anticryptococcal protective response (Buchanan and Murphy, 1993, 1994, 1997), one might predict that IFN-γ present in the brain, as a result of crossing the BBB or being produced in the brain, may activate microglial cells, astrocytes, or infiltrating macrophages to contribute to anticryptococcal resistance in the brain.

In vivo studies on the role of cytokines in CNS clearance of *C. neoformans* are limited. Aguirre et al. (1995) reported that neutralizing IFN-γ and TNF with specific antibodies resulted in increased numbers of *C. neoformans* yeast cells in the brains of *C. neoformans*-immune mice compared to immune mice given control antibody at the time of infection. Using an intracerebral infection model, Buchanan and Doyle (2000) reported that IFN-γ was important in acquired host defense against *C. neoformans* in the CNS. Others have reported elevated levels of IL-1β and IL-6 mRNA in mouse brains following intracerebral injection of heat-killed cryptococci (Blasi et al., 1995a). Expression of IL-1β and IL-6 correlated with increased resistance to intracerebral challenge with viable organisms, and intracerebral injection of recombinant IL-1β and IL-6 reduced yeast cell growth following intracerebral challenge (Blasi et al., 1995a). Thus, as observed in the lungs and other peripheral organs, a protective anticryptococcal response in the brain is likely to involve a complex network of multiple cytokines working together to recruit and/or activate the appropriate effector cells to rid the brain of the pathogen.

In addition to cytokines, chemokines play an important role in anticryptococcal resistance (Huffnagle et al., 1995, 1997; Doyle and Murphy, 1997). In this regard, MIP-1α knockout mice had reduced leukocyte infiltration into *C. neoformans*-infected brains and significantly higher brain fungal burden compared to wild-type mice following intratracheal infection (Huffnagle and McNeil, 1999; Huffnagle et al., 1999). In addition, CCR5 knockout mice have a decreased ability for peripheral leukocyte migration into *C. neoformans*-infected brains (Huffnagle and McNeil, 1999; Huffnagle et al., 1999).

Additional studies are needed to identify the important components necessary for host defense against *C. neoformans* in the CNS such that immunomodulation therapies can be devised to treat patients suffering from cryptococcal meningoencephalitis, especially those individuals with immunodeficiency. Addition of exogenous cytokines to modulate immunity is a possible approach to such treatments. Attempts to modulate clearance in mouse models of systemic cryptococcosis have shown some promise (Clemons et al., 2001) even in immunocompromised mouse models (Lutz et al., 2000). However, it is important to keep in mind that while induction of inflammatory processes in the brain by administration of exogenous cytokines or other pharmacological reagents may be beneficial in inhibiting the growth of or killing CNS pathogens, the inflammatory responses induced by these reagents can also be damaging to critical nervous tissue.

4.4. Differences between Lung and CNS Host Defense in Cryptococcosis

There is evidence, albeit limited, that host anticryptococcal resistance mechanisms in the brain differ somewhat from or may be delayed in comparison to responses in other tissues (Salkowski and Balish, 1990; Clemons et al., 1994; Blasi et al., 1995a). First, administration of IL-12 to mice by gavage resulted in reduced cryptococcal CFU in the brain compared to controls, whereas, no differences were seen in spleen and lung fungal burden between IL-12-treated mice compared to controls (Clemons et al., 1994). Second, beige mice had a much delayed granulomatous-type (CMI) inflammatory response to *C. neoformans* in the brain compared to the lung, liver, and spleen (Salkowski and Balish, 1990); however, it is possible that beige mice, besides having defects in macrophages, natural killer cells, and granulocytes, also have additional unknown defects in the brain that may be responsible for the delayed reactivity. Results of Blasi et al. (1995a) suggest that immunization by intracerebral injection of heat-killed cryptococci may induce a response that is compartmentalized in the brain and does not aid in protection in other tissues. Huffnagle et al. (1999) showed that CCR5 knockout mice differ in leukocyte recruitment into lungs as compared to the brain following intratracheal infection with *C. neoformans*. CCR5 knockout mice were able to clear the cryptococci from the lungs and mount DTH responses to cryptococcal antigens whereas, brain fungal burden increased in CCR5 knockout mice, and they died sooner than mice with intact CCR5 (Huffnagle et al., 1999). Additional studies are needed to identify potential mechanisms of immunity in the CNS that may differ from extracerebral tissues.

5. Summary

Cryptococcus neoformans is an encapsulated yeast that causes cryptococcosis, a life-threatening disease that develops following inhalation and dissemination of the ubiquitous organisms. *C. neoformans* has a predilection for the CNS, and mortality is most frequently associated with meningoencephalitis. Individuals with deficiencies in cell-mediated immunity, such as AIDS patients, are more susceptible to cryptococcosis; thus, the incidence of cryptococcosis is increasing as a result of the growing number of immunocompromised individuals. Loss of $CD4^+$ T cells predisposes individuals to progressive infection with *C. neoformans*, further emphasizing the importance of cell-mediated immunity in host resistance to this organism and partially explaining the high incidence of cryptococcosis in AIDS patients. Although much has been learned about host defense mechanisms against *C. neoformans* in the lungs, less is known about host resistance in the CNS. Clearly, some of the same cells and mechanisms are involved in host defense in the lungs and the CNS; however, the CNS has unique features that suggest there might be some differences as well. In fact, experimental evidence indicates that many anticryptococcal reactions in the CNS are delayed in comparison to extracerebral tissues, which may be due to differences in immune mechanisms in the CNS compared to other tissues. More defined experimental studies are required to identify the critical components needed for appropriate anticryptococcal activity in the CNS that restricts growth of *C. neoformans* while at the same time does not cause harmful damage to the nervous tissue.

References

Aguirre, K.M. and Johnson, L.L. (1997). A role for B cells in resistance to *Cryptococcus neoformans* in mice. *Infect. Immun.* 65(2): 525–530.

Aguirre, K., Havell, E.A., Gibson, G.W., and Johnson, L.L. (1995). Role of tumor necrosis factor and gamma interferon in acquired resistance to *Cryptococcus neoformans* in the central nervous system of mice. *Infect. Immun.* 63(5): 1725–1731.

Aguirre, K.M., Sayles, P.C., Gibson, G.W., and Johnson, L.L. (1996). Resistance to *Cryptococcus neoformans* is associated with an inflammatory response to *Toxoplasma gondii* in the central nervous system of mice. *Infect. Immun.* 64(1): 77–82.

Aguirre, K., Crowe, J., Haas, A., and Smith, J. (2004). Resistance to *Cryptococcus neoformans* infection in the absence of $CD4^+$ T cells. *Med. Mycol.* 42(1): 15–25.

Ahluwalia, M., Brummer, E., Sridhar, S., Singh, R., and Stevens, D.A. (2001). Isolation and characterization of an anticryptococcal protein in human cerebrospinal fluid. *J. Med. Microbiol.* 50(1): 83–89.

Alspaugh, J.A. and Granger, D.L. (1991). Inhibition of *Cryptococcus neoformans* replication by nitrogen oxides supports the role of these molecules as effectors of macrophage-mediated cytostasis. *Infect. Immun.* 59(7): 2291–2296.

Barluzzi, R., Mazzolla, R., Brozzetti, A., Puliti, M., Mariucci, G., Mosci, P., Bistoni, F., and Blasi, E. (1997). A low virulent strain of *Candida albicans* enhances brain anticryptococcal defenses: Characterization of the local immune reaction by RT-PCR and histochemical analysis. *J. Neuroimmunol.* 79(1): 37–48.

Barluzzi, R., Brozzetti, A., Mariucci, G., Tantucci, M., Neglia, R.G., Bistoni, F., and Blasi, E. (2000). Establishment of protective immunity against cerebral cryptococcosis by means of an avirulent, non-melanogenic *Cryptococcus neoformans* strain. *J. Neuroimmunol.* 109(2): 75–86.

Bauman, S.K., Huffnagle, G.B., and Murphy, J.W. (2003). Effects of tumor necrosis factor alpha on dendritic cell accumulation in lymph nodes draining the immunization site and the impact on the anticryptococcal cell-mediated immune response. *Infect. Immun.* 71(1): 68–74.

Beenhouwer, D.O., Shapiro, S., Feldmesser, M., Casadevall, A., and Scharff, M.D. (2001). Both Th1 and Th2 cytokines affect the ability of monoclonal antibodies to protect mice against *Cryptococcus neoformans*. *Infect. Immun.* 69(10): 6445–6455.

Binion, D.G., Fu, S., Ramanujam, K.S., Chai, Y.C., Dweik, R.A., Drazba, J.A., Wade, J.G., Ziats, N.P., Ersurum, S.C., and Wilson, K.T. (1998). iNOS expression in human intestinal microvascular endothelial cells inhibits leukocyte adhesion. *Am. J. Physiol.* 275(3 Pt 1): G592–G603.

Blasi, E., Barluzzi, R., Bocchini, V., Mazzolla, R., and Bistoni, F. (1990). Immortalization of murine microglial cells by a v-raf/v-myc carrying retrovirus. *J. Neuroimmunol.* 27(2–3): 229–237.

Blasi, E., Barluzzi, R., Mazzolla, R., Mosci, P., and Bistoni, F. (1992). Experimental model of intracerebral infection with *Cryptococcus neoformans*: Roles of phagocytes and opsonization. *Infect. Immun.* 60(9): 3682–3688.

Blasi, E., Barluzzi, R., Mazzolla, R., and Bistoni, F. (1993). Differential host susceptibility to intracerebral infections with *Candida albicans* and *Cryptococcus neoformans*. *Infect. Immun.* 61(8): 3476–3481.

Blasi, E., Mazzolla, R., Barluzzi, R., Mosci, P., and Bistoni, F. (1994). Anticryptococcal resistance in the mouse brain: Beneficial effects of local administration of heat-inactivated yeast cells. *Infect. Immun.* 62(8): 3189–3196.

Blasi, E., Barluzzi, R., Mazzolla, R., Pitzurra, L., Puliti, M., Saleppico, S., and Bistoni, F. (1995a). Biomolecular events involved in anticryptococcal resistance in the brain. *Infect. Immun.* 63(4): 1218–1222.

Blasi, E., Barluzzi, R., Mazzolla, R., Tancini, B., Saleppico, S., Puliti, M., Pitzurra, L., and Bistoni, F. (1995b). Role of nitric oxide and melanogenesis in the accomplishment of anticryptococcal activity by the BV-2 microglial cell line. *J. Neuroimmunol.* 58(1): 111–116.

Bocchini, V., Mazzolla, R., Barluzzi, R., Blasi, E., Sick, P., and Kettenmann, H. (1992). An immortalized cell line expresses properties of activated microglial cells. *J. Neurosci. Res.* 31(4): 616–621.

Borton, L.K. and Wintroub, B.U. (1984). Disseminated cryptococcosis presenting as herpetiform lesions in a homosexual man with acquired immunodeficiency syndrome. *J. Am. Acad. Dermatol.* 10(2 Pt 2): 387–390.

Bottone, E.J. and Wormser, G.P. (1986). Poorly encapsulated *Cryptococcus neoformans* from patients with AIDS. II. Correlation of capsule size observed directly in cerebrospinal fluid with that after animal passage. *AIDS Res.* 2(3): 219–225.

Brosnan, C.F., Battistini, L., Raine, C.S., Dickson, D.W., Casadevall, A., and Lee, S.C. (1994). Reactive nitrogen intermediates in human neuropathology: An overview. *Dev. Neurosci.* 16(3–4): 152–161.

Buchanan, K.L. and Doyle, H.A. (2000). Requirement for CD4+ T lymphocytes in host resistance against *Cryptococcus neoformans* in the central nervous system of immunized mice. *Infect. Immun.* 68(2): 456–462.

Buchanan, K.L. and Murphy, J.W. (1993). Characterization of cellular infiltrates and cytokine production during the expression phase of the anticryptococcal delayed-type hypersensitivity response. *Infect. Immun.* 61(7): 2854–2865.

Buchanan, K.L. and Murphy, J.W. (1994). Regulation of cytokine production during the expression phase of the anticryptococcal delayed-type hypersensitivity response. *Infect. Immun.* 62(7): 2930–2939.

Buchanan, K.L. and Murphy, J.W. (1997). Kinetics of cellular infiltration and cytokine production during the efferent phase of a delayed-type hypersensitivity reaction. *Immunology* 90(2): 189–197.

Buchanan, K.L. and Murphy, J.W. (1998). What makes *Cryptococcus neoformans* a pathogen? *Emerg. Infect. Dis.* 4(1): 71–83.

Casadevall, A. and Perfect, J.R. (1998). *Cryptococcus neoformans*. ASM Press, Washington, DC.

Cauley, L.K. and Murphy, J.W. (1979). Response of congenitally athymic (nude) and phenotypically normal mice to *Cryptococcus neoformans* infection. *Infect. Immun.* 23(3): 644–651.

Chang, Y.C., Stins, M.F., McCaffery, M.J., Miller, G.F., Pare, D.R., Dam, T., Paul-Satyaseela, M., Kim, K.S., and Kwon-Chung, K.J. (2004). Cryptococcal yeast cells invade the central nervous system via transcellular penetration of the blood-brain barrier. *Infect. Immun.* 72(9): 4985–4995.

Chao, C.C., Lokensgard, J.R., Sheng, W.S., Hu, S., and Peterson, P.K. (1997). IL-1-induced iNOS expression in human astrocytes via NF-kappa B. *Neuroreport* 8(14): 3163–3166.

Chen, L.C., Goldman, D.L., Doering, T.L., Pirofski, L., and Casadevall, A. (1999). Antibody response to *Cryptococcus neoformans* proteins in rodents and humans. *Infect. Immun.* 67(5): 2218–2224.

Chen, S., Sorrell, T., Nimmo, G., Speed, B., Currie, B., Ellis, D., Marriot, D., Pfeiffer, T., Parr, D., and Byth, K. (2000). Epidemiology and host- and variety-dependent characteristics of infection due to *Cryptococcus neoformans* in Australia and New Zealand. Australasian Cryptococcal Study Group. *Clin. Infect. Dis.* 31(2): 499–508.

Chen, S.H.M., Stins, M.F., Huang, S.H., Chen, Y.H., Kwon-Chung, K.J., Chang, Y., Kim, K.S., Suzuki, K., and Jong, A.Y. (2003). *Cryptococcus neoformans* induces alterations in the cytoskeleton of human brain microvascular endothelial cells. *J. Med. Microbiol.* 52(11): 961–970.

Chretien, F., Lortholary, O., Kansau, I., Neuville, S., Gray, F., and Dromer, F. (2002). Pathogenesis of cerebral *Cryptococcus neoformans* infection after fungemia. *J. Infect. Dis.* 186(4): 522–530.

Clark, R.A., Greer, D., Atkinson, W., Valainis, G.T., and Hyslop, N. (1990). Spectrum of *Cryptococcus neoformans* infection in 68 patients infected with human immunodeficiency virus. *Rev. Infect. Dis.* 12(5): 768–777.

Clemons, K.V., Brummer, E., and Stevens, D.A. (1994). Cytokine treatment of central nervous system infection: Efficacy of interleukin-12 alone and synergy with conventional antifungal therapy in experimental cryptococcosis. *Antimicrob. Agents Chemother.* 38(3): 460–464.

Clemons, K.V., Lutz, J.E., and Stevens, D.A. (2001). Efficacy of recombinant gamma interferon for treatment of systemic cryptococcosis in SCID mice. *Antimicrob. Agents Chemother.* 45(3): 686–689.

Collins, V.P., Gellhorn, A., and Trimble, J.R. (1951). The coincidence of cryptococcosis and disease of the reticulo-endothelial and lymphatic systems. *Cancer* 4(4): 883–889.

Collins, J.V., Tong, D., Bucknall, R.G., and Warin, A.P. (1972). Cryptococcal meningitis as a complication of systemic lupus erythematosus treated with systemic corticosteroids. *Postgrad. Med. J.* 48(555): 52–55.

de Jesus-Berrios, M., Liu, L., Nussbaum, J.C., Cox, G.M., Stamler, J.S., and Heitman, J. (2003). Enzymes that counteract nitrosative stress promote fungal virulence. *Curr. Biol.* 13(22): 1963–1968.

Dev, D., Basran, G.S., Slater, D., Taylor, P., and Wood, M. (1994). Immunodeficiency without HIV. Consider HIV negative immunodeficiency in cryptococcosis. *B.M.J.* 308(6941): 1436.

Diamond, R.D. and Bennett, J.E. (1974). Prognostic factors in cryptococcal meningitis. A study in 111 cases. *Ann. Intern. Med.* 80(2): 176–181.

Dobrick, P., Miksits, K., and Hahn, H. (1995). L3T4(CD4)-, Lyt-2(CD8)- and Mac-1(CD11b)-phenotypic leukocytes in murine cryptococcal meningoencephalitis. *Mycopathologia* 131(3): 159–166.

Doyle, H.A. and Murphy, J.W. (1997). MIP-1 alpha contributes to the anticryptococcal delayed-type hypersensitivity reaction and protection against *Cryptococcus neoformans*. *J. Leukoc. Biol.* 61(2): 147–155.

Doyle, H.A. and Murphy, J.W. (1999). Role of the C–C chemokine, TCA3, in the protective anticryptococcal cell-mediated immune response. *J. Immunol.* 162(8): 4824–4833.

Dromer, F., Ronin, O., and Dupont, B. (1992). Isolation of *Cryptococcus neoformans* var. *gattii* from an Asian patient in France: Evidence for dormant infection in healthy subjects. *J. Med. Vet. Mycol.* 30(5): 395–397.

Dromer, F., Mathoulin, S., Dupont, B., and Laporte, A. (1996). Epidemiology of cryptococcosis in France: A 9-year survey (1985–1993). French Cryptococcosis Study Group. *Clin. Infect. Dis.* 23(1): 82–90.

Duncan, R.A., von Reyn, C.F., Alliegro, G.M., Toossi, Z., Sugar, A.M., and Levitz, S.M. (1993). Idiopathic $CD4^+$ T-lymphocytopenia—four patients with opportunistic infections and no evidence of HIV infection. *N. Engl. J. Med.* 328(6): 393–398.

Edson, R.S., Fernandez-Guerrero, M.L., Roberts, G.D., and Van Scoy, R.E. (1987). Clinical and laboratory features of cryptococcosis. A five-year experience. *Minn. Med.* 70(6): 337–342.

Ellis, D.H. and Pfeiffer, T.J. (1990). Ecology, life cycle, and infectious propagule of *Cryptococcus neoformans*. *Lancet* 336(8720): 923–925.

Ellis, D. and Pfeiffer, T. (1992). The ecology of *Cryptococcus neoformans*. *Eur. J. Epidemiol.* 8(3): 321–325.

Eng, R.H., Bishburg, E., Smith, S.M., and Kapila, R. (1986). Cryptococcal infections in patients with acquired immune deficiency syndrome. *Am. J. Med.* 81(1): 19–23.

Fabry, Z., Raine, C.S., and Hart, M.N. (1994). Nervous tissue as an immune compartment: The dialect of the immune response in the CNS. *Immunol. Today* 15: 218–224.

Facchetti, F., Vermi, W., Fiorentini, S., Chilosi, M., Caruso, A., Duse, M., Notarangelo, L.D., and Badolato, R. (1999). Expression of inducible nitric oxide synthase in human granulomas and histiocytic reactions. *Am. J. Pathol.* 154(1): 145–152.

Farhi, F., Bulmer, G.S., and Tacker, J.R. (1970). *Cryptococcus neoformans*. IV. The not-so-encapsulated yeast. *Infect. Immun.* 1(6): 526–531.

Franzot, S.P., Salkin, I.F., and Casadevall, A. (1999). *Cryptococcus neoformans* var. *grubii*: Separate varietal status for *Cryptococcus neoformans* serotype A isolates. *J. Clin. Microbiol.* 37(3): 838–840.

Freeman, W. (1931). *Torula* infection of the central nervous system. *J. Psychol. Neurol.* 43: 236–245.

Gal, A.A., Koss, M.N., Hawkins, J., Evans, S., and Einstein, H. (1986). The pathology of pulmonary cryptococcal infections in the acquired immunodeficiency syndrome. *Arch. Pathol. Lab. Med.* 110(6): 502–507.

Gal, A.A., Evans, S., and Meyer, P.R. (1987). The clinical laboratory evaluation of cryptococcal infections in the acquired immunodeficiency syndrome. *Diagn. Microbiol. Infect. Dis.* 7(4): 249–254.

Gallis, H.A., Berman, R.A., Cate, T.R., Hamilton, J.D., Gunnells, J.C., and Stickel, D.L. (1975). Fungal infection following renal transplantation. *Arch. Intern. Med.* 135(9): 1163–1172.

Garcia-Hermoso, D., Janbon, G., and Dromer, F. (1999). Epidemiological evidence for dormant *Cryptococcus neoformans* infection. *J. Clin. Microbiol.* 37(10): 3204–3209.

Gasque, P., Fontaine, M., and Morgan, B.P. (1995). Complement expression in human brain. Biosynthesis of terminal pathway components and regulators in human glial cells and cell lines. *J. Immunol.* 154(9): 4726–4733.

Gasque, P., Dean, Y.D., McGreal, E.P., VanBeek, J., and Morgan, B.P. (2000). Complement components of the innate immune system in health and disease in the CNS. *Immunopharmacology* 49(1–2): 171–186.

Gentry, R.H., Farrar, W.E. Jr., Mahvi, T.A., Prevost, A.E., and Gionis, T.A. (1977). Simultaneous infection of the central nervous system with *Cryptococcus neoformans* and

Mycobacterium intracellulare. *South. Med. J.* 70(7): 865–866.

Goldman, D., Lee, S.C., and Casadevall, A. (1994). Pathogenesis of pulmonary *Cryptococcus neoformans* infection in the rat. *Infect. Immun.* 62(11): 4755–4761.

Goldman, D.L., Casadevall, A., Cho, Y., and Lee, S.C. (1996a). *Cryptococcus neoformans* meningitis in the rat. *Lab. Invest.* 75(6): 759–770.

Goldman, D., Cho, Y., Zhao, M., Casadevall, A., and Lee, S.C. (1996b). Expression of inducible nitric oxide synthase in rat pulmonary *Cryptococcus neoformans* granulomas. *Am. J. Pathol.* 148(4): 1275–1282.

Goldman, D.L., Lee, S.C., Mednick, A.J., Montella, L., and Casadevall, A. (2000). Persistent *Cryptococcus neoformans* pulmonary infection in the rat is associated with intracellular parasitism, decreased inducible nitric oxide synthase expression, and altered antibody responsiveness to cryptococcal polysaccharide. *Infect. Immun.* 68(2): 832–838.

Goldman, D.L., Khine, H., Abadi, J., Lindenberg, D.J., Pirofski, L., Niang, R., and Casadevall, A. (2001). Serologic evidence for *Cryptococcus neoformans* infection in early childhood. *Pediatrics* 107(5): E66.

Gomes, N.G., Boni, M., and Primo, C.C. (1997). The invasive behaviour of *Cryptococcus neoformans*: A possibility of direct access to the central nervous system? *Mycopathologia* 140(1): 1–11.

Gross, N.T., Nessa, K., Camner, P., and Jarstrand, C. (1999). Production of nitric oxide by rat alveolar macrophages stimulated by *Cryptococcus neoformans* or *Aspergillus fumigatus*. *Med. Mycol.* 37(3): 151–157.

Gupta, S., Ellis, M., Cesario, T., Ruhling, M., and Vayuvegula, B. (1987). Disseminated cryptococcal infection in a patient with hypogammaglobulinemia and normal T cell functions. *Am. J. Med.* 82(1): 129–131.

Gupta, R.K., Khan, Z.U., Nampoory, M.R., Mikhail, M.M., and Johny, K.V. (2004). Cutaneous cryptococcosis in a diabetic renal transplant recipient. *J. Med. Microbiol.* 53(Pt 5): 445–449.

Hamilton, A.J. and Gomez, B.L. (2002). Melanins in fungal pathogens. *J. Med. Microbiol.* 51(3): 189–191.

Hamilton, A.J. and Holdom, M.D. (1999). Antioxidant systems in the pathogenic fungi of man and their role in virulence. *Med. Mycol.* 37(6): 375–389.

Heenan, P.J. and Dawkins, R.L. (1981). Cryptococcosis with multiple squamous cell tumors associated with a T-cell defect. *Cancer* 47(2): 291–295.

Hill, J.O. and Aguirre, K.M. (1994). $CD4^+$ T cell-dependent acquired state of immunity that protects the brain against *Cryptococcus neoformans*. *J. Immunol.* 152(5): 2344–2350.

Hill, J.O. and Harmsen, A.G. (1991). Intrapulmonary growth and dissemination of an avirulent strain of *Cryptococcus neoformans* in mice depleted of $CD4^+$ or $CD8^+$ T cells. *J. Exp. Med.* 173(3): 755–758.

Hoag, K.A., Street, N.E., Huffnagle, G.B., and Lipscomb, M.F. (1995). Early cytokine production in pulmonary *Cryptococcus neoformans* infections distinguishes susceptible and resistant mice. *Am. J. Respir. Cell Mol. Biol.* 13(4): 487–495.

Hoag, K.A., Lipscomb, M.F., Izzo, A.A., and Street, N.E. (1997). IL-12 and IFN-gamma are required for initiating the protective Th1 response to pulmonary cryptococcosis in resistant C.B-17 mice. *Am. J. Respir. Cell Mol. Biol.* 17(6): 733–739.

Hobbs, M.M., Perfect, J.R., Granger, D.L., and Durack, D.T. (1990). Opsonic activity of cerebrospinal fluid in experimental cryptococcal meningitis. *Infect. Immun.* 58(7): 2115–2119.

Huffnagle, G.B. (1996). Role of cytokines in T cell immunity to a pulmonary *Cryptococcus neoformans* infection. *Biol. Signals* 5(4): 215–222.

Huffnagle, G.B. and McNeil, L.K. (1999). Dissemination of *C. neoformans* to the central nervous system: Role of chemokines, Th1 immunity and leukocyte recruitment. *J. Neurovirol.* 5(1): 76–81.

Huffnagle, G.B., Yates, J.L., and Lipscomb, M.F. (1991a). Immunity to a pulmonary *Cryptococcus neoformans* infection requires both $CD4^+$ and $CD8^+$ T cells. *J. Exp. Med.* 173(4): 793–800.

Huffnagle, G.B., Yates, J.L., and Lipscomb, M.F. (1991b). T cell-mediated immunity in the lung: A *Cryptococcus neoformans* pulmonary infection model using SCID and athymic nude mice. *Infect. Immun.* 59(4): 1423–1433.

Huffnagle, G.B., Lipscomb, M.F., Lovchik, J.A., Hoag, K.A., and Street, N.E. (1994). The role of $CD4^+$ and $CD8^+$ T cells in the protective inflammatory response to a pulmonary cryptococcal infection. *J. Leukoc. Biol.* 55(1): 35–42.

Huffnagle, G.B., Strieter, R.M., Standiford, T.J., McDonald, R.A., Burdick, M.D., Kunkel, S.L., and Toews, G.B. (1995). The role of monocyte chemotactic protein-1 (MCP-1) in the recruitment of monocytes and CD4+ T cells during a pulmonary *Cryptococcus neoformans* infection. *J. Immunol.* 155(10): 4790–4797.

Huffnagle, G.B., Toews, G.B., Burdick, M.D., Boyd, M.B., McAllister, K.S., McDonald, R.A., Kunkel, S.L., and Strieter, R.M. (1996). Afferent phase production of TNF-alpha is required for the development of protective T cell immunity to *Cryptococcus neoformans*. *J. Immunol.* 157(10): 4529–4536.

Huffnagle, G.B., Strieter, R.M., McNeil, L.K., McDonald, R.A., Burdick, M.D., Kunkel, S.L., and Toews, G.B. (1997). Macrophage inflammatory protein-1alpha (MIP-1alpha) is required for the efferent phase of pulmonary cell-mediated immunity to a *Cryptococcus neoformans* infection. *J. Immunol.* 159(1): 318–327.

Huffnagle, G.B., McNeil, L.K., McDonald, R.A., Murphy, J.W., Toews, G.B., Maeda, N., and Kuziel, W.A. (1999). Cutting edge: Role of C–C chemokine receptor 5 in organ-specific and innate immunity to *Cryptococcus neoformans*. *J. Immunol.* 163(9): 4642–4646.

Huffnagle, G.B., Traynor, T.R., McDonald, R.A., Olszewski, M.A., Lindell, D.M., Herring, A.C., and Toews, G.B. (2000). Leukocyte recruitment during pulmonary *Cryptococcus neoformans* infection. *Immunopharmacology* 48(3): 231–236.

Idnurm, A., Reedy, J.L., Nussbaum, J.C., and Heitman, J. (2004). *Cryptococcus neoformans* virulence gene discovery through insertional mutagenesis. *Eukaryot. Cell* 3(2): 420–429.

Ishaq, C.M., Bulmer, G.S., and Felton, F.G. (1968). An evaluation of various environmental factors affecting the propagation of *Cryptococcus neoformans*. *Mycopathol. Mycol. Appl.* 35(2): 81–90.

Janzer, R.C. (1993). The blood–brain barrier: Cellular basis. *J. Inherit. Metab. Dis.* 16(4): 639–647.

Janzer, R.C. and Raff, M.C. (1987). Astrocytes induce blood–brain barrier properties in endothelial cells. *Nature* 325(6101): 253–257.

John, G.T., Mathew, M., Snehalatha, E., Anandi, V., Date, A., Jacob, C.K., and Shastry, J.C. (1994). Cryptococcosis in renal allograft recipients. *Transplantation* 58(7): 855–856.

Jong, A.Y., Stins, M.F., Huang, S.H., Chen, S.H.M., and Kim, K.S. (2001). Traversal of *Candida albicans* across a human blood–brain barrier in vitro. *Infect. Immun.* 69: 4536–4544.

Kaplan, M.H., Rosen, P.P., and Armstrong, D. (1977). Cryptococcosis in a cancer hospital: Clinical and pathological correlates in forty-six patients. *Cancer* 39(5): 2265–2274.

Kawakami, K., Kohno, S., Kadota, J., Tohyama, M., Teruya, K., Kudeken, N., Saito, A., and Hara, K. (1995). T cell-dependent activation of macrophages and enhancement of their phagocytic activity in the lungs of mice inoculated with heat-killed *Cryptococcus neoformans*: Involvement of IFN-gamma and its protective effect against cryptococcal infection. *Microbiol. Immunol.* 39(2): 135–143.

Kawakami, K., Tohyama, M., Teruya, K., Kudeken, N., Xie, Q., and Saito, A. (1996a). Contribution of interferon-gamma in protecting mice during pulmonary and disseminated infection with *Cryptococcus neoformans*. *FEMS Immunol. Med. Microbiol.* 13(2): 123–130.

Kawakami, K., Tohyama, M., Xie, Q., and Saito, A. (1996b). IL-12 protects mice against pulmonary and disseminated infection caused by *Cryptococcus neoformans*. *Clin. Exp. Immunol.* 104(2): 208–214.

Kawakami, K., Qureshi, M.H., Zhang, T., Okamura, H., Kurimoto, M., and Saito, A. (1997). IL-18 protects mice against pulmonary and disseminated infection with *Cryptococcus neoformans* by inducing IFN-gamma production. *J. Immunol.* 159(11): 5528–5534.

Kawakami, K., Qureshi, M.H., Koguchi, Y., Zhang, T., Okamura, H., Kurimoto, M., and Saito, A. (1999a). Role of TNF-alpha in the induction of fungicidal activity of mouse peritoneal exudate cells against *Cryptococcus neoformans* by IL-12 and IL-18. *Cell Immunol.* 193(1): 9–16.

Kawakami, K., Qureshi, M.H., Zhang, T., Koguchi, Y., Shibuya, K., Naoe, S., and Saito, A. (1999b). Interferon-gamma (IFN-gamma)-dependent protection and synthesis of chemoattractants for mononuclear leucocytes caused by IL-12 in the lungs of mice infected with *Cryptococcus neoformans*. *Clin. Exp. Immunol.* 117(1): 113–122.

Kawakami, K., Qureshi, M.H., Zhang, T., Koguchi, Y., Yara, S., Takeda, K., Akira, S., Kurimoto, M., and Saito, A. (2000). Involvement of endogenously synthesized interleukin (IL)-18 in the protective effects of IL-12 against pulmonary infection with *Cryptococcus neoformans* in mice. *FEMS Immunol. Med. Microbiol.* 27(3): 191–200.

Kawakami, K., Kinjo, Y., Yara, S., Uezu, K., Koguchi, Y., Tohyama, M., Azuma, M., Takeda, K., Akira, S., and Saito, A. (2001). Enhanced gamma interferon production through activation of Valpha14(+) natural killer T cells by alpha-galactosylceramide in interleukin-18-deficient mice with systemic cryptococcosis. *Infect. Immun.* 69(11): 6643–6650.

Kovacs, J.A., Kovacs, A.A., Polis, M., Wright, W.C., Gill, V.J., Tuazon, C.U., Gelmann, E.P., Lane, H.C., Longfield, R., Overturf, G., Macher, A.M., Fauci, A.S., Parillo, J.E., Bennett, J.E., and Masur, H. (1985). Cryptococcosis in the acquired immunodeficiency syndrome. *Ann. Intern. Med.* 103(4): 533–538.

Kozel, T.R. (1996). Activation of the complement system by pathogenic fungi. *Clin. Microbiol. Rev.* 9(1): 34–46.

Kwon-Chung, K.J. (1992). Cryptococcosis. In K.J. Kwon-Chung and J.E. Bennett (eds), *Medical Mycology*. Lea & Febiger, Philadelphia, pp. 397–446.

Kwon-Chung, K.J. and Bennett, J.E. (1984). High prevalence of *Cryptococcus neoformans* var. *gattii* in tropical and subtropical regions. *Zentralbl. Bakteriol. Mikrobiol. Hyg. [A]* 257(2): 213–218.

Lee, S.C. and Brosnan, C.F. (1996). Cytokine regulation of iNOS expression in human glial cells. *Methods* 10(1): 31–37.

Lee, S.C., Dickson, D.W., Brosnan, C.F., and Casadevall, A. (1994). Human astrocytes inhibit *Cryptococcus neoformans* growth by a nitric oxide-mediated mechanism. *J. Exp. Med.* 180(1): 365–369.

Lee, S.C., Kress, Y., Dickson, D.W., and Casadevall, A. (1995a). Human microglia mediate anti-*Cryptococcus neoformans* activity in the presence of specific antibody. *J. Neuroimmunol.* 62(1): 43–52.

Lee, S.C., Kress, Y., Zhao, M.L., Dickson, D.W., and Casadevall, A. (1995b). *Cryptococcus neoformans* survive and replicate in human microglia. *Lab. Invest.* 73(6): 871–879.

Lee, S.C., Dickson, D.W., and Casadevall, A. (1996). Pathology of cryptococcal meningoencephalitis: Analysis of 27 patients with pathogenetic implications. *Hum. Pathol.* 27(8): 839–847.

Levitz, S.M. (1991). The ecology of *Cryptococcus neoformans* and the epidemiology of cryptococcosis. *Rev. Infect. Dis.* 13(6): 1163–1169.

Lewis, J.L. and Rabinovich, S. (1972). The wide spectrum of cryptococcal infections. *Am. J. Med.* 53(3): 315–322.

Lipovsky, M.M., Gekker, G., Anderson, W.R., Molitor, T.W., Peterson, P.K., and Hoepelman, A.I. (1997). Phagocytosis of nonopsonized *Cryptococcus neoformans* by swine microglia involves CD14 receptors. *Clin. Immunol. Immunopathol.* 84(2): 208–211.

Lipovsky, M.M., Gekker, G., Hu, S., Hoepelman, A.I., and Peterson, P.K. (1998a). Morphine enhances complement receptor-mediated phagocytosis of *Cryptococcus neoformans* by human microglia. *Clin. Immunol. Immunopathol.* 87(2): 163–167.

Lipovsky, M.M., Juliana, A.E., Gekker, G., Hu, S., Hoepelman, A.I., and Peterson, P.K. (1998b). Effect of cytokines on anticryptococcal activity of human microglial cells. *Clin. Diagn. Lab. Immunol.* 5(3): 410–411.

Liu, Y., Wu, Y., Ramarathinam, L., Guo, Y., Huszar, D., Trounstein, M., and Zhzo, M. (1995). Gene-targeted B-deficient mice reveal a critical role for B cells in the CD4 T cell response. *Int. Immunol.* 7: 1353–1362.

Lovchik, J.A. and Lipscomb, M.F. (1993). Role for C5 and neutrophils in the pulmonary intravascular clearance of circulating *Cryptococcus neoformans*. *Am. J. Respir. Cell Mol. Biol.* 9(6): 617–627.

Lovchik, J.A., Lyons, C.R., and Lipscomb, M.F. (1995). A role for gamma interferon-induced nitric oxide in pulmonary clearance of *Cryptococcus neoformans*. *Am. J. Respir. Cell Mol. Biol.* 13(1): 116–124.

Lutz, J.E., Clemons, K.V., and Stevens, D.A. (2000). Enhancement of antifungal chemotherapy by interferon-gamma in experimental systemic cryptococcosis. *J. Antimicrob. Chemother.* 46(3): 437–442.

Mackenzie, D.W. (1989). Cryptococcosis in the AIDS era. *Epidemiol. Infect.* 102(3): 361–363.

MacMicking, J., Xie, Q.W., and Nathan, C. (1997). Nitric oxide and macrophage function. *Annu. Rev. Immunol.* 15: 323–350.

Martinez, L.R., Garcia-Rivera, J., and Casadevall, A. (2001). *Cryptococcus neoformans* var. *neoformans* (serotype D) strains are more susceptible to heat than *C. neoformans* var. *grubii* (serotype A) strains. *J. Clin. Microbiol.* 39(9): 3365–3367.

Mazzolla, R., Barluzzi, R., Brozzetti, A., Boelaert, J.R., Luna, T., Saleppico, S., Bistoni, F., and Blasi, E. (1997). Enhanced resistance to *Cryptococcus neoformans* infection induced by chloroquine in a murine model of meningoencephalitis. *Antimicrob. Agents Chemother.* 41(4): 802–807.

Merkel, G.J. and Scofield, B.A. (1993). Conditions affecting the adherence of *Cryptococcus neoformans* to rat glial and lung cells in vitro. *J. Med. Vet. Mycol.* 31(1): 55–64.

Merkel, G.J. and Scofield, B.A. (1994). Comparisons between in vitro glial cell adherence and internalization of non-encapsulated and encapsulated strains of *Cryptococcus neoformans*. *J. Med. Vet. Mycol.* 32(5): 361–372.

Mody, C.H., Lipscomb, M.F., Street, N.E., and Toews, G.B. (1990). Depletion of $CD4^+$ ($L3T4^+$) lymphocytes in vivo impairs murine host defense to *Cryptococcus neoformans*. *J. Immunol.* 144(4): 1472–1477.

Mody, C.H., Chen, G.H., Jackson, C., Curtis, J.L., and Toews, G.B. (1993). Depletion of murine $CD8^+$ T cells in vivo decreases pulmonary clearance of a moderately virulent strain of *Cryptococcus neoformans*. *J. Lab. Clin. Med.* 121(6): 765–773.

Mody, C.H., Chen, G.H., Jackson, C., Curtis, J.L., and Toews, G.B. (1994). In vivo depletion of murine CD8 positive T cells impairs survival during infection with a highly virulent strain of *Cryptococcus neoformans*. *Mycopathologia* 125(1): 7–17.

Mucci, A., Varesio, L., Neglia, R., Colombari, B., Pastorino, S., and Blasi, E. (2003). Antifungal activity of macrophages engineered to produce IFNgamma: Inducibility by picolinic acid. *Med. Microbiol. Immunol.* (*Berl*) 192(2): 71–78.

Mukherjee, J., Scharff, M.D., and Casadevall, A. (1992). Protective murine monoclonal antibodies to *Cryptococcus neoformans*. *Infect. Immun.* 60(11): 4534–4541.

Mukherjee, J., Pirofski, L.A., Scharff, M.D., and Casadevall, A. (1993). Antibody-mediated protection in mice with lethal intracerebral *Cryptococcus neoformans* infection. *Proc. Natl. Acad. Sci. USA* 90(8): 3636–3640.

Mukherjee, J., Nussbaum, G., Scharff, M.D., and Casadevall, A. (1995). Protective and nonprotective monoclonal antibodies to *Cryptococcus neoformans* originating from one B cell. *J. Exp. Med.* 181(1): 405–409.

Ndimbie, O.K., Dekker, A., Martinez, A.J., and Dixon, B. (1994). Prostatic sequestration of *Cryptococcus neoformans* in immunocompromised persons treated for cryptococcal meningoencephalitis. *Histol. Histopathol.* 9(4): 643–648.

Neilson, J.B., Fromtling, R.A., and Bulmer, G.S. (1977). *Cryptococcus neoformans*: Size range of infectious particles from aerosolized soil. *Infect. Immun.* 17(3): 634–638.

Nosanchuk, J.D., Valadon, P., Feldmesser, M., and Casadevall, A. (1999). Melanization of *Cryptococcus neoformans* in murine infection. *Mol. Cell. Biol.* 19(1): 745–750.

Nosanchuk, J.D., Rosas, A.L., Lee, S.C., and Casadevall, A. (2000). Melanisation of *Cryptococcus neoformans* in human brain tissue. *Lancet* 355(9220): 2049–2050.

Olszewski, M.A., Huffnagle, G.B., McDonald, R.A., Lindell, D.M., Moore, B.B., Cook, D.N., and Toews, G.B. (2000). The role of macrophage inflammatory protein-1 alpha/CCL3 in regulation of T cell-mediated immunity to *Cryptococcus neoformans* infection. *J. Immunol.* 165(11): 6429–6436.

Olszewski, M.A., Huffnagle, G.B., Traynor, T.R., McDonald, R.A., Cook, D.N., and Toews, G.B. (2001). Regulatory effects of macrophage inflammatory protein 1alpha/CCL3 on the development of immunity to *Cryptococcus neoformans* depend on expression of early inflammatory cytokines. *Infect. Immun.* 69(10): 6256–6263.

Olszewski, M.A., Noverr, M.C., Chen, G.H., Toews, G.B., Cox, G.M., Perfect, J.R., and Huffnagle, G.B. (2004). Urease expression by *Cryptococcus neoformans* promotes microvascular sequestration, thereby enhancing central nervous system invasion. *Am. J. Pathol.* 164(5): 1761–1771.

Perfect, J.R. and Casadevall, A. (2002). Cryptococcosis. *Infect. Dis. Clin. North Am.* 16(4): 837–874.

Perfect, J.R., Hobbs, M.M., Granger, D.L., and Durack, D.T. (1988). Cerebrospinal fluid macrophage response to experimental cryptococcal meningitis: Relationship between in vivo and in vitro measurements of cytotoxicity. *Infect. Immun.* 56(4): 849–854.

Persichini, T., Mancino, G., Cappelli, G., Colizzi, V., and Lauro, G.M. (1997). *Mycobacterium tuberculosis* enhances iNOS mRNA expression and HIV replication in human astrocytoma cells. *Neuroreport* 8(8): 1897–1901.

Polentarutti, N., Bottazzi, B., Di Santo, E., Blasi, E., Agnello, D., Ghezzi, P., Introna, M., Bartfai, T., Richards, G., and Montovani, A. (2000). Inducible expression of the long pentraxin PTX3 in the central nervous system. *J. Neuroimmunol.* 106(1–2): 87–94.

Porter, K.G., Sinnamon, D.G., and Gillies, R.R. (1977). *Cryptococcus neoformans*-specific oligoclonal immunoglobulins in cerebrospinal fluid in cryptococcal meningitis. *Lancet* 1(8024): 1262.

Powderly, W.G. (1992). Therapy for cryptococcal meningitis in patients with AIDS. *Clin. Infect. Dis.* 14(Suppl. 1): S54–S59.

Powell, K.E., Dahl, B.A., Weeks, R.J., and Tosh, F.E. (1972). Airborne *Cryptococcus neoformans*: Particles from pigeon excreta compatible with alveolar deposition. *J. Infect. Dis.* 125(4): 412–415.

Qureshi, M.H., Zhang, T., Koguchi, Y., Nakashima, K., Okamura, H., Kurimoto, M., and Kawakami, K. (1999). Combined effects of IL-12 and IL-18 on the clinical course and local cytokine production in murine pulmonary infection with *Cryptococcus neoformans*. *Eur. J. Immunol.* 29(2): 643–649.

Ring, A. and Tuomanen, E.I. (1997). Targeting bacteria to the central nervous system. In P.K. Peterson and J.S. Remington (eds.), *Defense of the Brain: Current Concepts in the Immunopathogenesis and Clinical Aspects of CNS Infections.* Blackwell Science, Malden, MA, pp. 90–106.

Rosas, A.L., Nosanchuk, J.D., Feldmesser, M., Cox, G.M., McDade, H.C., and Casadevall, A. (2000). Synthesis of polymerized melanin by *Cryptococcus neoformans* in infected rodents. *Infect. Immun.* 68(5): 2845–2853.

Rossi, G.R., Cervi, L.A., Garcia, M.M., Chiapello, L.S., Sastre, D.A., and Masih, D.T. (1999). Involvement of nitric oxide in protecting mechanism during experimental cryptococcosis. *Clin. Immunol.* 90(2): 256–265.

Ruiz, A. and Bulmer, G.S. (1981). Particle size of airborn *Cryptococcus neoformans* in a tower. *Appl. Environ. Microbiol.* 41(5): 1225–1229.

Ruiz, A., Fromtling, R.A., and Bulmer, G.S. (1981). Distribution of *Cryptococcus neoformans* in a natural site. *Infect. Immun.* 31(2): 560–563.

Sabetta, J.R. and Andriole, V.T. (1985). Cryptococcal infection of the central nervous system. *Med. Clin. North Am.* 69(2): 333–344.

Salkowski, C.A. and Balish, E. (1990). Pathogenesis of *Cryptococcus neoformans* in congenitally immunodeficient beige athymic mice. *Infect. Immun.* 58(10): 3300–3306.

Salkowski, C.A., Bartizal, K.F., Balish, M.J., and Balish, E. (1987). Colonization and pathogenesis of *Cryptococcus neoformans* in gnotobiotic mice. *Infect. Immun.* 55(9): 2000–2005.

Santangelo, R., Zoellner, H., Sorrell, T., Wilson, C., Donald, C., Djordjevic, J., Shounan, Y., and Wright, L. (2004). Role of extracellular phospholipases and mononuclear phagocytes in dissemination of cryptococcosis in a murine model. *Infect. Immun.* 72(4): 2229–2239.

Schwartz, D.A. (1988). Characterization of the biological activity of *Cryptococcus* infections in surgical pathology. The budding index and carminophilic index. *Ann. Clin. Lab. Sci.* 18(5): 388–397.

Shrikant, P. and Benveniste, E.T. (1996). The central nervous system as an immunocompetent organ: Role of glial cells in antigen presentation. *J. Immunol.* 157: 1819–1822.

Sowa, G., Gekker, G., Lipovsky, M.M., Hu, S., Chao, C.C., Molitor, T.W., and Peterson, P.K. (1997). Inhibition of swine microglial cell phagocytosis of *Cryptococcus neoformans* by femtomolar concentrations of morphine. *Biochem. Pharmacol.* 53(6): 823–828.

Speed, B. and Dunt, D. (1995). Clinical and host differences between infections with the two varieties of *Cryptococcus neoformans*. *Clin. Infect. Dis.* 21(1): 28–34 [discussion 35–26].

Speed, B.R. and Kaldor, J. (1997). Rarity of cryptococcal infection in children. *Pediatr. Infect. Dis. J.* 16(5): 536–537.

Spitzer, E.D., Spitzer, S.G., Freundlich, L.F., and Casadevall, A. (1993). Persistence of initial infection in recurrent *Cryptococcus neoformans* meningitis. *Lancet* 341(8845): 595–596.

Staib, F., Seibold, M., and L'Age, M. (1990). Persistence of *Cryptococcus neoformans* in seminal fluid and urine under itraconazole treatment. The urogenital tract (prostate) as a niche for *Cryptococcus neoformans*. *Mycoses* 33(7–8): 369–373.

Tabone, M.D., Leverger, G., Landman, J., Aznar, C., Boccon-Gibod, L., and Lasfargues, G. (1994). Disseminated lymphonodular cryptococcosis in a child with X-linked hyper-IgM immunodeficiency. *Pediatr. Infect. Dis. J.* 13(1): 77–79.

Taylor, B.S. and Geller, D.A. (2000). Molecular regulation of the human inducible nitric oxide synthase (iNOS) gene. *Shock* 13(6): 413–424.

Trajkovic, V., Stepanovic, S., Samardzic, T., Jankovic, V., Badovinac, V., and Mostarica Stojkovic, M. (2000). *Cryptococcus neoformans* neutralizes macrophage and astrocyte derived nitric oxide without interfering with inducible nitric oxide synthase induction or catalytic activity—possible involvement of nitric oxide consumption. *Scand. J. Immunol.* 51(4): 384–391.

Truelsen, K., Young, T., and Kozel, T.R. (1992). In vivo complement activation and binding of C3 to encapsulated *Cryptococcus neoformans*. *Infect. Immun.* 60(9): 3937–3939.

Tuomanen, E. (1996). Entry of pathogens into the central nervous system. *FEMS Microbiol. Rev.* 18(4): 289–299.

Uicker, W.C., Doyle, H.A., McCracken, J.P., Langlois, M., and Buchanan, K.L. (2005). Cytokine and chemokine expression in the central nervous system associated with protective cell-mediated immunity against *Cryptococcus neoformans*. *Med. Mycol.* 43(1): 27–38.

van Beek, J., Elward, K., and Gasque, P. (2003). Activation of complement in the central nervous system: Roles in neurodegeneration and neuroprotection. *Ann. NY Acad. Sci.* 992: 56–71.

Vecchiarelli, A. and Casadevall, A. (1998). Antibody-mediated effects against *Cryptococcus neoformans*: Evidence for interdependency and collaboration between humoral and cellular immunity. *Res. Immunol.* 149(4–5): 321–333 [discussion 500–503].

Vecchiarelli, A., Pietrella, D., Bistoni, F., Kozel, T.R., and Casadevall, A. (2002). Antibody to *Cryptococcus neoformans* capsular glucuronoxylomannan promotes expression of interleukin-12Rbeta2 subunit on human T cells in vitro through effects mediated by antigen-presenting cells. *Immunology* 106(2): 267–272.

Wang, Y., and Casadevall, A. (1994a). Growth of *Cryptococcus neoformans* in presence of L-dopa decreases its susceptibility to amphotericin B. *Antimicrob. Agents Chemother.* 38(11): 2648–2650.

Wang, Y. and Casadevall, A. (1994b). Susceptibility of melanized and nonmelanized *Cryptococcus neoformans* to nitrogen- and oxygen-derived oxidants. *Infect. Immun.* 62(7): 3004–3007.

Wang, Y., Aisen, P., and Casadevall, A. (1995). *Cryptococcus neoformans* melanin and virulence: Mechanism of action. *Infect. Immun.* 63(8): 3131–3136.

Yip, S.K., Cheng, C., Wong, M.Y., Tan, B.H., Sim, C.S., and Lim, S.H. (1998). Cryptococcal prostatic abscess in an immunocompromised patient: A case report and review of the literature. *Ann. Acad. Med. Singapore* 27(6): 873–876.

Yuan, R., Casadevall, A., Spira, G., and Scharff, M.D. (1995). Isotype switching from IgG3 to IgG1 converts a nonprotective murine antibody to *Cryptococcus neoformans* into a protective antibody. *J. Immunol.* 154(4): 1810–1816.

Yuan, R.R., Casadevall, A., Oh, J., and Scharff, M.D. (1997). T cells cooperate with passive antibody to modify *Cryptococcus neoformans* infection in mice. *Proc. Natl. Acad. Sci. USA* 94(6): 2483–2488.

Yuan, R.R., Spira, G., Oh, J., Paizi, M., Casadevall, A., and Scharff, M.D. (1998). Isotype switching increases efficacy of antibody protection against *Cryptococcus neoformans* infection in mice. *Infect. Immun.* 66(3): 1057–1062.

Zebedee, S.L., Koduri, R.K., Mukherjee, J., Mukherjee, S., Lee, S., Sauer, D.F., Scharff, M.D., and Casadevall, A. (1994). Mouse-human immunoglobulin G1 chimeric antibodies with activities against *Cryptococcus neoformans*. *Antimicrob. Agents Chemother.* 38(7): 1507–1514.

Index